WHICH? MEDICINE

About the Author

Rosalind Grant MRPharmS is Head of Medicines Management in a primary care trust in south-west England. She has worked with Consumers' Association for over 20 years, contributing to books and articles on medicines and pharmaceutical matters. She was Managing Editor of *Drug and Therapeutics Bulletin* before becoming Pharmaceutical Adviser to a health authority, where she was responsible for providing prescribing advice to doctors and nurses and developing the role of pharmacists. A pharmacist for over 30 years, she has also specialised in medicines information in the National Health Service and the pharmaceutical industry.

Acknowledgements

The author and publishers wish to thank Andrea Tarr MRPharmS for checking the text; Jean Blake MRPharmS MSc for proof-reading the book; the members of the editorial board and advisory council of *Drug and Therapeutics Bulletin* and other medical and pharmaceutical advisers who helped with this book; and also the Department of Health for help with the table 'Useful sources of folate/folic acid'.

WHICH? MEDICINE

Rosalind Grant MRPharmS

CONSUMERS' ASSOCIATION

Which? Books are commissioned by
Consumers' Association and published by
Which? Ltd, 2 Marylebone Road, London NW1 4DF
Email: books@which.net

Distributed by The Penguin Group:
Penguin Books Ltd, 80 Strand, London WC2R 0RL

First edition August 1992
Reprinted October 1992
Revised edition August 1993
Revised edition September 1995
Revised edition May 1997
Reprinted October 1999
Revised edition March 2000
Revised edition March 2004

British Library Cataloguing in Publication Data
A catalogue record for Which? Medicine is available from the British Library.

ISBN 0 85202 967 5

Editorial and production: Robert Gray, Mary Sunderland
Index: Marie Lorimer
Typographic design: Dick Vine
Original cover concept: Sarah Harmer
Cover photograph: R-Zscharnack/A1PIX

Typeset by Saxon Graphics Ltd, Derby
Printed and bound in Wales by Creative Print and Design

CONTENTS

*An asterisk next to the name of an organisation in the text indicates that contact details for it can be found in this section, on page 482

FOREWORD

by Dr Andrew Herxheimer MB, FRCP

Founding Editor of *Drug and Therapeutics Bulletin*

Participant in the Cochrane Collaboration Consumer Network

Co-founder of DIPEx

(Database of personal experiences of illness – *www.dipex.org*)

I have taught students and doctors about medicines for most of my life, but I write this Foreword as an experienced patient.

I think the biggest problem with medicines is that they are too easy for doctors to prescribe and for patients to take. They seem so straightforward and uncomplicated, but actually to use them to the best effect requires knowledge, skill and care, both from the doctor and the patient – you and your doctor need to work together.

Which? Medicine can help you both to do that. I hope you will use it before you go to your doctor, to clarify what you want to discuss and what questions to ask in the consultation. When the pharmacist has given you the medicine, and later, when you are using it, the book will remind you what to look out for and what to do in various circumstances. Equally, it will help you to focus on what matters to you personally in conversations with the pharmacist and the nurse.

The book tells you what the most important medicines do in the great majority of people, but every person differs in some ways from the majority. Each of us needs to learn what is unusual about ourselves, and that applies particularly to medicines. We will learn things about how medicines affect us that may not be mentioned in books, and that doctors cannot know if we don't tell them. We will discover what medicines and what doses work well for us, which ones do not help us, and which ones cause trouble. We should note this for our families and our doctors: such experiences can be important for our and our doctors' future choices of medicines and their advice on how we use them.

Here are some examples of what I have learnt about myself. Either paracetamol 1,000mg or ibuprofen 200mg will relieve an occasional headache and cause no problems, but a higher dose of ibuprofen can give me indigestion. If I drink coffee or take caffeine after about 3pm, I find it difficult to sleep that night. Loratadine 10mg suppresses and relieves my hayfever and occasional urticaria – it suits me. If I use diazepam I shall probably get a nettle-rash, so I avoid it and other drugs like it. Simvastatin, which I used to lower the lipids in my blood, caused muscle weakness and pains. I discussed with my GP what we might do instead, and it was decided to drop simvastatin while keeping an eye on the blood lipids.

It really is worth paying attention to your medicines. Notice how well they work for you, and ask advice if anything puzzling or unexpected happens.

INTRODUCTION

Most of us today expect to enjoy good health. Indeed, we may even regard it as a right. If we are ill, we assume that a medicine will ease the symptoms or effect a cure. We use medicines extensively, particularly if we are among the growing population of older people, on whom around half of the National Health Service (NHS) drugs bill is spent. The use of a medicine is the most common health care intervention made in the NHS. Over 617 million NHS prescriptions worth around £6.8 billion were dispensed in England alone in 2002.

The reasons why we take so many medicines are complex: the desire to take something – anything – to make us feel better is deep-rooted, like the sense that eating will overcome hunger, and for both patients and doctors a prescription often seems the most satisfactory outcome of a consultation. The high media profile of drugs, and vigorous marketing by their manufacturers, increase the pressure to search for a medicinal cure for every problem, whether or not it is appropriate.

But how much do we know about the medicines we take? What do they contain? How are they supposed to help us? How will they affect our bodies? Do they have any unwanted effects? If we are to participate effectively in our own health care, we need the answers to these questions and many more besides. *Which? Medicine* endeavours to supply them. The book provides information, independent of government and the drug industry, so that you the consumer can begin to make informed choices.

KNOWLEDGE ABOUT MEDICINES

In Britain when you visit your doctor the consultation may finish with the handing over of a prescription, marking the end of your discussion. The doctor may assume that the instructions with the medicine will be crystal clear to you and require no further explanation or guidance. The pharmacist dispensing your medicine, who does not know what the doctor has told you, may not be aware that you are not fully confident about how to take the medicine, or that you may have queries. In any case, the pharmacist cannot always tell from the prescription what complaint it has been prescribed for. This scenario is still too common, but doctors, nurses, pharmacists, dentists and other health professionals should tell you about the medicines they prescribe or recommend and that you take, and you should feel confident in asking questions about them.

Knowledge of medicines and their potential to prevent illness and cure or relieve discomfort is increasing, but perhaps only when there is a need to know, such as when you fall ill. The advent of more information on medicines through newsletters, telephone helplines, the media and the Internet is creating a new consumer awareness. More information can increase confusion, especially with biased or inconsistent messages, and more information does not equal better understanding or decision-making.

Consumers' Association's report *Patient Information: What's the prognosis?* recommends that education on health, illness and medicines should be part of the school curriculum so that everyone has the chance to learn how to manage their own health effectively. Learning to be discerning about the details you find is another essential skill, if you are to navigate the vast amounts of information. As a consumer you are most vulnerable when you cannot exercise an informed choice about the products you become aware of and use. You need to know which product is safest, most effective and most reliable, why and how you should use it, and what to do if something goes wrong. *Which? Medicine* aims to tell you about medicines in a straightforward manner and to facilitate informed discussion with health professionals.

AVAILABILITY OF MEDICINES

Unlike many other commodities that can be bought, medicines have to be regulated because they have the potential to do harm as well as good. Any medicine, whether available on prescription or sold over the counter, becomes available only after it has been recommended for licensing by the relevant government body, either the Medicines and Healthcare products Regulatory Agency (MHRA), or the European Medicines Evaluation Agency (EMEA), which is responsible for appraising a product's safety, efficacy and quality. Access to prescription medicines is controlled under the Medicines Act 1968, mainly through doctors and dentists, although as part of the government strategy to improve access to health services, the Act has been amended to allow other health professionals, such as nurses and pharmacists, to take responsibility for prescribing or supplying certain prescription medicines.

Successive governments have encouraged consumers to treat minor self-limiting ailments (ones that clear up with time, such as coughs and colds) by buying a non-prescription medicine over the counter rather than seeing a doctor. Being able to do this means that consumers have access to treatments quickly and conveniently and can follow the pharmacist's guidance when necessary.

Increasingly, medicines for minor ailments can be bought in pharmacies or from other retail outlets; *Which? Medicine* includes information about many of them. Examples include cimetidine for heartburn, and treatments for vaginal thrush, cold sores and allergic conjunctivitis. Although vast numbers of branded products are available, the range of drugs used in them (i.e. the active ingredients of medicines) is in fact limited. For example, the many branded pain-relievers all contain one or more of only three analgesics that can be sold over the counter – paracetamol, aspirin, and ibuprofen. A fourth, codeine, is often added in low dosage. Brand-name pain relievers are no more effective than the ingredients sold simply as the generic version, but they are much more expensive.

SAFETY OF MEDICINES

Taking a medicine to effect a cure appears to be a simple part of everyday life, but swallowing a tablet is just the beginning of a complex biochemical process which may affect your body in a number of ways. Many medicines are unlikely to cause serious unwanted effects and not everyone is at risk from those that do, but medicine-taking is not without hazard. Major scares about medicines continue to hit the headlines: for example, those concerning paroxetine (Seroxat), an antidepressant that may worsen symptoms at the start of treatment or cause withdrawal problems on stopping the drug, and oral contraceptives linked to the increased risk of blood clots.

Medication errors unfortunately happen and fatalities occasionally occur with medicines given incorrectly or the wrong dose taken. The dangers are not restricted to prescription medicines but also apply to familiar remedies such as aspirin and paracetamol. Used according to their instructions these pain relievers are safe and effective, but not when misused or taken in overdose. Any delay in seeking medical advice will put the patient's health, and perhaps life, at risk.

Concerns about the safety of medicines have to be balanced with allowing reasonable access to established treatments. Over the years deaths and injuries have led the government to reduce the amount of aspirin and paracetamol that can be bought over the counter to a maximum of 16 tablets from non-pharmacy outlets or 32 from a pharmacy. Research has shown that people are likely to take fewer tablets or not take them at all if the number of tablets available in a pack for sale is restricted. Since lower pack sizes were introduced, the number of deaths and hospital admissions from paracetamol poisoning appears to have fallen.

Here, then, is the paradox about medicines: they are widely used commodities which can be life-saving, but their effectiveness and safety are often taken for granted by the public. Each year more and more medicines are prescribed or sold over the counter, but consumers need to be clear about how any medicine they take might contribute to improved health.

INFORMATION ON MEDICINES

The NHS Plan and other government initiatives for giving patients information encourage you to be an active participant in your own health care: you can become more involved by exercising choice about your medication. Research has shown that some patients want to share in decisions about their treatment and care, and that this can improve health outcomes. The burden of responsibility for your health and treatment must then shift towards being an equal partnership between you and your doctor or other health professional, and this means letting your doctor know about your health beliefs and whether or not you intend to pursue the recommended treatment.

Patient information leaflets

The pharmaceutical industry is responsible for providing and presenting patient information for both prescription and over-the-counter products. A patient information leaflet (PIL) must be supplied with all medicines in addition to the standard information on the label (page 28). This provides a ready source of instruction about a medicine. PILs are not intended to take the place of advice from your doctor, nurse or pharmacist but to remind you of what has been said and enable you to ask questions. However, there are concerns about the presentation and bias of these leaflets, including the accuracy of information about a medicine's unwanted or side effects.

Consumers' Association has consistently highlighted the shortcomings of PILs in communicating key concepts about medication that will enable patients to use their medicines safely and effectively. Because the choice of how to present the information is up to the company, PILs often emphasize brand names rather than the active ingredients and little mention is made of alternative sources of information. Layouts are variable, often downgrading information about potential side effects, and tiny print in leaflets is a challenge to read for those with failing eyesight. There are, however, proposals that PILs should be tested on patients so these problems may lessen.

Patient information leaflets are published on the industry's Medicines Compendium website at *www.medicines.org.uk*.

PROMOTION OF MEDICINES TO CONSUMERS

In the UK the pharmaceutical industry is allowed to promote only over-the-counter products directly to the public. However, drug companies can inform patients about prescription medicines in a number of ways. Examples include patient education material – discussing conditions such as asthma, diabetes and stomach ulcers, say – which may be published as free booklets, information on the Internet or as video and audio tapes. Specific medicines are not mentioned, but these materials build the company's image and insidiously strengthen the patient's association with its products. More recently, celebrities are being drawn into this type of promotion. The MHRA has published guidelines on how such disease awareness campaigns should be conducted. It is also charged with disciplining Internet service providers who breach advertising regulations.

Advertising prescription medicines direct to the consumer is permitted in the USA and New Zealand. Doctors in New Zealand have called for a ban because this has caused problems for patients, doctors and the economy. For example, pressure from patients to switch to a new asthma inhaler after it was advertised on television cost the country around £940,000 over nine months. The new inhaler was not necessarily appropriate for all patients, but because it had been advertised, patients demanded it. Doctors are concerned about the misleading content of many advertisements and the resulting commercial pressure to prescribe drugs. New is not necessarily better; usually some unwanted effects remain to be discovered following a product's launch (page 55).

The industry is permitted to sponsor patients' self-help organisations. Many patient groups are voluntary bodies, hard-pressed for resources, which welcome funding. Drug companies perceive the usefulness of patient groups in getting new developments discussed and known by patients, even before the medicine is marketed. It has been suggested that this kind of activity can feed patient demand for medicines which may not be proven to be the most clinically- and cost-effective treatment. This leaves doctors embattled in coping with rising requests for specific treatments which can divert resources away from other areas of need in the NHS.

Consumers' Association considers that the role of informing patients about medicines should be taken by an independent central agency that can act as a gateway directing people to trustworthy, impartial and unbiased information on medicines.

PROMOTION OF MEDICINES TO PRESCRIBERS

The drug industry spends about £516 million a year on marketing medicines to the NHS. The increasing numbers of patients who may benefit from new, expensive treatments for a wider range of conditions, some previously untreatable, have fuelled debates about the appropriateness of treatments and the impact on the NHS budget.

Doctors are the main target for the pharmaceutical industry's activities in promoting medicines, usually through company representatives but also through extensive advertising in the medical press. Commercial sponsorship supports research in a variety of ways, for example funding posts, professional development, conferences, buildings and equipment. Concerns are growing that the industry has been too successful in underpinning the activities of doctors and others in the health service. Industry rules ban the use of inappropriate gifts or incentives to prescribe. However, key journals such as *The Lancet* and *British Medical Journal* have published independent studies of industry-sponsored research where bias and distortion are evident. The Department of Health has issued guidance to NHS staff about accepting commercial sponsorship, and many hospitals and primary care trusts have their own guidelines for working in partnership with the industry.

THE INTERNET

Services offered by the Internet include medical information and the opportunity to purchase medicines.

Information

Over half the UK population has access to the Internet, which gives the individual immediate access to a wealth of global medical information via search engines, chat rooms for patient support groups, and pharmaceutical company, charity and university websites. Consumers' Association supports the aim of empowering patients with good-quality information, but while the knowledge gap between health professionals and patients is narrowing, access to professionals remains important for specific advice and to facilitate decision-making.

The explosion of medical information on the Internet is not without drawbacks, because the quality of information can be variable and is unregulated. Consumers need to be discerning, and assess the source and credibility of information. For example, who gives the information? Is it fact or opinion? Is the site up to date and supported by references? Who is the site for, and is it easy to use?

Consumers' Association proposes that ten core principles should underpin all information on health and medicines, including that available at websites. These principles are: accessibility, accuracy, appropriateness, consistency, up-to-date, evidence-based, non-biased, timeliness, transparency and understandability.

Buying medicines on the web

The sale of prescription-only medicines through the Internet seems an attractive proposition for consumers who wish to self-diagnose and avoid having to wait to see a doctor. However, consumers who buy medicines over the Internet or by mail order bypass the system and take risks when they use unregulated distributors. Treatment could be inappropriate and, in the absence of monitoring, there is no way of assessing the impact of the medicine on the patient's health. Many medicines are available only on prescription because their use needs to be supervised by a health professional, who must assess their effectiveness, safety and appropriateness in each patient. This requires a diagnosis of the condition, usually including a physical examination and access to the patient's medical history. These services cannot be provided adequately via the Internet yet. Furthermore, the Internet is not completely secure for transferring data, and confidential patient information needs to be safeguarded through encryption techniques. Another key issue is quality, because pharmaceuticals may be marketed fraudulently and are a major target for counterfeiters. The system for licensing and regulating medicines in the UK has been carefully built up over 40 years since the thalidomide disaster, when severe abnormalities occurred in the babies of pregnant women who took the drug. The burgeoning access via the Internet to medicines intended for prescription only breaches the UK Medicines Act and is a potential threat to individual safety. In addition, consumers can pay considerably more for medicines purchased from overseas Internet companies than through the NHS. In time the NHS will develop access to mail-order prescriptions and an electronic pharmacy.

EVIDENCE-BASED PRACTICE

The overwhelming and ever-growing volume of medical literature means that health professionals are hard-pressed to access, and then to implement, the results of research. All health professionals should base their practice on good-quality published evidence, so-called 'evidence-based practice'. Yet it is clear that in some parts of the NHS the care provided is inconsistent and of poor quality. The government has declared its determination that quality and efficiency must underpin the delivery of health services, and has set a national programme of standards and targets to improve performance. National Service Frameworks (NSFs), in which the patterns of care and levels of service are defined for certain conditions, such as heart disease or diabetes, or for a group such as children or older people, should increase consistency. The National Institute for Clinical Excellence (NICE), funded by the Department of Health, examines the evidence for the clinical- and cost-effectiveness of medicines (for example, antiviral medicines for flu) and other forms of treatment such as replacement hips and hearing aids. Its clinical guidelines (for example for heart failure) and audit programmes are setting standards of good practice. GPs and nurses can also access information known as PRODIGY – Prescribing RatiOnally with Decision support In General Practice studY – a computerised information system to help them decide on appropriate treatments, which provides evidence-based patient information on those treatments. NHS hospitals and PCTs have to have programmes of clinical governance – a framework for ensuring that clinical standards are met and the quality of service is continuously improved. NHS performance is reviewed by the Commission for Healthcare Audit and Inspection (CHAI).

HOW TO USE *WHICH? MEDICINE*

Before you take a medicine you should at the very least know broadly how it will act in the body and how it will help. You have a right to understand what happens in your own body and should do so for the sake of your own safety and well-being. This book discusses the medicines in the context of the diseases they are used to treat or prevent, by comparing different treatments and their risks and benefits. It will promote active discussion with health professionals and answer questions you forgot or were embarrassed to ask, or that did not occur to you while you were in the surgery.

Which? Medicine does not offer extensive information about all of the thousands of medicines available in Britain, nor is it a dictionary of medicines. It contains detailed profiles of over 80 of the most commonly used drugs (pages 16–18). Most drug profiles are representative of a particular 'family' of medicines, so that one drug serves as a model for that type of medicinal product. For example, there are over 20 anti-arthritis drugs, most of which are chemically related and have similar effects. One detailed profile of a drug from each class has been compiled and the remaining products listed at the end of the profile. Notes on many more preparations are included throughout the text, but it has not been possible to look at all the medicines available in Britain – there are around 5,000.

Finding out about your body is an important step towards being in control of your health – don't wait until you fall ill. Each chapter in the second part of the book looks at a particular body system and the medicines developed for the disorders that affect that group of organs. These sections broadly follow the classification used by the *British National Formulary (BNF)*, a comprehensive handbook for doctors, nurses and pharmacists describing the uses, unwanted effects and interactions of the majority of drugs used in Britain. It is produced twice-yearly by the British Medical Association and the Royal Pharmaceutical Society of Great Britain, and is available online.

You can use *Which? Medicine* to look up a drug you have been prescribed – there's an index of generic and brand names at the back to help you find the relevant section quickly. Remind yourself of what the doctor said, find out more about your illness and make sure you're happy with the consultation. Discuss any doubts or further questions with your doctor. Better still, use this book before a prescription is written or to help choose a medicine bought over the counter. Ask the questions listed on the medicine record sheet (see 'How to improve your use of medicines') and raise any points mentioned in the relevant drug profile. Read about your condition and discuss treatment with your doctor, nurse or pharmacist; do not start a course of treatment until you feel fully informed about it.

HOW YOU CAN HELP YOURSELF

Medicines may relieve symptoms, provide comfort and cure, but you can also take other measures to help yourself. Many sections include common-sense suggestions for helping you to take an active part in overcoming illness or disorder. For people with long-term conditions, there may be a self-help group.

Ideas in the 'How you can help yourself' sections do not replace taking a medicine if drug treatment is needed, but are intended to supplement treatment so you can do everything possible to help your health. Some illnesses can be managed without drug treatment: for example, by careful control of diet or taking up regular exercise.

EVALUATION OF MEDICINES

Wherever possible the book gives an indication of the medicines that are preferred and those that are considered a poor choice because the evidence for their use is inadequate. This selection is based on recommendations made in *Drug and Therapeutics Bulletin* and *Treatment Notes* from Consumers' Association plus other sources of independent information such as the *British National Formulary (BNF)*, PRODIGY (page 12), and the National Prescribing Centre *MeReC Bulletin*.

Words used in this book

The words medicine and drug are used interchangeably, although strictly speaking a **drug** is a chemical substance and the active ingredient of a medicine, while a **medicine** contains a drug and other substances (inactive ingredients), which help to deliver the drug to the body. It is more important to remember that a medicine is not necessarily a liquid and that the word drug does not necessarily mean an illicit substance such as heroin.

Medical terms have been explained wherever possible throughout the book, and you will also find a glossary in the reference section at the back.

DRUG NAMES

At the start of a drug's life in the laboratory, it is given a **chemical name** and a research number. Later in its development the drug is given a **generic name** – its official medical name, also called the approved name or non-proprietary name – according to World Health Organization (WHO) principles.

When a medicine is marketed, it has already been patented, so that the manufacturer has the sole right to develop and market it and the brand name is protected. Other companies may not copy this medicine or infringe the patent. Once a medicine's patent has expired, another company is free to make a generic copy. It can do so more cheaply because it does not have to fund development and initial marketing of the medicine. However, generic copies are not made for all branded medicines, even after the patent has expired.

Doctors are encouraged to prescribe generically because generic versions are just as effective and usually cheaper than brands. You should always know the generic name of any medicine you are taking to avoid confusion and duplication. Read the ingredients of any branded products you buy for the same reasons. For example, one week you might be prescribed diclofenac, a drug for pain relief and reducing inflammation, and then later see another doctor, perhaps at a hospital clinic, who prescribes you Voltarol, a brand name of diclofenac. You now have two supplies of the same medicine with different names and may end up taking double the dose without realising.

The licensing requirements for generic medicines are just as stringent as they are for branded products. The same medicine produced by separate manufacturers may differ in shape, size, colour or taste, but these differences are rarely significant; the active ingredient of the medicine is the same. A pharmacist must usually dispense exactly what the doctor has indicated on the prescription. If the prescription has a particular brand name, then you will receive that brand, but if the prescription has the generic name then the pharmacist only has to dispense a medicine containing that active ingredient: you may receive a generic version or any of the branded versions.

You should find out the active ingredients of any preparations you buy over the counter by looking at the information on the packaging. It is easy to buy apparently different cold remedies which turn out to have the same pain-relieving ingredient. Taking several medicines together can mean taking an excessively high dose of one drug; in extreme cases this has led to death.

Generic names, particularly for newer drugs, tend to be standard throughout the world wherever international agreements can be reached through the recommended international non-proprietary names (rINN) WHO scheme. This helps when you travel to other countries, although you will find some differences, especially with older drugs. For example, paracetamol is known as acetaminophen in the USA.

These older drugs with British approved names (BANs) will be renamed using the rINN scheme. Both old and new drug names have been used inconsistently in the UK recently, increasing the risk of medication errors. Drugs with possible safety risks will be targeted first, and manufacturers have two years in which to make changes to product literature. For example, amoxycillin (old) changes to amoxicillin (new). Two drug names will remain unchanged from the BAN system: adrenaline (rINN – epinephrine) and noradrenaline (rINN – norepinephrine). These drugs are used for emergency treatment and renaming them may increase the risk of medication errors. *Which? Medicine* uses the new names but the old names appear in brackets.

The brand name is chosen by the manufacturer alone, intended to be easily pronounced, remembered and written. There may be several brands of the same generic substance, each produced by a different company. The names may bear no resemblance to the generic name.

In *Which? Medicine* generic names are given in bold type before brand names in order to help you to become familiar with the active ingredient(s) of your medicine. A branded product may contain two or three active ingredients, but you cannot tell this from the name on the label. Furthermore, some medicines that doctors prescribe can also be bought over the counter, but they have different brand names, one for prescription and one for sale over the counter. For example, mebeverine has the brand name Colofac on prescription, but is sold over the counter under the brand names Colofac 100, Colofac IBS and Equilon. Using the generic name helps you to know the medicine you are taking and avoids confusion and duplication.

☐ **chemical name** 1-isopropylamino-3-*p*-(2-methoxyethyl) phenoxypropan-2-ol
☐ **generic name** metoprolol
☐ **brand names** Lopresor; Betaloc

DRUG CLASSES

All drugs are given a legal category to control how they can be supplied to the public. You may see the abbreviations on the packaging.

Prescription-only medicines (POM) can be obtained only with a health professional's prescription. Many medicines fall into this category because of the complexity of deciding when and how they should be used and their potential for harm if used improperly.

Medicines sold over the counter are split into two categories. **Pharmacy medicines (P)** may be sold only in a pharmacy and the sale must be supervised by the pharmacist – for example, antihistamines for the relief of hay fever symptoms. **General sale list medicines (GSL)** are sold in other stores, such as supermarkets, as well as pharmacies.

Drugs are also classified according to what they do, in groups such as antidepressants or antacids. These categories can include several families of drugs.

▼ *'BLACK TRIANGLE' MEDICINES*

All new prescription medicines are marked with an inverted black triangle (▼) in the *BNF* and other reference books, as well as in advertisements. The triangle is a device alerting health professionals to report any suspected adverse reaction to the new medicine to the Committee on Safety of Medicines. It does not appear in information leaflets for patients and so you cannot tell whether you have been prescribed a new medicine without asking your doctor.

Reading the drug profiles

Each chapter contains drug profiles, which are boxed. These begin with the name of the generic drug, followed by a list of the products which contain it. The list is split into prescription and non-prescription products, and any products considered a poor choice are listed separately. If there are no headings the products are all prescription-only. A brief description of the drug's uses and how it works follows.

In the lists of drug names, drugs that manufacturers produce under generic names are shown in **BOLD CAPITAL LETTERS**, while drugs produced under the manufacturers' own brand names are in ORDINARY CAPITALS. Names in **SMALL BOLD CAPITALS** underneath the brand names of similar preparations show what the active ingredient is. The different formulations – tablets, capsules, liquids, etc. – are given too. For example, in the profile of cimetidine, a drug used to heal ulcers, you will see:

CIMETIDINE – Tablets	This is a generic drug available under its own name.
DYSPAMET – Liquid	This is one manufacturer's product which contains cimetidine.
ZANTAC – Capsules **RANITIDINE**	Ranitidine is similar in action to cimetidine, so it is included in the same profile; Zantac is the brand name of a product which contains ranitidine

You will also see in the profiles the headings *From a pharmacy* and *Over the counter*. 'From a pharmacy' means exactly what it says and you will be unable to obtain the medicine anywhere else, while 'Over the counter' refers to medicines that can be bought in a pharmacy or elsewhere – for example, in a supermarket or garage.

Before you use this medicine

This section lists what you should tell your doctor, nurse or pharmacist when he or she is proposing the medicine as a treatment. You may not be a suitable candidate for treatment because of allergies or other conditions you have, or other medication you are on. Some medicines are unsuitable for pregnant or breastfeeding women.

How to use this medicine

Your doctor, nurse or pharmacist should give specific instructions for using a medicine, including any special storage instructions. **Over 65** details any special instructions for older people, who may be more sensitive to the effects of many drugs.

Interactions with other medicines

Medicines interact in many ways. The effects of two drugs may combine usefully but often they will disrupt or modify each other's action in a way which means your treatment must be adjusted in some way. This section lists only the important interactions; tell your doctor, nurse or pharmacist if you are using any prescription or over-the-counter preparations, including complementary therapies.

Unwanted effects

Reading a list of a medicine's unwanted effects can be an unnerving experience. You may wonder whether the drug will really cause all these problems as well as making you better. But you should be aware of the range of unwanted effects so that you can take action if a serious, usually rare, effect occurs. Your doctor or pharmacist can help put the benefits and unwanted effects in perspective.

Similar preparations

Many drugs are part of a family of preparations, which all work in a similar way. The drug profile applies broadly to all the members of the family listed; your doctor or pharmacist will be able to tell you about the minor differences and some are mentioned in the text preceding and following the profile.

The Selected List Scheme

In 1985 the government restricted some of the medicines that doctors could prescribe on the NHS in order to save money. The Selected List Scheme has reduced duplication and the numbers of less effective medicines, and it promotes prescribing by generic name. Medicines restricted by the first blacklist included antacids, laxatives, cough and cold remedies, analgesics for mild to moderate pain relief, vitamins and tonics and the benzodiazepine sedatives and tranquillisers. Further blacklisting has occurred over the years, most notably sildenafil (Viagra).

Medicines in most categories remain available for NHS prescription (the White List). Most blacklisted medicines can still be obtained on a private prescription and you can buy others over the counter. A doctor in the NHS cannot charge for writing a prescription for a blacklisted medicine, but you will have to pay for the medicine and probably a dispensing fee to the pharmacist.

• *DRUG LISTS* •

Of the hundreds of products available, most doctors have, in practice, prescribed from a personal list of around 200–300 medicines. Drug selection is influenced by a number of factors. These include the doctor's training at medical school, the latest medical research, continuing professional development and current medical opinion, what the specialist recommends at the local hospital, and also the activities of the pharmaceutical industry in developing and promoting medicines.

The government has taken measures to encourage quality- and cost-effective prescribing based on robust evidence. Doctors are encouraged to review their prescribing regularly and to develop formularies based on medicines selected for their effectiveness, safety, convenience and cost. Increasingly, hospitals and GP surgeries are developing joint formularies across local health communities to help manage the choice of medicines and the introduction of new ones, reduce drug wastage and to ensure consistency in treatment between hospital and community.

• *IMPORTED MEDICINES* •

Your medicine may sometimes come from another country in the European Union. The medicine and packaging may look familiar except that the wording on the pack will not be in English. The medicine will be exactly the same as the British product and the pharmacist will label the medicine with the required instructions.

The current system for buying pharmaceuticals varies throughout the European Union, which leads to discrepancies in prices. This has led to a brisk trade in some pharmaceuticals, known as 'parallel imports'. Parallel imports are the only form of competition to brand medicines and they annoy the pharmaceutical industry considerably, because they reduce profits.

OBTAINING MEDICINES ABROAD

A medicine may be available on prescription in one EU country but sold over the counter in another. For example, antibiotics cannot be bought from a pharmacy in the UK but can in some other EU countries. Codeine for pain relief is sold in a pharmacy as an ingredient in many headache remedies in the UK, but is carefully controlled through a doctor's prescription in Greece.

The way a medicine is used also varies from one country to another. For example, abroad you might be offered an antibiotic for the treatment of diarrhoea, whereas simple rehydration measures with glucose and salt solution are preferred in the UK.

Regulations on the sale and supply of medicines differ from country to country outside the EU and knowing the name of the active ingredient of the medicine will help. If you fall ill while on holiday and need to buy a medicine, check the label carefully of any product purchased over the counter. Quality and standards may not be assured in some countries. Otherwise, take your own first aid kit, over-the-counter and prescription medicine supplies and carry a letter from your doctor giving details of any prescription medicines, in both brand and generic names.

What isn't in *Which? Medicine*

Medicines that are used mainly in hospital have not been included – for example, general anaesthetics, some antibiotics and specialised medicines including those for children that are usually started in hospital – nor have treatments for cancer, HIV, multiple sclerosis and dementia, such as Alzheimer's disease. Other areas not covered include wound dressings, appliances, vaccines and immunological products.

There is little mention of exact dosages because these vary so much depending on who is being treated and for what condition. Drug abuse is not discussed except with reference to drugs normally used for a medical purpose. Alternative treatments are beyond the scope of this book, although some, particularly relaxation techniques, have a bearing on the 'How you can help yourself' sections.

HOW TO IMPROVE YOUR USE OF MEDICINES

During the last 50 years, many potent medicines have been developed. Patients have received these medicines, often quite passively, and sometimes with little understanding about how the medicine should work in the body and what to do if unwanted or adverse effects occur. In the past medicines were labelled merely as 'The Tablets' or 'The Mixture', instructions were often limited to 'One tablet to be taken three times a day' or 'One tablespoonful to be taken four times daily'. You were not required to think or question the advisability of taking a medicine. Much more information on medicines is available nowadays from a variety of sources, but this does not necessarily fulfil your particular needs as a patient. Surveys among patients continue to show that about a third of people think that they have not been given enough information about their medicines, especially about what unwanted effects to expect. Your right to information implies taking responsibility for your own health, and working in partnership with healthcare professionals in order to take a shared approach to decision-making. To improve the service your doctor, pharmacist or nurse gives you, and your use of medicines, consider the following:

- ☐ **take an active part in understanding the illness and its treatment**
- ☐ **assume nothing**
- ☐ **ask questions**
- ☐ **seek a second opinion if questions are not answered to your satisfaction**
- ☐ **become a full partner with the doctor or nurse in managing your illness and in medicine-taking**.

Only you can feel and experience a painful condition or an illness; try to be as accurate as you can in describing what is wrong with you or where it hurts and how long you have had the complaint. This will improve the accuracy of the diagnosis and choice of treatment. If your doctor follows the list of basic duties below, problems with drug treatment will be kept to a minimum.

1. **Restricting the use of drugs** Has your doctor taken a proper decision that drug therapy is warranted? Is there another possible way of treating you? Would the best thing (for mild symptoms) be just to wait and see?
2. **Making a careful choice** of an appropriate drug and dosage. Has your doctor taken into account your own needs and how susceptible you may be to unwanted effects? And the balance of likely benefits and unwanted effects of any drug? And the alternative drugs available?

3. **Consultation and consent** Has your doctor consulted you about the treatment that is proposed? Do you understand it? Have you given your informed consent to treatment?
4. **Explanation** A doctor should explain to you how a course of treatment will be given, and what your role in that course of treatment is going to be. Do you know?
5. **Prescription and recording** Your doctor should prescribe with care, and should make sure a record of the prescription is kept.
6. **Supervision** While you are on a course of drugs, the doctor who prescribed them should be looking out for any developments or changes, and altering or adapting the treatment if need be.
7. **Ending drug therapy** when it is no longer needed.
8. **Keeping within the law** as it relates to prescribing and using medicines.

The questions on page 22 are relevant when you buy or are prescribed any medicine. They also appear on the medicine record sheet, which can be copied or cut out so that you can take it with you to the doctor and jot down the answers to the questions. If you take a medicine every day you should know the answers to most of the questions.

Compliance moving to concordance

Health professionals now realise that if they explain what they expect a medicine to do – both the wanted and the unwanted effects – then a patient is more likely to take that medicine correctly and to benefit from treatment. Professionals talk about patients *complying* with treatment and define compliance as the extent to which a person's behaviour coincides with medical or health advice.

Compliance is not a one-way process, however, as it involves you, your doctor, nurse and your pharmacist. It is the quality of the relationship between you and them that will help you to understand and follow recommendations to take a particular medicine or pursue a special diet. Your doctor's responsibility is to share information with you to help you make informed choices about the diagnosis and treatment and to understand your concerns. This partnership approach, known as *concordance*, allows the patient and doctor or other health professional to exchange views frankly, agree a course of action together or agree to differ. You can use the list of 20 questions during a consultation to help you assess why a medicine might help (see box).

The government is committed to strengthening the patient–health professional partnership approach. It has introduced medicines management services (encompassing medicines review, drug monitoring, management of repeat prescribing, services to care homes and patient education) to the NHS and set up an Action Team to advise on redesigning local services around patients. The Department of Health also funds the Medicines Partnership, which aims to help patients get the most out of medications by involving them as partners in prescribing decisions (see *www.medicines-partnership.org*).

Medicines management services are being set up in primary care trusts to enable GP practices and pharmacies to work more closely together so that treatment is optimised and waste reduced. The value of unused medicines returned to pharmacies is estimated as more than £100 million a year. About five per cent of prescriptions are never dispensed and up to 50 per cent of medicines are only half-taken or remain untaken. This represents a mismatch of ideas between you, health care professionals and the pharmaceutical industry.

20 QUESTIONS TO ASK ABOUT YOUR PRESCRIPTION

Before the prescription is written

- ☐ Is there an alternative to treatment with medicines for my condition?
- ☐ How can I help myself apart from taking the medicine?
- ☐ What kind of medicine is it?
- ☐ How will it help me?
- ☐ How important is it to take this medicine?
- ☐ Is this a new medicine? If so, what advantages does the new medicine have over older products?

Before the consultation ends

- ☐ How and when should I take the medicine?
- ☐ How can I tell if it is working?
- ☐ For how long should I take the medicine?
- ☐ What may happen if I do not take it?
- ☐ What should I do if I miss a dose?
- ☐ Is the medicine likely to have any unwanted effects? If so, how can I recognise them and how serious might they be?
- ☐ What should I do if unwanted effects occur?
- ☐ Will I need to see you again?
- ☐ What will you need to know from me then?

When the prescription is dispensed

- ☐ Can I take other medicines with it?
- ☐ Are there any foods or drinks I should avoid, and if so why?
- ☐ Can I drive a car after taking the medicine?
- ☐ Where should I keep my medicine?
- ☐ What should I do with any leftover medicine?

REVIEW YOUR MEDICINES

Review your medicines regularly with your doctor, nurse or pharmacist, especially if you take medicines routinely. Sort out which you still need to take, which you need to take only occasionally and whether there are any you can stop. It is best to take as few medicines as necessary and at the lowest dose that is effective in order to minimise the risks of unwanted effects and interactions between the medicines. You need to have as simple a treatment plan as possible, particularly if you are over 65. The National Service Framework (NSF) for Older People advises that if you are aged over 75 years of age, you should have the medicines you take reviewed once a year; if you take four or more medicines routinely then six-monthly reviews are appropriate.

Make an appointment to see your doctor. Collect all the medicines, both prescribed and those bought over the counter, including herbal remedies, that you are taking at present or have taken within the last month. Using the medicine record sheet from the back of this book, list the medicines. This will help you and your doctor to see exactly what you take every day as well as the preparations that you take occasionally. Your doctor or nurse should never prescribe a medicine or renew a prescription for an old one without knowing exactly which medicines you are taking.

Your local pharmacist can help you fill in the medicine record sheet. Many pharmacies hold records of your medicines on computer (patient medication records). If you go to the same pharmacy each time to have your prescriptions dispensed, the pharmacist can, with your permission, list the medicines you take on the pharmacy computer. Some pharmacists can also record over-the-counter medicines that you buy and alert you to any potential interactions with your prescribed medicines.

Medicines in nursing homes

If you look after an elderly person – for example, someone who is confused – you might like to get the doctor, pharmacist or member of the nursing home staff to complete the medicine record sheet. Ask if you may discuss the medicines, finding out what each one is for and why it is being taken. Patients in nursing homes are particularly vulnerable to over-use of medicines. It is important to find out if all the medicines are really necessary. For older people, in particular, stopping a medicine may be more beneficial than starting one.

REPEAT PRESCRIBING

Repeat prescribing is the re-writing of a previous prescription without the doctor seeing you for a consultation. Surveys have shown that older people and women have a high proportion of repeat prescriptions. Prescriptions most commonly repeated without seeing the doctor are medicines for rheumatic complaints, nervous and sleeping disorders, oral contraceptives and medicines for conditions that require long-term treatment, such as thyroid disease and high blood pressure. Repeat prescribing may save you time and is certainly convenient for older people who cannot or may prefer not to travel to the surgery. It saves both you and your doctor time. However, each time a repeat prescription is issued an opportunity to review treatment is lost. Although some diseases and their treatments may not change much over the years, the doctor is less likely to find out if the medicine is acting properly, or if there are adverse effects or interactions. Medicines may be continued for longer than necessary and repeat prescriptions may lead to over-prescribing.

Repeat prescribing needs to be managed well in GP surgeries and many have reviewed their systems to build in safety, convenience and regular reviews for patients. However, repeat dispensing in pharmacies provides greater convenience for some patients. This enables you to have repeat prescriptions from the GP dispensed in instalments at suitable intervals at the pharmacy for up to a year. Your pharmacist can check and review your medication at each dispensing until it is time for a follow-up appointment with your doctor, perhaps once a year. This service is suitable if you are stabilised on regular medication.

The medicine record sheet

The *medicine record sheet* at the back of this book will help you record details of the medicines you take, whether you are reviewing existing treatment or starting the first course of a new medicine. If you do not wish to use the record, you may like to make notes based on it.

- ☐ **Name of the medicine** List the generic and brand name as both are commonly used, and record over-the-counter medicines, including herbal or homoeopathic remedies. The approximate daily amount of tea and coffee (for caffeine) and the quantity of alcohol and tobacco you consume should also be noted. This information is important as it will help you to avoid drug interactions.
- ☐ **Date started** Recording the date you start taking the medicine may help you later to relate any unwanted effects to particular medicines.
- ☐ **Why prescribed** Make sure you understand why the doctor is prescribing each medicine or altering your prescription and make a brief note. For example, 'an ACE inhibitor for heart failure – to improve the efficiency of the heart'.
- ☐ **How taken** Record the dose that you take each time, how many times a day and at what time of day. For example, one 500mg tablet, three times a day before breakfast, lunch and supper. Always check whether you should take your medicine before, with or after meals as this timing is critical for the absorption of some drugs.

  Dose It is important to note the exact dose rather than just the number of tablets as a drug may be available in different strengths.

  Times per day Taking medicines three, four or more times a day is difficult to remember, especially if the routine involves more than four different drugs. Ask your doctor to make the routine as simple as possible. Many manufacturers have incorporated drugs into modified-release preparations so that you need to take only one dose a day. However, a treatment may be seriously disrupted if you forget that one dose. Taking a medicine twice a day may be easier to remember and it may not matter quite as much if you forget one dose out of the two for the day.

  When Wherever possible, medicine taking should be linked with daily activities, such as mealtimes or at bedtime when you brush your teeth. When a medicine must be taken four times a day, be sure you understand what the doctor intends. Generally, four times daily means during your waking hours rather than spread over the full 24 hours, but you should always check this with the doctor, nurse or pharmacist and work out a convenient routine for taking your medicine.
- ☐ **How long for** Always find out how long your doctor intends you to take the medicine and record the length of time. When should there be a review to gauge the success or failure of treatment? Drug treatment

should be for as short a time as possible, unless there is evidence that the medicine must be taken for a long time or for lifetime problems such as diabetes or high blood pressure.

- ☐ **Problems to watch out for** Here you can summarise possible unwanted effects. It is particularly important for you to know about these effects in order to be able to recognise them and report them to your doctor. If you have your suspicions about a medicine's unwanted effects, you can always check with a pharmacist to see whether you should return to your doctor or not.

Some medicines very rarely cause an allergic or hypersensitivity reaction that calls for urgent medical help. You can use the medicine record sheet to note any drugs that have caused allergic reactions in the past. You must tell your doctor if you are allergic to any medicines.

Other unwanted effects may be less dramatic, but contact your doctor if you are concerned. Some unwanted effects fade in severity as you continue to take the medicine, and your doctor should tell you if this is the case.

Include interactions with other medicines, food or alcohol. List any food or medicines that you should avoid when starting a medicine. Always tell your doctor, pharmacist or nurse if you are already taking a medicine, whether bought over the counter or prescribed.

- ☐ **How are you taking the medicine?** Be honest with your doctor or nurse and say whether or not you are taking the medicine and how often. You should not feel bad about stopping treatment, even if you did not have a strong reason to stop. If you cannot tolerate the drug, say so; perhaps a lower dose could be tried. Not telling your doctor, pharmacist or nurse about treatment problems can lead to mistaken conclusions about dosages and which drugs work.
- ☐ **Any new problems?** Once you have started a medicine you should assume that any worsening of your condition is an unwanted effect of the medicine until proved otherwise. A recent study showed that as

AIDS TO MEDICINE TAKING

Many medicines are now supplied in the manufacturers' packs and many of these are in monthly calendar packs with the days of the week marked. This helps you to see whether you have taken your daily dose. If you have to take more than one or two medicines a day, a daily dose organiser may help to remind you to take your medicine. An alarm set to remind you when to take a medicine can also be useful.

A medicines organiser is a device that has compartments for each medicine and the times of day they must be taken. Pharmacists can supply and fill these boxes, some of which can take a week's supply of medicines or longer; Braille labels are available with some systems. Organisers are now in use in some nursing homes where the supply of medicines to individual patients needs careful control.

many as one in ten unwanted effects is not picked up because patients do not realise that they might experience them. Friends and relatives often notice change where you may not. Older people are more likely to blame many of their problems on old age rather than on drug effects. If you look after an older person it is especially important to think about unwanted effects of drugs and to talk to the doctor about your concerns.

- ☐ **Is the medicine working?** If not, ask your doctor what should be done.

Where to find information

You may get spoken information about a medicine when you see your doctor, nurse or pharmacist. Written information is provided on the label of the medicine and you should receive the manufacturer's patient information leaflet (PIL), in the pack or from the pharmacist (page 28). Other sources of information may also be available such as PRODIGY (page 12), *Treatment Notes* from *Drug and Therapeutics Bulletin* or leaflets from the government, self-help organisations or pharmaceutical industry.

FROM YOUR DOCTOR AT THE TIME THE PRESCRIPTION IS WRITTEN

Your doctor can give you all the information you need about your medicines although it can be difficult to communicate properly or to make time for it. Writing and giving a prescription to a patient is only part of the consultation and sometimes the doctor appears too busy to talk about the medicines being prescribed. Anxiety about your illness may cloud what you remember of what the doctor says about the diagnosis and the type of illness and what tests, investigations and treatment will be necessary. Studies have shown that many people remember the diagnosis, the tests needed and when to return to the doctor, but not the explanations of the illness or the instructions for treatment.

Doctors sometimes use unfamiliar technical terms. If you have your own ideas about illnesses these may differ from the doctor's, but you may fit the doctor's explanation into your own framework of ideas. Although it is very important that you should understand what the doctor is saying, many people who do not understand hesitate to ask. You can use the medicine record sheet to prompt questions – they can help put you and the doctor on the same wavelength.

FROM PRACTICE OR SPECIALIST NURSES

Many GPs employ practice nurses who assist in running clinics such as those for people with diabetes, asthma or high blood pressure, or people with weight problems. Nurses who specialise in the management of long-term illnesses such as diabetes can, for example, demonstrate how to use insulin and tell you what you need to know about your medicines. Nurses can prescribe a range of medicines and dressings as independent prescribers in their own right or as supplementary prescribers, after a doctor has prescribed initially. The nurse must have completed the relevant training course, gained a certificate and registered with the Nursing and Midwifery Council before gaining the right to prescribe.

FROM THE PHARMACIST

When the pharmacist dispenses your prescription, the medicine will be labelled with directions for use. Every time you take a dose of medicine, read the label to double-check that you are following instructions carefully and that you have not picked up the wrong medicine. The label should tell you:

- ☐ the name of the medicine – either generic or brand name, sometimes both
- ☐ the form of the medicine – tablets, capsules, mixture or ointment, etc.
- ☐ the strength of the medicine – how much of the active ingredient is in each tablet or in a 5ml spoonful
- ☐ the dose – how much medicine to take or use each time
- ☐ the frequency – how often to use the medicine
- ☐ how to take the medicine – for example, with meals or after meals
- ☐ your name
- ☐ the name and address of the pharmacy
- ☐ the date the medicine was dispensed
- ☐ special storage instructions
- ☐ to keep the medicine out of the reach of children.

For medicines used on the body rather than taken into the body the words 'for external use only' must appear. There are many other cautionary and advisory instructions: for example, 'Dissolve or mix with water before taking' or 'Warning. Causes drowsiness which may continue the next day. If affected do not drive or operate machinery. Avoid alcoholic drink'. Although the wording of these labels has been carefully thought out, labels can sometimes be confusing. Check with the pharmacist if you are unsure.

Some drugs are used to treat more than one condition, but the prescription does not tell the pharmacist what you are being treated for; it gives only the details about the medicine and the instructions for use. If you discuss your treatment with the pharmacist, you may need to say what the medicine is for so that you can put your treatment in context. A number of pharmacies now have a room or an area where you can speak to the pharmacist privately. Like nurses, some pharmacists are starting to qualify as supplementary prescribers which will mean that consumers have easier, more convenient access to treatment.

The pharmacist will always include on the label whatever instructions the doctor has given on the prescription. Labels saying 'As before' or 'Take as directed' are no longer acceptable and prescribers should give specific instructions for every medicine on each occasion, even for repeat prescriptions. Labels on medicines, especially those dispensed in brown bottles, should have precise details of the contents and instructions for use. Mistakes in the type and amount of medicine to be taken can occur when patients transfer from home to hospital and *vice versa*. Although you may have had the same treatment for years and know the instructions well, it is good practice to have these recorded on the label. Ask the pharmacist to put the instructions on the label if they do not appear on the prescription form.

All labels on medicines dispensed by pharmacists must be typed or mechanically printed. Many labels are generated using a computer and most should be readable. However, some patients – for instance, those whose first language is not English – may not read and understand instructions with medicines. Some foreign-language labels or leaflets are available. For the partially sighted, some labels can be printed in larger print size and for the blind some labels are available in Braille.

Some health professionals print information leaflets from their computers, and you may be given these when your medicine is prescribed or dispensed. These may provide additional information to the manufacturers' leaflets.

PATIENT INFORMATION LEAFLETS

Patient information leaflets (PILs) explain what the medicine is, how it can help you, how to use it and what the possible unwanted or side effects are. The leaflets are not intended to take the place of explanation given to you by your doctor, nurse or pharmacist, but to remind you of what has been said. The information on the leaflet should also enable you to discuss your treatment and ask questions. Each leaflet should have the following information:

- ☐ names of the medicine – brand and generic
- ☐ what is in the medicine
- ☐ the form of the medicine – whether tablets, capsules or liquid – and the amount by weight or volume
- ☐ how the medicine works and the class of medicine
- ☐ who makes the medicine – the product licence-holder
- ☐ important points to note before taking the medicine – precautions and warnings about interactions
- ☐ how to take the medicine
- ☐ what to do if you miss doses or stop the medicine
- ☐ what to do if an overdose is taken
- ☐ what might happen while you are taking the medicine – unwanted effects
- ☐ storing the medicine.

Pharmaceutical companies now provide leaflets with all medicinal products and must comply with the EU directive on labelling and patient information since 1999.

WHAT MEDICINES DO

Nature provides a wealth of chemicals in plants, fungi, animals, bacteria and even minerals. Ancient civilisations used many remedies, particularly those derived from plants, and some of these are still in use today, especially in China, where 1,700 herbal remedies remain popular from a catalogue of over 5,000 plants. Many substances were used crudely: for instance mercury, used as a treatment for syphilis in the sixteenth century, would have been quite harmful to the body as well as to the microorganism causing the disease. Advances in chemistry through the nineteenth century led to a better understanding of the structure of chemicals and eventually to the understanding of a relationship between a chemical substance and its specific effects on the body (*pharmacology*). Early in the twentieth century, the idea developed that chemicals could kill disease-causing organisms without seriously hurting the human body and scientists have been aiming to achieve ever greater precision with drugs since then. However, the 'magic bullet', a medicine that can deal with the disease without affecting the body in any way, has yet to be found. Twentieth-century research also advanced our knowledge about how the body's own chemicals work (*biochemistry*) and how drugs interact with the body at cell and tissue level in different ways to alter normal body responses (*physiology*). In the twenty-first century we will realise the potential of gene-based therapies and genetic testing as new treatments are applied to the very basis of life.

Five uses of medicines

• *TO PREVENT* •

Thanks to the efforts of some far-sighted Victorians, much of the improvement in health this century has come from better nutrition, sewage and rubbish disposal and cleaner drinking water, which have greatly reduced people's susceptibility and exposure to many diseases. *Vaccines* further improve public health by protection against specific diseases. A vaccine contains a tiny amount of a substance which usually causes the disease. Your body responds to it by making *antibodies* for that particular disease; these are chemicals made by special white blood cells to combat invading organisms. You are then immune to the disease: if you subsequently come into contact with it, your body will recognise it and produce antibodies to kill the disease-causing organism.

The use of vaccines to prevent killer or disabling diseases, such as diphtheria, tetanus and polio, has revolutionised medicine. Doctors qualifying today will rarely see these diseases in the developed world.

Other examples of preventive medicine include *antimalarial* tablets, *antiseptics* used to keep wounds clean and *antibacterials* used to prevent serious infections that can complicate surgical operations. Oral contraceptives alter the balance of sex hormones in a woman's body to prevent pregnancy.

• *TO CURE* •

Medicines are used, sometimes with dramatic effect, to cure diseases caused by microscopic organisms (*micro-organisms*) which get into the body and start infection. These micro-organisms – *bacteria*, *fungi*, *viruses* and *protozoa* – are parasites which live off healthy body cells, multiply and eventually cause disease in the body. Once this pattern of disease was understood in the late nineteenth century, researchers looked for chemicals to kill invading micro-organisms without harming the *host*, the human body. An antibacterial drug destroys invading bacteria either by stopping their multiplication or by destroying bacterial cells, allowing the body to return to health.

• *TO ADD TO BODY CHEMICALS* •

Medicines are sometimes used to replace or increase quantities of the body's own chemicals, such as *hormones*, which are vital for the proper working of the body. The pancreas makes insulin, the hormone responsible for regulating the breakdown of sugar (glucose). If the insulin supply fails or does not work correctly, you become diabetic and may then need a daily supply of externally manufactured insulin.

• *TO RELIEVE SYMPTOMS* •

Headache, an upset stomach, raised temperature, skin rashes, sneezing and coughing are all signs that you are not well. Often these symptoms indicate an illness which is *self-limiting* – that is, your body will get better of its own accord in time. You may take a medicine such as an *analgesic* or a *decongestant* to relieve the symptoms, perhaps together with a day or two resting in bed – you are the best person to judge your treatment. If you do not start feeling better after a few days and your symptoms do not improve, you must decide whether to see your doctor.

• *TO CONTROL DISEASE STATES* •

Some diseases are long-term (*chronic*) conditions and do not get better; they are not self-limiting. The disease may have phases when it is either more or less active, such as rheumatoid arthritis, or you may have the condition all the time, such as raised blood pressure (*hypertension*). A disease can be kept under control by the continuous or intermittent use of a medicine to maintain health, but without achieving a cure.

How medicines work

THE STRUCTURE OF THE BODY

The body is a collection of millions of microscopic units called *cells*. Each type of cell has a distinct job to do. For example, red blood cells carry oxygen around the body, while nerve cells send messages of pain and feeling to the brain. Cells group together to form *tissues*, such as skin and muscle. Groups of tissues form *organs*, for example the heart, lungs, liver and stomach. Groups of organs which work together are called *systems*. The heart, arteries and veins together form the *cardiovascular* system, which keeps blood flowing round the body. To keep the systems, organs and tissues working together, the body has chemicals which act as messengers: for instance, a nerve cell produces a chemical called a *neurotransmitter*, which is part of the chain taking messages from the brain and nerves to muscles.

When you take a medicine, the drug reaches the bloodstream and is then carried to many parts of the body. A non-selective drug acts widely in many places in the body and is likely to cause many unwanted effects, although these are not necessarily troublesome. A selective drug works on the part of the body where its action is wanted and so there are fewer unwanted effects.

CELL INTERFERENCE

Some drugs work by interfering with the workings of the cell, either on the cell's surface, within or across it. Most drugs work on one of several types of body protein. For example, there are special sites on the cell called *receptors* into which the body's own chemicals (for example hormones, neurotransmitters) lock to produce specific effects. A cell has different types of protein receptors so that different effects can be produced, depending on which chemical has arrived at the cell.

Other drugs work by interfering with the activity of enzymes (body chemicals that facilitate a biochemical pathway) or by interfering with the flow of minerals such as sodium or calcium, for example calcium channel blockers. Others work on proteins that transport body chemicals across the cell wall, preventing the body's usual action, for example loop diuretics, which act in the kidneys.

A drug can increase the cell's activity by adding to one of the body's chemicals or decrease activity by blocking receptors to prevent the body's chemicals from working. A drug which enhances cellular activity is called an *agonist* and a drug which dampens the activity down an *antagonist*. For example, the hormones adrenaline (epinephrine) and noradrenaline (norepinephrine) produced by the body's adrenal gland prepare the body for 'flight or fight' when it is challenged in some way. Adrenaline stimulates certain cells by locking into receptors called *adrenoceptors* to prepare the body to defend itself from an unpleasant external event. Beta blockers are antagonists which block beta adrenoceptors, dampening down the stimulating effect of the hormones and slowing the heartbeat. They are used to lower high blood pressure and to treat various other heart disorders, such as angina.

REPLACEMENT OF A BODY CHEMICAL

When the body's glands produce adequate amounts of hormones, the body works well and you feel healthy. If for some reason one of your glands fails to produce sufficient quantities of a hormone, you become ill. If a gland fails gradually you may not realise why you feel under the weather, but there may be a dramatic episode with the immediate loss of hormonal control, such as the onset of diabetes mellitus in a young person when the body's supply of insulin fails suddenly. Regular supplies of insulin from an external source enable a diabetic person to lead a normal active life.

OVERCOMING DIETARY DEFICIENCY

Food supplies the body with other chemicals such as vitamins and minerals. If you lack a particular vitamin for a long period, you suffer from a deficiency disease. Sailors used to suffer from scurvy on long voyages until it was realised that lack of vitamin C caused their symptoms. Lack of vitamin B results in beri-beri, a disease rife during times of famine in developing countries. Taking an external source of vitamin C or B, respectively, cures these diseases. Only small amounts of vitamins and minerals are needed each day to maintain good health, and a balanced diet with plenty of protein, fruit and vegetables usually supplies them.

ACTION ON AN INVADING ORGANISM

Many illnesses are caused by micro-organisms – bacteria, protozoa, viruses and fungi – often referred to as 'germs'. There are micro-organisms around us everywhere and a few can cause harm if they get into the body and overwhelm its defences. Micro-organisms can enter the body through a variety of routes, principally the skin, mouth, nose, vagina and rectum, but also the eyes and ears, and via broken or damaged skin. Medicines used to combat these infections disrupt the micro-organism, either by killing its cells or by stopping it multiplying.

Entering the body

MEDICINES BY MOUTH

In Britain medicines are most commonly taken by mouth (the oral route). The medicine (either as a tablet, capsule or liquid) passes down the gullet, through the stomach to the intestines, where it is absorbed into the bloodstream. A tablet or capsule contains a measured and therefore consistent dose of the drug. A liquid contains many doses and each time you need a dose you have to measure it yourself. Tablets and capsules are convenient to take and to carry around, but some people – children, for example – find them difficult to swallow.

Most tablets are designed to disintegrate in the stomach and to release the drug for absorption in the small intestine. These tablets should be swallowed with a tumblerful of water. Other tablets may need to be chewed before swallowing or dispersed in water. The activity of some drugs is destroyed by the gastric juices in the stomach, so tablets containing these drugs are covered with a special film called *enteric coating*, to stop the medicine breaking down before it has passed through the stomach. Some medicines taken by mouth dissolve there – either under the tongue (sub-lingual tablets or spray) or between the cheek and teeth (buccal tablets). These medicines release drugs in the mouth which can be absorbed directly into the bloodstream without passing through the stomach and intestines. These drugs get into the body quickly and are useful when rapid action is needed, for example for pain relief in an attack of angina.

A capsule contains the drug in a hard or soft gelatin shell. The shell breaks open after it has been swallowed to release the contents. Capsules are cylindrical-shaped to make them easier to swallow than many tablets, and can mask an unpleasant-tasting drug. *Modified-release* capsules contain tiny pellets that gradually release a drug.

Some medicines have to be taken three or four times a day to maintain the desired effect. Some can be mixed with ingredients which prolong or even out their activity. By varying these ingredients, the manufacturer can change the rate or the place at which the drug is released from the preparation into the intestine and thus affect absorption into the bloodstream. Taking the medicine once or twice a day is more convenient than three or four times daily. Tablets and capsules in sustained-release or controlled-release form are all types of *modified-release products*. They may not look different from an ordinary tablet or capsule, but you should know whether you are taking a modified-release product and understand a few points about them.

- ☐ Do not break or cut the medicine, unless told to do so.
- ☐ Do not chew or hold the medicine in the mouth.
- ☐ Take the medicine after a meal with a full glass of water.
- ☐ Do not worry if you notice the remains of a tablet or capsule in your faeces – the drug will have been absorbed.

THE RECTAL ROUTE

A drug can reach the body's systems from the rectum when given by suppository or rectal solution (*enema*). This method avoids the stomach's digestive juices and is also useful, for example if a person is too sick to take a medicine by mouth.

Drugs are also used for their local effect in the rectum to soothe painful piles or as enemas for ulcerative colitis.

INJECTIONS

Giving a medicine by injection (*parenteral* administration – implying not by the mouth or rectum) allows the drug to get into the body without passing through the stomach where it may be destroyed by digestive juices. The drug can have an effect on the whole body (*systemic* effect) which can be rapid, depending on the type of injection used. If the injection is made straight into the vein (*intravenously*) the body's response to the drug is almost instantaneous. This route is usually reserved for people who are severely ill. Drugs can also be injected into a muscle (*intramuscularly*), under the skin (*subcutaneously*), or into the skin (*intradermally*), but it takes longer for a drug to work by these routes than if given intravenously. A *depot* injection deep into a muscle releases a drug gradually into the body over a specified period. Medicines given this way include antipsychotics, contraceptives, corticosteroids and hormones.

A drug may also be injected for a local effect, for instance to deaden a nerve before dental work or to relieve an inflamed and painful arthritic joint.

PATCHES

Some drugs are absorbed through the skin in amounts which are intended to reach the bloodstream and have a therapeutic effect in the body. This is the *transdermal* route where the drug is incorporated in an adhesive base on one side of a patch or formulated in a gel. When the patch or gel is applied to the skin, the drug is gradually released into the bloodstream. This form of modified-release preparation achieves longer-lasting blood levels of drugs. Examples of transdermal patches include nicotine replacement therapy to help with stopping smoking and oestrogen and/or progestogen for hormone replacement therapy or contraception.

IMPLANTS

A tiny pellet is placed under the skin in fatty tissue from where it gradually releases the drug into the body. Some hormones are given this way when long-term treatment is needed.

TOPICAL ADMINISTRATION

When a medicine is used *topically*, it is applied to a body surface and put directly on the skin for a local effect to clear up a rash, infection or other skin condition. Preparations used topically on the skin include creams, ointments, pastes, gels, and lotions. A topical medicine should work only at the place where it is applied, that is remain a local treatment, and should not get into the body. Emollient creams and ointments soothe the skin and act directly there, for example to relieve eczema. However, sometimes the drug component of the topical medicine can be absorbed, causing unwanted effects in other parts of the body, for example corticosteroids.

Some medicines are used on the moist skin surfaces of the body (*mucous membranes*) for a local effect – in the mouth (oral gel), the nose (drops), vagina (pessaries or vaginal tablets) and rectum (suppositories). A drug acting on the eye has a very specific local effect, although sometimes the drug enters the body via the tear ducts or through the blood vessels.

INHALATION

A medicine is breathed into the lungs where the drug can have a local effect (an aerosol for asthma) or a general effect on the body (a general anaesthetic).

Acting and leaving

INACTIVE INGREDIENTS

The words 'drug' and 'medicine' are often used interchangeably, but strictly speaking a medicine is the whole preparation whereas the drug is the active ingredient which is mixed with other substances to form the medicine. These other substances are called inactive ingredients or *excipients* and they help to carry the drug into the body and determine the way in which it is absorbed. Medicines designed to produce a local effect only – for example, products for the skin, nose, ears and eyes – also need inactive ingredients or vehicles to help deliver the drug to its site of action.

Inactive ingredients may be added to a drug to improve the taste and appearance – 'sugar-free' preparations have a sweetening agent. Liquid preparations often need a preservative to stop bacterial growth. The number of inactive ingredients in a medicine varies and depends on the form of medicine and type of drug. For example, if the amount of drug per dose is small, a tablet or capsule may need a filler or bulking agent, such as lactose or sucrose. In a tablet a drug may need an inactive ingredient to bind it together (such as gum, gelatin or sucrose) and a disintegrating agent, such as starch or sodium bicarbonate, to help it break down once the tablet is in the stomach. A tablet formulation generally contains more inactive ingredients than either a capsule or liquid.

Inactive ingredients should not produce a noticeable pharmacological effect, but some do. For example, tartrazine, the orange-yellow colourant E102, or quinoline yellow (E104) can cause sensitivity such as skin reactions and asthma, especially if you are sensitive to aspirin. Although tartrazine has been removed from many medicines, related chemical products may cause a problem for some people. Some preservatives in skin preparations can cause allergic reactions and the ointment base lanolin (wool fat) commonly causes skin problems. Purified lanolin has recently overcome this latter problem.

REACHING THE SITE OF ACTION

If you take a tablet, it has to reach the stomach, disintegrate and dissolve before the drug is released. How well the manufacturer mixes the drug with inactive ingredients to make the medicine has a bearing on how easily the drug reaches its site of action. This also depends on the characteristics of the drug itself, for instance the size of drug particles and how readily they dissolve. Most drugs pass across the small intestine wall into the bloodstream, a process known as absorption. The rate of drug absorption varies from person to person, but may also depend on whether the stomach is empty or processing food. Some medicines must be taken on an empty stomach (for example, one hour before a meal) because food and gastric acid reduce absorption. As the drug passes through the intestinal wall, it gets into the bloodstream and is taken to the liver and around the body through the network of blood vessels (the circulation).

DRUG ACTION

Each drug has its own duration of action, which depends on the nature of the drug, how it is distributed within and how it leaves the body and by which route the drug is given. A drug taken by mouth takes longer to get into the bloodstream than when it is injected as a solution directly into a vein. A drug in liquid form, such as a mixture taken by mouth, is absorbed more rapidly than a drug in solid form.

Knowing how long certain drugs remain in the bloodstream helps doctors and pharmacists work out how often someone has to take a medicine for it to reach optimum effect. This is known as the half-life of a drug. With repeated dosing, a drug reaches an optimum blood level (the steady state) in the body. For example, the antidepressant fluoxetine has a half-life of between 96 to 144 hours (four to six days). However, it takes between 5 to 20 days before the drug works optimally with regular dosing, although some effects may be experienced before then. Conversely it takes between 5 to 20 days for fluoxetine to be eliminated from the body after stopping treatment. Other drugs like penicillin or aspirin (when used for pain relief) enter the bloodstream quickly, act and then leave the body rapidly. They have to be taken four times a day to be effective. Some drugs attach themselves to blood proteins and remain bound for prolonged periods. Other drugs are fat-soluble and are stored in the body's fat, from which they are gradually released back into the bloodstream.

Once in the bloodstream the drug reaches the body's organs and tissues where it starts to exert an effect. The strength and variety of the effects of a drug depend on the size of the dose and on how selective the drug is. Generally the desirable effects provide the benefits of the drug and the undesirable effects cause the unwanted effects, but sometimes the desirable effects can become excessive and therefore unwanted – for example, lowering blood pressure too far can cause dizziness.

INACTIVATION AND ELIMINATION

The liver is the main site for dealing with foreign substances in the body. Liver *enzymes* process food and drugs, breaking them down to *metabolites* – products of the group of chemical reactions known as *metabolism*. An *inactive* metabolite has no further effect on the body, but an *active* metabolite may have a similar, but perhaps weaker, effect to the chemical from which it is derived. The drug leaves the body mainly in urine produced in the kidneys. Blood passes through the kidneys where some of the drug and its metabolites are removed in urine. Although the kidneys are the main site for eliminating a drug from the body, it can leave in faeces, sweat and other body fluids, and even on breath.

Why effects vary

How the active ingredient of a medicine works in your body depends on you and your environment as well as the medicine and dose you take. Many factors such as your age, weight, genetics, and the state of your health are important. A drug may agree with one person whereas another cannot tolerate it.

AGE AND WEIGHT

Children need lower doses of medicines than adults. Weight is an important factor, but so is the distribution of body fat and water, because drugs get into them. The liver and kidneys of children, especially newborn babies, are not as developed as those of adults. A drug may not be broken down as quickly in the liver or removed from the body by the kidneys so efficiently. The drug dosage should not be just a proportion of an adult dose based on weight, but carefully worked out to take account of the body surface area and age, particularly for children under one year.

As you grow older, your kidney and liver function start to decline. By the age of 75 there is a reduction of approximately 50 per cent in the kidney filtration rate as the blood flow to the kidneys and liver and to other parts of the body slows. In old age the total body-water decreases, but there is an increase in body-fat, particularly in men; and certain parts of the body, such as the brain, become more sensitive to medicines. It may be difficult to separate the effects of ageing from the effects of disease on the body or from the unwanted effects of some medicines. Older people may need less than the usual adult dose of a medicine. The weight of a person is particularly important for certain medicines, such as antibiotics for injection during severe infection. The larger the body the higher the dose needed to achieve a specified concentration of the drug throughout the body.

GENETIC DIFFERENCES

Although the same building blocks and biochemicals are used in the make-up of each human, the codes for the way the materials are put together vary. We are 99.9 per cent the same but our uniqueness is down to small differences in the remaining 0.1 per cent of our genetic material. The codes are carried on genes and the differences in genetic material which account for obvious differences between people can also affect individuals' responses to different drugs. A standard dose of a medicine given to 100 people will produce a variety of responses which may range from no response to extreme sensitivity, with most people experiencing some effect in between the two extremes. Individual variation in response to a medicine is a very important factor in drug treatment. The Human Genome Project has identified the 30,000 or so human genes, which is leading to a greater understanding of genetics within a cell at molecular level and how groups of genes interact. This is unlocking the genetic basis of human disease and response to drug treatment and is leading to the development of new tests and treatments (pages 39–41).

HEALTH

The effects of a drug in your body depend on how healthy you are. Illness can alter your response to a medicine. For example, if you suffer from chronic lung disease or severe asthma you will be at risk from drugs like morphine which depress the breathing control centre in the brain. You should mention any long-term problems whenever you see a new doctor.

A reduction in liver or kidney function can affect drug treatment. As many drugs are broken down in the liver, any liver disease, such as cirrhosis or hepatitis, will alter the effectiveness of the drug. The kidneys remove most of a drug or its metabolites from the body in urine. If kidney function is reduced either through illness or old age then the body's response to drug treatment is altered, as more of the drug remains in the body. If you have liver or kidney disease or a degree of impairment, the dose or how often you take it is modified. A smaller dose of drug is generally given or the number of doses you take a day reduced. Some drugs must be avoided altogether, particularly in severe disease.

ENVIRONMENT

Response to medicines can be altered by climate and altitude. In hot places, body functions increase in activity and the body loses more water. In severe cold, there will be less blood flowing to the skin and limbs. At high altitudes less oxygen is available. These sorts of changes may modify drug effects.

Drugs and chemicals in the environment may affect some people. For instance, the general anaesthetic halothane in the air of an operating theatre has caused miscarriages in female staff who experience repeated exposure to the drug. The use of antibiotics and growth promoters in the feeds of animals which people eat is a cause for concern: antibiotic use in animals may produce drug-resistant bacteria and allow the spread of disease to humans. DDT, an insecticide now banned in Britain, accumulates in animals and in humans and modifies drug effects. DDT increases the rate at which enzymes break down some drugs so that the medicine has less time to work in the body. Smoking and alcohol have the same effect.

DOSAGE

The standard dose of a drug may not produce the expected response because not all people react to a medicine in the same way. If the dose proves ineffective, increasing it may well increase the intensity of the effect, but there is a limit. A bigger dose might produce a better effect on the disease or symptoms but it is more likely to cause unwanted effects. Beyond a certain level increasing the dose does not have a greater beneficial effect, and unwanted effects become a nuisance, even a danger. For example, an ordinary dose of aspirin (600mg) will relieve a moderate headache, but may not be adequate for a severe one. A dose of 900mg may help, but perhaps only partially. Taking an even bigger dose will not help because the drug cannot achieve greater relief. However, the bigger dose is more likely to cause unwanted effects such as symptoms of indigestion or ringing in the ears.

The aim of drug treatment is to achieve a concentration of drug in the blood or tissues that lies somewhere between the minimum effective dose and the maximum safe dose. The difference between these two is known as the *therapeutic range* or *margin* and is unique to each drug. A drug with a narrow therapeutic range, such as digoxin, must be used with care because there is a fine line between effective treatment and risk of serious unwanted effects.

Before a medicine is marketed the manufacturer tries to find the best dose of the product. The dose of the drug that produces an effect in 90 per cent of people in the early clinical studies is usually selected. This means that some patients will find this dose too high for comfort and may experience adverse reactions. Some people may find the dose too low and the drug ineffective. Sometimes the medicine is marketed in too high a dose. This is discovered only once the drug has been in general use, sometimes for three or four years, as experience with it accumulates. The blood pressure-lowering drug captopril was introduced in 1981 at a daily dose of 300mg (maximum dose 450mg), but by 1985 the dose was lowered to a maximum daily dose of 150mg because some patients had suffered adverse reactions to the drug.

Taking too little of a drug may also have consequences – for example, taking too low a dose of an antibacterial for a serious infection. Underdosage may also occur when one drug interacts with another, reducing the efficacy of the second medicine. For example, the antibacterial rifampicin reduces the effectiveness of the combined oral contraceptive pill. Similarly, relative overdosage can occur when one drug is added to another, increasing its effects: for example, the lipid-lowering drug simvastatin increases the blood-thinning effects of the anticoagulant warfarin.

Beyond the maximum safe dose overdosage and poisoning can occur, although this is not dangerous for all medicines. Taking one extra dose of a medicine is unlikely to cause problems but if you are unsure about how much you might have taken, contact your doctor or pharmacist and ask for advice. Taking more than the recommended dose or taking the medicine more often than recommended does not help you to get better more quickly.

BELIEF IN MEDICINE

Believing in the healing power of the medicine you take plays an important part in the restoration of your health. The actions of the doctor or nurse giving you a prescription and of your taking a medicine or using any treatment adds to the effectiveness of the drug. This is known as the placebo response. It is particularly prominent with drugs taken to relieve pain or anxiety. Approximately one person in three responds in this way to medicine. The placebo response may be subtle, but can be surprising because you can experience unwanted effects in the same way.

Biotechnology and gene technologies

Biotechnology describes the application of biology, using living organisms such as bacteria, to produce new drugs to treat diseases, some of which have been untreatable using conventional medicines. Biotechnological techniques are now used to manufacture pharmaceuticals such as insulin, growth hormone and vaccines. The process for producing these biopharmaceuticals entails using recombinant DNA (deoxyribonucleic acid) technology, where, for example, an extract of human insulin is inserted into bacterial cells which then multiply rapidly in controlled conditions and synthesise large amounts of the human protein. Recombinant technology involves the synthesis and purification of human proteins from cloned genes, that is genetic engineering. Before the use of this technology, replacement hormones were extracted from animal or human tissues. The pharmaceutical industry is developing new genetically-based therapies. New ways of delivering the genetically engineered proteins – large, fragile molecules which at present have to be given by injection – are also being developed.

Gene technologies

In 1953 Watson and Crick discovered the double helix structure of DNA and from then onwards our understanding of molecular and cell biology advanced rapidly. Genetic research has shown that some diseases have genetic and environmental components. Bacterial infections such as cholera have environmental causes while some diseases, such as cystic fibrosis, are clearly genetic in origin. Diseases such as cancer and heart disease involve changes at cellular level but environmental factors such as infection, exposure to toxins, diet, smoking and drinking habits are also influential. The Human Genome Project is unleashing new approaches to the management of disease and inherited disorders through genetic testing and gene-based treatments.

Genetic testing

Genetic testing is currently used to screen babies before and at birth for genetic disorders, to confirm a diagnosis where symptoms already exist (*diagnostic tests*) and to indicate whether someone is likely to develop an inherited disease, such as Huntington's, or whether parents will pass on a condition such as cystic fibrosis (*predictive tests*). Rare variants of cancers such as breast and colorectal cancer can be caused by a single defective gene which can be inherited. Genetic testing may help to predict the chance of healthy family members developing the disease in future (*susceptibility tests*). If symptoms have developed already then genetic testing may one day be able to assist in targeting appropriate treatment (*pharmacogenetic tests*). Genetic tests are available for about 200 of the 10,000 or so single-gene disorders.

As research progresses it may be increasingly possible to identify those who are susceptible and then to tailor treatment and to manage environmental factors. Pharmacogenetic testing will be able to answer questions about why some people metabolise certain medicines more quickly or more slowly than others, why some people experience hypersensitivity or severe adverse reactions to some medicines, and why some people fail to respond to a medicine at all. Tests will become commonplace which will shift medical management from 'diagnose and treat' to 'predict and prevent'.

Genetic testing is not widely available on the NHS yet, but the government is committed to supporting research and development. Information, advice, appropriate safeguards (i.e. to prevent genetic discrimination) and support will be needed to help people place the results of gene tests (and particularly susceptibility tests) in context.

Gene therapy

Gene therapy is like a form of pharmaceutical therapy, only with DNA as the drug molecule that is deliberately targeted at a patient's cells with the aim of treating or preventing a disease.

Gene therapy may have several applications, for example gene replacement to correct defective genes such as the inherited disorders muscular dystrophy and cystic fibrosis. Secondly, gene therapy is starting to be used to transfer biological products known as cytokines and growth factors into the body. Treatments based on cytokines are likely to be important in inflammatory, immune and infective conditions, for example in ulcerative colitis and rheumatoid arthritis. Finally, gene therapy could help with cell remodelling, to make the cell more resistant or more susceptible to disease – for example, cancer.

Progress with gene therapy has been much slower than anticipated, with little clinical application after almost a decade of research. No 'magic bullet' or 'surgical strike' has emerged, but unfortunately some serious adverse effects, a death and gene mutation have occurred in early trials. Nevertheless major advances are expected this century. The government has established the Human Genetics Commission to assist in addressing the ethical, legal and social issues arising from potential advances in human genetics, for which informed and public debate is needed.

THE HAZARDS OF TAKING MEDICINES

There is no such thing as a safe medicine: almost all medicines can cause unwanted effects.

Unwanted effects (also called adverse, undesirable or side effects) can generally be predicted from the drug's pharmacological activity and are usually known by the time the medicine is marketed. These effects may be inconvenient, such as a slight feeling of sickness or a dry mouth, but they often fade to a 'non-worrying' level as treatment continues. Predicting who will experience unwanted effects is difficult because drug trials seldom provide sufficient information to ascertain the true level of risk. Your doctor, who has to balance the unwanted effects and benefits of prescribing a medicine for you should tell you what effects to expect, so that you recognise them and are not concerned. Treatment choices depend on weighing the evidence, for example the clinical findings, physical examination, results of any tests, and the severity of your condition. If you have disabling asthma then the use of a medicine with unwanted effects, such as a corticosteroid to control inflammation in the lungs, is a risk worth taking. Your doctor should place a medicine's potential unwanted effects in context for you.

If unwanted effects are a nuisance and do not seem to fade with time, you need to discuss this with your doctor. A lower dose or taking the medicine less often may reduce them, or it may be necessary to change to another preparation and stop it altogether.

Serious unwanted effects

Serious adverse reactions to drugs may cause a reversible illness, permanent disability or even death. Such reactions are much rarer and sometimes unpredictable. They may not have been predicted from the drug's action or noted during clinical trials and may not be detected until many thousands of people have used the medicine once it is on the market. An individual may be affected unusually because of the way his or her body deals with the drug or its breakdown products (*metabolites*), perhaps due to an inherited disorder or some extreme sensitivity, for instance sudden collapse and shock (*anaphylaxis*) after a dose of penicillin. Many allergic reactions to drugs involve the skin and these range from non-serious rashes to severe eruptions with skin peeling (*exfoliation*) that can occasionally be fatal. Certain medicines can also trigger blood disorders; a range of blood cells may be affected.

REVERSIBLE ILLNESS

Drugs can mimic disease. It can be difficult to know whether a condition is occurring naturally or whether it is caused by a drug or even worsened by it. As an example, confusion, a common problem in very old people, may fluctuate from time to time.

Any variation, particularly a worsening of the condition, may be attributed to the condition rather than the medicine(s) being taken. However, pain-relievers, the heart drug digoxin, corticosteroids in high doses, anti-anxiety drugs and antidepressants can all exacerbate confusion. Other conditions aggravated by medicines that may be mistaken for the progression of natural disease include heart conditions – heart failure, abnormal rhythms, angina and high blood pressure – diabetes, gout, asthma, epilepsy and depression. For example, fluid retention, a potential unwanted effect of the anti-arthritis drugs (NSAIDs) can exacerbate heart failure or even trigger the condition in older people. Other medicines commonly associated with adverse events include corticosteroids taken by mouth, antidiabetics and diuretics.

Many adverse reactions are reversible once the drug has been identified as the culprit. A medicine which makes you more ill should be stopped, but discuss this with your doctor.

PERMANENT DISABILITY

This may occur because a medicine has been used in too high a dose and/or used for prolonged periods.

The antibiotic gentamicin is used to treat serious infections and is usually given by injection in hospital. The unwanted effects of deafness and kidney injury are dose-related; with careful control they are not generally a problem but if high doses have to be used, or if the drug is given to an elderly person or to someone with reduced kidney function, it may accumulate in the body. If deafness results it is not reversible, although kidney function is usually restored.

Chloroquine, primarily used against malaria, also affects rheumatic disease. It has to be taken for long periods and may damage the cornea (usually reversible) and the retina (generally not reversible) of the eye. Blindness can result. However, damage to the retina is rare provided the dosage is kept within recommended limits. Eye damage is more likely to occur if chloroquine treatment exceeds two years.

A corticosteroid, taken to reduce inflammation of the arteries just under the temple (temporal arteritis – a condition that can lead to severe headache and even blindness) – relieves the headache and controls this serious disease. Taken long-term the corticosteroid can cause the bones to crumble (*osteoporosis*) unless they are protected by another medicine, such as a bisphosphonate (page 347).

DEATH

Death can occur as a result of overdosage, whether intentional or non-intentional, as a result of medication errors, or in individuals who are very susceptible to the effects of a drug.

With drugs that have a narrow therapeutic range, such as lithium and some antiepileptics, the difference between the desired effects and harmful ones is small. For example, barbiturates, used for inducing sleep and widely prescribed until the 1970s, were found to be toxic just over the maximum dose.

Susceptible individuals may without knowing take a medicine that causes very little upset in other people. Aspirin, for instance, relieves millions of peoples' headaches a year, and through its blood-thinning properties at lower dose prevents stroke, but in some people it can cause severe ulceration and bleeding in the stomach, which may be fatal if not detected. Chloramphenicol, an antibiotic, frequently and safely used as drops in the eye to clear up infections such as conjunctivitis, can cause irreversible blood disorders, resulting in death, if used by mouth or injection for severe infections. Warfarin, an effective anticoagulant, can cause death through internal bleeding if blood is thinned too much and the effects of the medicine are not monitored appropriately.

Drug interactions

A drug interaction occurs when the effects of one drug (A) are modified by the effects of another drug (B). This can happen by one of two main mechanisms: firstly by A altering the amount of B available for drug action and secondly where A affects the drug action of B without altering B's amount in the body. Some foods, for example grapefruit juice, and alcohol, can also interact with specific drugs. A few drug interactions are beneficial. For example, probenecid, a drug previously used to control gout, helps to prevent kidney toxicity when given with cidofovir, an antiviral drug. Many drug interactions are dose-related, and altering the dose of one of the medicines deals with the problem. Other drugs interact with each other but do not cause problems in practice. However, most significant drug interactions are adverse reactions and the more drugs you take, the greater the chance of an interaction.

In the first type of interaction, the absorption, distribution, metabolism and elimination of one drug may be altered by another drug. For example, metoclopramide, the antiemetic, reduces the absorption of the heart drug digoxin from the gut, thus reducing its effectiveness. Rifampicin, a drug for treating tuberculosis, interferes with the metabolism of warfarin, a drug which thins the blood and affects clotting, to diminish the effect of warfarin, which could allow blood clots to form again.

In the second type, the effects of two drugs may interact at the site of action. For example, sildenafil (Viagra – for erectile dysfunction) and nitrates (for angina) both work at the same site which can lead to severe a drop in blood pressure. Alcohol depresses brain function and interacts with any drug that also dampens down brain function. Alcohol should not be taken at the same time as a sleeping tablet because it enhances the effect of the medicine; the combined effects of the two may lead to excessive sleepiness and even coma.

Most medicines come with a patient information leaflet (PIL – page 28) that will tell you about significant drug interactions, and the pharmacist may add a further warning label when dispensing the medicine. For instance, antibacterials such as ciprofloxacin or doxycycline should not be taken at the same time as iron or zinc preparations or indigestion remedies because these substances reduce the antibiotics' absorption and therefore their effectiveness. You should allow two to three hours between taking one of these antibiotics and an antacid or iron preparation.

Some interactions may be life-threatening and if you are prescribed one of the following groups of medicines you should be given a treatment card which lists important drug interactions, and in some cases, drug and food/alcohol interactions. You will then know which combination of medicines to avoid. Always check with your doctor or pharmacist before stopping, or taking any other medicine with:

- antiepileptics
- oral corticosteroids
- monoamine oxidase inhibitor antidepressants
- lithium
- rifampicin, an antibiotic
- warfarin, an anticoagulant.

Examples of food interactions include grapefruit juice, which significantly increases the blood levels of many calcium channel blockers, such as nifedipine and verapamil, by decreasing the amount of a body enzyme which breaks down these drugs. Anticoagulant control with warfarin can be reduced by vitamin K in green vegetables, particularly with a sudden change of diet (dosage can be adjusted to take account of this – green vegetables do not need to be avoided altogether!) Cranberry juice and warfarin appear to interact leading to changes in control, although the exact mechanism is currently unknown. It is therefore best to limit or avoid taking cranberry juice whilst on warfarin.

Not only do some prescription medicines interact, but medicines bought over the counter can also cause problems. Monoamine oxidase inhibitor antidepressants, now less used, interact with certain constituents of some cold remedies, resulting in a dangerous rise in blood pressure. Herbal remedies interact with many medicines. For example St John's wort, an antidepressant, reduces the effectiveness of the oral contraceptive pill. Always check with your doctor, nurse or pharmacist before you start taking a herbal remedy or over-the-counter preparation with other medication. Similarly, tell him or her if you are taking any over-the-counter remedy before a prescription is written.

COMBINATION PREPARATIONS

Combinations of some drugs can be taken together safely and sometimes they are mixed together in one medicine. A combined preparation can be useful if one drug enhances the activity of another or moderates its unwanted effects. It is easier to take, and to remember to take, one tablet rather than several different medicines, particularly if treatment is for long periods. Furthermore, if you pay a prescription charge, you pay only one charge for a combination product but several charges for the ingredients dispensed separately.

The disadvantage of combination products is that the individual drug dosages are fixed and cannot be adjusted to suit your needs during a course of treatment. Drugs may be combined inappropriately in medicines – some combination cough and cold remedies even contain ingredients with opposing effects. Certain combination analgesic preparations, often promoted as additionally effective, are no more effective than the main ingredient, such as aspirin or paracetamol, used alone. Caffeine, for instance, adds nothing to the pain-relieving properties of aspirin and may even worsen headache or any gastric irritation.

It is difficult enough for doctors and pharmacists to remember the individual ingredients of a combination preparation, let alone the patient, but a manufacturer's brand name masks the presence of several ingredients. Patient information leaflets are more informative and give the generic name of your medicine as well as the brand name. Generic names beginning with 'co' contain two drugs in fixed proportion, for example the analgesic co-codamol 8/500 contains codeine phosphate (8mg) and paracetamol (500mg) per tablet.

Missed doses

It is important to take medicines in the right dose, at the right times, by the right route and in the right way whenever you can. It may not matter if you do not take every dose of your medicine, but you must find out how important it is to do so from your doctor. Underdosing can lead to ineffective therapy. For certain conditions it is especially important to sustain drug levels in the body – for example, antiepileptic treatment for controlling seizures. If you have high blood pressure you will need to take medicine every day. If you have a hormone imbalance, such as thyroid disease, you may need to take medicine for ever, and it will certainly be important to take treatment regularly. You may need treatment for a particular length of time to prevent the risk of a relapse. Find out what to do if you miss a dose of your medicine as the advice varies depending on the type of drug. Patient information leaflets also provide guidance.

Polypharmacy and overprescribing

The use of several different medicines at the same time (usually four or more) is known as polypharmacy. Certain diseases or conditions, for example chronic obstructive lung disease, asthma, heart failure, high blood pressure and epilepsy, may require daily treatment with several medicines, particularly when someone has more than one medical problem at the same time. The doctor should balance the effects and the dosages of the medicines to provide the best treatment for the patient.

However, inappropriate or irrational use of several medicines – for example using two medicines of the same class, such as the benzodiazepines temazepam for sleep and lorazepam for its daytime tranquillising effect – can be a danger. Both drugs act in the body in a similar way and are likely to enhance each other's effects.

Polypharmacy can occur when the unwanted effects of a medicine are treated with a second medicine, which in turn produces unwanted effects requiring treatment with a third. This produces a vicious circle or cascade of unnecessary and harmful drug treatment when what is needed is a thorough assessment of all the medicines taken by the patient. Successful treatment may involve reducing or increasing the number of medicines taken, reducing or increasing the dosage, choosing alternative medicines, stopping some drug treatment and then ensuring that any changes made are monitored. Some conditions, such as giddiness, are not helped by a medicine, and other medicines such as antidepressants may contribute to falls. Stopping drug treatment may be the best option but your progress without medicines should still be checked.

Older people in nursing homes are particularly vulnerable to unnecessary treatment with many medicines if they are not reviewed regularly – for example, routine doses of laxatives and sedatives may be given along with any specific treatments.

Some medicines may be used in too high a dose, particularly in older people, for example benzodiazepines and antidepressants which act on the brain and nervous system. Medicines for removing excess fluid from the body (diuretics) are sometimes used at too high a dose and for unnecessarily long periods. In older people with fluid on the legs, a few days' treatment with a diuretic may be all that is needed to remove the fluid, followed by gentle exercise and then resting with the legs up. Yet many people are prescribed diuretics for months.

Medication errors

In the past the NHS has underestimated the scale of unintended harm or injury experienced by patients as a result of medical errors and adverse events in hospital and other areas of health care. Examples of medication errors in hospital have included failure to dilute potassium chloride solution, which causes abnormal heart rhythms, before injecting it into the patient; or injecting the anticancer drug vincristine into the spine, where it is toxic, instead of the veins.

In primary care most errors relate to prescribing decisions, how patients take their medicines and the lack of proper monitoring of medicines. Examples include a doctor's failure to monitor lithium blood levels, which can result in toxic symptoms in the patient; a patient's failure to take essential medication regularly (such as asthma medication); or failure by health professionals and the patient to recognise adverse reactions to medicines. The National Patient Safety Agency aims to ensure better healthcare systems, clearer labelling and packaging, the purchase of products with the best safety profile, and that health professionals report errors or 'near misses' routinely in a blame-free culture and learn from them.

Herbal remedies, vitamins and supplements

A wide range of vitamins, minerals and herbal products can be bought from pharmacies, supermarkets and health food shops. Some are licensed medicines but others are classed as food products and can be advertised as being dietary supplements or functional foods (*nutraceuticals*). The manufacturer is not allowed to make claims either on the label or in the advertising that the product can prevent, treat or cure a disease, otherwise the supplement would have to be licensed as a medicine. However, leaflets, books and magazines placed alongside dietary supplements are free to suggest how a product might help, and the claims may be misleading. Some supplements contain excessive doses of vitamins and minerals or are herbal remedies with established pharmacological effects. Although vitamin supplements cause few problems for many people, there is no firm evidence that they provide any benefit, unless the person taking them has a specific vitamin deficiency. Some vitamins and minerals actually cause unwanted effects in excessive doses, and food supplements containing, for example, herbal laxatives or ginseng do cause adverse reactions. Always tell a health professional about other medicinal or dietary products, including vitamins, that you are taking in addition to conventional medicines.

Herbal remedies and how they are licensed are under review by the European Commission following concerns about the safety and quality standards of some herbal medicine products. Aristolochia, a plant species used in Chinese herbal medicine, sometimes an un-named ingredient, has been associated with end-stage kidney failure in two UK cases and many more worldwide. Medicinal products containing it have now been banned. Kava-kava (Piper methysticum), a member of the pepper family found on South Pacific islands, is used to relieve anxiety and tension. Products containing Kava-kava have also been banned in the UK as it can cause severe liver toxicity. Drug interactions with the antidepressant St John's wort have also been highlighted – a factsheet on these can be downloaded from the Committee on Safety of Medicines website (*www.mca.gov.uk*).

The use of an unlicensed remedy as a medicine needs careful thought before you adopt it as regular treatment. Variability of quality between different sources or batches of the same herbal preparation can occur: some Chinese herbal medicines have been found to contain prescription-only medicines, such as corticosteroids. Unlicensed remedies are not usually as supported by evidence for efficacy, safety, quality and consistency of preparation as are officially endorsed medicines. There may be some evidence for effectiveness – for example, glucosamine in osteoarthritis of the knee – but a lack of robust evidence on long-term safety issues. Other products such as 'natural' progesterone creams for menopausal symptoms or for protection against post-menopausal bone loss have only weak evidence to support their use. Occasionally some products that your doctor has been able to prescribe in the past are no longer recommended. For example, product licences for gamolenic acid products, Efamast and Epogam, were withdrawn in 2002 by the Medicines and Healthcare products Regulatory Authority (MHRA) because long-term efficacy in the conditions for which they were used – breast pain and also eczema – was questionable.

Who is most at risk from medicine-taking?

The effects of a medicine depend on many factors. Although all people vary in their response to drugs, certain groups are more vulnerable when taking medicines than others.

BABIES AND CHILDREN

Age, weight and maturity of the liver and kidneys are important factors in drug treatment of the young. Not only do babies and children need smaller doses than adults, but a medicine which may not cause any problems in an adult may adversely affect a young baby. Pseudoephedrine, a decongestant drug for drying up colds, may cause sleep disturbances and nightmares and young children seem quite sensitive to this effect. Antihistamines, also in cough and cold remedies, help the child to sleep, but many are long-acting and the effects continue the next day, interfering with muscle control, co-ordination and balance.

A baby's immune system is immature and therefore it takes time to build up resistance to every sort of infection. Immunisation against serious diseases, starting at two months of age, prevents major illness, but otherwise the child develops immunity to common infections as contact occurs with other children in playgroups and school. Repeated infections, such as colds, coughs, diarrhoea and skin complaints, are quite normal in childhood: a child may well have had over 30 episodes of illness by the age of six years. Simple remedies, such as simple linctus for coughs, or paracetamol syrup for fever and pain relief, may be all that is needed.

Some medicines used for children may not have been tested specifically for use in such young patients, particularly for rarer conditions. A number of difficulties have been identified in carrying out clinical trials in children such as recruiting adequate numbers of children, obtaining consent, and the cost of developing suitable formulations of drugs to give to babies and young children. Many medicines are used unlicensed or 'off label' for children, which is not ideal. Greater awareness of the problems however means that the medicines' regulatory bodies are beginning to address the issues.

PREGNANT WOMEN

Most women now understand that it is best to avoid taking any non-essential medicine during any stage of a pregnancy because drugs can cross the placenta and enter the baby's bloodstream. During the first three months of pregnancy some drugs can interfere with the development of the baby and cause abnormalities. Such drugs are called *teratogens*. Few drugs are proven teratogens, but no drug is beyond suspicion in early pregnancy. After the first three months of pregnancy, drugs may affect the growth and further development of the baby. It is difficult for doctors to assess whether a baby's abnormality is due to chance or to the effect of a particular drug.

The thalidomide tragedy prompted much stricter testing of drugs so that now all pharmaceutical companies must make a statement about a medicine's use in pregnancy at the time the medicine is marketed and promoted. However, it is sensible to avoid taking any medicine unless absolutely necessary before you plan to conceive or during pregnancy.

If you have a permanent condition such as diabetes, drug treatment will be essential during your pregnancy, so you should see your doctor to discuss management of the pregnancy even before you conceive. Screening tests during pregnancy are available. If you are planning to become pregnant or are pregnant, check with your doctor or pharmacist before taking any medicine, either prescribed or over-the-counter, including herbal remedies. Even vitamins which might seem beneficial during pregnancy must be treated with care. High doses of vitamin A can affect the unborn baby and cause abnormalities. Smoking and alcohol should also be avoided as they may affect the developing baby.

• *BREAST-FEEDING WOMEN* •

Some drugs can pass through the mother's milk into the baby where they may act. Some may cause toxicity, whereas others have little effect on the baby. Certain drugs can inhibit the flow of milk. Breast milk concentrates some drugs so that the baby may get a toxic dose even though the mother is taking a normal dose. Other drugs, such as antibiotics, may in theory cause an allergic reaction, even though the drug concentration in the baby's blood may be low. Tranquillisers may make the baby drowsy and less able to feed. For many drugs there is inadequate information, but these examples illustrate that it is best to avoid taking medicines while breast-feeding unless absolutely necessary. Check with your doctor or a pharmacist before taking any medicine.

• *OLDER PEOPLE* •

Medicine use increases substantially in people over the age of 65 and with it the potential for unwanted effects and drug interactions. Four out of five people aged over 75 take at least one medicine, with over a third taking four or more medicines. Problems can occur not just in taking medicines but also with services, for example poor communication between hospital and the doctor's surgery.

As you grow older, your body and the way it works gradually changes. The body's regulatory mechanisms, such as the control of temperature or blood pressure, become less efficient. This is part of the normal ageing process and is separate from the effects of diseases which become increasingly commonplace with age. Elderly people's response to treatment with medicines and the way the body handles drugs changes. The liver and kidneys become less efficient. In particular, the decline in kidney function means that drugs are removed from the body more slowly. The brain and nervous system become more susceptible to drugs; the immune system may not protect the body reliably and drug treatment may set off an unusual response.

All these physical changes mean that drug treatment of elderly people must be approached with care. Conditions which are commonly treated include heart and blood pressure problems, nervous disorders, rheumatic diseases and digestive complaints. Older people take more medicines and for longer periods, because many diseases, such as arthritic conditions, last for a long time. The more medicines that are taken, the greater the risk of drug interactions and other unwanted effects. The standard adult dose of some medicines may be higher than necessary; with some medicines, treatment should be started with a lower dose than that used for younger adults.

The ageing process can be mistaken for disease and inappropriate drugs may be prescribed. For example, dizziness is common in older people because of the change in the blood pressure control mechanism. Prochlorperazine has been used to treat this sort of giddiness, but the drug can cause mental confusion and symptoms similar to Parkinson's disease (uncontrolled movements, particularly of the face, rigidity and tremor) which may not develop until the medicine has been taken for weeks or even months. Because drugs can mimic diseases and worsen them, the patient's deterioration might not be credited to the adverse effects of the medicine, but to the condition itself. When the adverse effects of medicines are not recognised, further drug treatment might then be prescribed to deal with the patient's new symptoms. See 'Polypharmacy and overprescribing', page 46.

DRIVERS AND OTHER DECISION-MAKERS

Any skill which requires judgement and co-ordination can be affected by a medicine which acts on the brain and nervous system. This type of medicine can affect car and train drivers, airline pilots, machine operators and many others who have to make quick decisions. Many drugs can interfere with driving skills, particularly during the first few days of treatment when the extent of unwanted effects is unknown. It is an offence to drive or be in charge of a vehicle when your ability to drive is impaired by medicines.

The following groups of prescribed medicines can affect performance of skilled tasks, mostly by causing drowsiness: most antihistamines; anti-anxiety drugs; antidepressants; antipsychotics; some pain-relievers; some blood pressure-lowering drugs; some drugs for epilepsy; some drugs to control vomiting; and some muscle relaxants.

You can become tolerant to the effects of some of these drugs, but until you are sure about your reaction to the medicine, you should avoid driving. Other medicines that affect vision (for example eye drops for glaucoma), or cause nausea or dizziness, can also impair driving ability. Ask your doctor if you can drive. Sleeping tablets can have 'hangover effects' the next day, particularly in older people, which can affect driving. You should not drive for 24 hours after a general anaesthetic. If you have diabetes and you are on insulin you should not drive just before a meal is due unless you take extra carbohydrate. Always carry a supply of snacks in the car to deal with symptoms of low blood sugar.

You have a legal duty to tell the Driver and Vehicle Licensing Agency (DVLA)* of any medical condition or disability which affects your fitness as a driver – for example, epilepsy, visual problems caused by glaucoma, or diabetes. Some heart conditions or the insertion of a pacemaker can lead to stopping temporarily, while you must stop driving in certain circumstances – for example, if you have the sleep disorder obstructive sleep apnoea syndrome – until your condition is controlled. Your doctor can advise you on fitness to drive. The DVLA is legally responsible for deciding whether a person is medically unfit to drive, but doctors have clear guidelines about how to manage situations if a person continues to drive after being advised to stop. Ultimately if you do not stop driving, your doctor must notify the DVLA and then tell you that a disclosure has been made.

Over-the-counter medicines, such as preparations for hay fever, and cough and cold remedies, contain antihistamines and decongestants. These can cause drowsiness, impair judgement and affect driving skills. The effect of alcohol on driving performance is well known and even a small quantity will enhance the effects of drugs that cause drowsiness.

Putting the risks into perspective

Medicines have enormous potential benefit: lives have been saved by antibiotics; the existence of a person with diabetes might depend on regular insulin injections. But some of the medicines described in this book have dramatic adverse effects. All medicines, even those sold in supermarkets, provide some benefits but also a risk of some harm.

Estimates vary but adverse drug reaction problems may account for two to three per cent of consultations in general practice and five to seven per cent of hospital admissions. Six to 17 per cent of hospital inpatients are thought to experience adverse drug reactions. These often seriously ill patients are likely to be treated with powerful medicines which carry greater risks of adverse reactions. It is difficult to get accurate figures because the reported incidence of adverse reactions varies depending on how the information has been collected.

The most common reactions to drugs involve the skin (rashes, eruptions, photosensitivity), then the nervous system, followed by the digestive system. Non-steroidal anti-inflammatory drugs (NSAIDs) cause serious and life-threatening reactions, particularly in older people, with bleeding and perforation of the intestines. Fortunately other medicines, such as a proton pump inhibitor, can protect the gut from these serious effects.

Medicines can cause death and a serious amount of drug-induced (iatrogenic) disease and discomfort, but the overall reported risk of dying from a serious adverse drug reaction has remained at less than one in a million for most years since records began in the 1960s.

Balancing the benefits and unwanted effects of a medicine needs to be done in context of the disease being treated. Generally, more serious diseases are treated with more powerful medicines. Treatment of cancer with medicines that can make you feel very ill may be worthwhile if they prolong life. Taking aspirin for a fleeting headache is not worthwhile for people who suffer serious unwanted effects. Arthritic patients are usually prepared to put up with some of the unwanted effects of NSAIDs which relieve joint pain and swelling in order to remain active and mobile. Many people are prepared to tolerate the unwanted effects of medicines so long as they understand that they will happen and know what to look out for.

Your doctor must choose the right medicine, weighing the evidence for and against in discussion with you. You should expect to know about the expected outcomes of treatment and have time for questions, and the doctor must take into account the patient's views in a concordant approach. It is then up to you to use the medicine correctly.

Monitoring adverse reactions

A medicine is licensed after testing in 2,000 to 3,000 people – both those who need treatment and healthy volunteers. However the rarer, unpredictable adverse reactions and who will be at risk cannot be determined until larger numbers have taken the medicine, usually after several years.

Licensed medicinal products have checks inbuilt for safety, quality and efficacy. Once a drug has been marketed, all suspected adverse reactions or unexpected events attributed to a new medicine should be reported to the Committee on Safety of Medicines (CSM), which monitors adverse drug reactions. New medicines are marked with a black triangle to indicate that health professionals should supply evidence (page 16). The assessment of these reports by the MHRA can eventually lead the CSM to publish guidance to health professionals – for example, a warning of a specific adverse reaction or drug interaction, or notification of a drug withdrawn from the market.

CLINICAL TRIALS

A *clinical trial* should be a carefully and ethically designed experiment with the aim of answering some precisely framed question. The trial should involve equivalent groups of patients treated at the same time, but in different ways. The patients should be randomly allocated to one treatment or another.

Tests of the medicine must be carried out in adequate numbers of patients to establish the true effect of a medicine. The effect must be statistically valid, so there is enough certainty that the result is not due to chance. This is particularly important because of the placebo effect.

Ideally, a clinical trial aims to show:

- ☐ the value of the treatment
- ☐ whether the treatment is better than existing treatments
- ☐ the type of patient who will benefit
- ☐ in what form the drug should be taken
- ☐ the dose and how often it should be taken
- ☐ the nature of any unwanted effects and adverse reactions.

A new drug may be tried against an established standard treatment or it may be tested against a placebo. For example, one group of patients may take the test drug for a particular period while another group takes the comparison treatment or placebo. The groups then swap to treatments they have not yet had. In a *double-blind randomised controlled trial* neither the

WHAT IS A PLACEBO?

Placebo is Latin for 'I shall please'. A placebo can be a medicine which is given more to please than to benefit the patient, who believes that taking a drug will help. The word is also used to describe a 'dummy drug', an inactive substance which has no pharmacological effect on the body and which is used in clinical trials to test the effects of a medicine. A placebo helps to sort out the true response to a medicine from the belief in medicine-taking. You can experience both beneficial and unwanted effects from a placebo, even though it does not act the same measurable way as the medicine. This is particularly so when you do not know whether you are taking a placebo or the active drug in a clinical trial.

doctor nor the patient knows whether the trial drug or placebo is being taken until the trial has ended.

Detailed information about the trial should be supplied to those taking part. Consent must almost always be sought from potential trial participants or legal representatives, for example on behalf of an adult who is incapable of giving consent. Parents or guardians can give consent for children under 16 years.

A clinical trial may take several years to set up, to find the correct number of patients, to collate and interpret the results and to publish the findings. At every stage of a trial it is possible to introduce error and bias, even quite unintentionally. A trial costs a large amount of money to conduct. Many are now supported by pharmaceutical companies and are also conducted globally as multicentre trials across a number of countries. Unfortunately, some trials do not provide clear-cut answers, although the results may be presented in optimistic and glowing terms, a tendency with some company-sponsored trials. The effects of a product can be exaggerated, for example, by reporting results as the *relative risk reduction*, that is the relative health gain or reduction in events between the treatment and the placebo groups. The relative risk reduction can inflate small differences in effect. The *absolute risk reduction*, that is the arithmetic difference in absolute risk between the treatment and placebo groups provides a more accurate treatment effect. For example, in a placebo-controlled trial of a drug taken for four years to slow bone loss, prevent osteoporosis and fractures of the vertebrae in women, the incidence of these fractures was 3.8 per cent in the placebo group and 2.1 per cent in the treatment group. This amounted to a 44 per cent relative risk reduction but an absolute risk reduction of only 1.7 per cent.

A systematic review (i.e. a collation) of the original evidence from all trials which attempted to answer the same question using reproducible methods provides more robust evidence. The mathematical technique of aggregating these trial results is known as meta-analysis. One of the skills your doctor needs is interpreting clinical trials. Meta-analyses and systematic reviews help doctors deal with the huge growth in medical literature. Much emphasis is being placed on the quality of medical evidence, and doctors are encouraged to practise evidence-based medicine. They must have reliable information on the effects and hazards of treatment which they can then apply to their own practice.

Once a medicine is licensed, the Medicines and Healthcare products Regulatory Agency (MHRA) and the European Medicines Evaluation Agency (EMEA) monitor reports of serious unwanted effects. Information comes from a variety of sources.

VOLUNTARY REPORTING BY HEALTH PROFESSIONALS

Health professionals including doctors, dentists, coroners, pharmacists and nurses are asked to report all cases of suspected adverse reactions to new medicines and serious or unusual reactions only with older established products. They fill in details on a special adverse reaction card (also known as a Yellow Card) and send it either electronically or by post to the MHRA or to one of five regional centres which collect adverse reaction information on behalf of the Committee on Safety of Medicines (CSM). Around 17,000 adverse drug reaction reports are sent to the MHRA each year. The Yellow Card scheme, which has been operating for 40 years, serves as an early warning system to alert prescribers to adverse drug reactions and potential problems in prescribing. The CSM advises when a drug should be withdrawn from the market for safety or efficacy reasons.

The main drawback of this scheme is that the true incidence of a drug's adverse effects cannot be obtained because the scheme is voluntary and is underused by health professionals. The Department of Health is therefore reviewing the Yellow Card scheme. Recent research suggests that the way in which adverse drug reactions are classified by the CSM can lead to inconsistency, confusion and may not highlight patients' problems adequately. The scheme, however, is being extended to include patients' reports of adverse drug reactions via NHS Direct centres.

PHARMACEUTICAL COMPANIES

The Medicines Act requires manufacturers to report any suspected adverse reactions to their products whether in Britain or overseas.

WORLD HEALTH ORGANIZATION

The MHRA has an on-line link to the World Health Organization's database which collects information from 71 countries, giving a worldwide perspective on drug safety matters. See *www.who-umc.org*

POST-MARKETING SURVEILLANCE SCHEMES

The Drug Safety Research Unit (DSRU), an independent group, monitors prescriptions on selected, usually new medicines prescribed by general practitioners. Prescription Event Monitoring (PEM) can identify adverse drug reactions that might occur in around 1 in 3,000 patients, a more accurate approach than reports via the Yellow Card scheme. The prescriber is asked to provide a detailed report and say whether he or she considers the event represents an adverse drug reaction. These reports are assessed for possible associations between the reported events and exposure to the drug being monitored: potential adverse reactions are thus identified.

Many general practitioners now store on computer details of patients, records of illnesses and any medicines prescribed. Several independent companies operate a record linkage scheme where the prescriptions for the selected medicine can be linked to clinical reports and a search made for specific reactions.

Once a medicine is marketed, a pharmaceutical company might set up a study to monitor its safety in everyday use. Guidelines for operating these studies, Company Sponsored Safety Assessment of Marketed Medicines (SAMM), are agreed by representatives from doctors' organisations (the British Medical Association and the Royal College of General Practitioners), from the government (as the MHRA and the CSM), and from the industry (as the Association of the British Pharmaceutical Industry). In spite of the existence of these guidelines, some studies are thinly veiled promotional studies, encouraging the doctor to prescribe the medicine which patients may then continue to take for many years. Doctors are paid per person to recruit patients for these studies. Sometimes the results remain unpublished, particularly if they are unfavourable to the company, or perhaps only selective results are reported. If your doctor is considering entering you into a trial of a new medicine, you may like to ask:

- ☐ Why is this the best drug for me?
- ☐ Are there options other than drug treatments?
- ☐ Is there a more established drug that will work as well?
- ☐ What are the possible unwanted effects?
- ☐ What should I do if I think I am experiencing or have experienced an unwanted effect?

What if treatment goes wrong?

Health professionals do not intend to harm patients with medicines, but accidents and mistakes do occur. If you suffer permanent disability from the adverse effects of a medicine or you are the relative of someone who dies as a result of taking a medicine, redress can be difficult to obtain, expensive and time-consuming; although you may be entitled to Legal Aid. You have to prove that the doctor (or the drug company for medicines marketed before 1 March 1988) was negligent and that it was this negligence that caused your present condition. Under the Consumer Protection Act, you have to prove that the drug was defective. It can be very difficult to prove that medical negligence caused your injuries. Proving that a drug was defective is also hard because a company can claim that potential risks were unknown at the time the medicine was developed.

Consumers' Association research has shown that people want to know the risks involved in any treatment. If you have suffered avoidable harm through a prescribing error, you should expect a prompt explanation of the facts. You may be confused, angry and worried. You will want to know what went wrong, what compensation you are entitled to, and to have an assurance that all appropriate steps will be taken to prevent a repetition in other patients. It would be helpful if the doctor offered an apology, but many fear that to do so would be an admission of liability.

Various 'no fault' compensation schemes have been suggested but the adoption of a comprehensive scheme seems unlikely. In 2003 the Chief Medical Officer published proposals for the reform of how clinical negligence cases are dealt with in the NHS, which were under consultation at the time of writing. The proposals in *Making Amends* include 19 reforms that should, if implemented, reduce the costs and the time taken for claims to be settled.

The NHS is developing a culture of quality improvement through risk management and clinical governance. Adverse events and 'near misses' should be reported routinely in NHS organisations and information fed back to ensure that people learn from their mistakes. The National Patient Safety Agency, a special health authority, is starting to co-ordinate NHS reports including errors resulting from drug administration (which are treated anonymously), and is managing the national reporting system. All health professionals must keep up to date through continuing professional development, regular appraisal and re-accreditation.

If, however, you have problems with your NHS care, you should complain first of all directly at the place where you received the service, such as the doctor's surgery, pharmacy or hospital, to attempt local resolution. The Patient Advice and Liaison Service (PALS) in main NHS hospitals and primary care trusts can deal with minor problems and tell you about the complaints process. Local Independent Complaints Advocacy Services (ICAS) may also be able to help. If you are not happy with how your complaint is handled at local level or you consider there is unreasonable delay, you can ask for an independent review. At the moment this is organised by the local hospital trust or PCT, but in future this will move to the Commission for Healthcare Audit and Inspection. If you are still not satisfied, you can consider taking your complaint to the Health Service Ombudsman.

If you have NHS treatment in a private hospital, you can use the NHS complaints procedure. Otherwise private hospitals, clinics and surgeries should have their own complaints procedures. You can also complain to the professional body that regulates the particular health professional, such as the General Medical Council for doctors, General Dental Council for dentists, Nursing and Midwifery Council for nurses, or the Royal Pharmaceutical Society of Great Britain for pharmacists.

1

DIGESTIVE SYSTEM

Indigestion Peptic ulcers
Diarrhoea Constipation
Piles and anal disorders

The digestive system (also known as the gut or *gastrointestinal* system) includes the gullet (*oesophagus*), stomach, small and large intestines, the rectum and anus. Chewed food passes from the mouth into the oesophagus, down into the stomach where digestive juices (including hydrochloric acid and the enzyme *pepsin*) break down the food into smaller particles; these pass into the small intestine, where more enzymes break them down (digest them) into molecules small enough to be absorbed through the intestinal wall into the bloodstream. These molecules go to the liver, which sorts them and breaks them down further (*metabolises* them) into nutrients for the body to use. The remnants of digestion pass to the large intestine (*colon*) where water is absorbed into the bloodstream leaving stools (or faeces), which are passed out of the body through the anus.

Indigestion

Indigestion (*dyspepsia*) is a symptom popularly attributed to difficulty with digesting food: you may experience bloating, pain under the ribs or heartburn – a sharp or burning pain in the centre of the chest which you sometimes also feel in the throat; you may have an acid taste in the mouth, burp a lot or feel sick. You may feel a burning pain after swallowing hot drinks. Symptoms tend to come and go and may be worse after a meal. Indigestion during pregnancy, especially in the later stages, is common.

Your stomach may be irritated or inflamed because you have eaten or drunk too much. Some medicines, particularly aspirin and other non-steroidal anti-inflammatory drugs (NSAIDs), can irritate the stomach and cause indigestion or even ulceration. Indigestion can be due to a condition called *hiatus hernia* – a weakness of the muscle between the gullet and the stomach which is supposed to stop food and acid leaking into the gullet. This type of indigestion (also called *oesophagitis*, *reflux oesophagitis* or *gastro-oesophageal reflux disease*) is particularly noticeable after meals and when stooping or lying down, and is more likely if you are overweight. Occasionally, symptoms can mimic other conditions, such as hoarseness or persistent night-time cough which are sometimes mistaken for asthma but can be due to refluxed acid irritating the windpipe. Severe chest pain from indigestion can be mistaken for a heart attack (page 125) or vice versa.

A few medicines seem to relax the muscle between the gullet and stomach, which worsens acid reflux into the oesophagus. Medicines that act in this way include **nitrates** and **calcium channel blockers** for heart problems and also **theophylline** for breathing problems.

Indigestion is a common symptom and may occur only occasionally, but if you have indigestion which persists for more than a few weeks or keeps recurring, or the pattern of symptoms changes, particularly if you are over the age of 55 years, you should see your doctor. If you have lost weight recently for no obvious reason, cannot swallow food, do not feel like eating or have anaemia then discuss these symptoms with your doctor. Indigestion sometimes has serious causes, such as cancer of the upper part of gastrointestinal system, which occurs in less than 2 people in 100. Long-term symptoms can be caused by an ulcer (page 64), although the lining of the stomach may not be damaged as it is by a full-blown ulcer. You should see your doctor immediately if you feel sick or vomit matter that looks like coffee grounds, suffer from stomach cramps or pain, or if you have black, tarry or speckled stools. These are signs of a bleeding ulcer. Other causes of indigestion include *irritable bowel syndrome* (pages 77–79), but indigestion for which there is no clear explanation is called *non-ulcer dyspepsia*.

– HOW YOU CAN HELP YOURSELF –

- ☐ Lose weight if you are overweight.
- ☐ Cut down on alcohol.
- ☐ Give up smoking or at least cut down: any form of tobacco can irritate the digestive system.
- ☐ Sit upright when you eat your food, so that you are not pressing down on your stomach.
- ☐ Eat at regular intervals, avoiding large meals late at night
- ☐ Avoid stooping forwards, especially after meals, and avoid reclining after meals.
- ☐ If you have heartburn or reflux symptoms sleep with the bed-head raised by about 20cm (8in).
- ☐ Avoid coffee, and spicy foods if you are not used to them.
- ☐ Avoid foods and drinks you know cause you problems.
- ☐ Eat a sensible balanced diet, with not too many fried and fatty foods – these can aggravate indigestion.
- ☐ Avoid medicines that irritate the stomach: use paracetamol instead of aspirin, for example.

Medicines for indigestion

Many people try one of the indigestion remedies available over the counter, particularly for the occasional relief of indigestion. These are mainly antacids but H_2-receptor antagonists (page 66) can also be bought. If you consult your doctor about indigestion you will need to discuss what type of over-the-counter medicine you have taken (for example antacid with alginate), the dose and how often you took it. Sometimes a trial of an antacid taken regularly can relieve symptoms. H_2-receptor antagonists can be prescribed at higher doses than the over-the-counter products. Your doctor may want to try a stepwise approach to managing your symptoms, starting with an antacid and then, if needed, progressing to an H_2-receptor antagonist. If symptoms persist then your doctor may want to test for the presence of *Helicobactor pylori*, a bacterium that lives in the stomach and duodenum. Eliminating *Helicobactor pylori* may get rid of your symptoms (page 65). Proton pump inhibitors (page 70) can be used for severe symptoms of gastro-oesophageal reflux disease or for protecting the stomach and duodenum from the unwanted effects of NSAIDs. Referral for endoscopy (page 66) may also be considered.

Antacids

Antacids neutralise stomach acid. They are useful once you have indigestion or if you expect symptoms. Many antacids can be bought over the counter (often for less than the cost of a prescription), but you should avoid using them continuously for long periods without seeking advice from a doctor or pharmacist. Unsupervised use of up to two weeks' treatment is reasonable, and prolonged use of an antacid when monitored by your doctor is acceptable. Some antacids contain sodium compounds, which are used to make liquid and tablet preparations, because sodium, commonly called salt, dissolves readily. If you have heart or kidney disease you should keep your salt intake as low as possible. Some preparations are sugar-free which is helpful for diabetics.

Liquid preparations work better than tablets, although tablets are more convenient. You could use liquid or powder preparations at home and take tablets with you when you go out. Liquids must be shaken before use and tablets must be chewed well. Antacids need to be taken four or more times daily – about an hour after meals and at bedtime.

ALUMINIUM AND MAGNESIUM ANTACIDS

Most antacid preparations are based on **aluminium** or **magnesium salts** or mixtures of both (**co-magaldrox**), sometimes with additional ingredients. Aluminium- and magnesium-containing antacids stay in the digestive system and are not much absorbed into the body. Aluminium preparations (**aluminium hydroxide** liquid or tablets) may cause constipation whereas magnesium-containing antacids, such as **magnesium trisilicate** mixture, tend to have a laxative effect: preparations containing both aluminium and magnesium may suit you better. Occasionally aluminium hydroxide is prescribed in capsule form (Alu-Cap) for removing high levels of phosphate in the body which have formed kidney stones. Antacids should not be taken at the same time as other medicines – for example, antibiotics and antifungal medicines – if possible. This is because antacids reduce the absorption of other medicines, rendering them less effective. Antacids may damage the coating of enteric-coated tablets, used to delay the release of a drug from a tablet into the gut.

Additional ingredients

Manufacturers often add extra ingredients to aluminium and magnesium antacids. **Alginic acid** is a mucus-like substance derived from seaweed which helps to protect the lining of the stomach and oesophagus. Little evidence exists that other extras, such as activated **dimeticone** (dimethicone; simethicone) to relieve flatulence, make the basic antacid work any better. Because these preparations are generally more expensive than simple antacids and have no clear advantages, many complex antacids are no longer available on prescription: your doctor only prescribes the most cost-effective.

ALGINIC ACID/ANTACID MIXTURES

On prescription/over the counter
ALGICON* – Liquid, tablets
GASTROCOTE – Liquid, tablets
GAVISCON – Liquid, tablets 500mg, oral powder for children
GAVISCON ADVANCE – Liquid
PEPTAC – Liquid
TOPAL* – Tablets

Over the counter (not NHS)
ASILONE HEARTBURN – Liquid, tablets
BISODOL HEARTBURN – Tablets
BOOTS HEARTBURN RELIEF – Tablets
GAVISCON – Tablets 250mg

* low salt content

Alginic acid and related compounds sodium and magnesium alginates are mucus-like substances derived from seaweed, which protect the lining of the oesophagus and stomach from acid. They are usually mixed with antacids, aluminium and magnesium compounds and with sodium bicarbonate and calcium carbonate. Alginic acid or alginates combine with stomach acid to form a thick gel or 'raft', which floats on the stomach contents, forming a barrier and preventing acid from attacking the gut lining. Alginic acid/antacid mixtures are used for relieving indigestion and heartburn, but are particularly useful for gastro-oesophageal refluxdisease, where stomach acid leaks back into the oesophagus, a condition often associated with hiatus hernia.

Alginic acid/antacid combinations have few unwanted effects, but the amounts of alginic acid, antacid, sugar and salt (sodium) content vary between products. Liquids come in a range of flavours such as aniseed, lemon and peppermint, while tablets may be lemon- or peppermint-flavoured.

Before you use this medicine

Tell your doctor or pharmacist if you are:
□ pregnant or breast-feeding – alginic acid/antacids are useful for relieving heartburn in pregnancy and can also be taken during breast-feeding □ taking any other medicines, including vitamins and those bought over the counter □ on a low-salt diet – alginic acid/antacids contain variable amounts of salt (sodium). Products with a high salt content should be avoided in heart and kidney disease; those marked* have a low salt content □ diabetic – some preparations are sugar-free.

Tell your doctor or pharmacist if you have
□ severe or prolonged stomach pain □ blood in stools □ prolonged diarrhoea □ heart disease or high blood pressure □ kidney disease.

See your doctor immediately if you feel sick or vomit matter that looks like coffee grounds, suffer from stomach cramps or pain or if you have black, tarry or speckled stools. These are signs of a bleeding ulcer.

How to use this medicine

Liquid preparations are more effective than tablets, although tablets are more convenient to carry around. It is a good idea to use a liquid preparation at home and take tablets with you when you go out. Take them four times daily about an hour after meals and at bedtime. See your doctor if you take an antacid continuously for more than two weeks and feel no better. Liquids must be shaken before use; tablets must be chewed thoroughly before swallowing.

Over 65 No special requirements.

Interactions with other medicines

Antacids, particularly in large doses, may affect the absorption of other drugs if taken at the same time.
Tablet coatings Antacids may damage the enteric coating, used to delay the release of a drug from a tablet into the gut.

Avoid taking an antacid at the same time as any other medicine if possible.

Unwanted effects

Less likely Aluminium-containing antacids may cause constipation, whereas magnesium-containing antacids may cause loose stools or diarrhoea. Most alginic acid/antacid preparations contain a mixture of aluminium and magnesium compounds, which should avoid either problem.

Similar preparations

On prescription/over the counter

Antacids containing aluminium or magnesium

ALUMINIUM HYDROXIDE – Liquid
AROMATIC MAGNESIUM CARBONATE – Liquid
MAGNESIUM TRISILICATE – Mixture

Antacids containing aluminium and magnesium

ALUMINIUM-MAGNESIUM COMPLEX – HYDROTALCITE* – Liquid
MAGNESIUM TRISILICATE COMPOUND – Tablets
CO-MAGALDROX – A mixture of aluminium and magnesium hydroxides
MAALOX* – Liquid
MUCOGEL* – Liquid

Aluminium and magnesium with other ingredients

With dimeticone:
ALTACITE PLUS* – Liquid
ASILONE* – Liquid
KOLANTICON – Liquid
MAALOX PLUS* – Liquid

* low salt content

SODIUM BICARBONATE

Taken as powder or tablets this works more quickly than either aluminium- or magnesium-containing antacids and is effective and cheap for relieving occasional indigestion. However, if taken in large doses for long periods it is absorbed into the body, where it can upset the blood chemistry. Like other carbonate-containing antacids, it releases carbon dioxide gas, which causes burping. This does not mean that the antacid is working more effectively; the gas it forms may be trapped in the stomach and add to discomfort. You should not use sodium bicarbonate if you have heart, liver or kidney problems or are on a low-salt diet.

CALCIUM AND BISMUTH

Some over-the-counter products contain either **calcium** or **bismuth** (see Box below). Short courses of a calcium-containing antacid or occasional doses are fine but high doses for long periods may rarely increase blood-calcium and upset the acid balance in the stomach. Calcium-containing antacids can also result in the stomach producing more acid after treatment, although in practice this is rare.

Bismuth-containing antacids (although not **bismuth chelate**) are best avoided, especially for prolonged use, because bismuth absorbed into the body can damage nerves. They also tend to cause constipation.

POPULAR OVER-THE-COUNTER ANTACIDS

These antacids cannot be prescribed, but are cheap. Most contain several ingredients, such as **sodium bicarbonate + magnesium carbonate + calcium carbonate**. Here they are listed under their main ingredient.

Sodium bicarbonate-containing

ANDREWS ORIGINAL SALTS – Powder
BOOTS GRIPE MIXTURE 1 MONTH PLUS
ENO'S – Powder

Calcium carbonate-containing

ANDREWS ANTACID – Tablets
BISODOL – Tablets
DE WITTS – Tablets, powder
MACLEAN – Tablets
NULACIN – Tablets (contains gluten)
OPAS – Tablets
*RAP-EZE – Tablets
*REMEGEL – Tablets
RENNIE – Tablets
*SETLERS – Tablets

Bismuth-containing (not recommended)

MOORLAND – Tablets
PEPTO-BISMOL – Liquid

* contain calcium carbonate only

Other medicines for indigestion

ANTISPASMODIC MEDICINES

These relax control of the muscle around the stomach. They are sometimes used with other treatments for non-ulcer dyspepsia and irritable bowel syndrome (page 77). They have been used for treating ulcers but the high doses needed to stop gastric acid production cause unwanted effects such as dry mouth, blurred vision, constipation and difficulty in passing urine. Older people are particularly sensitive to these effects, even at a lower dosage. If you have the eye problem *closed-angle glaucoma*, *myasthenia gravis*, an enlarged prostate or a condition known as *paralytic ileus* you should not take these medicines.

Antispasmodic medicines have been superseded by ulcer-healing drugs (pages 65–72) which are much more effective for treating gastro-oesophageal reflux disease and ulcers and have fewer unwanted effects. Products include **dicycloverine** (**dicyclomine**) (Merbentyl), and **propantheline** (Pro-Banthine). Dicycloverine, combined with antacids aluminium and magnesium as Kolanticon gel, is used for indigestion accompanied by muscle spasm. **Hyoscine** tablets (Buscopan) are not recommended.

MOTILITY STIMULANTS

Medicines that enhance or stimulate the movement of the intestine (*motility stimulants*) are sometimes used for treating non-ulcer dyspepsia and gastro-oesophageal reflux disease. **Metoclopramide** and **domperidone** speed emptying of the stomach and increase the movement of the intestines thereby helping the flow of contents along the gut. They also help to enhance the narrowing of the muscle between the stomach and gullet and control acid leaking from the stomach into the gullet. Both drugs also act on the central nervous system as anti-emetics and so are used for controlling nausea and vomiting (pages 221–226).

Metoclopramide and occasionally **domperidone** can cause unwanted *parkinsonian* effects (similar to the symptoms of Parkinson's disease), such as spasms of the facial muscles and abnormal movements of the eyes. Contact your doctor if these effects occur. The effects are more common in younger people (especially girls and young women) and the very old. They usually happen just after starting treatment, but will fade a day or so after stopping the drug.

Peptic ulcers

A peptic ulcer is a damaged section, rather like a small crater, in the lining of the stomach or intestine wall. It is caused by the irritant action of stomach acid which has broken through the layer of mucus that protects the tissue from harm. Peptic ulcers are known specifically as *gastric* or *duodenal* ulcers depending on whether they occur in the stomach or in the first part of the small intestine (*duodenum*). If an ulcer is left untreated it can burst (perforate), causing a great deal of pain, or it can bleed – sometimes so severely as to be life-threatening. Most of the symptoms of indigestion can be caused by an ulcer, particularly if they go on for several weeks without relief. However, the pain from an ulcer can start suddenly and severely. A bleeding ulcer will cause you to vomit blood or matter that looks like coffee grounds or to have black, tarry stools; you should see your doctor immediately if you have either of these symptoms. The causes of an ulcer (as opposed to a perforated ulcer) are thought to include smoking, stress and alcohol; while some drugs – particularly aspirin and other non-steroidal anti-inflammatory drugs (NSAIDs) – and stomach infection with a bacterium, *Helicobacter pylori*, are definitely associated with peptic ulceration. Some people are prone to developing ulcers. Food, milk or antacids may relieve the pain, but you should see your doctor if you have indigestion for more than a few weeks or if it recurs regularly. Avoid alcohol. For other suggestions on how to help yourself, see the box on page 59.

NSAID-ASSOCIATED ULCERS

Non-steroidal anti-inflammatory drugs (NSAIDs) are widely prescribed for the treatment of arthritis and other painful conditions. If you take an NSAID by mouth you may experience indigestion, which is a common unwanted effect. This does not necessarily mean that you will develop an ulcer, although it is more likely if you are over 60 or have had a peptic ulcer previously. NSAID-induced ulcers can develop and even bleed or perforate without causing pain or any other warning symptom. An ulcer-healing drug, either a H_2-receptor antagonist, proton pump inhibitor or **misoprostol** (pages 69–70), is usually prescribed to heal the ulcer. It is best to stop taking the NSAID, but if you have to continue, then your doctor will prescribe a proton pump inhibitor such as **omeprazole,** or other ulcer-healing medicine such as misoprostol, to take as well.

HELICOBACTER PYLORI INFECTION

Helicobacter pylori (H. pylori) is a bacterium that lives in the acidic environment of the stomach, unlike most bacteria that are killed by the acid. It can infect the lining of the stomach and duodenum and lead to peptic ulceration. Most peptic ulcers that are not associated with taking an NSAID are caused by H. pylori. Your doctor can test for the presence of the bacterium, usually by a breath test (the carbon urea breath test) or from a sample of blood. If your doctor finds that you have H. pylori infection then you will need to have treatment with a short course of triple therapy, a combination of antibiotics and an acid suppressant, such as a proton pump inhibitor (page 70). This treatment usually heals the ulcer. Many people are infected with H. pylori but do not have any symptoms, in which case no treatment is needed. H. pylori is also found in about half of people who have non-ulcer dyspepsia, that is, indigestion without an identifiable cause, and treatment to eradicate infection may help to relieve symptoms in around 1 in 15 people. However eradication therapy is not recommended routinely for people with non-ulcer dyspepsia, nor is it helpful for reflux symptoms.

Ulcer-healing medicines

Some ulcer-healing medicines work by reducing the amount of acid in the digestive system; others form a protective layer over the ulcer. High doses of an antacid can promote ulcer-healing, but the amount of medicine that you have to take every day may be unacceptable. To overcome this, better medicines have been developed to heal ulcers, although relapse may occur when you stop treatment. These include H_2-receptor antagonists, misoprostol (a prostaglandin-type drug) and the proton pump inhibitors (page 70). An antacid and an H_2-receptor antagonist may be used together – your doctor will advise you about this. An H_2-receptor antagonist can be used for minor digestive disorders, such as occasional dyspepsia or heartburn.

Before the introduction of ulcer-healing medicines, many gastric ulcers were treated by surgical operations, but these are generally unnecessary now. Your doctor may need to make sure that you do indeed have an ulcer and that there are no other underlying conditions, such as cancer, particularly if you are middle-aged or older, which may involve attending a hospital outpatient clinic to have an *endoscopy* (also called *gastroscopy*). This procedure involves swallowing a thin fibre-optic tube passed down the back of your throat into your stomach and duodenum, through which the ulcer can be seen. You do not need an anaesthetic for this, but you will be given a mild sedative.

• H_2-RECEPTOR ANTAGONISTS •

These are *antihistamines* which block histamine receptors in the stomach to limit the flow of gastric acid (see 'Allergies and hay-fever', pages 174–175). The H_2-receptor antagonists **cimetidine**, **ranitidine**, **famotidine** and **nizatidine** can all heal gastric and duodenal ulcers in one to two months and there is little to choose between them. They have few unwanted effects and can now be bought from a pharmacy for the relief of indigestion (dyspepsia) and heartburn.

Although H_2-receptor antagonists heal ulcers, an ulcer may recur once you finish a course of treatment. Your doctor may decide to treat you with further courses of an H_2-receptor antagonist each time this happens, or put you on a lower dose for a longer period. The profile of cimetidine, below, is an example of how you should use any of this group of medicines.

CIMETIDINE

On prescription
CIMETIDINE – Tablets
DYSPAMET – Liquid
TAGAMET – Tablets

Over the counter
TAGAMET 100 – Tablets
CIMETIDINE

Cimetidine is an H_2-receptor antagonist, which blocks the release of stomach acid by binding to histamine receptors in the cells of the stomach wall. Histamine is a body chemical that triggers the body's response to an allergen (H_1-receptor) and controls the rate and the amount of stomach acid (H_2-receptor) produced to aid digestion. Excess acidity and another body chemical, pepsin, cause duodenal ulceration, whilst gastric ulceration may develop if the lining of the stomach wall is damaged. The bacterium H. pylori is also associated with the development of peptic ulcers. Cimetidine can heal ulcers in the oesophagus, stomach and duodenum. It can also be bought from a pharmacy to treat short-term symptoms of dyspepsia, heartburn and excess acidity and to prevent night-time symptoms of heartburn.

Before you use this medicine

Tell your doctor if you are:
☐ pregnant or breast-feeding ☐ taking any other medicines, including vitamins and those bought over the counter.

See your doctor immediately if you vomit blood or matter that looks like coffee grounds or if you have black, tarry stools. These are signs of a bleeding ulcer.

How to use this medicine

Your doctor will tell you how long you need to take cimetidine – it will be for at least a month, often two. Do not alter the dose without talking to your doctor. Avoid drinking alcohol or smoking. Do not stop taking this medicine before you finish the course of treatment, even if you feel much better.

Take the tablets twice a day, with breakfast and at bedtime; sometimes the dose may be increased to four times daily. If you have a duodenal ulcer, for example caused by a non-steroidal anti-inflammatory drug (NSAID), you should take the whole dose at every bedtime for eight weeks.

Over 65 You may need less than the adult dose if your kidney function is very poor. Older people or the very ill are more at risk of rare side effects.

Interactions with other medicines

Oral anticoagulants (e.g. **warfarin**), **antiarrhythmics** (e.g. **amiodarone**), **antiepileptics** (e.g. **carbamazepine**), **theophylline**, **aminophylline**, **antipsychotics** (e.g. **chlorpromazine**), the immunosuppressant **ciclosporin** and the peripheral vasodilator **cilostazol** Cimetidine increases the effects of these, so your doctor may need to adjust the dose. Other H_2-receptor antagonists, **ranitidine**, **famotidine** and **nizatidine**, do not interact with these medicines.

Unwanted effects

Less likely Diarrhoea, rash, dizziness, tiredness, headache.
Rare but serious Blood disorders, acute pancreatitis, muscle or joint pain, irregular heartbeat, confusion, depression and hallucinations, hypersensivity reactions, swollen breasts. These usually occur only with high dosage and generally cease when you stop taking cimetidine.

Similar preparations

On prescription

AXID – Capsules, injection
NIZATIDINE

FAMOTIDINE – Tablets

NIZATIDINE – Capsules

PEPCID – Tablets
FAMOTIDINE

PYLORID – Tablets
RANITIDINE BISMUTH CITRATE

RANITIDINE – Tablets, soluble tablets, liquid

ZANTAC – Tablets, soluble tablets, liquid, injection
RANITIDINE

From a pharmacy

BOOTS EXCESS ACID CONTROL
FAMOTIDINE

PEPTID AC – Tablets, chewable tablets, combined with antacid
FAMOTIDINE

RANZAC – Tablets
RANITIDINE

ZANTAC 75 – Tablets
RANITIDINE

H2-receptor antagonists over the counter

Ulcer-healing drugs can be bought from a pharmacy – for example, cimetidine (Tagamet 100), famotidine (Pepcid AC), ranitidine (Zantac 75) and nizatidine (Axid) can be purchased in smaller pack sizes and at lower doses than those on prescription. They can be used for the short-term relief of indigestion or dyspepsia, heartburn and excess acidity associated with the consumption of food and/or drink. Famotidine, nizatidine and ranitidine may also be used to prevent heartburn and indigestion; cimetidine may be used to prevent night-time symptoms of heartburn.

In lower doses the over-the-counter H_2-receptor antagonists are probably as effective as antacids. They may have a longer-lasting effect, but have a slower onset of action than antacids. They are considerably more expensive.

The pharmacist or trained assistant should assess whether an over-the-counter H_2-receptor antagonist will suit you and help your symptoms before you buy one of these products. In some cases it is better to see your doctor and not to self-medicate. Contact your doctor if:

- ☐ you are under 16 years of age
- ☐ you are pregnant or breast-feeding
- ☐ you are being or have been treated for a peptic ulcer
- ☐ you are middle-aged or older and experience dyspepsia for the first time
- ☐ your symptoms have changed in nature or intensity or you have difficulty in swallowing
- ☐ you have lost weight suddenly
- ☐ you have liver or kidney disease
- ☐ you are already being treated for other conditions by a doctor, e.g. with a non-steroidal anti-inflammatory drug (NSAID)
- ☐ you are taking any other medicines, specifically cimetidine and anticoagulants (e.g. warfarin), the antiepileptic drug phenytoin or the anti-asthma drug theophylline
- ☐ you are sensitive to any of the ingredients of an H_2-receptor antagonist medicine.

See your doctor immediately if you feel sick or vomit matter that looks like coffee grounds, suffer from stomach cramps or pain or if you have black, tarry or speckled stools. These are signs of a bleeding ulcer.

PROSTAGLANDIN-TYPE MEDICINE

Misoprostol is related to a family of body chemicals, the prostaglandins. It promotes healing of peptic ulceration but is used mostly for treating or preventing gastric or duodenal ulceration associated with the anti-inflammatory pain relief medicines, the NSAIDs (page 236). Misoprostol will not treat indigestion caused by an NSAID unless you have an ulcer. It is available with an NSAID to help to protect the stomach and intestine and prevent ulcers; this combination is useful for frail and elderly people who need gastric protection and must continue to take an anti-inflammatory drug.

MISOPROSTOL

ARTHROTEC 50/75 – **Diclofenac** (an NSAID) and misoprostol in a combination tablet
CYTOTEC – Tablets
NAPRATEC – **Naproxen** tablets (an NSAID) and misoprostol tablets in one pack

Misoprostol works in a different way to the H_2-receptor antagonists. It is related to a prostaglandin, one of a range of body chemicals, which acts in the stomach specifically to reduce the production of acid, promote mucus formation and repair damaged cells. Misoprostol can be used for treating ulcers, whether or not these are caused by an NSAID. It can also prevent ulcers forming if taken with an NSAID, but does not relieve indigestion. Misoprostol and **diclofenac** in one tablet as Arthrotec 50 or 75 tablets are suitable only if the doses of the individual ingredients have already been shown to be satisfactory for you.

Before you use this medicine

Tell your doctor if you are:
☐ pregnant or planning to become pregnant – misoprostol must not be taken during pregnancy; if you have monthly periods, you must take effective contraceptive measures to make sure that you do not become pregnant during treatment ☐ breast-feeding – avoid ☐ taking any other medicines, including vitamins and those bought over the counter.

If you have low blood pressure, heart disease, narrowing of the arteries or have had a stroke, see your doctor for regular check-ups.

How to use this medicine

The usual dose is four tablets a day: you can either take **two** tablets **twice** a day with breakfast and at bedtime or you can take **one** tablet **four** times a day with or just after meals. If you develop diarrhoea whilst on misoprostol, taking one dose four times a day after meals may help this problem. Treatment for existing ulcers usually lasts for one or two months.

Avoid drinking alcohol or smoking. Do not stop taking this medicine until you have finished the course of treatment, even if you feel much better. If you miss a dose take it as soon as you remember, but skip it if it is almost time for your next dose. Do not take double the dose.

Over 65 No special requirements.

Interactions with other medicines

Avoid magnesium-containing antacids, especially if diarrhoea is a problem.

Unwanted effects

Likely Loose stools or diarrhoea – if the diarrhoea is severe, you must contact your doctor, who will decide whether you should continue treatment. Other effects include feeling sick, indigestion, excess wind and stomach cramps.
Less likely Vomiting, dizziness, skin rashes.
Rare but serious There have been occasional reports of women experiencing heavier than usual monthly periods and bleeding in between periods, and of women who have stopped menstruating experiencing bleeding. See your doctor if you suffer any of these effects.

PROTON PUMP INHIBITORS

These medicines stop stomach acid production completely by blocking an enzyme system (hydrogen-potassium adenosine triphosphatase) within a special type of cell (*parietal*) lining the stomach. The enzyme system, known as the 'proton pump', aids stomach acid formation.

The proton pump inhibitors, omeprazole, esomeprazole, lansoprazole, pantoprazole and rabeprazole sodium, heal gastric and duodenal ulcers – including those associated with taking an NSAID (such as aspirin) – by mouth. A proton pump inhibitor is the most effective treatment for severe oesophagitis, particularly where the gullet lining has become ulcerated and damaged.

A proton pump inhibitor is the drug of choice for managing a rare condition known as Zollinger-Ellison syndrome where a pancreatic tumour causes excess production of gastric acid and severe peptic ulceration. Treatment with a proton pump inhibitor is generally well tolerated, but long-term acid suppression may increase the risk of microbial gut infections. Stomach acid is one of the body's defences against microbial invasion, and suppressing it seems biologically unnatural. However, long-term treatment with a proton pump inhibitor has not revealed major problems.

OMEPRAZOLE

LOSEC – Capsules, tablets, injection
NEXIUM – Tablets
ESOMEPRAZOLE (a close relative or isomer of omeprazole)

Omeprazole blocks stomach acid production completely by binding to an enzyme which is necessary for acid manufacture. It is used for treating and preventing peptic ulcers, including those caused by NSAIDs, as a short course for severe symptoms of erosive oesophagitis (gastro-oesophageal reflux disease) and other rarer conditions such as Zollinger-Ellison syndrome. An ulcer will heal while you take omeprazole, but may recur after you stop treatment. Eradication of *Helicobacter pylori*, the gut bacterium that plays a role in peptic ulcer formation, has reduced the recurrence rate of ulcers. Omeprazole or another proton pump inhibitor is used with two antimicrobials as triple therapy for one week to eradicate H. pylori (see below). Omeprazole works rapidly and very specifically in the body, and people generally tolerate it well. Related medicines lansoprazole, pantoprazole and rabeprazole sodium are similar to omeprazole.

Before you use this medicine

Tell your doctor if you are:

☐ pregnant or breast-feeding, taking any other medicines, including vitamins and those bought over the counter.

Tell your doctor if you have or have had:

☐ kidney or liver disease.

How to use this medicine

The usual dose is one capsule or tablet daily for one to two months, although treatment can be for shorter periods for H. pylori eradication or for longer periods for other situations, such as protecting the gut from NSAID-induced ulcers. Three strengths are available: 10mg, 20mg and 40mg; the usual treatment dose is 20mg daily, which can be reduced to a maintenance dose of 10mg if circumstances allow. If you have severe reflux oesophagitis you may be given the higher dose. Take the capsule or tablet at a regular time each day.

Avoid drinking alcohol or smoking. Do not stop taking this medicine until you have completed the course of treatment, even if you feel much better. If you miss a dose take it as soon as you remember, but skip it if it is almost time for your next dose. Do not take double the dose.

Over 65 No special requirements.

Interactions with other medicines

Diazepam Possible increased effects. Omeprazole and esomeprazole may prevent breakdown of diazepam.
Cilostazol, a peripheral vasodilator Effects increased by omeprazole. Avoid these two drugs together.
Phenytoin, **warfarin** Effects enhanced by omeprazole and esomeprazole, so the doses may need reducing.

Unwanted effects

Likely Feeling and/or being sick, headache, diarrhoea, constipation, excess wind, abdominal pain.
Less likely Dizziness, faintness, itching, tingling in the limbs, severe skin reactions and rashes, increased sensitivity to sunlight, hypersensitivity (urticaria, angioedema, bronchospasm, anaphylaxis), muscle and joint pain, swollen ankles, blurred vision, swollen breasts, baldness, insomnia, changes to liver function, blood disorders.
Rarely In a person who is severely ill, mental confusion (reversible on stopping treatment), agitation, depression and hallucinations.

Tell your doctor if diarrhoea or headache are severe.

Similar preparations

PARIET – Tablets
RABEPRAZOLE SODIUM

PROTIUM – Tablets, injection
PANTOPRAZOLE

ZOTON – Capsules, liquid
LANSOPRAZOLE

HELICOBACTER PYLORI ERADICATION

A proton pump inhibitor is used in combination with a variety of antibacterials to get rid of the bacterium *Helicobacter pylori* (H. pylori), which is now known to cause peptic ulceration by invading the stomach and intestine lining. Both duodenal and gastric ulcers (not caused by an NSAID) can be healed by one- or two-week courses (sometimes at high doses) of combinations of three medicines; these can include an ulcer-healing medicine (a proton pump inhibitor) or **ranitidine bismuth citrate** plus the antibacterials **amoxicillin** and **clarithromycin**, and an antimicrobial, usually **metronidazole**. Occasionally **tinidazole** or **tetracycline** are used with a proton pump inhibitor and other antibacterials. Combinations of three medicines ('triple therapy') give better results than two medicines together ('dual therapy'), and are preferred. It is important to take the course as directed and to finish it.

H. pylori eradication usually results in long-term healing of the ulcer. It should avoid the need to continue taking an ulcer-healing medicine indefinitely and the nuisance of repeat medication. Occasionally, H. pylori infection can recur – possibly because of antibacterial resistance or failure to complete the course. Further eradication treatment with a different combination of medicines may be required. Unwanted effects of antibacterial treatment include indigestion, feeling sick, diarrhoea and headaches. Antibiotic-induced colitis, where the colon becomes inflamed and diarrhoea occurs, is an uncommon risk of eradication therapy.

MEDICINES THAT PROTECT THE STOMACH

Both tripotassium dicitratobismuthate, a **bismuth chelate** (De-Noltab) and **sucralfate** (Antepsin) are less used now. The bismuth in De-Noltab is bound in a complex, unlike bismuth antacids, which means that very little is absorbed into the body. It is usually reserved for resistant cases of H. pylori infection when it is taken with a proton pump inhibitor plus two antibacterials. One notable unwanted effect is discoloration or blackening of the tongue and faeces.

Sucralfate is an aluminium complex. The tablets are large, but can be dispersed in a little water. You must not take sucralfate at the same time as other medicines, particularly phenytoin, tetracyclines, ciprofloxacin and similar antibacterials, cimetidine or digoxin; allow two hours in between taking sucralfate and any other medicines. Constipation is a common unwanted effect.

OTHER ULCER-HEALING MEDICINES

Carbenoxolone (Pyrogastrone) can promote ulcer-healing but adverse effects are difficult to manage, especially for people aged over 65. These include salt and water retention, and a lowering of blood-potassium. It is not recommended.

Acute diarrhoea

Diarrhoea is an increase in the frequency and looseness of your bowel movements. Water is normally absorbed from the remnants of digested food in the large intestine and the waste left over from this water-recycling process becomes stools, which are then passed out of the body at regular intervals. If this absorption process is upset, less water is taken back into the body and the remainder is passed out in liquid stools. Serious loss of water is called *dehydration*; it causes thirst, dry mouth, dry skin, reduction in quantity and darkening of urine, fast breathing and fever.

Sudden (acute) diarrhoea generally lasts only a few days and may get better whether you treat it or not. However, for babies, young children, and frail or elderly people, diarrhoea can be serious and must be treated with glucose and salt solution (page 75) to replace the body's lost water and salts if it causes dehydration or lasts for more than a few hours.

– HOW YOU CAN HELP YOURSELF –

• *ACUTE DIARRHOEA* •

- ☐ Avoid dairy products, spicy or fatty foods, fresh fruit and vegetables or any other food you do not tolerate well; do not drink milk, coffee or concentrated fruit juices.
- ☐ Drink plenty of clear liquids (at least four glasses every 12 hours) – weak tea without milk, for example; children should be given extra liquids immediately – the glucose and salt solution described on page 75 is ideal.
- ☐ Monitor your temperature.
- ☐ Depending on the severity of the attack, you may need to stay in bed and rest.
- ☐ If you have to remain active, you can avoid inconvenience and embarrassment by taking an antidiarrhoeal medicine (not for young children).
- ☐ Always wash your hands after you have been to the toilet and before handling or eating food to prevent the spread of infection.
- ☐ When you begin to feel like eating again, re-introduce food gradually; start with, say, dry toast or cracker biscuits with a clear soup and leave out dairy products and fatty food until later.

Contact your doctor if:

- ☐ a baby or young child, a frail person (someone who is weak and ill already) or an elderly person has acute and severe diarrhoea
- ☐ diarrhoea lasts for more than three days
- ☐ you have a fever: temperature above 38.5°C (101°F)
- ☐ severe, disabling stomach pains accompany diarrhoea
- ☐ there is blood in your stools or they are black and tarry
- ☐ you have dehydration, characterised by dizziness while standing, confusion or drowsiness
- ☐ a medicine may be the cause of diarrhoea.

Common causes include viral or bacterial infections in the digestive system (food poisoning) or a change of country and climate when your body is not yet immune to a new set of bacteria and viruses (often called 'traveller's diarrhoea'). Traveller's diarrhoea is defined as the passage of three or more unformed stools over 24 hours, which is often accompanied by abdominal pain, cramps and urgency in visiting the toilet, feeling or being sick, and occasionally fever. If diarrhoea develops while you are abroad and continues on your return for more than 14 days, see your doctor. Persistent diarrhoea can occur with bacterial or protozoal diseases such as dysentery (page 294).

Anxiety, alcohol, food intolerance and some medicines (for example some antibiotics, magnesium-containing antacids, the ulcer-healing drug misoprostol, stimulant-laxatives, some medicines for high blood pressure and those for regulating the heartbeat) can also cause acute diarrhoea.

Prolonged (chronic) diarrhoea usually has other causes and does not clear up like acute diarrhoea. Your doctor will need to diagnose and treat it; pages 77–84.

Medicines for diarrhoea

In an acute attack of mild to moderate diarrhoea, you can replace the water and salts lost from your body with a glucose and salt solution. Glucose increases the amount of water absorbed in the large intestine, which allows the salts in the solution to get into your body, too. This process is called *rehydration*. The aim of the treatment is to prevent dehydration developing, particularly in babies and the elderly, both of whom should be seen by a doctor.

The diarrhoea is the body's way of getting rid of harmful substances and it may be unhelpful to interfere with this natural response. Most people with acute but mild diarrhoea get better so quickly using oral rehydration salts and a light diet that the use of any other medicine is unnecessary. However, antidiarrhoeal medicines may sometimes be useful; they are discussed briefly after the profile of oral rehydration salts, below.

ORAL REHYDRATION SALTS

On prescription/from a pharmacy
DIORALYTE – Soluble powder, effervescent tablets
DIORALYTE RELIEF – Soluble powder (contains rice powder)
ELECTROLADE – Soluble powder
REHIDRAT – Soluble powder

A mixture of salts and glucose powder must be dissolved in water and made into a solution for drinking. There are several recipes for oral rehydration salts but the formula that is used most in the UK is based on sodium chloride, potassium chloride, sodium bicarbonate and glucose, or sometimes rice starch. You can buy sachets of ready-prepared, flavoured powders in a pharmacy.

If the diarrhoea is not too severe or you do not have a ready-prepared powder to hand, you can make your own mixture (page 75). The commercial solutions can be substituted as soon as possible if the attack is prolonged, if you are more severely ill or if dehydration has already started. Extra water can be taken in as required between drinks of the rehydration solution, depending on the severity of dehydration.

Before you use this medicine

Tell your doctor or pharmacist if you are:
☐ diabetic – the glucose (sugar) content of the solution should not cause a problem ☐ taking any medicines, such as laxatives or magnesium-containing antacids ☐ pregnant or breast-feeding.

Always contact your doctor if diarrhoea does not get better within three days or if you have severe vomiting. People aged over 70, frail people, babies and children under three years must be seen by a doctor.

How to use this medicine

The powder in one sachet or the tablets should be dissolved in 200–250ml (7–8fl oz) of drinking water, depending on the instructions given with the particular product. Do not add extra salt, sugar or glucose: make up the solution exactly as instructed. A weaker than specified solution will not be effective. The solution should be made just before it is needed, but can be kept in a refrigerator for up to 24 hours. If it cannot be stored in a fridge, the solution must be thrown away after one hour. For babies and children under three use freshly boiled and cooled water, but do not reboil the prepared solution.

An adult usually needs around 200–400ml (half to one pint) of prepared solution after liquid stools are passed; a child needs approximately 200ml. If you feel sick or are being sick, take sips of the solution as frequently as possible.

Over 65 No special requirements.

Unwanted effects

Likely Feeling sick; flavoured solutions can be more palatable.

ANTIDIARRHOEAL MEDICINES

Treating diarrhoea with an antidiarrhoeal medicine is of less importance than rehydration and should not distract you from fluid replacement measures. For adults, it can help to overcome some of the inconvenience and embarrassment associated with an acute attack. Babies, young children, frail people and elderly people must always be rehydrated with glucose and salts solution; they should avoid antidiarrhoeal medicines.

HOME-MADE SALT AND GLUCOSE SOLUTION

Use one small level teaspoon (3.5g) of salt and eight large level teaspoons (40g) of sugar – or four large level teaspoons (20g) of glucose powder – to one litre of water. A small amount of fruit juice or squash can be added to flavour the solution.

You can get a two-ended spoon, the large end for sugar and the small end for salt from Teaching Aids at Low Cost*.

Absorbent medicines

These form bulk in the intestines; mixtures of chalk and kaolin are sometimes used in mild chronic diarrhoea. They are not recommended for acute diarrhoea.

Antimotility medicines

These slow down intestinal movement (*peristalsis*). Although these medicines relieve diarrhoea symptoms, they can prolong contact between harmful micro-organisms and the intestinal cells. Opioids (derivatives of the poppy plant) have long been used: these include liquid mixtures of **opium** or **morphine** (such as Kaolin and Morphine mixture BP) or tablets. Over-the-counter products include Diocalm, Opazimes and Collis Browne's. **Codeine** (Kaodene) and **co-phenotrope** (Lomotil) are also used. These products are of limited use in controlling acute diarrhoea.

They can reduce breathing and cause constipation and even dependence after prolonged use of high doses. Lomotil was an important cause of accidental poisoning in young children before oral rehydration was introduced and symptoms of overdosage can occur after as little as one dose; children under four must not be given Lomotil.

– HOW YOU CAN HELP YOURSELF –

TRAVELLER'S DIARRHOEA

- ☐ Avoid drinking tap water, and even using it for cleaning teeth, unless you are sure that it is fit to drink. Use bottled or treated water; add chemical water-purifying tablets or ten drops of weak iodine solution to a litre of water in parts of the world where water supplies are suspect. In areas where amoebic dysentery is likely, boiling water for half an hour will kill the organisms and any amoebic cysts satisfactorily.
- ☐ Avoid ice cubes in your drinks unless you are sure of the water.
- ☐ Avoid eating unwashed salads and vegetables and unpeeled fruit (even in drinks).
- ☐ Avoid eating dishes containing uncooked eggs, shellfish, unpasteurised dairy products and food from street traders that is not freshly prepared or hot.
- ☐ Wash your hands or use an antiseptic wipe after going to the toilet and before you handle food or eat.
- ☐ Take with you a supply of salt and glucose sachets and an antidiarrhoeal medicine.
- ☐ Do not buy or use an antibiotic to treat diarrhoea, unless under guidance from a doctor.

For general advice on how to stay healthy when going overseas contact the Medical Advisory Service for Travellers Abroad (MASTA)*, or look up their website at *www.masta.org*. Other useful websites are: *www.doh.gov.uk/traveladvice/eatdrink.htm* and in Scotland *www.fitfortravel.scot.nhs.uk*

Loperamide (Imodium; Arret; Diasorb; Diocalm Ultra; Normaloe) works more specifically on the intestinal wall and does not have so many unwanted effects. It is the most useful medicine for temporarily suppressing acute diarrhoea in adults.

ANTIBIOTICS

Antibiotics were used to treat acute diarrhoea until it was realised that they seldom helped, even when a micro-organism was involved. A doctor will sometimes prescribe an antibiotic, usually after investigation of a stool sample. For example, **ciprofloxacin** may reduce the severity and duration of traveller's diarrhoea; **metronidazole** is used for amoebic dysentery and *giardiasis* (page 294). Medicines for use abroad in case of illness are not covered on the NHS but you can buy them with a private prescription.

Chronic diarrhoea

Chronic diarrhoea is a long-term condition where the stools are loose or watery, and sometimes bloody or fatty. The diarrhoea does not clear up with the usual treatment for acute diarrhoea, and can eventually result in weight loss, anaemia and various forms of malnutrition. Your doctor will need to investigate your condition carefully, because some of the causes of chronic diarrhoea are serious, and include bowel cancer.

Irritable bowel syndrome

Irritable bowel syndrome (IBS) is a very common disorder of bowel movement. Its symptoms include griping, colicky pain across the lower abdomen, bloating and a disturbed bowel habit with frequent, loose stools and/or constipation with hard, 'rabbit-pellet' stools. Diarrhoea often occurs at the onset of pain, but the pain is reduced once you have had a bowel movement. You may pass mucus and feel that you have not emptied your bowel completely. You may feel sick or have flatulence, heartburn, wind or fatigue. These symptoms can be intermittent or you may experience them all the time. Sometimes other symptoms, such as back pain, urinary frequency and generalised muscle and joint pains may also be associated with IBS.

Although the cause of IBS is not clear, symptoms often start after an acute intestinal infection or after a course of antibiotics. Stress, lifestyle changes and intolerance to some foods (although not on an allergic basis) can trigger IBS. Women aged under 40 seem to suffer most from IBS, and symptoms are often worse before a menstrual period. You should see your doctor if you are worried or have severe, persistent and recurrent symptoms – particularly if you have rectal bleeding, a family history of bowel cancer or are aged over 50 when you develop symptoms. You may need to have some tests in hospital, particularly if the first treatment has not worked.

Diverticulitis and diverticular disease

Diverticulitis is an acute inflammatory condition of the large intestine or colon. Small pockets of the inside of the intestine (mucosa) bulge through the outer muscular wall at weak points along the colon. These are called diverticula, but exactly how and why they form are not fully understood. The presence of diverticula without symptoms is known as *diverticulosis*. Diverticula occur in middle age and are present in most old people, but seldom cause problems. Occasionally, a diverticulum becomes infected and inflammed (diverticulitis), resulting in appendicitis-like pain but usually on the left side of the abdomen. You may need an antibiotic to control the infection, but this requires specialist advice. Chronic diverticulitis may develop if inflammation persists, leading to changes in bowel habit. Constipation is common but diarrhoea can also occur. These symptoms are similar to bowel cancer and must be discussed with your doctor. Symptoms of diverticular disease – colicky pain and altered bowel habit – are managed by increasing fibre and fluid in the diet, although symptoms may worsen in the first few weeks before settling. Bran-based products can be tried, but if symptoms continue after three to four weeks then taking bran should be stopped. A bulk-forming preparation may also help (page 86). An antispasmodic (not the antimuscarinic type) such as **mebeverine** may help colicky pains and **paracetamol** may also be useful for pain relief. Antidiarrhoeal medicines containing **codeine**, **co-phenotrope**, **loperamide** or **morphine** cause constipation which can exacerbate symptoms, and should not be used.

Ulcerative colitis and Crohn's disease

Ulcerative colitis and *Crohn's disease* are uncommon inflammatory bowel diseases, the causes of which are unknown. The wall of the intestine becomes inflamed, causing bouts of colicky pain and frequent diarrhoea with blood. You may feel unwell, lose your appetite and lose weight

– HOW YOU CAN HELP YOURSELF –

Ulcerative colitis and Crohn's disease

- ☐ Make sure you have a healthy diet with plenty of fluids, high in fibre and with foods that suit your body – a high-fibre diet is the most helpful treatment for irritable bowel syndrome.
- ☐ Some people find that milk aggravates their system – it might be worth avoiding cow's milk to see if it helps your condition.
- ☐ Reduce stress in your life as far as possible, for example by taking regular exercise and using relaxation techniques – excessive stress is known to aggravate these diseases.
- ☐ Rest in bed during acute attacks.
- ☐ In cases of ulcerative colitis and Crohn's disease see your doctor regularly for checks – you will probably have to see a hospital doctor as well as your GP.

The IBS Network* offers advice and support to people with irritable bowel syndrome. Their website is *www.ibsnetwork.org.uk*. The National Association for Colitis and Crohn's Disease (NACC)* provides information on irritable bowel syndrome and Crohn's disease at *www.nacc.org.uk*.

because food is not properly absorbed. Ulcerative colitis involves only the large intestine, while Crohn's disease can also affect other parts of the digestive system but most commonly the small intestine. *Proctitis* is a similar condition which affects only the rectum and is seldom severe.

These inflammatory bowel diseases cannot be cured, but medicines can suppress the inflammation, control the symptoms and prevent complications, such as anaemia or perforation of the intestine. The aim of treatment is to bring about (induce) remission with medication in the acute phase, and then to prevent relapse, so prolonged 'maintenance' treatment is often needed plus nutritional care. Surgery may be necessary to remove damaged parts of the intestine.

Malabsorption syndromes

Sometimes the body cannot absorb one or more nutrients from the digestive system (*malabsorption syndrome*), and chronic diarrhoea may result. The stools are often fatty. Once the offending nutrient is known you can avoid it, thereby relieving the diarrhoea, but you may need to take particular replacement products. For example, a child who is lactose-intolerant will have to avoid cow's milk as this is high in lactose, but may then need a substitute milk product which is lactose-free. *Coeliac disease* is caused by an allergy to gluten, which is found in wheat, and requires a very strict diet supplemented with special gluten-free products. Your doctor can prescribe a range of these special products and gluten-free foods can be purchased in supermarkets.

Medicines for chronic diarrhoea

IRRITABLE BOWEL SYNDROME (IBS)

It may not be necessary to take a medicine to control your symptoms if they are mild and intermittent or related to foods that you can avoid such as wheat or dairy products, or you benefit from a high-fibre diet. Wheat bran can worsen symptoms in some people and you will need to decide what kind of fibre helps your particular symptoms. An explanation of IBS by your doctor, to help you obtain a thorough understanding of your condition, can be very valuable. However, your doctor may decide that drug treatment can help relieve your symptoms, particularly at first while you are improving your diet. Bulk-forming preparations (page 86) are used to improve the consistency and regularity of bowel movements. An *antimotility* medicine such as **loperamide** reduces stool frequency and urgency. It can help diarrhoea and can be used preventatively in certain situations, for example when going out. Opioid antidiarrhoeal medicines, such as **codeine**, should be avoided because they cause drowsiness and increase the risk of dependence.

Antispasmodic medicines work either by slowing down intestinal movement or by exerting a direct relaxant effect on intestinal muscle; **dicycloverine (dicyclomine)** (Merbentyl) appears to work both ways. Antispasmodics relieve stomach cramps and colicky abdominal pain. Those based on **atropine** have a limited use because of their unwanted effects (pages 63–4). **Alverine** (Spasmonal), **peppermint oil** and **mebeverine** (Colofac) in particular are of some value because they act only on the digestive system. Mebeverine and alverine are also available in combination with bulk-forming granules as Fybogel Mebeverine (with ispaghula) or Spasmonal Fibre (with sterculia). Peppermint oil in capsules (Colpermin; Mintec) can be taken three times a day, half to one hour before food with a little water. Persistent symptoms may need treatment for two to three months. The capsules must be swallowed whole, otherwise oil released into the mouth and gullet will cause irritation. Unwanted effects include heartburn and irritation around the anus.

Medicines to relieve depression (particularly tricyclic antidepressants) used at lower dosage than for depression are used occasionally. They may help relieve symptoms of IBS whether or not you are depressed, but can cause or worsen constipation.

MEBEVERINE HYDROCHLORIDE

COLOFAC – Liquid, tablets, modified-release capsules
FYBOGEL MEBEVERINE – Granules
MEBEVERINE + ISPAGHULA HUSK – pages 86–7

From a pharmacy
COLOFAC 100, COLOFAC IBS – Tablets
MEBEVERINE
EQUILON – Tablets
MEBEVERINE
IBS RELIEF – Tablets
MEBEVERINE

Mebeverine has a direct relaxant effect on intestinal smooth muscle. It is used for the relief of colicky abdominal pains, stomach cramps and spasm associated with irritable bowel syndrome and similar conditions. Mebeverine has few unwanted effects and does not cause the atropine-like effects of some other antispasmodics.

Before you use this medicine

Tell your doctor if you are:
□ lactose- or sucrose-intolerant – mebeverine tablets contain these sugars, but the liquid does not □ pregnant or breast-feeding □ taking any medicines, including vitamins and those bought over the counter.

Tell your doctor if you have:
□ Paralytic ileus – like all anti-spasmodics, mebeverine should not be taken if you have this condition □ porphyria – mebeverine should be avoided □ reduced kidney function – mebeverine + ispaghula granules should be avoided because of a high salt content.

How to use this medicine

Take one tablet three times a day or one capsule twice daily with a glassful of water, 20 minutes before meals. Shake the liquid suspension well before taking the dose (three 5ml spoonfuls). Your doctor will tell you for how many weeks you need to take the medicine. You may be able to reduce the dose gradually once the symptoms are under control. If you miss a dose, take it as soon as you remember, but skip it if it is almost time for your next dose. Do not take double the dose.

Over 65 No special requirements.

Unwanted effects

Mebeverine can aggravate irritable bowel syndrome (IBS) if there is underlying constipation, which is commonly the case; you may be constipated even if you defecate every day.
Rare Allergic reactions including inflamed or reddened skin, itching or rash.

ULCERATIVE COLITIS

For acute attacks your doctor may prescribe a rectal *corticosteroid* or an *aminosalicylate* as an enema, foam or suppositories to be inserted into the rectum at bedtime or twice daily. A corticosteroid (steroid), **prednisolone**, **budesonide** or **hydrocortisone**, reduces inflammation of the intestinal wall and brings the symptoms under control. Administering a corticosteroid directly into the bowel (locally) avoids some of the adverse effects such as moon face, thinning of the skin and weight gain that can occur with a corticosteroid taken by mouth for long periods. Treatment is usually limited to three- or four-week courses, so the corticosteroid does not cause unwanted effects throughout the body (*systemically*). Some absorption can occur with prolonged treatment, should this prove necessary, and then you may need additional doses of a corticosteroid in times of major stress, such as surgery. Liquid and foam preparations are equally effective. Foam products are easier to use and more convenient, especially if you have difficulty retaining a liquid enema. Suppositories are prescribed for proctitis.

Sometimes it may be necessary to take a course of an aminosalicylate and/or **prednisolone** by mouth. A corticosteroid is not taken all the time and the dose will be tapered off gradually once the disease is under control. In acute flare-ups you may need to be admitted to hospital.

The aminosalicylates, **sulfasalazine** (Salazopyrin) or one of the other related drugs, **mesalazine** (Asacol; Ipocol; Salofalk; Pentasa) or **olsalazine** (Dipentum) and **balsalazide sodium** (Colazide) are also taken by mouth to reduce bowel inflammation. They prevent relapse and are the standard maintenance treatment for ulcerative colitis. Each of these medicines has its own pattern of unwanted effects. Olsalazine may cause diarrhoea which can be confused with an exacerbation of the underlying disease.

SULFASALAZINE

SULFASALAZINE – Tablets, enteric-coated tablets
SALAZOPYRIN – Tablets, enteric-coated tablets, liquid, suppositories, retention enema

Sulfasalazine is used for reducing intestinal inflammation in ulcerative colitis and Crohn's disease. It is used for treating active ulcerative colitis to achieve remission and as maintenance treatment once the disease has been controlled. Sulfasalazine splits into two chemicals in the body: the active drug, 5-aminosalicylic acid and sulfapyridine, a sulfonamide which acts as a carrier to deliver the drug to the bowel. Unwanted effects are caused by both parts. Some of these effects can be diminished by a gradual increase in the daily dose to the full dosage, but in high doses unwanted effects are common. If you cannot tolerate sulfasalazine, you may be prescribed an alternative aminosalicylate – mesalazine, olsalazine or balsalazide sodium; each has different unwanted effects. Rarely, all can cause potentially serious blood disorders.

Sulfasalazine is also used for treating rheumatoid arthritis, if NSAIDs have not controlled the condition (page 387) as it has an anti-inflammatory effect and suppresses the disease process.

Before you use this medicine

Tell your doctor if you are:
☐ pregnant – sulfasalazine should be used with caution, although there is no evidence of risk to the fetus ☐ breast-feeding ☐ taking any other medicines, including vitamins and those bought over the counter.

Tell your doctor if you have or have had:
☐ kidney or liver disease ☐ lack of glucose-6-phosphate dehydrogenase (G6PD) ☐ a blood disorder ☐ allergy to *sulfonamides* or *salicylates* (for example, aspirin) ☐ porphyria.

How to use this medicine

Take the tablets or liquid regularly four times a day. *Enteric-coated* tablets may be tolerated better; they should be swallowed whole and not be crushed or broken. The night-time interval between doses should be no more than eight hours. During an acute attack a corticosteroid may be prescribed alongside sulfasalazine. For ulcerative colitis treatment may be needed for several years to prevent relapse.

Suppositories may be used for treating inflammatory disease in the rectum, either alone or in conjunction with tablets. They are inserted into the rectum in the morning and at bedtime after defecation. Enemas should be used once a day towards bedtime and the liquid retained in the rectum for at least one hour.

Drink plenty of fluids while you are taking sulfasalazine. Eat plenty of green vegetables as sulfasalazine can reduce the absorption of folic acid and iron. Most unwanted effects occur early in treatment, within the first six months of therapy. Your doctor should check your blood cell count before treatment and monthly during the first three months of taking sulfasalazine, but you should also know how to recognise blood disorders (see below). Liver function should also be checked every month during the first three months of treatment.

It is usually safe to drive with sulfasalazine, but until you know how you react to it, do not drive or do other activities that require alertness.

Do not stop taking sulfasalazine suddenly except on the advice of your doctor: take the full course of treatment even if you feel better. If you miss a dose take it as soon as you remember. If your next dose is due within two hours, take the missed dose immediately and omit the next dose.

Over 65 No special dosage requirements. Aminosalicylates should be avoided if you are hypersensitive to aspirin or another salicylate, and in moderate to severe impairment of kidney function.

Interactions with other medicines

The absorption of **digoxin** may be reduced by sulfsalazine.

Unwanted effects

Likely Headache, feeling or being sick, loss of appetite, rash and fever.
Less likely Flare-up of the bowel disease, temporary sterility in men – reversible on stopping treatment or changing to an alternative treatment.
Rare Blood disorders, generalised skin eruptions, sensitivity to sunlight, tinnitus, dizziness, hypersensitivity reactions, inflammation of the pancreas, liver or kidney, other kidney problems.

Report any unexplained bleeding or bruising, sore throat, unexplained fever or malaise, or swollen ankles immediately to your doctor. A blood cell count should be performed and if it is abnormal you should stop taking the medicine. This also applies to related medicines mesalazine, olsalazine and balsalazide.

Sulfasalazine may colour the urine orange-yellow and extended-wear soft contact lenses may stain permanently. Daily-wear soft and gas-permeable contact lenses should respond to routine cleansing.

Similar preparations

ASACOL – Tablets, suppositories, foam enema
MESALAZINE

COLAZIDE – Capsules
BALSALAZIDE

DIPENTUM – Capsules, tablets
OLSALAZINE

IPOCOL – Tablets
MESALAZINE

PENTASA – Modified-release tablets, modified-release granules by mouth, enema, suppositories
MESALAZINE

SALOFALK – Tablets, suppositories, enema, rectal foam
MESALAZINE

Other medicines

The symptoms of mild ulcerative colitis can be controlled with an antidiarrhoeal medicine (pages 79–80), such as **codeine** or **loperamide**, but not for long periods. An antidiarrhoeal should not be used alone for treating colitis because it does not reduce the inflammation and may cause constipation, which aggravates the disease. Antispasmodic medicines (pages 63–4) are not helpful in ulcerative colitis. A high-fibre diet and a bulk-forming agent (page 86) may be needed to adjust the consistency of stools.

Second-line treatments

Sometimes your doctor may consider trying a medicine that affects the immune system (*immune-modifying*), such as **azathioprine** (Imuran) or **mercaptopurine** (Puri-Nethol), if other measures have not been successful in maintaining remission. Azathioprine reduces the need to give as much corticosteroid and may even allow it to be stopped. Other immune-modifying drugs include **methotrexate**, given by mouth or by weekly injection, and **ciclosporin** to induce remission. These second-line treatments are not official or licensed uses, but clinical evidence for their use in inflammatory bowel disease, both ulcerative colitis and Crohn's disease, is accumulating.

Infliximab (Remicade) is another new approach to inducing remission in people who have severe Crohn's disease and when treatment with a corticosteroid or immune-modifying drug has not worked or when surgery is not appropriate. Infliximab is a genetically modified monoclonal antibody that stops the tumour necrosis factor from working. Unwanted effects of infliximab include an increase in the likelihood of infection, such as tuberculosis. All patients must be screened before starting treatment, during and after a course, because it takes six months for the drug to leave the body. Infliximab must not be used in moderate to severe heart failure. The use of all these second-line medicines requires close hospital supervision.

CROHN'S DISEASE

If the large intestine is inflamed then treatment is similar to ulcerative colitis. Active disease of the small intestine is usually treated with a corticosteroid such as **prednisolone**, **hydrocortisone** or **budesonide** (Entocort) to damp down the inflammation. Sometimes an antibacterial may be prescribed to control bacterial overgrowth in the small intestine.

Both ulcerative colitis and Crohn's disease can cause general ill health because your body may not absorb nutrients and water properly through the intestinal wall. You may need food, mineral and vitamin supplements and rehydration treatment to prevent malnutrition. Your doctor will advise you about the supplements you need; you should not buy them over the counter without taking advice.

Constipation

Constipation is the difficult, infrequent and sometimes painful passage of hard stools which is different from your usual pattern. Water and salts are absorbed into the body from the remnants of digested food in the bowel (large intestine or colon). The residue in the bowel becomes stools and as the bowel fills up, the urge to defecate develops. If the movement of digested food through the intestines is too slow, too much water is absorbed in the bowel and the stools become hard and dry and difficult to pass.

Healthy people can have anything from two bowel movements a week to three movements a day. If there is a change in the frequency of your bowel movement, from every day to less than twice a week, for example, or you are having difficulty passing stools, then you are constipated. However, you do not need to treat yourself with a laxative: the commonest cause of constipation is a lack of roughage, fibre and fluid in Western diets. It is essential to include in your diet high-fibre food and plenty of liquids.

Irritable bowel syndrome (page 77) often involves underlying constipation, even when loose, watery stools are being passed.

HOW YOU CAN HELP YOURSELF

- ☐ Eat a balanced diet high in fibre to maintain health and prevent constipation.
- ☐ Take daily exercise to help maintain regular bowel movements.
- ☐ Do not ignore the body's urge to pass stools.
- ☐ Try to develop a regular time to defecate – after a meal for instance.
- ☐ Do not become preoccupied with your bowel function.
- ☐ If you do become constipated, increase your daily intake of fibre and non-alcoholic liquids such as fruit juice.
- ☐ A change in bowel habit may not necessarily be simple constipation: if you have pain, notice bleeding when you pass stools, or you are worried, see your doctor.

Laxatives

Medicines for relieving constipation are known as laxatives. They are broadly grouped as *bulk-forming medicines*, *stimulants*, *softeners* and *osmotic laxatives*, but some drugs act in more than one way. A laxative may be needed to relieve constipation or painful passage of stools when:

- ☐ you have an illness which causes temporary constipation (a feverish illness or one that keeps you in bed, for example)
- ☐ straining when defecating might worsen a condition such as angina, haemorrhoids or anal fissure
- ☐ constipation is an unwanted effect of a medicine, such as the pain-relievers morphine, codeine and related opioids, anti-muscarinics, antidepressants, verapamil and aluminium antacids
- ☐ an elderly person develops constipation due to poor mobility.

A laxative may also be used to prepare the bowel for surgery or radiological procedures.

A laxative should be used only for a short period and once your normal bowel movement is re-established you should maintain the routine with additional roughage in your diet. If a laxative is taken every day, your bowel will become dependent on it to function. Long-term use of regular doses of a powerful laxative will make the bowel insensitive to it. This results in constipation again. In some cases the nerves controlling the bowel muscles are destroyed and the bowel ceases to work on its own.

If a laxative is needed, bran or another bulk-forming agent is best for long-term use and is particularly suitable for people aged over 60. If a bulk-forming agent is ineffective or difficult to take then a stimulant laxative, such as senna, could either be added or substituted for a short time.

Children, especially young ones, should not be given laxatives unless supervised by a doctor. Dietary adjustments, such as the addition of fruit (puréed for babies) can regulate bowel action. If dietary changes do not make any difference, discuss your child's problem with your doctor.

BULK-FORMING MEDICINES

These retain water and increase the mass of stools and residue in the bowel, which stimulates bowel movement (*peristalsis*). They are useful for relieving constipation and in conditions where the consistency of stools needs to be improved, such as irritable bowel syndrome, and for patients with *colostomy* and *ileostomy*. Bulking agents take some days to have an effect.

All the bulk-forming agents must be taken with plenty of water or other liquids to lubricate the bowel and to prevent them from becoming jammed in the intestine. If you have an intestinal stricture or the muscles of your bowel are damaged, you should not take a bulk-forming agent. All the products are effective and there is little to choose between them. However, there are differences in presentation and taste, so you should find a product that suits you.

Raw, unprocessed bran is slightly more effective than fine, processed bran but you may find the finer, cooked bran more palatable. You need 10 to 30g a day of raw bran, which can be added to any food at the table. You should increase the amount of bran you eat gradually until the passage of stools is comfortable. Do not take a whole day's dose with one meal. If you have a high requirement for calcium, iron or zinc you should take processed bran because these minerals can be removed from the intestine by coarse bran. Bran can cause excess wind and bloating, which you may find unpleasant. Do not take bran if you are gluten-sensitive or have coeliac disease.

Many cereals, breads and biscuits contain bran – you may find these as effective as raw bran and more acceptable.

ISPAGHULA HUSK

On prescription/over the counter

FYBOGEL – Granules
ISOGEL – Granules
ISPAGEL – Powder
KONSYL – Powder
REGULAN – Powder

Ispaghula husk is a general term for preparations containing ground seed husks of the Plantago species (plantain). The seeds swell on contact with water.

Ispaghula is a bulk-forming laxative which is used to treat constipation and other long-term conditions where stool consistency requires regulating, such as irritable bowel syndrome, diverticular disease, ulcerative colitis, haemorrhoids and patients with colostomy or ileostomy.

While taking ispaghula you must take plenty of water or other liquids so that the bulking agent passes down the digestive tract and does not stick or cause an obstruction.

Before you use this medicine

Tell your doctor or pharmacist:

☐ whether your constipation happens often or was a sudden change.

Tell your doctor or pharmacist if you are:

☐ pregnant or breast-feeding ☐ diabetic – some preparations contain sugar – ask your doctor or pharmacist to check which are suitable □ taking any medicines, including vitamins and those bought over the counter.

Ispaghula and other bulking agents must not be used when any part of the intestine is blocked or when the stools are hard, dry and blocking the bowel (impacted). They cannot be used if the bowel's nerves and muscles are destroyed.

How to use this medicine

Take the recommended dose in half a glass of water, stir the granules or powder briskly and drink immediately. Carbonated water can be used for non-effervescent preparations. Orange- and lemon-flavoured preparations are available, or you can flavour the water with a fruit squash. Take ispaghula at meal times or just after, but not immediately before going to bed; you may need to take a dose once, twice or three times a day depending on your bowel action.

Always drink plenty of non-alcoholic drinks while you are on a course of ispaghula, so that the bulking agent passes down the digestive tract and does not stick or cause an obstruction.

Over 65 No special requirements. This is the best choice of laxative.

Unwanted effects

Likely Excess wind, flatulence, bloating.
Rare but serious Intestinal obstruction if liquid intake is insufficient.

Similar preparations

On prescription/over the counter

CELEVAC – Tablets
METHYLCELLULOSE

NORMACOL – Granules
STERCULIA

NORMACOL PLUS – Granules
STERCULIA + FRANGULA

STIMULANT LAXATIVES

Stimulant laxatives speed up intestinal movement (increase *motility*). Most take eight to twelve hours to work and can be taken at bedtime. When the bowel is loaded and a bulking agent is ineffective, a short course of stimulant laxative can be helpful. Stimulant laxatives must not be taken for long periods, as they can destroy the nerves to the bowel and so prevent the normal defecation process. They must not be used if there is an intestinal obstruction and should be avoided in pregnancy.

Stimulant laxatives can cause stomach cramps and griping. If the dose is too high, diarrhoea may occur. You should start with a low dose and increase it gradually until you feel comfortable passing stools.

Senna, an established laxative since ancient times, is a good choice and is cheap to buy over the counter.

STIMULANT LAXATIVES

On prescription

DANTRON (danthron – only for constipation in patients who are terminally ill) – available in combination with **POLOXAMER** as **CO-DANTHRAMER** capsules and liquid, or combined with **DOCUSATE** as **CO-DANTHRUSATE** as capsules and liquid.

On prescription/over the counter

BISACODYL – Tablets, suppositories

DIOCTYL – Capsules
DOCUSATE SODIUM

DOCUSOL – Liquid
DOCUSATE SODIUM

DULCOLAX (not on prescription) – Tablets, suppositories
BISACODYL

FLETCHERS' ENEMETTE – Enema
DOCUSATE SODIUM + GLYCEROL

GLYCEROL – Suppositories

MANEVAC – Granules
SENNA + ISPAGHULA HUSK

NORGALAX MICRO – Enema
DOCUSATE SODIUM

SENNA – Tablets

SENOKOT – Granules, liquid, tablets (not on prescription)
SENNA

Not recommended

Other over-the-counter preparations containing:

☐ **CASCARA, FRANGULA, RHUBARB, SENNA** – they are unstandardised, so the laxative effect is unpredictable

☐ **COLOCYNTH, JALAP** – these are strong purgatives ☐ **ALOES** (CALSALETTES) ☐ **PHENOLPHTHALEIN** (KEST) – its laxative effect may continue for several days as it is recycled in the liver; it can cause skin rashes and colour urine pink

☐ **CASTOR OIL** – now obsolete.

STOOL SOFTENERS

Any effective laxative softens stools, in particular bulk-forming agents, and **glycerol** and **docusate**. Enemas (page 90) containing **arachis oil** lubricate and soften stools. **Liquid paraffin** has been a popular lubricant and stool softener. Once widely available, it can now be bought only from a pharmacy in small bottles because it should not be used regularly for long periods to relieve constipation. Long-term use has caused adverse effects, such as skin irritation, changes to the bowel wall due to absorption of small quantities of the paraffin, interference with the absorption of certain vitamins, and a form of pneumonia. **Liquid paraffin** emulsion should also be avoided.

OSMOTIC LAXATIVES

These work by retaining liquid, mostly water, in the bowel. They also soften stools. Commonly used osmotic laxatives include **magnesium salts**, **lactulose solution** (page 89) and **macrogols**, inert polymers of polyethylene glycols (Idrolax; Movicol). **Sodium phosphate** or **sodium citrate** enema solutions are used for urgent relief of constipation.

Magnesium salts

These are used to relieve constipation and when rapid bowel evacuation is needed. **Magnesium hydroxide** mixture is effective within about four hours. Repeated use of the mixture is not recommended. **Magnesium sulphate** (Epsom salts) has a rapid effect, particularly if a dose is taken on an empty stomach before breakfast, followed by a glass of warm water. This should not be used routinely for a laxative effect. **Liquid paraffin and magnesium hydroxide** mixture is no longer recommended.

Magnesium salts should be used only occasionally by elderly people. If you have poor kidney function, you should avoid magnesium-based laxatives. If you have poor liver function, you should avoid magnesium sulphate.

LACTULOSE

On prescription/over the counter
LACTULOSE SOLUTION – Liquid
DUPHALAC – Liquid (not on prescription)

Lactulose is a sugar which, when broken down by bacteria in the bowel, increases stool bulk and stimulates intestinal movement. Softer stools are then passed. Lactulose solution may take up to two days to work at the start of treatment.

Before you use this medicine

Tell your doctor or pharmacist if you are:
☐ sensitive to the sugar galactose – lactulose breaks down to galactose and fructose ☐ sensitive to lactose, a similar sugar ☐ pregnant or breast-feeding – lactulose can be used ☐ taking any other medicines, including vitamins and those bought over the counter.

How to use this medicine

Take three 5ml spoonfuls twice a day to start with, then reduce the dose to suit your needs; you can take lactulose with water or fruit juice. You should take plenty of water or other liquids whilst taking an osmotic laxative and, as with all laxatives, you should not take lactulose if you have an intestinal blockage. If you are diabetic, you can still use lactulose: a daily dose of 15ml provides 14 kcal.

Over 65 No special requirements.

Unwanted effects

Likely Flatulence, cramps and feeling sick, especially in the first few days of treatment.
Less likely Bloating and diarrhoea can occur if the dose is too high. These should ease if you reduce the dose.

SEVERE CONSTIPATION

Stools in the rectum and bowel which are very hard, dry and difficult to move are *impacted*. The intestinal tract may be temporarily blocked and you may feel uncomfortable. You may also pass loose stools which leak around the impaction and are not true diarrhoea. Faecal impaction can occur in frail, elderly people and those who are seriously ill and immobile.

Your doctor may prescribe a stimulant suppository, such as **bisacodyl** or **glycerol**, or an enema. An enema is a solution of salts – of **sodium** or **magnesium**, for example – in a disposable pack which has a nozzle for inserting into the rectum. An enema produces a speedy response and is therefore used in emergencies or to clear the bowel before an operation.

Piles and anal disorders

Piles occur when the veins in the anus and rectum become swollen or irritated. Piles, also called haemorrhoids because the haemorrhoidal veins are involved, may be *external* (at the anus) or *internal* (within the rectum). They are purple in colour and may look like a bunch of grapes. Internal piles may not cause much trouble, but can bleed, cause occasional discomfort and itch. Sometimes during defecation the piles are pushed down through the anus but return again spontaneously. Severe piles come down readily and need to be pushed back into the rectum.

Piles appear to occur because of prolonged local pressure on the haemorrhoidal veins. Pregnant women are prone to develop them and they are made worse by constipation and straining to pass stools. Occasionally blood clots form in the piles, which causes severe pain. Blood around the stools, or bleeding before or after defecation are commonly caused by piles, but you should always see your doctor to confirm this, as bleeding is also a symptom of bowel cancer. Your doctor will need to examine you and may use an instrument called a *sigmoidoscope* to look into your rectum.

Sometimes surgery may be needed to relieve painful and persistent haemorrhoids. They can also be treated by *rubber band ligation*, where the haemorrhoid is tied off from the vein.

Other anal disorders include anal fissure, painful tears around the anus, and anal itching (*pruritus ani*). All these are relieved by attention to cleanliness and diet.

HOW YOU CAN HELP YOURSELF

- ☐ Increase the amount of fibre in your diet and drink plenty of water or non-alcoholic drinks.
- ☐ Use a bulk-forming laxative if necessary to soften stools.
- ☐ Whenever possible, wash your anus carefully after defecation; soap is irritant and should be avoided in conditions such as anal fissure; dry the area gently.
- ☐ Always see your doctor if you have a sudden change of bowel habit or blood mixed with your stools.

Medicines for anal discomfort

Medicines used to relieve anal discomfort and irritation are soothing preparations applied locally as creams, ointments, suppositories and dusting powders. Preparations may be bland and some include a local anaesthetic. A **corticosteroid** to reduce inflammation should not be used for long periods.

BLAND SOOTHING PREPARATIONS

Some are a mixture of astringents, which cause tissue to contract; others contain astringents plus an antiseptic, or a local anaesthetic, or a vasoconstrictor (which reduces the size of blood vessels) or a lubricant. A soothing preparation is used at night and in the morning, and also after a bowel movement. An unwrapped suppository is inserted into the rectum or the cream or ointment can be used with a special applicator. You can also use the cream or ointment externally around the anus.

Bismuth subgallate, **zinc oxide** and **hamamelis** (witch hazel) are astringents which may relieve itching and uncomfortable piles.

A local anaesthetic, **lidocaine** (**lignocaine**) can be used just before passing stools to relieve the pain associated with anal fissure. However, a local anaesthetic should only be used for a short period, no longer than two weeks, because it may cause skin sensitisation. Young children should not be treated with products containing a local anaesthetic: see your doctor about any problems your child has with defecation.

Other products contain a variety of ingredients which add little to their basic efficacy, such as **ephedrine**. **Heparinoid** is thought to relieve swelling. Always read the list of ingredients before you make a purchase.

BLAND SOOTHING PREPARATIONS

On prescription/over the counter

ANACAL – Suppositories, ointment
HEPARINOID

ANODESYN – Suppositories, ointment
LIDOCAINE + ALLANTOIN

ANUSOL – Suppositories, cream, ointment
BISMUTH + ZINC

LANACANE – Cream
BENZOCAINE

NUPERCAINAL – ointment
CINCHOCAINE

Over the counter

GERMOLOIDS – Cream, ointment, suppositories
LIDOCAINE + ZINC

HEMOCANE – Cream
LIDOCAINE + BISMUTH + ZINC

PREPARATION H – Suppositories, ointment
SHARK LIVER OIL + YEAST CELL EXTRACT

PREPARATION H – Gel
HAMAMELIS WATER

• *CORTICOSTEROIDS* •

Anti-inflammatory corticosteroids are combined with soothing preparations and local anaesthetics. These preparations are usually prescribed by your doctor, although some products can also be bought from a pharmacy. They should be used only for short periods of about five to seven days, once infection has been excluded as a cause of the complaint. If infection is present, a corticosteroid should not be used because it can make the infection worse.

CORTICOSTEROID-CONTAINING PREPARATIONS

All products contain several ingredients but we list the corticosteroid component only.

ANUGESIC-HC – Cream, suppositories
HYDROCORTISONE

ANUSOL-HC – Ointment, suppositories
HYDROCORTISONE

PROCTOFOAM HC – Aerosol foam
HYDROCORTISONE

PROCTOSEDYL – Ointment, suppositories
HYDROCORTISONE

SCHERIPROCT – Ointment, suppositories
PREDNISOLONE

ULTRAPROCT – Ointment, suppositories
FLUOCORTOLONE

UNIROID-HC – Ointment, suppositories
HYDROCORTISONE

XYLOPROCT – Ointment
HYDROCORTISONE

Over the counter

ANUSOL PLUS HC – Ointment, suppositories
HYDROCORTISONE

PERINAL – Spray solution
HYDROCORTISONE

2

HEART AND CIRCULATION

High blood pressure Angina
Heart attack Heart failure
Irregular heart rhythms Stroke
Circulatory problems Blood clots

The heart is a strong muscle which constantly pumps blood to all parts of the body, through thousands of miles of blood vessels called *arteries*. The blood fuels every cell, organ and system with oxygen and nutrients which the body needs to function. Blood from the main arteries flows into smaller and smaller vessels ending in the *capillaries*. This network of very fine blood vessels allows oxygen and nutrients to reach individual cells. The blood then takes the cells' waste products through veins back to the heart. Discovered by the English physician William Harvey in the seventeenth century, the body's network of arteries, capillaries and veins is known as the circulation. This closed system of blood vessels carries about eight pints of blood which the heart circulates continuously.

The heart has four chambers. There are two on the left and two on the right, each side operating as a separate pump yet working together harmoniously. Each of the smaller top chambers is called an *atrium* while the larger, lower parts are known as the *ventricles*. The right atrium receives blood from the veins which then passes into the right ventricle. From here the blood carrying waste gas (carbon dioxide) is pumped to the lungs, where the blood cells exchange it for oxygen; blood is returned to the left side of the heart for circulation to the rest of the body. (The heart receives its own blood supply through the coronary arteries.) Inside the heart and blood vessels there are valves which ensure that the blood flows in only one direction. The heart and circulation are known collectively as the cardiovascular system.

Heart and circulatory problems

The heart beats about 100,000 times every single day. Not surprisingly, problems can occur. Arteries and veins are like rubber tubing with good elasticity. Blood is constantly forced through the arteries at great pressure, but over time the artery walls gradually fur up, roughen and thicken, causing narrowing of the arteries and loss of elasticity (*arteriosclerosis*). Blood clots in blood vessels are more likely to form in narrowed arteries anywhere in the circulatory system. Alternatively, a blood clot formed in one part of the system can travel in the bloodstream to block either partially or completely another artery. A clot that blocks an artery in the brain suddenly and completely can cause a *stroke.* Blood vessels may also become blocked by fatty deposits (*atheroma*). A narrowing of the coronary arteries supplying blood, and therefore oxygen, to the heart results in chest heaviness and pain, usually on exertion, known as *angina* (page 120). A clot in the arteries supplying the heart is known as a *coronary thrombosis* and can lead to a heart attack (page 125) when the blood supply is blocked resulting in death of parts of the heart muscle (*myocardial infarction*). Conditions affecting the blood supply to the heart are referred to as *coronary heart disease* (also *ischaemic heart disease* or *coronary artery disease*). The term cardiovascular disease covers coronary heart disease and also stroke (page 144).

Further problems with arteries include weakness in an artery wall, known as an *aneurysm* – the wall balloons under the pressure of blood, thus increasing the likelihood of the artery bursting (requiring urgent surgical treatment). *Peripheral vascular disease* (page 146) results from a long-term reduction in blood flow to the arms and legs, particularly in the arteries, providing less oxygen and nutrients to feed the cells and tissues. Other conditions that affect the heart and circulation include irregular heart rhythms (page 139), for example following a heart attack, and heart failure (page 133) when the heart's ability to pump blood around the body is decreased, often as a consequence of coronary heart disease.

Risk factors for developing heart and circulatory problems

Although the death rate from coronary heart disease is falling, Britain still has one of the highest rates among developed countries. However, more people are living with coronary heart disease such as angina or following a heart attack. The key to tackling heart and circulation diseases is prevention, and this is now a national priority. A National Service Framework (NSF) for coronary heart disease not only sets standards of care for preventing heart problems but also for treating them. The main approach to preventing heart disease is through modifying lifestyle (reducing smoking); healthy eating; reviewing alcohol consumption; exercise; reducing weight and obesity) and treating medical risk factors – high blood pressure, diabetes and high cholesterol levels. See 'How you can help yourself', below. Other factors contributing to risk that cannot be modified are age, gender and a family history of heart disease. All of these factors are interrelated and more than one area is likely to need attention rather than changing a single risk factor, as doctors advocated previously, such as lowering high blood pressure or cholesterol. For example, if you have a raised cholesterol level (more than 5 millimoles/litre) but no other risk factors and are aged under 50 years, you are unlikely to need cholesterol-lowering treatment with a medicine, unless high cholesterol runs in the family; a change in diet may be all that is needed.

Some doctors have proposed that everyone over the age of 55 years should take a combination of six drugs and vitamins (the 'Polypill') each day regardless of their initial levels of blood pressure or cholesterol, to reduce cardiovascular risk factors. They have calculated that about a third of people aged over 55 would benefit from the strategy. However, this means that the other two-thirds of this population would be exposed to medicines that may not be needed, with the potential for adverse effects as well as benefits. At present the Polypill strategy remains an interesting theory.

– HOW YOU CAN HELP YOURSELF –

- ☐ **Lose weight** – the heart has to work much harder to pump blood around the body if you are overweight; losing weight can reduce your risk of heart and circulation disease, high blood pressure, heart failure and diabetes (type-2 or non-insulin dependent diabetes).
- ☐ **Eat a balanced diet** – more fruit and vegetables (five pieces a day), fish (especially oily fish), starchy foods such as bread, rice, pasta and potatoes – and reduce the amount of fatty foods (containing saturated fat).
- ☐ **Restrict salt** – reducing your daily salt intake may be all that is required to treat mildly raised blood pressure.
- ☐ **Reduce alcohol** – even in moderate quantitites, alcohol adds calories and can increase blood pressure; try to cut down and definitely stay within the recommended weekly limit (men: 21 units/week and women: 14 units/week).
- ☐ **Stop smoking** – smokers are in a high-risk category for heart attacks and strokes.
- ☐ **Avoid stress and take plenty of rest** – relaxation therapy may help some people with mild to moderately raised blood pressure.
- ☐ **Exercise regularly** – exercise helps the circulation, improves blood flow through the muscles and helps the efficiency of the heart; regular exercise may prevent the development of high blood pressure and it can lead to a reduction in blood pressure. It helps in heart failure. Avoid strenuous exercise if you are not used to it, but start gently with a brisk walk, cycling a few times a week or swimming. Ideally build exercise into your daily routine.

High blood pressure

Consistently raised blood pressure is a major risk factor for developing heart disease and stroke. Blood pressure is the force the heart uses to pump blood around the body. During each heartbeat pressure is highest when the heart muscle contracts to push blood through the system. Blood pressure is at its lowest when the heart then relaxes before the process is repeated. The higher force is known as the *systolic* pressure, the lower as the *diastolic* pressure; both are measured when you have your blood pressure taken.

Blood pressure also depends on the width of blood vessels and the volume of blood in circulation. It varies between individuals, although it generally increases with age because of natural ageing of the blood vessels and changes in lifestyle: as people grow older they tend to put on weight, take less exercise and become less tolerant to alcohol (their alcohol intake may also increase). An individual's blood pressure is partly hereditary, and so high blood pressure tends to run in families. Blood pressure varies throughout the day and depends on what you are doing. It will rise when you take exercise because blood needs to be pumped around the body faster; when you rest, sit or lie down your blood pressure will be lower. It is only when your blood pressure is consistently higher than it should be, no matter what you are doing, that you have high blood pressure (*hypertension*). If high blood pressure is left untreated, it will reduce your life-expectancy.

The increase in pressure puts an extra workload on the heart, making it more difficult for it to pump blood efficiently around the body, and the heart is gradually damaged. Kidney function can be reduced if high blood pressure persists and the walls of the arteries supplying blood to the kidneys thicken. A few people with high blood pressure suffer worsening eyesight because of damage to the blood vessels in the eye.

Many people have no obvious cause of high blood pressure, but a few have *secondary hypertension* caused by a disease or condition, such as kidney disease or pregnancy. Very high blood pressure (*malignant hypertension*) needs urgent hospital treatment. High blood pressure is common in people with type-2 diabetes (page 305); lowering blood pressure helps prevent some of the long-term complications of diabetes. Several lifestyle factors contribute to high blood pressure, such as being overweight and taking extra dietary salt – see 'How you can help yourself', page 95.

Measuring blood pressure

Many people with raised blood pressure have no symptoms at all. Measuring blood pressure is the only way to find out whether it is high or not. You should have your blood pressure measured on several different occasions while sitting to see if the reading is consistent; stress and anxiety (perhaps brought on by a visit to the doctor or hospital clinic) can increase blood pressure. Blood pressure should also be measured when standing if you are older and/or diabetic to rule out postural low blood pressure – low blood pressure that occurs when you change position. Your doctor may ask you to measure blood pressure over a number of days at home with a small electronic machine, which is increasingly used in place of the traditional mercury-containing sphygmomanometer, or to consider 24-hour blood pressure monitoring with a small machine attached to your body (ambulatory measurement). Even with the new electronic blood pressure measuring devices the values continue to be expressed in millimetres of mercury (mmHg) and as the systolic blood pressure over the diastolic blood pressure, for example 140/85 mmHg. Adults who have not had their blood pressure checked during the last five years should consider having a check-up.

When blood pressure needs treatment

Doctors generally advise drug treatment to reduce blood pressure for people whose systolic blood pressure is at or above 160 mmHg or whose diastolic blood pressure is at or above 100 mmHg on repeated measurements over one or two weeks. Drug treatment is also recommended for people whose systolic blood pressure is 140–159 mmHg or whose diastolic blood pressure is 90–99 mmHg on repeated measurement if they are at a high risk of developing coronary heart disease for other reasons (e.g. because of diabetes or high blood cholesterol) or have evidence of organ damage such as heart or kidney problems. If your blood pressure is only slightly raised (systolic 140–159 mmHg or diastolic 90–99 mmHg), you are at low risk of developing coronary heart disease and there is no evidence of organ damage, your doctor would probably suggest no drug treatment, but repeat blood pressure measurements annually.

Older people are at greater risk of heart and circulatory diseases and therefore benefit more from treatment to lower blood pressure. For people aged over 65, treatment is recommended if systolic blood pressure is at or above 160 mmHg or diastolic blood pressure at or above 95 mmHg on repeated measurement at several surgery visits and in spite of appropriate lifestyle changes (see page 95). Systolic blood pressure rises steadily with age and around half the population aged 65 years and over is likely to have high blood pressure. If your systolic blood pressure is raised (160 mmHg or more) but not the diastolic pressure (less than 95 mmHg) – a condition known as *isolated systolic hypertension* – then reducing the systolic blood pressure is also beneficial in terms of diminishing your cardiovascular risk. Benefit from blood pressure-lowering treatment is demonstrable until 80 years of age at least and if you started treatment before then, you should probably continue for the rest of life.

If you are diabetic, blood pressure control helps to reduce the risk of both cardiovascular and kidney disease.

Treatment is life-long for most people, unless high blood pressure has an obvious cause, for example during pregnancy. Some medicines can increase blood pressure, such as non-steroidal anti-inflammatory drugs (NSAIDs). If your blood pressure increases during NSAID treatment, it should decrease when you stop the medicine.

Low blood pressure rarely requires treatment. Faintness or dizziness may sometimes be troublesome, but most people do not experience any symptoms or health problems.

Medicines for high blood pressure

Lowering blood pressure, even if mildly raised, reduces the risk of stroke and cardiovascular problems. High blood pressure cannot usually be cured, but it can be kept under control. If your doctor diagnoses high blood pressure, the approach to treatment depends on how high it is and whether you have any underlying problems. Your doctor will aim to lower blood pressure to a systolic pressure of less than 140 mmHg and a diastolic pressure of less than 85 mmHg. If you are diabetic then the aim will be to reduce the systolic pressure to below 140 mmHg and diastolic pressure to below 80 mmHg. These measures apply in the clinic situation but ideally blood pressure should be marginally lower when you are at home or walking about.

Most people with high blood pressure will need to take one or more medicines, but modifying lifestyle – losing weight, controlling salt and alcohol consumption, increasing exercise and stopping smoking – is also important and part of the treatment. If you modify your lifestyle successfully you may delay or limit the need for medicines. For some people with mildly raised blood pressure these measures may be all that is needed. Even if you do not have to take a medicine, your doctor will still want to see you to check your blood pressure regularly.

The different types or classes of medicines used to treat high blood pressure act in different ways in the body. These medicines (*antihypertensives*) lower blood pressure by increasing the width of blood vessels (*vasodilators*) through a variety of mechanisms, or by reducing the volume of blood. The classes of blood pressure-lowering medicines, each of which is profiled in this chapter, are:

- ☐ diuretics
- ☐ beta blockers
- ☐ angiotensin-converting enzyme inhibitors (ACE inhibitors) and the related angiotensin-II receptor antagonists (ACE II)
- ☐ calcium channel blockers
- ☐ alpha blockers.

All lower blood pressure effectively and in general there are no important differences in their tolerability or effect on quality of life. For each class of medicine there is good-quality evidence to support its use, but you may find that you tolerate one type better than another. Most evidence for good results in blood pressure-lowering lies with the use of a beta blocker, such as **atenolol**, or low dose of a thiazide diuretic, such as **bendroflumethiazide**. Higher doses of thiazide offer no additional benefit, but may increase unwanted effects. A thiazide is best avoided if you have raised cholesterol levels or gout. If a thiazide diuretic does not control blood pressure adequately, your doctor may suggest an alternative type of blood pressure-lowering medicine such as a beta blocker, ACE inhibitor or a calcium channel blocker or may add one or more of them to the diuretic. Adding different types of blood pressure-lowering medicines together usually increases their effect. Slightly lower doses of two different drugs can lower blood pressure better, and with fewer unwanted effects, than the maximum dose of a single drug. If you are diabetic you are quite likely to need at least two blood pressure-lowering medicines. People respond differently to different classes of blood pressure-lowering medicine depending on their racial origin. For example, African-Carribean people may respond to treatment with just one medicine, such as a diuretic or a calcium channel blocker, but not to an ACE inhibitor or beta blocker.

Some blood pressure-lowering medicines treat other heart and circulation problems or other medical problems. For example an ACE inhibitor such as **enalapril** helps heart failure and also lowers high blood pressure; a calcium channel blocker such as **nifedipine** treats high blood pressure and chest pains (angina); an alpha blocker such as **doxazosin** reduces high blood pressure and is used for prostate problems. These medicines are useful, therefore, if you have several medical problems that one drug can treat. The dosage may vary depending on the condition.

Most of the medicines have unwanted effects and older people are especially susceptible to them. Your doctor will need to assess the benefits of treating high blood pressure against the likelihood of adverse effects from them. Some of the unwanted effects are quite subtle, because the medicines affect the body's metabolism; other people may notice a change in you that you do not, and it is worth noting these developments on the medicine record sheet. You must tell your doctor about any unwanted effects, especially if these effects put you off taking the medicine. You are likely to have to take a medicine for blood pressure control for the rest of your life, so it is important to find a treatment that suits you. You need to allow about four weeks to try out a new blood pressure-lowering medicine or different formulation (unless you cannot tolerate it at all) to see how it affects you. You should work in partnership with your doctor to try to achieve a sensible blood pressure level without taking the enjoyment out of life. This may not be the exact target level, but the lower your blood pressure, the lower your risks.

DIURETICS

Diuretics, sometimes called 'water tablets', remove water and salts from the body. Water, mineral salts (mostly sodium and potassium) and waste products are taken out of the bloodstream as blood flows through the kidneys. Some of the water and salts are recycled back into blood (a process called reabsorption) and the rest leave the body with the waste products as urine. Diuretics interfere with the recycling process in the kidneys to increase the amounts of mineral salts (electrolytes) and water lost from the body, which reduces blood volume and tension in the arteries. Diuretics also help the heart to work more efficiently and reduce extra fluid trapped in body tissues. A diuretic increases the frequency and the amount of urine you produce, particularly at the start of treatment.

There are several types of diuretic. The main classes are *thiazides*, *loop diuretics* and *potassium-sparing diuretics*. They work at slightly different places in the kidney, but all block sodium and water reabsorption. Loop diuretics are not generally used to lower high blood pressure, but they are used to remove excess water from the body, especially in heart failure (see **furosemide** (frusemide), pages 135–6).

The unwanted effects of diuretics are sometimes troublesome, although lower doses lessen them. Not only is there the inconvenience of more frequent and larger volumes of urine, but diuretics may also upset the balance of the body's chemistry. Older people are particularly sensitive to these effects; you may need lower doses and should not take a diuretic for long periods without your doctor reviewing the need for treatment.

Potassium in particular, but also sodium and magnesium, are lost from the body when you take a diuretic other than the potassium-sparing type. The body needs potassium for the proper functioning of muscle, especially heart muscle. The rhythm of the heart may be upset by low potassium levels, which can be dangerous. If blood levels of potassium fall, you may feel weak, dizzy, sick and even vomit. You must see a doctor if you get these symptoms.

Thiazide diuretics

Thiazide diuretics are very effective in low doses for controlling high blood pressure and have similar actions: **bendroflumethiazide** (bendrofluazide) is the most commonly prescribed.

BENDROFLUMETHIAZIDE

BENDROFLUMETHIAZIDE – Tablets
APRINOX – Tablets
NEO-NACLEX – 5mg Tablets

Poor choice: bendroflumethiazide with potassium (amount may be insufficient)
NEO-NACLEX K

Bendroflumethiazide (bendrofluazide) is a thiazide diuretic widely used in low doses, usually 2.5mg daily, to reduce high blood pressure. It is used on its own in mild cases and with other medicines when high blood pressure is more severe. Bendroflumethiazide is sometimes used in higher doses to remove excess fluid (*oedema*) from the body, for example in mild to moderate heart failure. It starts to act within one or two hours of taking it by mouth and is effective for 18–24 hours.

Bendroflumethiazide can upset the body's chemistry (e.g. potassium loss) and metabolism, particularly if taken for long periods, although low doses may avoid this. Older people are particularly sensitive to these metabolic effects. A combination of potassium and bendroflumethiazide in the same tablet as a modified-release product may not contain enough potassium for people who need supplementation. Many people taking a low dose of thiazide only need to take in potassium as part of their diet.

Before you use this medicine

Tell your doctor if you are:
☐ pregnant ☐ breast-feeding – large doses may stop milk production ☐ restricting salt or sugar in your diet – bendroflumethiazide affects salt and sugar levels ☐ taking any other medicines, including vitamins and those bought over the counter.

Tell your doctor if you have or have had:
☐ diabetes ☐ pancreatitis ☐ gout ☐ kidney disease ☐ liver disease ☐ sensitivity to any thiazide diuretic or a sulphonamide ☐ high blood-calcium levels ☐ the hormone disorder Addison's disease ☐ porphyria ☐ the arthritis-like condition systemic lupus erythematosus.

If you have to take bendroflumethiazide for long periods or in high doses, you should ask your doctor about potassium supplementation. Bendroflumethiazide removes potassium from the body as well as sodium and water (see 'Keeping potassium in balance', page 102).

How to use this medicine

Take the tablet in the morning with breakfast, so that night-time sleep is not interfered with by additional visits to the toilet: during the first few days of treatment, you will produce a larger volume of urine and need to go to the toilet more often than usual. If you are away from home, make sure you know where the toilet facilities are for emergencies.

Because a diuretic helps you to lose water, you may lose too much and become dehydrated. You may feel thirsty and your skin may look and feel dry. Check with your doctor to see that your daily fluid intake is appropriate. You will lose potassium from your body; make sure that you eat foods rich in potassium every day. If you reduce salt intake your body will lose less potassium, but discuss salt restriction with your doctor. Your doctor should check your blood potassium levels after about a month of treatment; if potassium is low discuss whether you can adjust this by dietary intake.

You may feel dizzy or faint when you get up from sitting or lying down, especially during the first few days of treatment. Get up slowly and stay beside the chair or bed until you are sure you are not dizzy.

Alcohol intake should be kept low: loss of body fluids increases the effects of alcohol.

Do not stop taking this medicine without discussing this with your doctor. If you miss a dose take it as soon as you remember, but no later than mid-afternoon. Otherwise skip this dose and take the next one as usual.

Over 65 You need as small a dose as possible.

Interactions with other medicines

Thiazide diuretics interact with a number of medicines, but only the important interactions are given here. Do not take any other medicines, such as those bought over the counter, without checking with your doctor or pharmacist.

Lithium Bendroflumethiazide stops lithium from leaving the body; the amount of lithium in the blood may increase to toxic levels.

Heart drugs If bendroflumethiazide causes low body levels of potassium, the adverse effects of certain heart drugs increase. These include **digoxin**, **amiodarone**, **disopyramide**, **flecainide** and **quinidine**. Similarly, low potassium levels increase the risk of irregular heart rhythms with **antipsychotics** such as **pimozide**, **amisulpride**.

Antihistamine terfenadine may cause irregular heart rhythms if there are low blood levels of potassium in the body.

NSAIDs may blunt the diuretic and blood pressure-lowering effect of bendroflumethiazide.

Corticosteroids and **acetazolamide** (for glaucoma) may exacerbate low body levels of potassium.

Carbamazepine, an antiepileptic, increases the risk of low body levels of sodium.

Other blood pressure-lowering drugs can be given with bendroflumethiazide but this will enhance its unwanted effects, such as dizziness and faintness.

Unwanted effects

Likely Dizziness, muscle cramps, weakness.

Less likely Feeling or being sick, loss of appetite, diarrhoea, impotence, skin rashes, photosensitivity, hypersensitivity, inflammation of the pancreas, blood disorders. Contact your doctor if you develop a rash. Problems of impotence should always be discussed.

Bendroflumethiazide may aggravate diabetes and increase blood-sugar levels. Symptoms may appear if you are on the threshold of developing diabetes. The blood sugar-lowering effect of antidiabetic medicines is opposed by bendroflumethiazide and this may upset the control of diabetes. Blood levels of uric acid may be increased, causing or aggravating gout. Bendroflumethiazide may cause or aggravate high blood-cholesterol levels (*hyperlipidaemia*).

You should have a yearly check, with blood and urine samples to check potassium levels and assess your kidney function.

Similar preparations

DIURETIC – Tablets
XIPAMIDE

HYGROTON – Tablets
CHLORTALIDONE

INDAPAMIDE – Tablets

METENIX 5 – Tablets
METOLAZONE

NATRILIX – Tablets, modified-release tablets
INDAPAMIDE

NAVIDREX – Tablets
CYCLOPENTHIAZIDE

Keeping potassium in balance

Potassium is an essential mineral for keeping the body healthy. Too little or too much potassium can trigger irregular heart rhythms. The mild loss of potassium that occurs with diuretic treatment usually has no symptoms, although elderly people may experience muscle weakness and confusion. However, you may need to change your diet if it is low in potassium.

POTASSIUM-RICH FOODS		
almonds	coconut	peas
apricots (dried)	dates and figs (dried)	pork
avocados	fish (fresh)	potatoes
bananas	ham	prunes (dried)
beans	lentils	raisins
beef	liver	shellfish
bran	melon	spinach
broccoli	milk	tomato juice
Brussels sprouts	oranges and lemons	turkey
carrots (raw)	peaches	veal
chicken	peanut butter	

For example, six halves of dried apricots, a glass of fresh orange juice and a medium-size banana per day should provide enough potassium to prevent low blood levels, but taking potassium in your daily diet may not be sufficient if your potassium loss is moderate to severe. Your doctor will need to assess blood-potassium levels and replacement treatment may be needed:

- ☐ for older people with a poor diet
- ☐ if you take high doses of a diuretic or the heart drug digoxin or an antiarrhythmic drug
- ☐ if the body's potassium control is disrupted – by severe liver disease, for example
- ☐ if you lose potassium in faeces through an illness such as chronic diarrhoea, or experience vomiting or diarrhoea while taking a diuretic.

Some drugs taken for long periods (corticosteroids, for example) produce further potassium loss, so replacement must be given.

Restricting your salt intake helps to maintain potassium levels while lowering body sodium. A salt substitute, such as Losalt, contains large amounts of potassium chloride and may be used as an additional source of potassium. However, you should not use a salt substitute if you have poor kidney function or you are already taking a potassium supplement, a potassium-sparing diuretic or an ACE inhibitor or related ACE II (angiotensin-II receptor antagonist).

Potassium replacement is usually given as potassium chloride in liquid form to minimise harmful effects on the lining of the stomach and intestines. Tablets should be dissolved in a tumblerful of water before swallowing the solution. Potassium chloride solution can be taken with or after food to lessen the effect on the stomach. Slow-release potassium chloride tablets have caused ulceration of the gullet and intestines and are not recommended. Some diuretics are combined with potassium, which is unnecessary in most cases and often too little to be useful when replacement is needed. It is better to take the diuretic and the potassium separately.

Potassium chloride can make you feel sick or be sick and you should tell your doctor if this happens. Your doctor may recommend a potassium-sparing diuretic as an alternative to a potassium supplement to overcome this problem.

POTASSIUM CHLORIDE PREPARATIONS

On prescription/from a pharmacy	*Not recommended*
KAY-CEE-L – Syrup (sugar-free)	Modified-release preparation:
KLOREF – Effervescent tablets	SLOW-K
SANDO-K – Effervescent tablets	

Potassium-sparing diuretics

Amiloride and **triamterene** are weak diuretics on their own and are therefore used in combination with thiazide or loop diuretics. They conserve the body's potassium supplies and must not be taken with potassium supplements as the body would then retain too much potassium. **Spironolactone**, also a potassium-sparing diuretic, is used to remove excess fluid in severe heart failure and also in liver disease.

Combination preparations

Many products combine a potassium-sparing diuretic with a thiazide, a loop diuretic such as **furosemide** (e.g. **co-amilofruse**) or a beta blocker in a fixed dose. Amiloride is combined in one tablet with the thiazide diuretic hydrochlorothiazide and this combination now has the generic name of **co-amilozide**. There are two tablet strengths of co-amilozide, amiloride/hydrochlorothiazide 2.5/25 and 5/50, but they do not allow for treatment with, say, a low dose of hydrochlorothiazide and a standard dose of amiloride. Ideally, your doctor should at first prescribe each drug separately, so that the dose of each can be adjusted to meet your needs.

Fixed-dose preparations seem an attractive way to improve reliability in medicine-taking by reducing the number of medicines a patient has to take. Although widely used now, these combinations may encourage the use of a potassium-sparing diuretic when a thiazide with a potassium-rich diet might be appropriate.

Some combinations contain three drugs – a potassium-sparing diuretic, a thiazide and a beta blocker. This combination should be used only when blood pressure has not been controlled by dietary measures and a thiazide or a beta blocker alone (see **atenolol**, pages 107–9).

AMILORIDE

AMILORIDE – Tablets

Combination preparations

CO-AMILOZIDE 2.5/25 – Tablets
AMILORIDE 2.5 mg + HYDROCHLOROTHIAZIDE 25 mg

CO-AMILOZIDE 5/50 – Tablets
AMILORIDE 5 mg + HYDROCHLOROTHIAZIDE 50 mg

AMIL-CO – Tablets
CO-AMILOZIDE 5/50

AMILAMONT – Liquid

MODURETIC – Tablets
CO-AMILOZIDE 5/50

MODURET 25 – Tablets
CO-AMILOZIDE 2.5/25

Amiloride is a weak diuretic with a potassium-conserving action. It may be used alone to remove excess fluid in heart failure or liver disease, such as cirrhosis. However, it is used more often in combination with a thiazide or loop diuretic to retain potassium in the body which would otherwise be lost during blood pressure-lowering treatment or in heart failure. Amiloride starts to work within two hours after you take it.

Before you use this medicine

Tell your doctor if you are:
☐ pregnant – not usually prescribed ☐ breast-feeding ☐ taking any other medicine that increases body levels of potassium – e.g. an ACE inhibitor or a salt substitute containing potassium.

Tell your doctor if you have or have had:
☐ long-term severe kidney problems ☐ diabetes ☐ gout.

How to use this medicine

Take the tablet in the morning, usually as a single dose. Sometimes your doctor may prescribe a twice-daily dose. Take the second dose of the day no later than mid-afternoon because night-time sleep may be disrupted by additional visits to the toilet. Amiloride can be taken at the same time as another diuretic.

Until you know how you react to amiloride, do not drive or do other activities that require alertness. Alcohol should not cause problems with amiloride.

Do not stop taking this medicine without discussing this with your doctor. If you miss a dose take it as soon as you remember, but no later than mid-afternoon. Otherwise skip this dose and take the next one as usual.

Over 65 Amiloride is likely to conserve more potassium in the body because the kidneys work less efficiently. Your kidney function and potassium levels should be checked before you start treatment. You may need less than the usual adult dose.

Interactions with other medicines

ACE inhibitors Increase blood pressure-lowering effect and blood potassium levels.
Ciclosporin Possibility of potassium levels becoming too high.

Unwanted effects

Less likely Feeling sick, dry mouth, dizziness or faintness, loss of appetite, stomach upsets, abdominal pain, flatulence, confusion, rashes, high blood levels of potassium (particularly if kidney function is reduced), low levels of sodium.

See your doctor if you develop a rash, muscle weakness or confusion. Too much potassium in the body causes irregular heartbeats, muscle weakness or heaviness, and numbness or tingling in the hands and feet.

Similar preparations

ALDACTIDE – Tablets
SPIRONOLACTONE + HYDROFLUMETHAZIDE

ALDACTONE – Tablets
SPIRONOLACTONE

CO-FLUMACTONE – Tablets
SPIRONOLACTONE + HYDROFLUMETHIAZIDE

CO-TRIAMTERZIDE – Tablets
TRIAMTERENE + HYDROCHLOROTHIAZIDE

DYAZIDE – Tablets
TRIAMTERENE + HYDROCHLOROTHIAZIDE

DYTAC – Capsules
TRIAMTERENE

DYTIDE – Capsules
TRIAMTERENE + BENZTHIAZIDE

KALSPARE – Tablets
TRIAMTERENE + CHLORTALIDONE

NAVISPARE – Tablets
AMILORIDE + CYCLOPENTHIAZIDE

SPIRONOLACTONE – Tablets, liquid

BETA BLOCKERS

Two main types of receptors in the body can be blocked by medicines to treat heart and circulation problems. These are alpha- and beta-adrenoceptors. Both alpha blockers (*alpha adrenergic* blocking drugs) and beta blockers (*beta adrenergic* blocking drugs) block these receptors to varying degrees, sometimes in different parts of the body, to dampen the effects of *noradrenaline* (*norepinephrine*), a neurotransmitter – one of the body's chemicals produced in the adrenal glands – which plays a part in controlling the heart, blood vessels, lungs and muscles. Together with adrenaline (epinephrine) it prepares the body for 'fight or flight', when the heart beats faster and more strongly, and other parts of the body are prepared for action. Beta blockers oppose the stimulating effect by slowing the heart rate and decreasing the force of the heartbeat. They lower blood pressure, but how they do so is not completely understood. Alpha blockers relax blood vessels, resulting in lower blood pressure (see doxazosin, page 118). Alpha blockers are also used for prostate problems (page 372).

All beta blocker preparations act in much the same way. They vary in their effect on the receptors and how long they work in the body, and different beta blockers suit different conditions and patients. **Oxprenolol**, **acebutolol**, **pindolol** and **celiprolol** stimulate beta receptors as well as block them; this lessens some of the unwanted effects, such as coldness in the hands and feet, but the heart is not slowed as much as with other preparations. **Carvedilol** (Eucardic) has a mixed mode of action with alpha- and beta-blocking properties. **Propranolol**, **metoprolol** and **pindolol** are lipid-soluble (they dissolve in body fat); others are water-soluble. Solubility affects a drug's distribution throughout the body systems and how it leaves the body. The most water-soluble beta blockers, **atenolol**, **celiprolol** and **nadolol**, cause less sleep disturbance because they are less likely to enter the brain than fat-soluble preparations. However, they stay in the body longer if kidney function is poor and the dosage must be reduced.

Beta blockers act throughout the body and are used to treat a range of conditions – high blood pressure, angina, in heart failure and after a heart attack, to control irregular heart beats, to relieve anxiety, prevent migraine, relieve pressure in the eye (*glaucoma*) and before surgery on the thyroid gland (*thyroidectomy*). Not all beta blockers are used for all the conditions and with some uses, the medicines are used outside their product licence, such as metoprolol (modified-release) for heart failure. The use of the medicines in this way has grown by clinical usage, often helping in difficult-to-manage areas. Some beta blockers are used for one condition only, such as **sotalol** for irregular heart beats. The choice of beta blocker depends on your condition and the evidence for its use, for example atenolol or metoprolol reduces the risk of a further heart attack occurring early after the first one, and **bisoprolol** or carvedilol helps in heart failure.

Some cautions with beta blockers

Beta blockers must not be used if you have asthma, chronic bronchitis, emphysema or any other breathing difficulties (respiratory disease) or have a history of obstructive airways disease: a beta blocker may narrow the airways in the lungs. Even the beta blockers that do not have such a marked effect on the lung should not be used. However, there may be a rare occasion when your doctor feels that a beta blocker is the only treatment for you, in which case special precautions (such as additional use of your relieving inhaler) must be taken.

Beta blockers make the heart pump blood through the body at a slower rate and less oxygen is required to do the work. This may worsen the effects of heart failure (although some beta blockers can help this when tried cautiously under specialist supervision) or heart block. A beta blocker will also worsen poor circulation to the hands and feet or Raynaud's phenomenon (page 147) because it constricts the blood vessels, preventing blood flow to your extremities. A beta blocker should be avoided in severe peripheral arterial disease, where the arteries in the limbs have narrowed. A beta blocker can affect diabetic control slightly, for example your response to low blood sugar (hypoglycaemia), but although you should avoid one if you experience frequent episodes of hypoglycaemia, a beta blocker can be used effectively in diabetes.

Other unwanted effects include dry mouth and digestive system disorders, tiredness, headaches, confusion, disturbed sleep, dizziness (particularly when you stand up quickly) and skin problems – psoriasis can worsen when you start **atenolol**. Depressive symptoms have been attributed to treatment with a beta blocker, but a thorough review of the evidence in over 35,000 people taking one, over periods of 6 to 59 months, has not revealed an increased risk of depression. Fatigue and sexual dysfunction such as impotence were also reported as unwanted effects, but the study showed only a small increase in these effects. Recent studies suggest that men taking beta blockers may be reacting psychologically; impotence can occur in older age and with smoking. A third of men who knew about the possibility of developing impotence on a beta blocker did so, compared with only 3 in 100 men who did not know that they were taking this class of medicine. Impotence is also reported with other blood pressure-lowering drugs. Beta blockers are effective medicines and studies show that people rarely stop taking them because of their unwanted effects.

If you take a beta blocker for a long time – for angina, for example – you must not stop taking it suddenly, as this has been known to worsen symptoms and even cause a heart attack. Your doctor will supervise a gradual withdrawal of the beta blocker if treatment needs to be stopped.

Combination preparations

Atenolol combined with a thiazide diuretic (**chlortalidone**) is available generically as **co-tenidone** in two different strengths. A combination of a beta blocker with a calcium channel blocker (**atenolol** and **nifedipine** – Beta-Adalat; Tenif) is also used only if one or the other has not controlled blood pressure. Several blood pressure-lowering medicines are used routinely together because blood pressure targets are now more stringent. However, combined preparations can increase the likelihood of unwanted effects and do not allow the dose of an individual drug to be varied.

ATENOLOL

ATENOLOL – Tablets

TENORMIN – Tablets, liquid, injection

Combined with a calcium channel antagonist

BETA-ADALAT – Capsules
ATENOLOL + NIFEDIPINE

TENIF – Capsules
ATENOLOL + NIFEDIPINE

Combined with a diuretic

CO-TENIDONE – Tablets
ATENOLOL + CHLORTALIDONE

TENORETIC – Tablets
CO-TENIDONE 100/25

KALTEN – Capsules
ATENOLOL + CO-AMILOZIDE

TENORET 50 – Tablets
CO-TENIDONE 50/12.5

Atenolol is a beta blocker used to treat high blood pressure, angina, and irregular heartbeats (*arrhythmias*). It prevents the heart from beating too quickly, although its exact effect in lowering blood pressure is not fully understood. Atenolol is also used to prevent further damage to the heart after a heart attack (*myocardial infarction*).

Atenolol starts to act within two to four hours of taking it by mouth and is effective for longer than a day (20–30 hours). It can therefore be taken once a day (some other beta blockers may need to be taken twice or three times daily). When used to lower blood pressure the dose of atenolol rarely needs to be more than 50mg as little further effect is obtained. Use in angina or heart arrhythmias may need dosing at 100mg a day. Atenolol stays in the body longer if kidney function is reduced; the dose needs to be reduced in moderate to severe kidney impairment.

Some beta blockers are also used for thyroid disorders, for preventing migraine and for relieving some of the symptoms of anxiety such as tremor and palpitations, although atenolol is not licensed for these conditions. A beta blocker such as timolol is also used locally in the eye in the management of glaucoma.

Before you use this medicine

Tell your doctor if you are:
☐ pregnant — avoid beta blockers: atenolol would be used only under close medical supervision ☐ breast-feeding – atenolol passes into the milk, but is unlikely to cause problems at normal doses ☐ taking any other medicines.

Do not use if you have:
☐ asthma ☐ wheezing e.g. bronchitis or other breathing problems ☐ heart failure that has not been treated ☐ acidosis – excess acid in the blood.

Tell your doctor if you have or have had:
☐ poor blood circulation ☐ Raynaud's phenomenon ☐ poor kidney function ☐ diabetes – atenolol may interfere with the body's response to low blood-sugar ☐ irregular heart rhythms ☐ low blood pressure ☐ phaeochromocytoma – a rare tumour, usually in the adrenal glands, that increases blood pressure (unless also given with an alpha blocker).

How to use this medicine

The tablets are usually taken once a day, or sometimes twice a day for angina. It may take one or two weeks of treatment before the full effect of atenolol is felt. A modest intake of alcohol will not cause problems. Some diabetics can take atenolol, but it would be unsuitable if you experience frequent episodes of low blood sugar (hypo).

If you miss a dose take it as soon as you remember. Skip the dose if your next dose is due within eight hours and take that as usual. Do not take double the dose. Do not stop taking this medicine suddenly, especially if you have ischaemic heart disease: to prevent a worsening of your condition your doctor will give you a schedule to decrease the dose of atenolol gradually if you are on long-term treatment. Make sure you do not run out of tablets.

Over 65 You may need a lower dose of atenolol, e.g. 25mg, especially if your kidney function is reduced.

Interactions with other medicines

Anaesthetics enhance the blood pressure-lowering effect of atenolol and other beta blockers. Tell your doctor or dentist that you take atenolol before you have surgery.
Heart drugs such as those for controlling the heart rhythm (e.g. **amiodarone** and **disopyramide**) increase the risk of reducing and slowing heart activity.
Calcium channel blockers: **diltiazem** affects heart activity; **nifedipine** may induce severe low blood pressure and heart failure; **verapamil** should not be used with a beta blocker.
Other blood pressure-lowering drugs enhance the effect of atenolol.

NSAIDs, e.g **ibuprofen** and **indometacin,** oppose atenolol's blood pressure-lowering effect.
Antidepressants, e.g. **monoamine oxidase inhibitors**, increase the blood pressure-lowering effect.
Tricyclic antidepressants, antihistamines and sotalol increase the risk of irregular heart rhythms.
Antimalarials, e.g **mefloquine** for preventing malaria, increase the risk of slow heart rhythm.

Unwanted effects

Likely Cold hands and feet, fatigue, slow heart rhythm, wheezing or breathing problems, worsening heart failure.
Less likely Sleep disturbances, skin rashes and/or dry eyes, depression and confusion, dizziness.

You should contact your doctor if you have severe breathing difficulties, a skin rash, or dizziness or confusion.

Similar preparations

BETALOC – Tablets, modified-release tablets
METOPROLOL

BETIM – Tablets
TIMOLOL

BISOPROLOL – Tablets

▼CARDICOR – Tablets
BISOPROLOL

CELECTOL – Tablets
CELIPROLOL

CELIPROLOL – Tablets

CORGARD – Tablets
NADOLOL

EMCOR – Tablets
BISOPROLOL

▼EUCARDIC – Tablets
CARVEDILOL

INDERAL – Tablets, modified-release capsules
PROPRANOLOL

KERLONE – Tablets
BETAXOLOL

LABETALOL – Tablets

LOPRESOR – Tablets, modified-release tablets
METOPROLOL

METOPROLOL –Tablets

MONOCOR – Tablets
BISOPROLOL

NEBILET – Tablets
NEBIVOLOL

OXPRENOLOL – Tablets

PROPRANOLOL – Tablets, liquid

SECTRAL – Tablets, capsules
ACEBUTOLOL

TRANDATE – Tablets
LABETALOL

TRASICOR – Tablets, modified-release tablets
OXPRENOLOL

VISKEN – Tablets
PINDOLOL

Combined with a diuretic

CO-BETALOC – Tablets, modified-release tablets
METOPROLOL + HYDROCHLOROTHIAZIDE

CORGARETIC – Tablets
NADOLOL + BENDROFLUMETHIAZIDE

INDERECTIC/INDEREX – Capsules
PROPRANOLOL + BENDROFLUMETHIAZIDE

MODUCREN – Tablets
TIMOLOL + CO-AMILOZIDE

MONOZIDE 10 – Tablets
BISOPROLOL + HYDROCHLOROTHIAZIDE

PRESTIM – Tablets
TIMOLOL + BENDROFLUMETHIAZIDE

SECADREX – Tablets
ACEBUTOLOL + HYDROCHLOROTHIAZIDE

TRASIDREX – Tablets
OXPRENOLOL + CYCLOPENTHIAZIDE

VISKALDIX – Tablets
PINDOLOL + CLOPAMIDE

ACE INHIBITORS

Angiotensin converting enzyme (ACE) inhibitors act on a complex system of body chemicals (the renin-angiotensin-aldosterone system) which are found in blood vessel walls, particularly in the kidneys and lungs. This system helps to regulate blood pressure and the body's mineral and fluid balance. ACE inhibitors dilate blood vessels by blocking an enzyme (angiotensin-converting enzyme) that helps produce a body chemical that normally narrows (constricts) the blood vessels and so increases tension. When the chemical (angiotensin II) is prevented from working, the blood vessels widen (dilate), reducing resistance to the flow of blood around the body, and blood pressure falls. ACE inhibitors are used for lowering blood pressure when a thiazide diuretic and beta blocker have not worked, are not tolerated or cannot be used. All 11 ACE inhibitors can be used for lowering blood pressure; some are also used for preventing and treating heart failure and when heart failure occurs after a heart attack. Treatment of severe heart failure with an ACE inhibitor is generally started in hospital under a doctor's close supervision and can be combined with a diuretic, and also with spironolactone which can lead to better symptom control. Kidney function and the body's potassium need careful monitoring. **Digoxin** can also be added to ACE inhibitor treatment, usually for controlling atrial fibrillation (page 140).

ACE inhibitors are a valuable class of drugs, especially for people with heart failure in whom they reduce symptoms and prolong life. They also help diabetics with early evidence of decline in kidney function (*microalbuminuria*), or where body protein spills into the urine (*proteinuria*) by slowing the deterioration in kidney function. Even if you do not have raised blood pressure as a diabetic, but have evidence of a decline in kidney function, an ACE inhibitor can help. There are few differences between the ACE inhibitors and all act in a similar way in the body. A persistent dry cough is a common unwanted effect which affects women and non-smokers more often, especially when an ACE inhibitor is used to lower high blood pressure.

All the ACE inhibitors can cause a sudden drop in blood pressure, particularly with the first dose – this should be taken at bedtime or when you can lie down for a few hours afterwards. Paradoxically, ACE inhibitors can sometimes damage kidney function by reducing or stopping the filtration process that produces urine in the kidneys. This effect is more likely if you have severe narrowing of the arteries leading to the kidneys (renal artery stenosis), in older people and anyone who already has poor kidney function or kidney disease. Before you start an ACE inhibitor, and routinely during treatment, your kidney function should be checked.

ACE inhibitors can be used with some diuretics to increase the blood pressure-lowering effect, but not generally with a potassium-sparing diuretic. An ACE inhibitor also keeps potassium in the body and the combination with a potassium-sparing diuretic increases the risk of heart arrhythmias. Some ACE inhibitors are combined with a thiazide diuretic (e.g. **hydrochlorothiazide**). However, it is better to take the individual drugs separately so that the dosages can be tailored to your needs. For example, **captopril** is normally given twice daily and hydrochlorothiazide once daily. A combination preparation is useful if you already take the individual drugs in those dosages. However, the combination of fixed doses of an ACE inhibitor with the calcium channel blocker, **verapamil** (Tarka) is not recommended, because this type of combination is not first-line treatment.

Angiotensin-II receptor antagonists, such as **losartan** (Cozaar), act in a slightly different way to ACE inhibitors by blocking the body's angiotensin II receptors, rather than preventing the production of angiotensin II in the chemical pathway. This results in a similar effect to ACE inhibitors with the prevention of the constricting action of angiotensin II on blood vessels. The effect of angiotensin-II receptor antagonists is not identical to that of ACE inhibitors. For example, they do not appear to cause the same unwanted effects (including irritating cough or the rare condition angio-oedema). All the angiotensin-II receptor antagonists are used for lowering blood pressure and some are used to delay kidney deterioration in diabetics. None is licensed for use in heart failure yet, although your doctor may decide to try one for this condition particularly if you cannot tolerate an ACE inhibitor – for example, because of unwanted effects.

ENALAPRIL

ENALAPRIL – Tablets INNOVACE – Tablets

Combined with a diuretic
INNOZIDE – Tablets
ENALAPRIL + HYDROCHLOROTHIAZIDE

Enalapril is an ACE inhibitor used for lowering high blood pressure when other methods such as dietary control, diuretics or beta blockers have not worked or cannot be used. In the treatment of heart failure enalapril is used often together with a diuretic. It is also used to prevent heart failure worsening if you have early symptoms and can help even before symptoms become apparent. Enalapril starts to work within an hour and its effect lasts about 24 hours. Like other ACE inhibitors, enalapril can produce a rapid drop in blood pressure (*hypotension*) in some people at the first dose, causing dizziness and fainting. Older people and those with poor kidney function should take a lower dose or avoid enalapril altogether. At the start of ACE inhibitor therapy, dosing is increased gradually to minimise unwanted effects.

Before you use this medicine

Tell your doctor if you are:
☐ pregnant – enalapril and other ACE inhibitors should not be used ☐ breast-feeding – unlikely to be harmful ☐ on a low-salt diet ☐ taking potassium supplements ☐ taking any other medicines, particularly diuretics, and including vitamins and those bought over the counter.

Tell your doctor if have or have had:
☐ severe kidney disease or poor kidney function ☐ narrowing of heart valve (aortic stenosis) ☐ narrowing of blood vessels to the kidneys ☐ hypersensitivity to an ACE inhibitor.

You should not take an ACE inhibitor if you have experienced hypersensitivity to one previously, you have severe narrowing of the blood vessels to both kidneys or you are pregnant. Your blood levels of sodium and potassium and your kidney function should be assessed before you start an ACE inhibitor, and once a year during treatment.

How to use this medicine

Take the tablets once or twice a day, with a glass of water; the first dose should be taken at bedtime or when you can lie down for a few hours afterwards. You may feel dizzy or faint when you get up from sitting or lying down, especially during the first few days of treatment. Get up slowly and stay beside the chair or bed until you are sure you are not dizzy. Alcohol and other medicines for lowering blood pressure enhance this effect.

If you have heart failure, are on a low-salt diet, are dehydrated (e.g. with severe diarrhoea) or on dialysis before or while taking enalapril, it may cause a sudden drop in blood pressure. If enalapril is added to existing treatment with a diuretic, this should be stopped, or the dose reduced greatly, before the ACE inhibitor is introduced. If you have poor kidney function, you should start treatment with a low dose. Until you know how you react to enalapril, do not drive or do other activities that require alertness.

Do not stop taking this medicine suddenly; your doctor will give you a schedule to decrease the dose gradually. If you miss a dose, take it as soon as you remember, but skip it if your next dose is due within eight hours. Do not take double the dose.

Over 65 or if you have kidney impairment You should start at half the usual adult dose.

Interactions with other medicines

ACE inhibitors can interact with a range of medicines, particularly those that affect blood pressure. The most important interactions are given here but you should always check with your doctor or pharmacist when you take an ACE inhibitor with another medicine.

Anaesthetics enhance the blood pressure-lowering effect of enalapril. Tell your doctor or dentist that you take an ACE inhibitor before you have surgery.

Ciclosporin, the immunosuppressant, increases the risk of higher blood levels of potassium, thus increasing the risk of irregular heart rhythms (pages 139–40).

Diuretics enhance the blood pressure-lowering effect. ACE inhibitors keep potassium in the body, so if enalapril is taken with a potassium-sparing diuretic, blood potassium levels can rise, thus increasing the risk of irregular heart rhythms (pages 139–40).

Lithium blood levels increase because ACE inhibitors prevent its removal from the body and it may reach toxic levels.

Non-steroidal anti-inflammatory drugs (NSAIDs) antagonise the blood pressure-lowering effects of ACE inhibitors; there is also an increased risk of kidney impairment when ACE inhibitors and NSAIDs are taken together.

Potassium salts, including low-sodium salt substitutes, and enalapril together increase the blood levels of potassium, thus increasing the risk of irregular heart rhythms (pages 139–40).

Unwanted effects

Likely Persistent dry cough, throat discomfort, headache, dizziness.

Less likely Feeling sick, diarrhoea (occasionally constipation), muscle cramps, skin rashes, lack of appetite, taste alteration, chest pain, fast or irregular heartbeat, hypersensitivity reactions, swelling of the face, lips and mouth, confusion, depression, drowsiness, sleeplessness, blurred vision, tinnitus, breathlessness, liver impairment.

Contact your doctor if these effects are severe or they do not fade as treatment continues. Contact your doctor immediately if you experience dizziness or faintness, indicating a severe fall in blood pressure, particularly at the start of treatment; hypersensitivity reactions (fever, joint/muscle pains, photosensitivity or other skin reactions), swelling of the face, lips and mouth (*angio-oedema*).

Similar preparations

ACCUPRO – Tablets
QUINAPRIL

ACEPRIL – Tablets
CAPTOPRIL

CAPOTEN – Tablets
CAPTOPRIL

CAPTOPRIL – Tablets

CARACE – Tablets
LISINOPRIL

COVERSYL – Tablets
PERINDOPRIL

GOPTEN – Capsules
TRANDOLAPRIL

LISINOPRIL – Tablets

ODRIK – Capsules
TRANDOLAPRIL

PERDIX – Tablets
MOEXIPRIL

RAMIPRIL – Capsules, tablets

STARIL – Tablets
FOSINOPRIL

TANATRIL – Tablets
IMIDAPRIL

TRITACE – Tablets
RAMIPRIL

VASCACE – Tablets
CILAZAPRIL

ZESTRIL – Tablets
LISINOPRIL

Combined with diuretic

ACCURETIC – Tablets
QUINAPRIL + HYDROCHLOROTHIAZIDE

ACEZIDE – Tablets
CAPTOPRIL + HYDROCHLOROTHIAZIDE

CAPOZIDE – Tablets
CAPTOPRIL + HYDROCHLOROTHIAZIDE

CARACE PLUS – Tablets
LISINOPRIL + HYDROCHLOROTHIAZIDE

COVERSYL PLUS – Tablets
PERINDOPRIL + INDAPAMIDE

CO-ZIDOCAPT – Tablets
CAPTOPRIL + HYDROCHLOROTHIAZIDE

Poor choice

TARKA
TRANDOLAPRIL + VERAPAMIL

▼TRIAPIN – Tablets
RAMIPRIL + FELODIPINE

LOSARTAN

COZAAR – Tablets

Combined with a diuretic

COZAAR-COMP – Tablets
LOSARTAN + HYDROCHLOROTHIAZIDE

Losartan is an angiotensin-II receptor antagonist which prevents angiotensin-II from tightening blood vessels, thus allowing them to relax and widen (*vasodilatation*). Widened blood vessels lead to a reduction in blood pressure. Losartan is used when an ACE inhibitor is not tolerated for lowering high blood pressure and also for slowing the progression of kidney disease in type-2 diabetes. Unlike ACE inhibitors, which have broader actions, angiotensin-II receptor antagonists do not block the body chemical bradykinin, which appears to be linked with coughing, an irritating unwanted effect of ACE inhibitors. Coughing can still occur with an angiotensin-II receptor antagonist, but the likelihood is reduced. Losartan starts to work within an hour and its effect lasts for 24 hours which allows once-daily dosing. The maximal blood pressure-lowering effect is achieved three to six weeks after the start of losartan treatment. Losartan is not licensed for the treatment of heart failure, but doctors may decide to try it when an ACE inhibitor is not tolerated. Research is under way to look at the effects of combining an ACE inhibitor with an angiotensin-II receptor antagonist in the management of heart failure.

Before you use this medicine

Tell your doctor if you are:
☐ pregnant – losartan and similar medicines should not be used, particularly in the second and third trimesters ☐ breast-feeding ☐ on a low-salt diet or taking potassium supplements ☐ taking any other medicines, particularly diuretics, and including vitamins and those bought over the counter.

Tell your doctor if you have or have had:
☐ severe kidney disease, poor kidney function or a kidney transplant ☐ hypersensitivity to an angiotensin-II receptor antagonist ☐ poor liver function ☐ problems with the heart valves or muscle (aortic or mitral valve stenosis or hypertrophic cardiomyopathy) ☐ narrowing of the blood vessels to the kidneys.

Your blood levels of sodium and potassium and your kidney function should be assessed before you start and during treatment.

How to use this medicine

Take the tablets once a day, usually at the same time each day, with a glass of water. The usual dose is 50mg daily, but this can be increased to 100mg after several weeks' treatment. You may feel dizzy or faint from rapid blood pressure lowering when you get up from sitting or lying down, especially during the first few days of treatment. Get up slowly and stay beside the chair or bed until you are sure you are not dizzy. Alcohol and other medicines for lowering blood pressure enhance this effect.

If you are on a low-salt diet or dehydrated (e.g. with severe diarrhoea) before or while taking losartan, it may cause a sudden drop in blood pressure. If you have poor kidney function or dehydration you should start treatment with a low dose (25mg daily).

Do not stop taking this medicine suddenly. If you miss a dose, take it as soon as you remember, but skip it if your next dose is due within eight hours. Do not take double the dose.

Over 65 You may need a lower dose at the start of treatment.
Over 75 A lower dose of 25mg daily is recommended.

Interactions with other medicines

Angiotensin-II receptor antagonists follow the pattern of interactions with ACE inhibitors (page 110). In particular:
Non-steroidal anti-inflammatory drugs (NSAIDs) can antagonise the effects of angiotensin-II receptor antagonists.

Potassium salts, including low-sodium salt substitutes, and angiotensin-II receptor antagonists together increase the blood levels of potassium.
Antituberculosis treatment, **rifampicin**, may reduce losartan's effectiveness
Antifungal fluconazole may reduce losartan's effectiveness.

Unwanted effects

Likely Dizziness, diarrhoea, muscle and joint pains, muscle cramps, skin rash, itching, migraine, taste disturbance, cough.
Less likely Liver problems, anaemia e.g. in severe kidney disease, hypersensitivity reactions, swelling of the face, lips and mouth, inflammation of blood vessels (vasculitis).

Contact your doctor if these effects are severe or they do not fade as treatment continues. Contact your doctor immediately if you experience dizziness or faintness, indicating a severe fall in blood pressure, particularly at the start of treatment; hypersensitivity reactions (fever, joint/muscle pains or other skin reactions), swelling of the face, lips and mouth (*angio-oedema*).

Similar preparations

AMIAS – Tablets
CANDESARTAN

APROVEL – Tablets
IRBESARTAN

DIOVAN – Tablets
VALSARTAN

MICARDIS – Tablets
TELMISARTAN

▼OLMETEC – Tablets
OLMESARTAN

TEVETEN – Tablets
EPROSARTAN

Combined with a diuretic

CoAPROVEL – Tablets
IRBESARTAN + HYDROCHLOROTHIAZIDE

MICARDIS PLUS – Tablets
TELMISARTAN + HYDROCHLOROTHIAZIDE

CALCIUM CHANNEL BLOCKERS

Calcium is an important mineral which the body needs for the proper functioning of muscles. Calcium channel blockers (calcium antagonists) widen the blood vessels by interfering with the flow of calcium through special channels in the cells of the heart and the smooth muscle of blood vessels, thereby relaxing them. This allows blood to flow more easily around the body and for more oxygen to reach the heart and other organs. **Verapamil** (pages 141–2) and **diltiazem** (pages 124–5) have more of an effect on the heart than the peripheral arteries (those furthest from the heart); they also help maintain the rhythm and pace of the heart. Diltiazem and verapamil are used for preventing and treating angina and also for high blood pressure, but must be avoided if you also have heart failure. **Nifedipine** and related medicines (dihydropyridines) do not act on the heart's rhythm, but have more effect on the blood flow to the peripheral circulation. Most are used for angina and all can be used for high blood pressure – sometimes at the same time as other medicines such as an ACE inhibitor or beta blocker.

NIFEDIPINE

Modified-release preparations recommended for high blood pressure or angina:

ADALAT LA – Tablets
ADALAT RETARD – Tablets
ADIPINE MR – Tablets
CARDILATE MR – Tablets
CORACTEN SR and XL – Capsules
CORODAY MR – Tablets
FORTIPINE LA – Tablets
HYPOLAR RETARD – Tablets
NIFEDIPRESS MR – Tablets
NIFOPRESS RETARD – Tablets
SLOFEDIPINE and XL – Tablets
TENSIPINE MR – Tablets

Combination preparations:

NIFEDIPINE + BETA BLOCKER – See **atenolol**, pages 107–9.

For Raynaud's phenomenon only:

ADALAT – Capsules
NIFEDIPINE – Capsules

Nifedipine is a calcium channel blocker which relaxes arterial smooth muscle of the heart and peripheral blood vessels (vasodilator). It is used in modified-release form for the control of high blood pressure, for the prevention and treatment of chest pain (angina) and in short-acting form for Raynaud's phenomenon. It can be taken with a beta blocker if you have both raised blood pressure and angina. Unlike beta blockers, nifedipine is suitable for treating asthmatics with high blood pressure.

Nifedipine starts to work in about half to one hour and its effects last up to about 12 hours. The once daily modified-release preparations are now preferred for managing angina or lowering blood pressure as they provide more sustained levels of the drug in the body throughout 24 hours. Minor unwanted effects – flushing, swollen ankles, headaches, palpitations, dizziness and tiredness – are quite common at the start of treatment and are more likely in older people.

Before you use this medicine

Tell your doctor if you are:

☐ pregnant – not usually prescribed, may inhibit labour ☐ breast-feeding – nifedipine passes into the milk but amounts are too small to be harmful ☐ taking any other medicines, such as the antibiotic **rifampicin**, including vitamins and those bought over the counter ☐ a regular grapefruit juice drinker.

Tell your doctor if you have or have had:

☐ heart failure ☐ low blood pressure ☐ diabetes ☐ poor liver or kidney function ☐ a heart attack within the last month ☐ severe narrowing of the aortic valve in the heart ☐ unstable or acute attacks of angina ☐ porphyria – an inherited metabolic disorder that affects the body's manufacture of blood.

How to use this medicine

For high blood pressure or to prevent angina Modified-release tablets or capsules are usually used, taken once or twice daily with or after food. Adalat LA modified-release nifedipine tablets are not suitable if you have liver disease, have narrowing of the gullet or intestines, inflammation of the intestines or bowel such as Crohn's disease because the type of formulation (a membrane containing the drug) may get caught in the gut. If it is suitable for you, the complete tablet may appear in faeces or the toilet but this does not mean that the drug has not been absorbed into the body or is not working. For **Raynaud's phenomenon** capsules are taken three times daily with or after food.

You may feel dizzy or faint when you get up from sitting or lying down, especially during the first few days of treatment. Get up slowly and stay beside the chair or bed until you are sure you are not dizzy. Avoid alcohol which may lower blood pressure further. Until you know how you react to nifedipine, do not drive or do other activities that require alertness. Grapefruit juice increases blood levels of nifedipine and related medicines, except **amlodipine** (Istin), and you should avoid the combination.

If you miss a dose, take it as soon as you remember. Skip the dose if it is almost time for your next dose and take that as usual. Do not take double the dose. Do not stop taking this medicine suddenly; your doctor will give you a schedule to decrease the dose gradually.

Over 65 You may need a lower dose, particularly if unwanted effects are troublesome. If you have poor liver function, you may need a lower dose.

Interactions with other medicines

Beta blockers Occasionally severe low blood pressure and heart failure.
The heart drug digoxin Blood levels of digoxin may rise, increasing its unwanted effects.
Antibacterials: **rifampicin** speeds up the metabolism or reduces blood levels of nifedipine and related medicines, rendering them less effective; **erythromycin** may increase the blood levels of **felodipine** (similar to nifedipine).
Antiepileptic carbamazepine reduces the effect of nifedipine and related medicines.
Antifungals itraconazole and **ketoconazole** increase the blood levels, particularly of **felodipine** and other related medicines.
Other blood pressure-lowering medicines enhance blood pressure-lowering effect.
Antivirals possibly increase the blood levels of nifedipine and related medicines.
Immunosuppressant ciclosporin may increase blood levels of nifedipine and increase the risk of unwanted effects, such as swollen gums; nifedipine increases blood levels of **tacrolimus** (used following transplants).

Unwanted effects

Likely Headache, a feeling of warmth, flushing, dizziness, swollen ankles, tiredness, palpitations, constipation.
Less likely Feeling or being sick, rashes, itching, stomach pain, swollen gums, dry mouth, leg cramps, fast heart beat.
Rarely increased desire to urinate, increased sensitivity to light, hypersensitivity, pins and needles, muscle and joint pains.

Contact your doctor if nifedipine makes you feel dizzy and this does not fade after the first few days of treatment, or if your chest pains (angina) get worse when you start taking nifedipine or any related medicines.

Similar preparations

CARDENE – Capsules, modified-release capsules
NICARDIPINE

ISTIN – Tablets
AMLODIPINE

MOTENS – Tablets
LACIDIPINE

NICARDIPINE – Capsules

PLENDIL – Tablets
FELODIPINE

PRESCAL – Tablets*
ISRADIPINE

SYSCOR – Modified-release tablets
NISOLDIPINE

ZANDIP – Tablets*
LERCANIDIPINE

* not used for angina

ALPHA BLOCKERS AND THER VASODILATORS

Calcium channel blockers and ACE inhibitors are both *vasodilators* – that is, they open up the blood vessels. This leads to an improvement in blood flow around the body and better oxygen supply. A calcium channel blocker acts directly on the muscle surrounding the blood vessel while an ACE inhibitor blocks an enzyme in the blood. Some other vasodilators affect the nerves which control blood vessel muscles, such as alpha blockers, whilst others have a direct effect on the muscles around the blood vessels, for example **hydralazine**. This is used occasionally to treat moderate to severe high blood pressure, usually with a beta blocker or a thiazide diuretic. If used on its own, hydralazine can cause rapid heart beat (*tachycardia*) and it also retains fluid in the body. Unwanted effects can be minimised if low doses are given. Long-term treatment is rarely appropriate now as an auto-immune, arthritis-like syndrome, systemic lupus erythematosus, may develop, although this usually disappears when hydralazine is stopped.

Other vasodilators act on the brain chemicals that play a part in controlling blood pressure. Many were in use before beta blockers, calcium channel blockers and ACE inhibitors were developed. **Methyldopa** (Aldomet) remains the drug of choice to control high blood pressure during pregnancy.

Moxonidine (Physiotens) is a newer treatment which may be added to other blood pressure-lowering treatments. A related, but older medicine **clonidine** (Catapres) is no longer recommended. Similarly, **guanethidine** (Ismelin) and **debrisoquine** cause too sudden a drop in blood pressure and are no longer recommended. Alpha blockers (**doxazosin**, **indoramin**, **prazosin** and **terazosin**) remain useful for lowering blood pressure and the newer, longer-acting ones, doxazosin and terazosin are better tolerated than prazosin. They are sometimes used on their own, but are more usually given with a thiazide diuretic or a beta blocker for additional control of blood pressure. Alpha blockers are also used to reduce the symptoms caused by an enlarged prostate gland (page 372).

DOXAZOSIN

DOXAZOSIN – Tablets

CARDURA – Tablets, modified-release tablets
DOXAZOSIN

Doxazosin is a vasodilator alpha blocker which blocks the nerve stimulus that tightens the muscles around blood vessels. As the muscles relax, the blood vessels widen, blood flow improves and blood pressure is reduced. Doxazosin can be used on its own or with other blood pressure-lowering medicines. It is also used to ease the symptoms caused by an enlarged prostate gland at lower doses used for lowering blood pressure. Doxazosin can cause a fall in blood pressure (*hypotension*) on starting treatment, resulting in dizziness and fainting.

Before you use this medicine

Tell your doctor if you are:

☐ pregnant or breast-feeding ☐ on a low-salt diet ☐ taking any other medicines, including vitamins and those bought over the counter.

Tell your doctor if you have or have had:
☐ heart failure ☐ poor liver function – monitoring advised.

How to use this medicine

Treatment starts with a low dose (1mg) once a day. The dose is gradually increased over a period of weeks depending on your response to treatment (maximum daily dose 16mg or 8mg for modified-release tablets). If you have liver disease or poor kidney function you may need a reduced dose.

The first dose should be taken at bedtime to avoid fainting and collapse. Take the tablets with a glass of water with food.

You may feel dizzy or faint when you get up from sitting or lying down, even after the first dose and especially during the first few days of treatment. Get up slowly and stay beside the bed or chair until you are sure you are not dizzy. Alcohol and other medicines for lowering blood pressure enhance this effect: avoid alcohol.

Until you know how you react to doxazosin do not drive or do other activities that require alertness, especially at the start of treatment.

Over 65 Older people are more susceptible to dizziness and fainting which may continue beyond the first dose.

Interactions with other medicines

Anaesthetics enhance the blood pressure-lowering effect of doxazosin. Tell your doctor or dentist that you take doxazosin before you have surgery.
ACE inhibitors, **beta blockers**, **calcium channel blockers** and **diuretics** enhance the blood pressure-lowering effect and increase the risk of dizziness or faintness with the first dose.
Antidepressants may enhance the blood pressure-lowering effect.
The antibacterial linezolid (Zyvox) enhances the blood pressure-lowering effect.
Moxisylyte (Opilon) for Raynaud's syndrome increases the risk of severe dizziness or faintness.

Unwanted effects

Likely Dizziness, fainting, headache, drowsiness, weakness, fatigue, lack of energy, vertigo, fluid retention, feeling sick, runny nose.
Less likely Skin rash, itchy skin, nose bleeds, bruising, inability to control urination, liver problems e.g. jaundice, blurred vision, impotence.

Dizziness, feeling sick and headache should fade. Contact your doctor if these effects are severe and they do not fade or if you develop a rash or palpitations.

Similar preparations

BARATOL – Tablets
INDORAMIN

DORALESE* – Tablets
INDORAMIN

FLOMAX* – Modified-release capsules
TAMSULOSIN

HYPOVASE – Tablets
PRAZOSIN

HYTRIN – Tablets
TERAZOSIN

HYTRIN BPH* – Tablets
TERAZOSIN

PRAZOSIN* – Tablets

TERAZOSIN – Tablets

XATRAL* – Tablets, modified-release tablets
ALFUZOSIN

*For treating an enlarged prostate (pages 372–3)

Angina

Chest pain or angina occurs when the supply of oxygen to heart muscle is restricted by a narrowing of the heart's own blood vessels, the coronary arteries (*ischaemic heart disease*). Angina usually strikes when you exert yourself – running for a bus, for example – or in times of emotional stress, when the heart has to beat faster. If you have angina, the narrowed arteries cannot supply sufficient blood and oxygen to the heart during periods of exercise or stress. When you rest, the heartbeat slows, less oxygen is needed and the pain disappears. This is known as stable angina.

During an angina attack, you may experience a tightening or choking feeling which lasts about five to ten minutes and then fades as you rest. You may feel a vice-like pain in the middle of the chest, or it may spread to your jaws and down your arms; you may get breathless, become pale and perspire. Your doctor will need to investigate the cause of your pain with blood tests for haemoglobin to identify anaemia (pages 464–5), for signs of diabetes and for cholesterol, and may suggest an electrocardiogram (ECG) and exercise testing.

Angina may warn of an approaching heart attack, which can occur if a narrowed artery becomes completely blocked. You must therefore see a doctor at the first sign of any symptoms. If the pattern of your angina changes and comes on suddenly and intensely or occurs when you are not exerting yourself, you must seek help immediately; this is known as unstable angina and may be a sign of an imminent heart attack, which requires emergency hospital attention. Another form of angina, known as variant or Prinzmetal's angina, occurs at rest, and in response to cold. The coronary artery goes into spasm and this often occurs at the same time each day or night. In older people fainting can occur with angina, an indication of severe coronary artery disease.

The coronary arteries tend to fur up with fatty deposits of cholesterol as you grow older – this is part of the normal ageing process, but the way we live, what we eat and drink and how much exercise we take all affect how quickly this happens. Ways to avoid or reduce some of the risk factors that encourage heart and circulatory diseases are given in 'How you can help yourself', see page 95. Your doctor will also want to identify and discuss the management of your risk factors. These include lowering cholesterol and blood pressure if these are raised, guidance on stopping smoking if appropriate, weight reduction and an exercise programme within your capabilities. The most important risk is smoking, which is a major cause of coronary artery narrowing. Smokers are more likely to have angina and stopping smoking reduces your risk of dying from ischaemic heart disease.

Medicines for angina

Medicines are used to relieve the discomfort of an attack of angina (**glyceryl trinitrate**, for example) or to prevent an attack (a beta blocker and/or calcium channel blocker, for example). If you have more than two anginal attacks a week on glyceryl trinitrate, you are likely to need regular medicines for prevention. For very severe angina that is not controlled by medicines and lifestyle changes, you may be referred for surgery; techniques such as coronary artery bypass grafting (CABG) and percutaneous transluminal coronary angioplasty (PTCA) improve blood flow to the heart. Although angina is not cured by taking a medicine, most people manage the condition successfully with a nitrate, a beta blocker and/or a calcium channel blocker such as **diltiazem**. If you take a beta blocker regularly, ensure that you always have a supply. A beta blocker must not be stopped suddenly because this may worsen your angina. An alternative type of vasodilator, **nicorandil** (Ikorel), can prevent or treat angina when standard treatment is inappropriate.

Other long-term treatments you are likely to need to reduce your risk of further cardiovascular disease include aspirin (e.g. 75mg daily), a statin to lower cholesterol, medicines to lower your blood pressure if it is raised and possibly an ACE inhibitor.

NITRATES

Nitrates are vasodilators with a direct effect on blood vessels and have been in use for well over a hundred years. They are still an important group of medicines for preventing angina before exertion and for relieving chest pain when angina occurs at rest. A nitrate compound such as glyceryl trinitrate may be used with other medicines or it can sometimes be used on its own, especially for older people with occasional symptoms. Glyceryl trinitrate works for a short time in the body but if a longer action is needed your doctor may prescribe modified-release forms of related compounds **isosorbide dinitrate** or **isosorbide mononitrate**.

Glyceryl trinitrate (also known as GTN, nitroglycerin, trinitroglycerin or trinitrin) can be taken by a variety of routes – a common way is under the tongue with tablets or spray or between the teeth and cheeks (buccal tablets). These methods provide almost immediate relief of symptoms and the effect lasts up to 30 minutes. Modified-release preparations have a longer effect, to prevent an attack. Skin preparations may be helpful if you have angina at rest, for example at night. However, ointment is messy to use and patches (transdermal patches) may have to be removed for part of the day or night because tolerance can develop, reducing the drug's effectiveness.

All the nitrates can cause tolerance and therefore their therapeutic effect lessens. This tends to happen more with isosorbide dinitrate or mononitrate in conventional tablets, some modified-release products (although not with once-daily isosorbide mononitrate preparations), and skin patches. The solution is to allow the body nitrate levels to fall between doses by not taking the tablets at regular intervals during the day or by taking the patch off for several hours each day. Your doctor will guide you on any dosage changes.

GLYCERYL TRINITRATE

On prescription/from a pharmacy
GLYCERYL TRINITRATE – Tablets
CORO-NITRO SPRAY – Spray
DEPONIT – Patches
GLYTRIN SPRAY – Spray
GTN 300mcg – Tablets
MINITRAN – Patches
NITRO-DUR – Patches
NITROLINGUAL SPRAY – Spray
NITROMIN – Spray
PERCUTOL – Ointment
SUSCARD – Modified-release tablets
SUSTAC – Modified-release tablets
TRANSIDERM-NITRO – Patches
TRINTEK – Patches

Prescription-only: injections
GLYCERYL TRINITRATE
NITROCINE
NITRONAL

Glyceryl trinitrate is a vasodilator acting directly on the veins and coronary arteries, widening the blood vessels to allow more blood and oxygen to reach the heart muscle. It relieves an attack of angina or prevents one developing and is also used by injection to treat heart failure. When the tablets are dissolved in the mouth under the tongue (sublingual) or the spray is used, glyceryl trinitrate starts to work almost at once and acts for about half an hour. One preparation (Suscard) can be dissolved in the mouth for immediate as well as longer-term relief. Modified-release tablets of **isosorbide mono-** or **dinitrate** are used for a longer action.

Before you use this medicine

Tell your doctor if you are:
□ pregnant or breast-feeding □ taking any other medicines, including vitamins and those bought over the counter.

Tell your doctor if you have or have had:
□ severe anaemia or malnutrition □ head injuries or internal bleeding □ severe liver or kidney impairment □ poor thyroid function □ hypothermia □ recent heart attack.

Do not use: □ closed-angle glaucoma □ hypersensitivity to nitrates □ low blood pressure.

How to use this medicine

To relieve an angina attack Always keep tablets or spray handy, for example before you start any activity. Dissolve a tablet slowly under the tongue. Do not chew, crush or swallow the tablet. You should feel the effects of glyceryl trinitrate in about five minutes. You can spit out the remains of the tablet as soon as the pain is relieved. If the pain does not go away in five minutes, take a second tablet. Alternatively, use the spray, applying one or two doses under the tongue and closing the mouth after each dose. Do not take more than three doses of the spray at one time or inhale it. **If you still have pain after 10 to 15 minutes, dial '999' for an ambulance.**

To prevent angina Take the tablets two or three times a day. Modified-release forms vary in their dosing, with isosorbide mono- or dinitrate taken once and twice daily respectively. Detailed instructions on how to apply skin preparations are supplied with the manufacturers' packs. Avoid putting the patch on the same part of the skin every time. The ointment must be carefully measured, put on the body without rubbing in, and dressed with a clean dressing.

You may feel dizzy or faint during the first few days of treatment. Try to sit down to take the dose of medicine. If you feel dizzy, lie down or put your head between your knees, breathe deeply and move your arms and legs about. Alcohol and other medicines for lowering blood pressure may make you feel more dizzy: avoid alcohol. Until you know how you react to glyceryl trinitrate do not drive or do other activities that require alertness. Do not stop taking this medicine suddenly; your doctor will give you a schedule to decrease the dose gradually without chest pains recurring.

Storage Glyceryl trinitrate tablets lose their strength once the bottle is opened to the air. The tablets must not be put into any other container and the bottle must always be kept tightly closed. Eight weeks after opening, replace any unused tablets with another supply. The spray preparation can be kept for up to three years and this might be better if you need glyceryl trinitrate only occasionally. However, the spray products are flammable and must not be used near a naked flame, or stored either in direct sunlight or near a radiator.

Over 65 You may be more susceptible to dizziness or fainting, especially if glyceryl trinitrate is given with a beta blocker. You may need a lower dose.

Interactions with other medicines

Anaesthetics enhance the blood pressure-lowering effects of glyceryl trinitrate. Tell your doctor or dentist that you take glyceryl trinitrate before you have surgery.
Blood pressure-lowering medicines enhance the effect of glyceryl trinitrate.
Drugs for erectile dysfunction e.g. **sildenafil** increase blood pressure-lowering effects and must not be used with glyceryl trinitrate.
Dry mouth Some medicines make your mouth dry (antidepressants, for example): glyceryl trinitrate may not dissolve so easily and may be less effective.

Unwanted effects

Likely Dizziness, lightheadedness, flushing of the face and neck, throbbing headache, palpitations.

Unwanted effects are quite common during the first few days of treatment, but usually fade with time. If any of the effects continue to trouble you, contact your doctor.

Similar preparations

On prescription/from a pharmacy

ISOSORBIDE DINITRATE
Brand names (short-acting tablets):
SORBICHEW; SORBITRATE
(modified-release tablets and capsules):
CEDOCARD RETARD; ISOKET RETARD (spray): ANGITAK (injection): ISOKET

ISOSORBIDE MONONITRATE
Brand names (short-acting tablets):
ELANTAN; ISMO; ISOTRATE; MONIT
(modified-release tablets and capsules):
CHEMYDUR 60XL; ELANTAN LA; IMDUR; ISIB 60XL; ISMO RETARD; ISODUR; ISOTARD; MCR-50; MODISAL XL; MONIT SR/XL; MONOMAX SR/XL; MONOSORB XL 60

With aspirin
IMAZIN XL
ISOSORBIDE MONONITRATE + ASPIRIN

DILTIAZEM

DILTIAZEM – Tablets
TILDIEM – Tablets

Modified-release preparations:
ADIZEM-SR/XL – Capsules, tablets
ANGITIL SR/XL – Capsules
CALCICARD CR – Tablets
DILCARDIA SR – Capsules
DILZEM SR/XL – Capsules
SLOZEM – Capsules
TILDIEM LA/RETARD – Capsules, tablets
VIAZEM XL – Capsules
ZEMTARD – Capsules
ZILDIL SR – Capsules

Diltiazem is a calcium channel blocker which has a direct effect on the electrical and mechanical properties of heart muscle, relaxes arterial smooth muscle of the heart and to some extent the peripheral blood vessels (vasodilator). It is used for the prevention and treatment of chest pain (angina). Diltiazem may be given with a beta blocker, with careful supervision to ensure that the heart does not slow too much on this combination. Response can vary and dosage requirements differ significantly. The modified-release preparations, which are longer-acting formulations taken once or twice daily, are also used to control high blood pressure when other medicines have not lowered blood pressure sufficiently or are not tolerated.

Diltiazem's effects last up to about eight hours in the standard three-times-daily formulation. The longer-acting preparations are popular because they can be taken once or twice daily depending on the medicine. To avoid confusion between the products your doctor should prescribe the modified-release preparations by their brand names.

Before you use this medicine

Tell your doctor if you are:
☐ pregnant – avoid, may inhibit labour ☐ breast feeding – avoid, significant amounts pass into the milk ☐ taking any other medicines, including vitamins and those bought over the counter.

Tell your doctor if you have or have had:
☐ heart failure ☐ slow heart beat (severe bradycardia) ☐ heart arrhythmias.

Do not use: ☐ poor liver or kidney function.

How to use this medicine

☐ **to prevent or treat angina** standard tablets are taken three times daily with water.

☐ the longer-acting formulations are used for angina or to lower **high blood pressure**. Take the tablet or capsule with water, swallowing it whole before or during a meal. Chewing the tablet or capsule destroys the modified-release mechanism.

☐ if you have poor liver or kidney function, you may need a lower dose.

You may feel dizzy or faint when you get up from sitting or lying down, especially during the first few days of treatment. Get up slowly and stay beside the chair or bed until you are sure you are not dizzy. Avoid alcohol, which may lower blood pressure further. Until you know how you react to diltiazem, do not drive or do other activities that require alertness.

If you miss a dose, take it as soon as you remember. Skip the dose if it is almost time for your next dose and take that as usual. Do not take a double dose. Do not stop taking this medicine suddenly; your doctor should give you a schedule to decrease the dose gradually.

Over 65 You may need to take the standard tablets twice daily initially; your heart rate should be monitored, and the dose not increased if the heart rate falls below 50 beats/minute. Some of the modified-release preparations will be used only after you have been stabilised on other dosage forms. You may also need a lower dose of the longer-acting diltiazem, especially if liver or kidney function is impaired. You are more likely to experience the vasodilator unwanted effects which include swollen ankles, flushing and headache.

Interactions with other medicines

Beta blockers – increased risk of slow heart beat and heart beat irregularities.
Amiodarone – increased risk of slow heart beat and heart beat irregularities.
Antiepileptics – increased risk of unwanted effects with **carbamazepine**; **phenytoin** and **phenobarbital** reduce the effectiveness of diltiazem.
Ciclosporin – diltiazem increases risk of ciclosporin unwanted effects.
Digoxin blood levels of this heart drug may increase to toxic levels.
Nitrates and blood pressure-lowering medicines, especially alpha blockers, increase the risk of lower blood pressure.
Rifampicin for tuberculosis reduces the effectiveness of diltiazem.
Theophylline – diltiazem increases risk of theophylline unwanted effects.

Unwanted effects

Likely swollen ankles, flushing, headache, loss of appetite, feeling sick, constipation, diarrhoea, malaise, dizziness, palpitations, heart beat irregularities, aggravation of heart failure.
Less likely rashes, photosensitivity, inflamed liver, swollen breasts, overgrowth of the gums, movement disorders.

Unwanted effects are generally mild and transient. If diltiazem makes you feel dizzy and this feeling does not fade after the first few days of treatment, you should contact your doctor.

Heart attack

Heart attack occurs when the blood supply to the heart is cut off because the coronary artery becomes blocked. In arteries that have already narrowed, a sudden blood clot can stop the blood flow (*coronary thrombosis*). Part of the heart muscle that has been starved of blood and oxygen then becomes permanently damaged (*myocardial infarction*). If you have stable angina, narrowing of the arteries restricts blood supply, but does not stop it completely and this leaves the heart undamaged.

Although angina may warn of a heart attack, it is possible to have chest pains for years without suffering an attack. Many people show no direct signs of an impending heart attack; some have a heart attack without realising (for example, the elderly and diabetics) – only tests show that the heart has been damaged. It is important to recognise the signs of a heart attack, to know what is happening to you or to someone who is with you:

there may be crushing pain in the middle of the chest which extends to the jaw and down the left arm; you may look pale, feel faint and unwell and you may be breathless and perspire. You should get help immediately. Dial 999 for an ambulance and tell them you think it may be a heart attack. Chewing an aspirin (one 300mg tablet) or dispersing it in water before swallowing is helpful but the ambulance and hospital teams need to know if you or a carer have done this.

After an attack there is a high risk of complications and treatment will be needed urgently. Once the heart is damaged, its cells often generate erratic electrical impulses, disrupting the heart's beat and rhythm. These *arrhythmias*, particularly *ventricular fibrillation*, prevent the heart from working properly. At this stage the heart may stop suddenly (*cardiac arrest*), causing death (see 'Could you save a life?', below). A defibrillator, a machine that delivers an electric shock to the heart, can halt ventricular fibrillation and restore normal rhythm.

COULD YOU SAVE A LIFE?

Many people die in the first minutes after a heart attack. Once the heart is damaged, the regular rhythm and pace may be disrupted and the heart may suddenly stop beating. Without adequate blood flow, the organs, particularly the brain, are damaged by lack of oxygen. In about 25 to 30 per cent of heart attacks, the person dies before reaching hospital. The prompt action of a bystander could save the person's life. Emergency life support skills can be taught in just two hours and are applicable to a wide range of emergencies. The most important life-supporting measure is cardiopulmonary resuscitation, which is easily learned and performed by lay people with no special medical knowledge. Heartstart UK, a national initiative co-ordinated by the British Heart Foundation★, promotes and develops emergency life support skills training throughout the UK. Courses in resuscitation techniques are also run by The British Red Cross Society★, St John's Ambulance★, The Royal Life Saving Society★ and St Andrew's Ambulance Association★ in Scotland. The Resuscitation Council UK★ produces a variety of publications on resuscitation and life support.

When medical help arrives, you will usually have an *analgesic*, a pain-relieving injection of **diamorphine**, which continues in hospital. You may feel sick and vomit, which may be treated with an anti-sickness medicine (*anti-emetic*) such as **metoclopramide**. You should have a dose of dispensible or chewable aspirin for its anti-clotting effect) either at home or in hospital. *Fibrinolytic* drugs, also called *thrombolytics*, break up blood clots (*thrombi*) in the coronary artery and minimise long-term damage to the heart muscle. They are used as early as possible after a heart attack, preferably within an hour of the start of the heart attack. Urgent surgery to re-open the blocked coronary artery (primary angioplasty) is sometimes an option.

In hospital you should start a beta blocker to help stabilise the heart which should be continued indefinitely (or for at least one year) by your general practitioner, unless you cannot tolerate one. An ACE inhibitor reduces the work the heart has to do after a heart attack, especially if you have signs of heart failure. ACE inhibitor treatment should be reviewed four to six weeks after your attack and continued indefinitely, particularly if the left side of the heart is failing to work normally (*left ventricular dysfunction*). Other medicines such as nitrates and calcium channel blockers may be needed as second-line treatments in hospital. Aspirin is essential for preventing the blood from clotting in arteries and should be taken indefinitely, usually at a dose of 75mg/day. A lipid-lowering medicine such as a statin may also be prescribed if your cholesterol is raised (pages 130–33). If you are diabetic you are likely to need intensive insulin treatment whilst in hospital and thereafter control of blood glucose levels needs to be meticulous, as does that of blood pressure.

A heart attack is serious, but on recovery you should be able to lead an active life. Initially you should have a rehabilitation plan and support to help you recover physically, socially and adapt mentally to life after a heart attack. You may need to change your lifestyle – eating a balanced diet, taking regular exercise and giving up smoking.

Reducing the risk of heart attack

The UK has one of the highest rates of coronary heart disease in the world. It is the most common cause of premature death, accounting for 26 per cent of deaths in men and 16 per cent of deaths in women. The difference in the rates can be explained in part by the presence of the female hormone oestrogen, which gives women some natural protection against heart disease. However, this protection disappears after the menopause, leaving women as vulnerable to a heart attack as men.

Risk factors for coronary heart disease include smoking, high blood pressure, high blood cholesterol levels, diabetes, being overweight and inactive and family history, and the risk of developing it is further increased if you have more than one of these risk factors. The best way to prevent heart disease and also stroke and circulation problems from developing is to reduce the number of risk factors you have by making healthy lifestyle choices. If you have a family history of heart disease, or any of the other risk factors, it is a good idea to talk about this with your GP, who may then want to do some simple tests, such as blood pressure and blood cholesterol measurements, and will assess the likelihood of your having a heart attack or stroke in the future.

Assessing your risk of heart disease

The risk of developing heart and circulation disease is influenced by the combination of factors that you have. Your doctor will be able to assess your absolute risk, or the **probability** that you as an individual will experience an event during a specified period. Risk assessment tools, charts and computer programmes have been developed and the these are identified in the National Service Framework. Risk assessment calculations are based on the North American study, the Framingham Heart Study, which has been running for over 50 years in Massachusetts where characteristics of the mainly Caucasian population, such as blood pressure, diabetic and smoking status, are documented. The risk assessment tools may be less useful for other racial groups, such as African-Caribbean or South Asian people, as the tools may wrongly or incorrectly estimate the risks. Other studies have confirmed the benefits of modifying factors to reduce heart and circulation disease risk. Some risk assessment tools measure the risk of coronary heart disease occurring, not the total cardiovascular risk, which includes the risk of peripheral vascular disease and stroke. As part of your assessment your doctor will need to measure your blood pressure and cholesterol. These measures, together with your age, gender, whether you smoke or have ever smoked, and whether you are diabetic, form the risk assessment. Risk assessment charts can be used only if you have no obvious symptoms yet of coronary heart disease (or of diabetes or kidney disease), or you are already being treated for high blood pressure or high cholesterol, as they predict the likelihood of an event or condition occurring in the future. If your calculated risk is greater than 30 per cent over 10 years, then your doctor is likely to suggest lifestyle changes and/or appropriate drug treatment to modify your risks. This is known as *primary prevention*. If you have established cardiovascular disease, such as angina or have had a heart attack, you should be known to your doctor already and be receiving appropriate advice and treatment to prevent further events. This is known as *secondary prevention*.

● *Stop smoking*

Stopping smoking is very important. Each cigarette contains over 3,000 chemicals of which nicotine and carbon monoxide are the most significant causes of cardiovascular disease. Nicotine increases the heart rate, raises the blood pressure and slowly tightens the blood vessels, so reducing blood flow around the body, especially to the hands and feet. Carbon monoxide gas binds tightly to haemoglobin (a constituent of blood) to form carboxyhaemoglobin. This decreases the amount of oxygen circulating in the blood so that all parts of the body, including the heart, receive less oxygen. Carboxyhaemoglobin and nicotine significantly increase the risk of angina and heart attacks. Circulatory problems lead to peripheral vascular disease which may result in gangrene and ultimately limb amputation.

The best thing you can do for your heart is to stop smoking. Although lung cancer is a well-known adverse effect of smoking, you are just as likely to suffer cardiovascular disease. Smokers are twice as likely to have a heart attack as non-smokers and if you are aged under 50, you are ten times more likely to die from a heart attack than a non-smoker of the same age. If you have high blood pressure or raised blood-cholesterol levels, smoking adds to the risk of a heart attack. It is never too late to give up smoking: the heart and blood vessels start to recover immediately and the risk of heart disease diminishes. Help with stopping smoking is available – ask at the doctor's surgery or a pharmacy. **Nicotine replacement therapy** or **bupropion** (▼Zyban) can be used to help you stop if you smoke more than ten cigarettes a day.

Reduce high blood pressure

The risks of high blood pressure have already been discussed; see 'How you can help yourself', page 95.

Reduce blood cholesterol

Inappropriate diet and in particular high blood levels of cholesterol (a type of fat, also known as a lipid) are important risk factors for heart disease. Lowering high levels of cholesterol reduces the risk of developing coronary heart disease and can slow its progress. Cholesterol plays an essential part in the body's control of fat, its use and storage. Eating too much fat, especially saturated fat, stimulates the liver to produce more cholesterol than the body needs. This additional cholesterol is carried around in the blood and eventually deposited in the arteries as *atheroma*. Although these deposits break off from time to time without causing harm, as the process (*atherosclerosis*) continues over a long period, the arteries narrow and the blood flow can become restricted (*ischaemia*) and slower. When blood flows less freely and has to be squeezed through narrow vessels it is more likely to form abnormal clots. It is these abberrant clots that can trigger a heart attack or stroke if the blood vessel becomes blocked completely.

Cholesterol is produced in the liver and is also absorbed from the intestine; it is transported in the blood by two main kinds of carriers. *Low-density lipoproteins* (LDL) take cholesterol from the liver to the arteries and deposit it along the walls of the blood vessels. *High-density lipoproteins* (HDL) carry cholesterol from the arteries to the liver where it is broken down. High levels of HDL are therefore associated with a lower risk of heart disease, whereas high levels of LDL increase the risk. Some people have inherited disorders of lipid metabolism which cause them to have too much of these body fats and to need lipid-lowering treatment.

Cutting down on fatty foods and replacing saturated fats with unsaturated fats can help to reduce blood levels of cholesterol. Do not cut fat out of your diet altogether: a small amount is necessary for a healthy diet. Saturated fat is found in butter, hard margarine, milk, hard full-fat cheeses, lard, cream, palm oil, sausages, pies and red meat. Unsaturated fat is found in polyunsaturated margarines, in corn, sunflower and safflower oils, and in oily fish, such as tuna, herring and mackerel. Eating oily fish such as mackerel or herring, which contain particular unsaturated fatty acids (*omega-3 marine triglycerides*), may help to prevent heart disease. A fish-oil product (Maxepa), which is rich in omega-3 marine triglycerides or an omega-3 fatty acid taken daily is useful for lowering raised triglyceride levels. Replacing saturated fats with monosaturated fats, such as olive oil, and increasing your intake of soy protein, plant sterols (phytosterols) found naturally in grains, nuts (such as almonds) seeds, vegetables and vegetable spreads (Benecol; Flora Pro-activ) can also reduce LDL-cholesterol levels. Eating a diet rich in foods known to lower cholesterol may reduce your risk of heart disease by up to one quarter.

LIPID-LOWERING MEDICINES

People who have high blood-fat levels in spite of dieting, stopping smoking and reducing high blood pressure may need treatment with a fat- (lipid-) lowering medicine. They may have a condition that puts them at risk, such as diabetes or an inherited disorder of fat metabolism. A family history of coronary heart disease, especially if someone had a heart attack before the age of 50, puts young men at risk. Illness can disturb the body's handling of fat: your blood-fat levels may be altered for up to three months after a heart attack and during acute pancreatitis. Diabetics and people on long-term kidney dialysis may also have high blood-fats. If you have coronary heart disease (e.g. angina) or are at high risk of developing it, treatment with a lipid-lowering medicine combined with appropriate diet is likely to be necessary.

Treatment begins after blood tests to determine your blood-fat levels and which type of fat is raised. A lipid-lowering medicine will not affect existing cholesterol deposits, but may stop new ones forming. You may have to take the medicine for a long time: blood-fats usually return to a high level once you stop treatment.

Older medicines **colestyramine** (**cholestyramine**) (Questran) and **colestipol** (Colestid) are powdered resins taken in liquid that bind with cholesterol-containing bile acids which help with the digestion of fat in the intestine. As the drug plus cholesterol and bile acids are removed from the body, the liver converts more cholesterol into bile acids to replace the lost amount. These drugs increase the amount of LDL-cholesterol broken down in the liver resulting in lower blood-cholesterol levels. They are not absorbed into the body and can interfere with the absorption of vitamins (A, D and K) and other medicines in the gut. Fibric acid drugs (**bezafibrate**, **ciprofibrate**, **fenofibrate** and **gemfibrozil**) and the less-used nicotinic acid (Vitamin B) group (**nicotinic acid** (Niaspan) and **acipimox** – Olbetam) interfere with the conversion of fatty acids to different types of lipids in the liver. In the high doses used nicotinic acid is limited by its unwanted effects – widening of the blood vessels, resulting in flushing. The statins (**atorvastatin**, **fluvastatin**, **pravastatin**, **rosuvastatin** and **simvastatin**), block an enzyme in the cholesterol production process, mostly in the liver. The statins lower LDL-cholesterol effectively and are now preferred. Two different types of lipid-lowering medicine, for example the combination of a statin and a fibrate, may be needed in resistant cases, but this may increase the risk of unwanted effects such as muscle pain or weakness. However, a new medicine, **ezetimibe** (▼Ezetrol), is designed to be taken with a statin, to reduce cholesterol levels in the body, although it can also be used on its own. Ezetimibe prevents the absorption of cholesterol from the intestine into the body whilst a statin inhibits cholesterol formation in the liver. This two-pronged approach allows a dose reduction of the statin. Alternatively if you have reached the maximum dose of a statin, but further reductions in cholesterol are needed, then ezetimibe can be added to treatment. Unwanted effects of ezetimibe taken alone include headache, abdominal pain and diarrhoea; with a statin additional unwanted effects include fatigue, constipation, feeling sick, flatulence and muscle pain.

BEZAFIBRATE

BEZAFIBRATE – Tablets
BEZALIP – Tablets
BEZALIP-MONO – Modified-release tablets
ZIMBACOL XL – Modified-release tablets

Bezafibrate affects the blood-cholesterol levels by reducing LDL-cholesterol levels and increasing HDL-cholesterol. Its main action is to decrease blood levels of another type of fat, triglyceride. Bezafibrate should be used only if dietary measures have failed, for example in people who have inherited disorders of fat metabolism, and where high levels of blood fats are a risk, for example with coronary heart disease. Fibrates can cause muscle inflammation, with weakness and pain, especially if kidney function is impaired. Combined treatment of fibrate and statin increases the risk of serious muscle toxicity, although the actual occurrence is rare.

Before you use this medicine

Tell your doctor if you are:
☐ pregnant or breastfeeding – bezafibrate is not recommended ☐ diabetic –- bezafibrate may improve glucose control ☐ taking any other medicines, including vitamins and those bought over the counter.

Tell your doctor if you have or have had:
☐ gallstones ☐ gallbladder disease ☐ kidney or liver disease – bezafibrate is not recommended in severe cases ☐ hypersensitivity to a fibrate.

How to use this medicine

Take the tablets three times daily with or after meals. Modified-release tablets must be swallowed whole, not chewed, and can be taken once a day with an evening meal. You will need to continue on a low-fat diet.

If you have mild to moderate impairment of kidney function, you are at increased risk of muscle problems and need a lower dose of bezafibrate. You may need periodic blood tests to assess blood cholesterol levels, kidney and liver function. If you miss a dose take it as soon as you remember, otherwise skip this dose and take the next one as usual.

Over 65 No special requirements.

Interactions with other medicines

Anticoagulants (e.g. **warfarin**) Their effect is enhanced by bezafibrate and the dose of the anticoagulant will need to be reduced.
Statins Increased risk of severe muscle damage (*rhabdomyolysis*), especially with impaired kidney function and also with low levels of thyroid.
Ciclosporin, the immunosuppressant Increased risk of kidney function impairment.

Unwanted effects

Likely Feeling sick, loss of appetite, abdominal pains, bloating or discomfort, headache, dizziness.
Less likely Aching or muscle cramps and toxicity risk (especially if kidney function impaired), impotence, hair loss, skin rashes, photosensitivity, hypersensitivity.

Unwanted effects usually fade with time; increasing the dose gradually over one week may help to reduce these effects. Muscle pains should be discussed with your doctor. The use of the fibrate, **gemfibrozil** (Lopid) and a statin should be avoided.

Similar preparations

FENOFIBRATE – Capsules
GEMFIBROZIL – Capsules
LIPANTIL – Capsules
FENOFIBRATE
LOPID – Capsules
GEMFIBROZIL
MODALIM – Capsules
CIPROFIBRATE
SUPRALIP 160 – Modified-release tablets
FENOFIBRATE

SIMVASTATIN

SIMVASTATIN – Tablets
ZOCOR – Tablets

Simvastatin lowers blood levels of cholesterol and LDL-cholesterol by suppressing a liver enzyme (HMG CoA reductase) needed for their production. Simvastatin lowers high blood levels of cholesterol that have not responded to diet or other treatments. The higher the cholesterol levels, the greater your risk of developing or worsening heart and circulatory disease and stroke (cardiovascular disease), when considered in context with all the other risk factors (page 127). Simvastatin reduces cardiovascular disease and also premature death when used preventatively for people at high risk (primary prevention) and for people with established heart disease (secondary prevention). Diabetics are particularly at risk of cardiovascular disease and benefit from statin treatment. Blood levels of total cholesterol (below 5 millimoles/litre) or LDL-cholesterol (below 3 millimoles/litre), or percentage reductions if that produces lower levels, are target values that your doctor will aim for if you need statin treatment. Simvastatin is also used if you have inherited disorders of the fat metabolism. Unwanted effects of simvastatin include headache and stomach upsets. Statins can sometimes cause muscle inflammation with weakness and pain, and you should tell your doctor about this.

Before you use this medicine

Tell your doctor if you are:
□ pregnant or planning to become pregnant – do not take simvastatin; women of child-bearing age must use reliable contraception other than an oral contraceptive □ breast-feeding □ taking any other medicines, including vitamins and those bought over the counter.

Tell your doctor if you have or have had:
□ liver or kidney disease □ porphyria □ hypersensitivity to a statin.

How to use this medicine

For high cholesterol levels, simvastatin treatment is started at a low dose (10mg), which is increased gradually depending on blood-fat levels to a maximum of 80mg. If you have heart disease the starting dose is 20mg. The tablets are taken once a day in the evening to achieve maximum effect on cholesterol levels, as this is when the body produces most of its cholesterol. No more than 10mg a day will be needed if you take a lipid-lowering fibrate or nicotinic acid or the immunosuppressant, ciclosporin. You will need to continue on a low-fat diet and maintain a low alcohol intake. You should have periodic blood tests to assess blood-fat levels and liver function (all statins should be avoided in active liver disease).

If you miss a dose, take it as soon as you remember unless it is nearly time for your next dose, otherwise skip this dose and take the next one as usual. Do not take double the dose. A statin is very effective, life-saving treatment and once started you need to take it continuously long-term to realise its benefits in preventing death and disability.

Over 65 No special dose requirements – but increased risk of unwanted effects, e.g. muscle problems, particularly if poor kidney function or low thyroid levels.

Interactions with other medicines

When taken with simvastatin, the following may increase the risk of muscle problems, sometimes seriously, and dosages should be adjusted or use with simvastatin avoided:
Antiarrhythmic amiodarone
Antibacterials Erythromycin, **clarithromycin**.
Antifungals by mouth **Itraconazole**, **ketoconazole**, **miconazole**.
Calcium channel blockers Verapamil; **diltiazem** with simvastatin 80mg
Immunosuppressant ciclosporin Increased risk of muscle pains or weakness.
Lipid-lowering drugs Fibrates (e.g. **bezafibrate**) and **nicotinic acid**.
Avoid use of **gemfibrozil** together with a statin.
Anticoagulants warfarin and **acenocoumarol** (**nicoumalone**) Simvastatin may enhance their effect and their dosage may need altering.
Antivirals: Protease inhibitors for HIV.
Grapefruit juice in large quantities increases simvastatin in the body, but one glass (250ml) a day is unlikely to cause problems.

Unwanted effects

Likely Digestive disorders such as flatulence, indigestion, stomach pain, constipation, diarrhoea and feeling or being sick, weakness, headache.
Less likely Dizziness, liver disease, hair loss, skin rashes, hypersensitivity and allergic reactions, muscle pains, weakness and rarely severe muscle toxicity (estimated to occur in around one case in every 100,000 treatment years).

Contact your doctor if you have any muscle pains or weakness.

Similar preparations

▼CRESTOR – Tablets
ROSUVASTATIN

LIPITOR – Tablets
ATORVASTATIN

LIPOSTAT – Tablets
PRAVASTATIN

LESCOL – Capsules
FLUVASTATIN

Heart failure

Chronic heart failure is a gradual process which develops when the heart cannot pump blood efficiently. The left side of the heart pumps blood from the lungs to the rest of the body; if it cannot do this effectively, the lungs become congested, causing breathlessness, particularly during physical exertion, although this can also occur at rest, for example at night. In addition, the rest of the body does not receive all the oxygen it needs, which leads to severe tiredness and the accumulation of excess fluid (*oedema*), mainly in the ankles, feet and legs. Weight gain occurs because excess fluid remains in the lungs and tissues (congestion) – so-called congestive heart failure. High blood pressure, narrowing of the coronary arteries, heart attack or damage to the heart valves may cause the heart to fail. Acute heart failure is sudden and severe and must be treated urgently.

Heart failure is common, causes major disability and shortens life; two thirds of people die within six years of developing heart failure if it is not treated. National standards have therefore been introduced outlining the approach to diagnosis, drug treatment, monitoring and review, and support for patients and carers. Heart failure is a complex collection of symptoms that can sometimes be similar to those of other problems. For example, chest disease, obesity, severe anaemia or thyroid disease are conditions that can masquerade as heart failure. Fluid retention caused by medicines such as certain calcium channel blockers (e.g. nifedipine), or NSAIDs such as diclofenac, can also be mistaken for symptoms of heart failure; these should be avoided if you have existing heart failure. Your doctor will want to assess your symptoms, examine you and then arrange for an ECG and, if available, a blood test for the hormone brain natriuretic peptide (BNP), which increases in heart failure. If the ECG and blood test are normal then heart failure is excluded, but if one or both tests are abnormal then echocardiography, which looks at the functioning of the heart, can confirm or rule out heart failure.

Heart failure is graded from mild (grade 1), with no symptoms but evidence of heart disease, to severe (grade 4) depending on how much physical activity is possible without tiredness or shortness of breath. Although heart failure is progressive, better treatments with medicines can improve life expectancy and quality of life. You can also help yourself (page 95), for example with regular aerobic exercise (within your capabilities), stopping smoking, reviewing alcohol intake and weight reduction. You should also protect yourself against influenza (with an annual injection) and against pneumococcal disease (a one-off injection).

Medicines for heart failure

ACE inhibitors (page 110) are essential for managing heart failure, providing you can tolerate one. They improve symptoms, delay progression of the condition and hospital admission, and increase life-span. If the left side of your heart is damaged (e.g. left ventricular systolic dysfunction), following a heart attack for example, but symptoms of heart failure are not yet apparent, an ACE inhibitor slows their development. All ACE inhibitors appear to help heart failure, but need to be given in as high a dose as you can tolerate (sometimes above the usual maximum recommended dosage). ACE-II receptor antagonists, e.g. **losartan**, have been tried in heart failure in place of an ACE inhibitor or in addition to one, although they are not licensed for this. Their use in heart failure is still being researched, but they may offer an alternative if you cannot tolerate an ACE inhibitor.

If you have mild to moderate symptoms of heart failure, then a diuretic such as **furosemide** or **bumetanide** will be added to remove excess fluid. Adding a beta blocker (pages 105–9), in particular **bisoprolol** or **carvedilol**, improves the nervous control of the heart and extends life-span. A beta blocker is usually started in hospital and as with other drugs used in heart failure, dosages are started low and increased slowly according to symptom control. In moderate to severe heart failure when symptoms require further control, the potassium-sparing diuretic **spironolactone** may be added at low dose (12.5–50mg daily). Although potassium-sparing diuretics are not routinely recommended with an ACE inhibitor, this particular one is helpful in heart failure because it reduces the activity of a body chemical, aldosterone, that helps to regulate the body's fluid content. Blood potassium and kidney function need careful monitoring. Other medicines that may be added include **digoxin** (pages 137–9), particularly if you have heart failure and atrial fibrillation (a heart rhythm disorder). The combination of a nitrate (pages 121–3) by mouth and **hydralazine** (vasodilator) is an alternative treatment if you cannot take an ACE inhibitor because of severe kidney impairment. Calcium channel blockers are not recommended for heart failure, except **amlodipine**, which may help if you have co-existing high blood pressure and/or angina.

Hospital specialist interventions may be considered, including (rarely) a transplant, but otherwise the main approaches for managing heart failure are with medicines, rehabilitation and lifestyle changes. Other co-existing conditions also need to be treated: for example, high blood pressure or angina. With heart failure your condition fluctuates and repeated admission to hospital may be needed; good co-ordinated support and palliative care become important.

• *DIURETICS* •

A diuretic helps remove excess fluid from the body. This will reduce the pressure in the heart, ease congestion in the lungs and remove accumulated fluid from the ankles and feet. A loop diuretic, such as **furosemide** (frusemide) (Lasix), is generally used in both acute and chronic heart failure. A similar diuretic **bumetanide** (Burinex) is an alternative; sometimes furosemide is not as well absorbed into the body in heart failure. In severe chronic heart failure and when kidney function is impaired, your doctor may give you a thiazide (pages 100–102) or similar diuretic, **metolazone** (Metenix 5). This increases the diuretic effect, and also the potential for unwanted effects, and needs careful monitoring.

FUROSEMIDE

FUROSEMIDE – Tablets, liquid, injection
LASIX – Tablets, liquid, injection

Combined with potassium-sparing diuretic

CO-AMILOFRUSE – Tablets
FUROSEMIDE + AMILORIDE

FRUMIL – Tablets
FUROSEMIDE + AMILORIDE

FRUSENE – Tablets
FUROSEMIDE + TRIAMTERENE

LASILACTONE – Capsules
FUROSEMIDE + SPIRONOLACTONE

Poor choice – furosemide with potassium
LASIKAL – Tablets

Furosemide (frusemide) is a loop diuretic, so called because it acts on the looped part of the kidney tubule. It stops sodium, potassium and water being taken back into the body, so they are lost as urine. Furosemide is a powerful diuretic used to remove extra fluid from the heart, lungs, liver, kidneys and the periphery of the body (the ankles, for example). The tablet acts within an hour and continues working for up to six hours; the injection is used for emergencies when prompt and effective diuresis is needed. The body's salt and water balance may be upset, particularly with long-term treatment.

You should take extra potassium (page 106). **Co-amilofruse**, a potassium-sparing diuretic (amiloride) combined with furosemide in one tablet, avoids the need to take potassium separately and is now preferred.

Before you use this medicine

Tell your doctor if you are:
☐ pregnant or breast-feeding ☐ on a low-salt or low-sugar diet ☐ taking any other medicines, including vitamins and those bought over the counter.

Tell your doctor if you have or have had:
☐ diabetes ☐ gout ☐ kidney or liver disease (especially liver disease caused by alcohol) ☐ prostate trouble ☐ hearing loss ☐ porphyria ☐ hypersensitivity to furosemide or an antibacterial sulphonamide.

How to use this medicine

Take the tablet usually once a day in the morning. If you have to take another dose, try to take it by mid-afternoon, so that night-time sleep is not disturbed by extra visits to the toilet; during the first few days of treatment, you will produce a larger volume of urine and may need to go to the toilet more often than usual.

You will lose potassium while taking furosemide so eat plenty of potassium-rich foods (page 102). Your doctor may prescribe a potassium supplement or potassium-sparing diuretic that helps conserve the body's potassium. Because a diuretic helps you to lose water, you may lose too much and become dehydrated – you will feel thirsty and your skin may look and feel dry. Make sure that your daily fluid intake is adequate. Dehydration is likely to make you more susceptible to alcohol: drink only small quantities.

You may feel dizzy when you get up from sitting or lying down, especially during the first few days of treatment. Get up slowly and stay beside the chair or bed until you are sure you are not dizzy. Do not drive or do other activities that require alertness until you know how you react to furosemide.

Over 65 You may need a lower dose. Older people are more susceptible to the unwanted effects, such as dizziness and mental confusion.

Interactions with other medicines

Used without additional potassium or a potassium-sparing diuretic, furosemide causes low blood levels of potassium (*hypokalaemia*) and this increases the risk of unwanted effects of some medicines:
Digoxin, **antiarrhythmic drugs**, **antihistamines** (**terfenadine**), **antipsychotics**.
Other significant interactions include:
ACE inhibitors and **other blood pressure-lowering medicines** Their blood pressure-lowering effect is enhanced by furosemide.
Antibiotics, cephalosporins – increased risk of kidney toxicity, and **gentamicin** and **amikacin**, with furosemide or bumetanide, increase the risk of hearing loss.
Lithium stays in the body longer and may reach toxic levels.
NSAIDs The risk of kidney impairment increases.

Unwanted effects

Likely Dizziness, upset in body's salts – loss of sodium, potassium and calcium.
Less likely Feeling sick, digestive disorders, mental confusion, headache, muscle cramps, unusual tiredness or weakness, gout, high blood sugar.
Rarely rashes, photosensitivity, tinnitus and deafness (with injection).

If any of the unwanted effects are troublesome, discuss them with your doctor. If skin rash occurs, stop taking furosemide.

Similar preparations

BUMETANIDE – Tablets, liquid, injection
BURINEX – Tablets
BUMETANIDE

Combined loop and potassium-sparing diuretic
BURINEX A – Tablets
BUMETANIDE + AMILORIDE

Poor choice – bumetanide with potassium
BURINEX K – Tablets

TOREM – Tablets
TORASEMIDE

DIGOXIN

Digoxin, a cardiac glycoside, is an age-old remedy from a species of the foxglove family which was widely used to treat heart failure. It remains useful for this condition but is reserved for use if you have severe symptoms which need further treatment despite taking an ACE inhibitor, a diuretic and a beta blocker. Digoxin also controls heart rhythm disorders, particularly *atrial fibrillation* (and especially when this occurs with heart failure). It makes the heart beat more forcefully and simultaneously reduces the flow of electrical impulses which stimulate the heart to beat. It has a narrow therapeutic index where the margin between its helpful effects and harmful ones is small. When the levels of digoxin rise in the body, for example through a drug interaction or when kidney function is impaired and the dose has not been reduced, then potentially serious heart arrhythmias can occur. Unwanted effects limit digoxin's usefulness for treating heart failure, especially for older people.

DIGOXIN

DIGOXIN – Tablets, injection
LANOXIN – Tablets, injection

LANOXIN-PG – Liquid, tablets
(for children and elderly people)

Digoxin makes the heart muscle contract more forcefully and improves the pumping of blood through the heart. Digoxin slows the heart rate by affecting the nervous and electrical control of the heart. It can relieve heart failure and control certain types of irregular heart rhythm (particularly atrial fibrillation).

Digoxin must be used carefully because paradoxically it can also cause heart beat irregularities. It causes more unwanted effects if kidney function is impaired, and older people are especially susceptible to the toxic effects of digoxin.

Before you use this medicine

Tell your doctor if you are:
☐ pregnant or breast-feeding ☐ taking any other medicines, including vitamins and those bought over the counter.

Tell your doctor if you have or have had:
☐ Wolff-Parkinson-White syndrome (a particular type of heart rhythm irregularity) or other heart disorders e.g. heart block, some heart arrhythmias, heart muscle disorder (*myopathy*) ☐ a recent heart attack ☐ toxic effects from digoxin or other digitalis preparations ☐ thyroid problems ☐ poor kidney or liver function ☐ severe lung disease.

How to use this medicine

The dose and the timing of each dose may vary at the start of treatment depending on the heart's requirements. Take the tablets or liquid on an empty stomach. If digoxin makes you feel sick, then you can take it with food. Digoxin is usually taken once a day, but may be taken on alternate days. Eat plenty of potassium-rich foods (page 138); your doctor may prescribe a potassium-sparing diuretic or supplement, especially if you are taking a diuretic as well.

Do not drive or do other activities that require alertness until you know how you react to digoxin. Do not stop taking this medicine suddenly as symptoms may recur; your doctor will give you a schedule to decrease the dose gradually. If you miss a dose, take it as soon as you remember, but skip it if it is almost time for your next dose – do not take double the dose.

If you have kidney disease or poor kidney function, you will need less than the adult dose. You may need periodic blood tests to monitor digoxin and potassium blood levels.

Over 65 You are more likely to experience unwanted effects and adverse reactions with digoxin, so should have a reduced dose. Check with your doctor that you really need to take digoxin.

Interactions with other medicines

Digoxin interacts with many other medicines. Do not take other medicines without checking with your doctor or pharmacist, including those bought over the counter e.g. **St John's wort** which reduces digoxin's effectiveness. The following are the most important:
ACE inhibitors, **ACE-II receptor antagonists**, **antiarrhythmics**, **calcium channel blockers**, **ciclosporin, itraconazole, quinine** (and possibly **chloroquine**) increase the blood levels of digoxin and therefore the toxic effects. The dose of digoxin must be reduced.
Diuretics, corticosteroids Increased risk of low potassium which therefore increases the risk of digoxin toxicity.

Unwanted effects

Likely Loss of appetite, feeling or being sick, diarrhoea, irregular heartbeats.
Less likely Slow pulse, weakness, blurred vision or coloured 'haloes', confusion, headache, bad dreams, hallucinations, fatigue, depression.
Rarely Skin rash, swollen breasts (men), bruising, bleeding.

Unwanted effects may be due to an increase in the level of digoxin in the blood; contact your doctor to discuss them. Irregular heartbeats need emergency action.

Similar preparations

DIGITOXIN – Tablets

Irregular heart rhythms

The pumping action of the atria and ventricles is co-ordinated by electrical impulses generated by the nerves to the heart. Specialised heart cells act as pacemakers to control the flow of electrical impulses across the heart muscle cells. Irregular heart rhythms (*arrhythmias*) occur if the co-ordination of the heart's pumping action is upset or interrupted in any way. The heart may beat too slowly (*bradycardia*), too quickly (*tachycardia*) or irregularly. 'Missed beat', 'jumped beat' or palpitations which you feel are usually not serious; the occasional missed beat rarely needs treatment. Rhythm disturbances which you cannot feel, but which cause the heart to pump blood around the body less efficiently, usually do need medical treatment. They may cause sudden death, fainting, heart failure, dizziness, palpitations or no symptoms. Abnormal rhythms should be diagnosed accurately with an electrocardiograph (ECG) – a machine which measures the heart's electrical activity.

NORMAL HEART RHYTHM

An adult heart beats at the rate of 60–80 beats per minute at rest, whereas a child's heart rate may be 90 beats per minute. The rate of the heartbeat varies with activity so during hard exercise it may increase to 200 beats per minute or even more. Stress or anxiety also increase the rate, and while you are asleep or resting it decreases to around 60 beats per minute

Some babies are born with irregular heart rhythms, but for many people, abnormal rhythms develop when the heart is damaged or diseased. Other causes of irregular heart rhythms include caffeine in tea and coffee, alcohol, certain medicines (e.g. **amitriptyline**, **terfenadine**, **erythromycin**), smoking and thyroid disease. Arrhythmias can occur at any age and may not always need treatment.

Irregular heart rhythms are named after the part of heart they affect and the type of beat abnormality: *supraventricular* or *atrial arrhythmias* occur in the atria, *ventricular* in the ventricles; *tachycardia* is fast co-ordinated beating at more than 100 beats per minute; *fibrillation* or flutter is rapid unco-ordinated beating. *Bradycardia* is slow beating – below 60 beats per minute. Heart block (*atrioventricular block*) occurs when electrical impulses are not passed from the atria to the ventricles. The ventricles beat at a slower rate.

Technological devices have improved the management of heart beat irregularities, for example with pacemakers that can be fitted temporararily or permanently to improve irregular slow heart beats and conduction abnormalities. Implantable cardioverter-defibrillators (ICDs) detect ventricular abnormalities (tachycardia or fibrillation) and deliver a small electric shock to return the heart beat to normal rhythm (*cardioversion*). These devices are placed into the upper chest below the left shoulder from where they monitor the heart and control the rate of the beat. Radiofrequency catheter ablation, where selected abnormal electrical pathways in the heart are destroyed, is used for controlling tachycardia, such as the Wolff-Parkinson-White syndrome. Drug therapy is still useful, sometimes in combination with devices. Drugs help to control arrhythmias, although they may not completely abolish them.

Antiarrhythmic medicines

Antiarrhythmic medicines are grouped either according to their effects on the electrical activity of heart cells or, more usually, the arrhythmias they control. Antiarrhythmics may be given to treat a single episode of heart rhythm irregularities or, if these become established, to prevent them happening. Low levels of blood-potassium increase the antiarrhythmic effects of many of these medicines: a daily diet with some potassium-containing foods is advisable, but discuss this with your doctor. Most or all antiarrhythmics are also capable of provoking arrhythmias in certain circumstances and other unwanted effects, including interactions with other medicines, limit their usefulness. Antiarrhythmic treatment is usually started in hospital because the type of irregular heart rhythm must be diagnosed precisely before an appropriate medicine is prescribed.

Supraventricular arrhythmias

Atrial fibrillation occurs when the atria beat rapidly (300–600 per minute) and are not co-ordinated with the ventricles. Atrial fibrillation is common: up to 1 in 10 people over 65 years of age has the condition. It may be temporary, for example lasting less than a day (*paroxysmal*), persist for a while but be amenable to reversion, or become permanent. Atrial fibrillation can occur with for example heart disease, heart failure, high blood pressure, an over-active thyroid, alcohol excess, and acute infections such as pneumonia. When no underlying cause is found for atrial fibrillation, this is known as 'lone' atrial fibrillation. Some people do not know they have atrial fibrillation whilst for others it may be an emergency. Most people experience a deterioration in their capacity to exercise and feel unwell, but this may be appreciated only when normal rhythm is restored. You will have a very irregular pulse which continues during exercise.

The approach to treatment needs to be tailored to each person. It may include maintaining the normal (*sinus*) rhythm with antiarrhythmic medicines and cardioversion, a hospital procedure where a controlled electric shock is used to get the heart back into normal rhythm. You are likely to need anticoagulation treatment (page 150) before cardioversion if atrial fibrillation has lasted longer than two days. Drug cardioversion with the antiarrhythmics **flecainide** or **amiodarone** may also be an option. Relapse following cardioversion occurs and is commonest in the first month, but the procedure can be attempted again. Otherwise medicines are used to control the rate at which the ventricles beat and these include beta blockers, calcium channel blockers – **diltiazem** or

verapamil, and **digoxin**. Digoxin is used to control ventricular electrical activity, especially if atrial fibrillation is accompanied by heart failure.

Atrial fibrillation increases the likelihood of blocked blood vessels in the brain (*cerebral emboli*) and therefore stroke (page 144). Blood pools in the left atrium of the heart, allowing blood clots to form that can then travel in blood vessels to the brain. Anticoagulation with **warfarin** preferably (page 151) or **aspirin** (depending on risk factors such as age and other underlying conditions) will reduce this risk of stroke. As with other heart conditions you need to check with your doctor whether it is safe to drive.

Supraventricular tachycardia happens when extra electrical impulses arise in the heart's pacemaker region to stimulate the ventricles. The calcium channel blocker **verapamil** is sometimes used. A beta blocker slows the heart and dampens increased nervous activity to the heart.

Ventricular arrhythmias

Ventricular tachycardias range from minor to life-threatening problems. Various drugs, such as **lidocaine (lignocaine)** are given by injection in hospital to control abnormal rhythms. The underlying heart disorders that contribute to rhythm irregularities are treated, for example with **amiodarone**.

Supraventricular and ventricular arrhythmias

A variety of medicines is used when these two types of arrhythmia occur simultaneously – **amiodarone**, a beta blocker such as **sotalol, disopyramide,** and less commonly **flecainide, procainamide, propafenone** and **quinidine**.

VERAPAMIL

VERAPAMIL – Tablets, liquid
CORDILOX – Tablets, injection
SECURON – Tablets,injection

For high blood pressure and angina: modified-release preparations
HALF SECURON SR/SECURON SR – Tablets
UNIVER – Capsules
VERAPRESS MR – Tablets
VERTAB SR 240 – Tablets

Verapamil is a calcium-channel blocker which affects the flow of calcium across the cells of blood vessels and heart muscle. It can be used to lower high blood pressure and to treat and prevent angina or supraventricular arrhythmias. Verapamil causes constipation because of its calcium channel-blocking activity in the gut.

Before you use this medicine

Tell your doctor if you are:
□ pregnant or breast-feeding □ taking any other medicines, including vitamins and those bought over the counter.

Tell your doctor if you have or have had:
□ kidney or liver disease.

Do not take if you have or have had:
□ heart failure □ very slow heart rate (*bradycardia*) □ low blood pressure □ Wolff-Parkinson-White syndrome or heart block □ sick sinus syndrome □ porphyria.

How to use this medicine

Take the tablets two or three times daily; modified-release preparations may be taken once daily. You may be given the injection in hospital to control arrhythmias and then change to tablets. You may feel dizzy or faint when you get up from sitting or lying down, especially during the first few days of treatment. Get up slowly and stay beside the chair or bed until you are sure you are not dizzy.

Do not drive or do other activities that require alertness until you know how you react to verapamil. Alcohol and other blood pressure-lowering medicines increase verapamil's effect: avoid alcohol. Avoid grapefruit juice, which may increase blood levels of verapamil.

Do not stop taking this medicine suddenly as this may change the heart rhythm. Your doctor will give you a schedule to decrease the dose of verapamil gradually. If you miss a dose, take it as soon as you remember. If your next dose is due within three hours take the missed dose and skip the next one. Do not take double the dose.

If you have poor liver function, you will need a reduced dose.

Over 65 Take the same as the normal adult dose, unless your liver or kidney function is reduced.

Interactions with other medicines

General anaesthetics Verapamil enhances the blood pressure-lowering effects; tell your doctor or dentist that you take verapamil before you have surgery.
Antiarrhythmics amiodarone, **disopyramide**, **flecainide** Increased risk of irregular heart rhythms and depressed beat.
Beta blockers used with verapamil may cause irregular heartbeats, a severe drop in blood pressure and heart failure. Careful monitoring required.
Carbamazepine Effect enhanced through increased blood levels.
Ciclosporin Blood levels increase, with a risk of toxicity.
Digoxin Blood levels increase, with a risk of toxicity.
Quinidine may interact with verapamil to cause a severe drop in blood pressure.
Theophylline (used for asthma) Blood levels increase, with a risk of toxicity.

Unwanted effects

Likely Constipation.
Less likely Headache, feeling or being sick, dizziness, tiredness or weakness, ankle swelling, flushing of face or neck.
Rare but serious Allergic reactions and skin rashes, reversible impairment of liver function, muscle and joint pains, pins and needles. Long-term treatment can cause reversible breast-swelling in elderly men and overgrowth of the gums. Low blood pressure, heart failure and heartbeat problems can occur with high doses or injection.

Contact your doctor if you feel dizzy whilst taking verapamil. Discuss troublesome unwanted effects with your doctor.

AMIODARONE

AMIODARONE – Tablets, injection CORDARONE X – Tablets, injection

Amiodarone is used for the treatment of irregular heart rhythms, especially the Wolff-Parkinson-White syndrome, where extra electrical impulses travel from the atria to the ventricles and upset the rhythm. Amiodarone can be used to control supraventricular and ventricular tachycardias, atrial fibrillation (including after cardioversion, page 140) and recurrent ventricular fibrillation. It is generally used when other medicines cannot be used or have proved ineffective. When taken by mouth amiodarone's effects develop gradually, but it may stay in the body for up to three months after treatment is stopped. Intravenous amiodarone acts quite rapidly. Because amiodarone can cause a number of adverse effects, such as thyroid problems and eye, liver and lung damage, treatment is usually started by a specialist although the GP may continue to prescribe it under shared care management.

Before you use this medicine

Tell your doctor if you are:
☐ pregnant or breast-feeding – you should not use amiodarone ☐ taking any other medicines, including vitamins and those bought over the counter.

Tell your doctor if you have or have had:
☐ liver disease ☐ heart failure ☐ reduced kidney function ☐ eye problems ☐ lung conditions, such as asthma ☐ thyroid problems ☐ heart block ☐ extremely low heart rate ☐ porphyria.

How to use this medicine

The tablets are taken on a long-term basis to prevent attacks. To begin with they are taken three times a day, then the dosage is reduced to twice a day and finally once a day or every other day. You should have the lowest possible dose to control arrhythmias and to minimise unwanted effects. If you miss a dose and the next dose is due within 12 hours, do not take it. Do not take double doses: take your next scheduled dose as usual.

If you have poor liver function, you may need a lower dose. You should have periodic tests to assess liver function. Your doctor will also monitor thyroid function. Amiodarone can cause both high and low thyroid levels in the body. It also interferes with some of the tests for thyroid function and so you should be alert for changes in how you feel while you take amiodarone.

Over 65 You may need less than the usual adult dose. You are most likely to experience unwanted reactions. There may be another antiarrhythmic drug that is more suitable to take than amiodarone.

Interactions with other medicines

Many drugs, including **other antiarrhythmics**, **antibacterials** (**co-trimoxazole, erythromycin**), **antihistamines** (**mizolastine**, **terfenadine**), **antimalarials**, **antipsychotics** (**amisulpride**, **haloperidol**, **phenothiazines**, **pimozide**, **sertindole**), **antivirals** (**nelfinavir**, **ritonavir**), **pentamidine** and **tricyclic antidepressants** increase the risk of ventricular arrhythmias – avoid combinations.
Anticoagulants (**nicoumalone**, **phenindione**, **warfarin**). Effects increased by amiodarone.

Heart drugs (**digoxin**, **beta blockers** and **calcium channel blockers**) Amiodarone increases the risk of very low heart rate and heart block.
Phenytoin Effect increased by amiodarone.

Unwanted effects

Likely Sensitivity to light – you should protect your skin from sunlight with a reliable sunscreen preparation. During long-term treatment tiny spots appear on the cornea; they rarely interfere with sight, although occasionally may cause 'haloes'. Drivers may be dazzled by headlights at night. These spots fade when amiodarone is stopped. Routine eye examinations are advisable.
Less likely Slate-grey or bluish discoloration of the skin, skin rashes, numbness and tingling in the limbs, shortness of breath, thyroid problems, feeling or being sick, headache, heart problems, lung problems, liver damage, metallic taste, nightmares, dizziness, tiredness, impotence.

While you are taking amiodarone you will need to see your doctor for routine checks. Low doses minimise unwanted effects which usually disappear once you stop taking amiodarone. You should contact your doctor if you develop any of these effects.

Stroke

Stroke, or 'brain attack' as it is starting to be described, is damage to the brain caused by bleeding (*haemorrhagic stroke*) or more usually by a blocked blood vessel in the brain (*ischaemia*). If the blood supply to a part of the brain is interrupted for longer than 24 hours, a stroke has occurred. If the blood supply is cut off for a shorter time, this is known as a *transient ischaemic attack* or 'mini stroke'. Most people who have a transient ischaemic attack begin to improve within minutes and have often recovered by the time they see a doctor; there is no lasting damage to the body. If you suffer a stroke, you may not recover completely. When fatty deposits build up inside blood vessels and cause them to narrow, a blood clot (*thrombus*) may block a vessel. Other parts of the brain may not be able to compensate for the lost brain cells because the remaining arteries are also likely to be diseased. Part of a blood clot or collection of blood cells may break off from a blood vessel and travel round the bloodstream until it gets stuck in a smaller artery. If the collection of cells (*embolus*) is very small, it may disperse, letting the blood flow return to normal. This happens in a transient ischaemic attack.

Haemorrhage occurs when a blood vessel ruptures and blood leaks out into the brain. The blood starts to clot and pressure from the clot also damages the brain. Unlike thrombosis, which may develop over some hours or days, a brain haemorrhage usually happens suddenly.

Prompt recognition of the symptoms and management as a medical emergency can influence recovery following stroke. The symptoms vary and can include loss of consciousness, paralysis, dizziness, intense headache, seizures and incontinence. The right side of the brain controls the functions of the left side of the body and vice versa. The part of the body controlled by the damaged area of the brain will be affected. Weakness or paralysis of one side of the body is common, although other faculties may be lost – for example, control of mental and emotional processes or the ability to speak or understand language. Sight, sound, smell, taste and touch may be affected. If brain cells die, then other areas of the brain try to compensate and take over their role. Recovery depends on how well the brain can do this and it may take several months before you know what parts of the body have been affected permanently.

Stroke is a leading cause of death in the UK and the risk of having a stroke increases if you have other medical conditions such as atrial fibrillation (page 140), diabetes (pages 301–8) or have had previous transient ischaemic attacks. It is associated with high blood pressure, certain types of 'the Pill' (oral contraception) and can occur in any age group, although it is primarily a condition of old age. The National Service Framework for Older People has set standards of care for stroke, recommending in particular that people should receive hospital care in a stroke unit from a specialist team. Twenty per cent of stroke victims die within a month and just over half die or become dependent on others after a year. Around 300,000 people are living with the effects of stroke. Stroke care varies widely and currently many hospital services are poorly organised. If stroke is managed effectively then you should expect rapid evaluation from a multidisciplinary team including a brain scan or image (computed tomography – CT or magnetic resonance imaging – MRI) to identify what has happened to the brain, ECG, chest X-ray, and a barrage of other tests including blood cell counts, electrolytes, testing for diabetes, kidney function, lipids and an assessment to see if swallowing is affected. Management of other medical conditions that occur alongside a stroke also need attention, for example stabilising heart and lung function.

HOW YOU CAN HELP YOURSELF

PREVENTING STROKE

- ☐ Lose weight – reduce fat and salt intake.
- ☐ Stop smoking.
- ☐ Take regular exercise.
- ☐ Review alcohol consumption.
- ☐ Reduce high blood pressure. If taking blood pressure-lowering medicine(s), take them regularly.
- ☐ Treat raised cholesterol with a statin to reduce the level to less than 5 millimoles/litre or a 20–25 per cent reduction – whichever produces the lowest level of cholesterol in the blood.
- ☐ Aim for good diabetic control, where appropriate.
- ☐ If you have atrial fibrillation, keep taking warfarin to prevent blood clots forming in the heart. Have regular blood tests to assess your clotting time.
- ☐ A daily dose of aspirin prevents a recurrence of stroke; discuss this with your doctor.

Treatment for stroke

Medicines cannot cure a stroke once it has happened, but if the stroke is caused by a blood clot then aspirin should be given immediately. 'Clot busters' (*thrombolytics*) that break up blood clots (pages 148–9) may be helpful, providing one is given within three hours of the stroke. They are not used routinely because a reliable diagnosis with a brain scan must be made before one is given, as they can cause bleeding in the brain. It is important that doctors distinguish between a stroke caused by ischaemia and one caused by bleeding. Anticoagulants and clot-busting drugs increase the risk of bleeding and therefore must not be used in haemorrhagic stroke. Other drug treatment will be used in the management of a person after a stroke – for example in maintaining regular bowel movement or in managing muscle spasms.

If you have a transient ischaemic attack or a stroke your doctor should prescribe an antiplatelet drug to reduce the risk of further ischaemic attacks or strokes occurring (secondary prevention). Aspirin in low dosage (75mg) is very effective and should be taken long-term. Other antiplatelet medicines include **clopidogrel** and **dipyridamole** (page 150).

The success of rehabilitation depends on your physical and mental condition and social circumstances, and not on the type of stroke. Good nursing and co-ordinated remedial therapy help early recovery and can prevent disablement. Morale is important in achieving the best recovery and planning for a worthwhile future is important. A hopeful, but realistic approach from nurses, therapists and doctors towards the patient can prevent depression. Treatment with an antidepressant medicine may help but you must have a chance to vent anger, frustration or misery and to ask questions.

For the relatives of stroke victims, the aftermath of stroke is a difficult and worrying time. The Stroke Association* in England and Wales, Chest, Heart and Stroke Scotland* and the Northern Ireland Chest, Heart and Stroke Association* have information which will help patients and their relatives to understand the illness better. These organisations also run the Volunteer Stroke Service, which helps people with speech difficulties. There are also pilot schemes running which aim to ease the change from hospital to home, from professional to family care and to improve support for the families of stroke victims.

Circulatory problems

PERIPHERAL ARTERIAL DISEASE

As people grow older, the arteries narrow, harden and lose their elasticity (*arteriosclerosis*). The process causes reduced blood flow to many parts of the body, but most noticeably the arms and legs. The arteries may 'silt up' with fatty deposits (*atherosclerosis*) leading to sluggish blood flow. A blood clot or part of one may block the artery and prevent blood flow. If this happens suddenly the arm or leg becomes pale, painful and pulseless. More usually, the restriction of blood supply happens gradually, to produce a long-term (chronic) condition. This can range from muscle pain when walking which is relieved by rest (*intermittent claudication*), to pain even when the limb is at rest, to non-healing ulcers on the legs. A completely obstructed blood flow may cause gangrene. Severe, extensive limb disease or signs of gangrene require hospital referral.

The most significant contributor to peripheral arterial disease is smoking, but other risk factors include untreated high blood pressure, raised cholesterol and triglyceride levels, diabetes and lifestyle problems of being overweight and lack of exercise. The approach to managing peripheral arterial disease is therefore to address the underlying risk factors. Your doctor will encourage you to stop smoking and suggest an exercise programme to increase the distance that you can walk without pain. These two approaches improve outcomes in intermittent claudication. A daily dose of aspirin (usually 75mg) helps to lessen the stickiness of blood and if appropriate medicines can be taken to lower raised blood pressure (page 95) and cholesterol (page 130), and to control diabetes mellitus (page 301). Losing weight, good foot care and avoiding tightly fitting footwear are also important measures.

Treatment of intermittent claudication is not usually helped directly by medicines although there may be a marked placebo effect with treatment. There are a number of drugs which increase the blood flow to the skin, particularly when the limb is at rest. The peripheral vasodilator **naftidrofuryl oxalate** (Praxilene) may improve symptoms, including pain; your doctor should check every three to six months whether the drug is causing an improvement. Other peripheral vasodilators – **cinnarizine** (Stugeron; Stugeron Forte), **nicotinic acid** preparations (Hexopal), **pentoxifylline** (**oxpentifylline**) (Trental) and **moxisylyte** (**thymoxamine**) (Opilon) – are not recommended because evidence of their effectiveness is not well established. The unwanted effects of peripheral vasodilators include flushing, dizziness, nausea and headache. Similarly, **rutosides** or **oxerutins** (Paroven) have been used for various circulatory disorders such as leg cramps. There is little evidence that rutosides are effective and they are not recommended. Unwanted effects include headaches, flushing, skin rashes and gastro-intestinal upsets. **Cilostazol** (▼Pletal) may improve pain-free walking distances if you have intermittent claudication without pain at rest or damage to peripheral tissue. It is taken twice daily, but the unwanted effects, such as headache, diarrhoea, feeling or being sick, dyspepsia and less commonly dizziness, heart attack, heart failure and hypersensitivity reactions, plus many potential interactions with other medicines, may limit its use. Stopping smoking and keeping active are the best treatments for peripheral arterial disease.

RAYNAUD'S PHENOMENON AND RAYNAUD'S DISEASE

These are conditions of the hands and sometimes the feet in which the small blood vessels (*arterioles*) constrict or squeeze together and restrict blood flow. The fingers become pale, then blue and finally red as the attack passes. It is sometimes painful and you may have pins and needles, numbness and a burning sensation. Cold or emotion are the most common triggers for an attack. **Raynaud's phenomenon** is associated with many other disorders, such as rheumatoid arthritis or atherosclerosis. People in certain occupations are prone to develop the condition, for example chainsaw or pneumatic drill operators and pianists. Excessive vibration may be the cause in these cases. When there is no underlying disease, the condition is known as **Raynaud's disease**. This occurs mostly in young women and more commonly affects the hands.

Severe symptoms may be helped by **nifedipine** (pages 116–17). You should not take a beta blocker as this will worsen the condition. **Naftidrofuryl** (Praxilene) and **nicotinic acid** preparations may be helpful.

HOW YOU CAN HELP YOURSELF

- ☐ Avoid exposure to cold, and wear warm clothing including gloves.
- ☐ Avoid working with vibrating machinery.
- ☐ Stop smoking.

Blood clots

When you cut yourself, the blood flow stops eventually because the blood clots. Special blood cells called *platelets* act as a plug to stem the initial blood flow; they activate clotting factors to form *fibrin* which meshes in with red blood cells to form a clot. A blood clot (*thrombus*) that forms inside a blood vessel, where it is not wanted, does so either because of **injury to the vessel wall**, for example when a fatty deposit breaks off (*atheroma*), or **when blood flow alters**, for example with an irregular heart rhythm such as *atrial fibrillation*. An unwanted blood clot can also form if **the blood clotting process alters**, for example during immobility or pregnancy, or with an inherited disorder, such as increased clotting (*coagulability*) of the blood (*thrombophilia*). The blood-clotting process can be affected by medicines, for example there is a small risk of blood clots developing in women taking HRT or the combined oral contraceptive pill (pages 337 and 354). Other medicines, antiplatelets and anticoagulants are used to prevent clots forming.

In the arteries blood clots that form are made up of clumps of platelets with little fibrin. These blood clots are usually associated with a build up of fatty deposits in the arteries (*atherosclerosis*). They can interrupt blood flow causing lack of oxygen (*ischaemia*) or death (*infarction*) of the tissues, as in stroke and heart attacks. A blood clot is a danger not only because it affects the flow of blood, either in an artery or vein, but also because a piece of the blood clot (*embolus*) may break off and travel to other parts of the body, such as the brain, heart or lungs where it may cause damage if it blocks the blood supply to an organ. For example, an embolism on the lungs (*pulmonary embolism*), a rare condition, can cause breathlessness, chest pain and in severe cases collapse.

Blood moves more slowly back to the heart through the veins. A clot in the veins therefore differs from one in the arteries; it consists of a fibrin web with platelets and red cells. A clot in the veins (*venous thrombus*) is usually associated with slowed blood flow or stasis which can occur for example after prolonged inactivity. Clots within a leg vein (*deep vein thrombosis*) or the abdomen can occur after an operation, injury, childbirth or periods of immobility. If a clot forms deep in a leg vein, part of the leg below the clot swells as fluid is retained. Pain, tenderness and reddening of the skin may also develop. Deep vein thrombosis can develop during any form of long-distance travel where you remain immobile, sitting for long periods without exercise. You can be at risk on air flights lasting longer than five hours, particularly if you do not exercise or are already at increased risk of deep vein thrombosis. The Department of Health provides advice on travel-related deep vein thrombosis at *www.doh.gov.uk/blood/dvt/index.htm*.

Antiplatelet medicines

Antiplatelet drugs such as aspirin stop clot formation in arteries by lessening platelet stickiness through effects on one of the body's chemical pathways involved in activating platelets. When blood vessel walls become damaged, platelets become activated and then clump and stick together (*aggregation*). This in turn assists fibrin formation and ultimately blood clots. Aspirin, known for its pain-relieving properties (page 299), has become widely used to prevent platelet activation and hence the formation of blood clots and their potential to obstruct arterial blood flow. Research has shown that just one tablet of aspirin a day can prevent heart attacks and stroke in people at risk. A once-daily dose (ranging from 75–150mg) ensures that platelets are prevented from sticking together permanently and blood is less thick. Higher doses are used (150–300mg) after a heart attack or stroke.

Unfortunately aspirin has unwanted effects; potentially serious bleeding from the digestive tract and other places, such as the brain. For this reason aspirin is recommended only if you are at high risk of having a heart attack or stroke for the first time or for preventing further events. Aspirin is best taken dispersed in water and at the low dose (75mg) unwanted effects should be minimised. Enteric-coated preparations do not avoid unwanted effects of aspirin because these develop mainly through modification to the biochemical pathway and not through a direct effect on the gut wall. Aspirin should be used cautiously in people who have high blood pressure that is uncontrolled and in those have had a peptic ulcer. An ulcer-healing medicine, such as a proton pump inhibitor or misoprostol (page 69), can help to protect the gut from aspirin's effects. You must not take aspirin if you have an active peptic ulcer or have the bleeding disorder, haemophilia or a similar problem. Aspirin can also cause allergic reactions, for example acute breathing difficulties (*bronchospasm*), and because it can worsen asthma, you need to see how you react to it, making sure that you have your reliever (bronchodilator) to hand. Other less common unwanted effects include constipation and kidney impairment.

Clopidogrel (Plavix) and related medicine **ticlopidine** (▼Ticlid) also prevent platelets sticking together. Clopidogrel is an alternative option if you cannot tolerate aspirin at all but it also causes very similar unwanted effects to aspirin, including gastric upsets, peptic ulceration and bleeding. Some doctors recommend the use of aspirin and clopidogrel together, and this will increase the risk of adverse effects. Clopidogrel should not be taken with warfarin. **Dipyridamole** (Persantin) is used with an anticoagulant to stop clots forming on artificial heart valves. Modified-release dipyridamole (Persantin Retard) or combined with low-dose aspirin (25mg) (Asasantin) is used to prevent ischaemic stroke or transient ischaemic attack after the first occurrence.

Fibrinolytic drugs, or 'clot-busters', dissolve blood clots once they have formed. They are also known as thrombolytics and activate a body chemical, *plasminogen*, to form *plasmin* that breaks down fibrin in the the blood clot. The drugs **streptokinase** (Streptase), **alteplase** (Actilyse), **reteplase** (Rapilysin) and **tenecteplase** (▼Metalyse) have to be injected into the vein and are therefore used mainly in hospital. They are useful for dissolving blood clots immediately after a heart attack and the sooner they are given, the more effective they are. **Streptokinase**, also used in life-threatening venous thrombosis or embolism in the lung, generates antibodies to itself, making it less effective in subsequent treatment. You will need to ensure that doctors treating you in the future know this, for example by carrying a card stating that you should not be given this drug again. Unwanted effects of fibrinolytics include feeling or being sick and bleeding.

Anticoagulants

Anticlotting medicines (*anticoagulants*) are used to prevent blood clots forming – for example during surgery – or from getting bigger in the veins, lungs, or on artificial (prosthetic) heart valves or if you have atrial fibrillation. They cannot dissolve blood clots once formed and have little effect on clotting in the arterial circulation.

Deep vein thrombosis in the legs is sometimes a serious complication of surgery, but it can be prevented by an anticoagulant. Patients suffering from major trauma, a heart attack, heart failure, stroke or cancer and people who are overweight, aged over 40 or have a family history of blood clots or inherited clotting tendency or have had previous deep vein thrombosis are particularly at risk. Lengthy operations, including those on the pelvis, hips or knees, are especially likely to lead to deep vein thrombosis. Before you have an operation, ask the surgeon whether you need anticoagulant cover during and after surgery. Other measures, such as anti-embolism stockings, are also used.

Heparin is used to start anticoagulation treatment. It acts rapidly in the body to prevent clots from forming, but it is effective for only a short time and has to be given by injection. Heparin treatment is generally given in hospital and has to be carefully supervised: too much causes bleeding, such as nose bleeds, blood in the urine and bruising. These effects are soon reversed by stopping the drug or by giving a specific antidote – **protamine sulphate**. At the same time as heparin is started, an anticoagulant is given by mouth. Heparin is used for an immediate effect because oral anticoagulants take time to work in the body (48–72 hours).

Vitamin K is absorbed from the digestive system in fats and is essential for the formation of certain clotting factors. Oral anticoagulants interfere with certain stages of the clotting factor formation in the liver. **Warfarin** is commonly used because unwanted effects are low, although bleeding is a risk; **acenocoumarol** (**nicoumalone**; Sinthrome) and **phenindione** are rarely used.

Discovered through a change in agricultural policy in North America in the 1920s, warfarin, an acronym – Wisconsin Alumni Research Foundation – was first used as rat poison. It is often life-saving, but its use has to be monitored carefully. At the start of treatment this involves frequent blood tests to measure its effect on clotting time, the prothrombin time expressed as the International Normalised Ratio or INR; the dosage is adjusted during this phase. Regular monitoring will be required while you are taking warfarin because the therapeutic effect of thinning blood has to be balanced and the dose altered in response to blood tests. Too little means that blood continues to coagulate and treatment is not effective. Too much can lead to bleeding, warfarin's main adverse effect. This usually requires a dose reduction, by omitting doses until clotting time is back in range. You may require hospital treatment if bleeding is severe. Your doctor should give you an emergency plan of what to do in the event of bleeding. You may need to stop the drug for a day or two and possibly have a vitamin K injection or a transfusion of fresh frozen plasma in hospital.

Many drugs either enhance or reduce the effect of anticoagulants, including those bought over the counter – such as St John's wort and ginseng, which reduce the anticoagulant effect. Illness, such as diarrhoea, may reduce the body's intake of vitamin K, which in turn affects the clotting factors. Liver or kidney damage alters the body's response to warfarin and a dose reduction will be required. Eating large amounts of green vegetables, such as broccoli, cabbage, spinach, salad or liver can reduce the effect of warfarin as they contain vitamin K; this requires an increased dose of warfarin. Alcohol in large amounts increases the blood-thinning effect of warfarin so the dose should be lower. If you are on long-term oral anticoagulation treatment it is essential to carry an anticoagulation treatment card – this gives advice about the treatment and will be given to you by your doctor or your pharmacist.

WARFARIN

WARFARIN – Tablets MAREVAN – Tablets

Warfarin is an oral anticoagulant used for treating or preventing the development of blood clots deep in the leg veins and fragments of clot in the lungs. Warfarin is used to prevent blood clots forming in people with rheumatic heart disease, atrial fibrillation and after operations to insert artificial heart valves.

Warfarin takes 36–48 hours to work in the body, but continues to act for 48 hours after it is stopped. The dosage must be carefully adjusted for each person and tablet strengths (500 micrograms, 1mg, 3mg and 5mg) help with flexible dosing. You should see your doctor, nurse or pharmacist regularly to monitor progress and to have blood tests. Self-monitoring is now possible with the CoaguChek machine; test strips are available on prescription.

Before you use this medicine

Tell your doctor if you are:
☐ pregnant – you should not take warfarin in the first three months nor during the last few weeks of pregnancy ☐ breast-feeding ☐ taking any other medicines, including vitamins and those bought over the counter. Vitamin and mineral supplements containing vitamin K and/or ginseng and herbal remedies containing the antidepressant St John's wort reduce warfarin's effectiveness.

Tell your doctor if you have or have had:
☐ severe liver or kidney impairment –– avoid warfarin ☐ recent surgery ☐ peptic ulcer ☐ severe high blood pressure ☐ infection of the heart (bacterial endocarditis) ☐ blood disorders ☐ hypersensitivity or resistance to warfarin.

How to use this medicine

Take the tablets exactly as directed. The dosage will be adjusted from time to time, depending on the clotting (prothrombin) time (INR). Eat a well-balanced diet. Do not change your diet or weight, or take nutritional supplements or vitamins without checking with your doctor or pharmacist. Avoid alcohol – the anticlotting activity may be increased, particularly with large amounts or 'binge drinking'. Be careful doing activities that may cause bruising or bleeding, including falling over.

Carry an anticoagulation card stating that you take warfarin. A medical identification bracelet may also be helpful. If you have to have an operation, tell your doctor or dentist that you take warfarin.

Do not stop taking this medicine suddenly as this may cause a worsening of your condition. Your doctor should give you a schedule to reduce dosage gradually. Regular blood tests are essential to monitor coagulation. If you miss a dose take it as soon as you remember.

Over 65 You may need less than the adult dose, especially if your liver or kidney function is impaired.

Interactions with other medicines

Warfarin interacts with many medicines. Do not take any other medicines, including over-the-counter remedies such as aspirin, cold remedies, antacids, laxatives, vitamin supplements and herbal remedies. Do not change the dose of any medicine you are taking without checking with your doctor or pharmacist.

Warfarin's anticlotting effect is enhanced by (therefore dose reduction may be needed):

☐ **anabolic steroids**
☐ **analgesics and antirheumatics**, especially aspirin, azapropazone (avoid with warfarin); possibly dextropropoxyphene (in co-proxamol), celecoxib, diclofenac, diflunisal, etoricoxib, flurbiprofen, ibuprofen, mefenamic acid, meloxicam, piroxicam, rofecoxib, sulindac and some other NSAIDs. Paracetamol used regularly can prolong warfarin's anticoagulant effect
☐ **antiarrhythmics** amiodarone, propafenone, quinidine
☐ **antibacterials**, such as ciprofloxacin, ofloxacin, co-trimoxazole, erythromycin, clarithromycin, metronidazole, sulphonamides possibly enhanced by trimethoprim, tetracyclines and ampicillin, for example
☐ **antidepressants** Possibly enhanced by SSRI type such as fluoxetine, paroxetine; venlafaxine

- ☐ **antiepileptic sodium valproate** Possibly enhanced effect
- ☐ **antifungals**, such as fluconazole, itraconazole, miconazole
- ☐ **antiplatelets**: aspirin, clopidogrel, dipyridamole and ticlopidine increase the risk of bleeding
- ☐ **antivirals** Possibly ritonavir
- ☐ **hormone blockers**: danazol, flutamide, tamoxifen; possibly bicalutamide, toremifene
- ☐ **lipid-lowering medicines**: fibrates, e.g. bezafibrate, and statins e.g. simvastatin; colestyramine may both enhance or reduce anticoagulant effect
- ☐ **methylphenidate** (for ADHD) Possibly enhanced anticoagulant effect
- ☐ **alcohol dependence treatment**: disulfiram
- ☐ **Parkinson's disease**: entacapone
- ☐ **gout treatment**: sulfinpyrazone
- ☐ **thyroid supplement**: thyroxine
- ☐ **ulcer-healing drugs**: cimetidine, including over-the-counter Tagamet 100, possibly omeprazole, esomeprazole
- ☐ **vaccines**: influenza may occasionally enhance anticoagulant effect.

Warfarin's anticlotting effect is reduced by (therefore dose increase may be needed):

- ☐ **acitretin for psoriasis** Possibly reduced effect
- ☐ **antibacterial rifampicin** and related drugs
- ☐ **antiepileptics**, such as carbamazepine, phenobarbital (phenobarbitone), primidone; phenytoin may enhance or reduce effects
- ☐ **antifungal**: griseofulvin
- ☐ **barbiturates**
- ☐ **corticosteroids** Anticlotting effect altered
- ☐ **herbal remedies**: the antidepressant St John's wort – avoid use together; ginseng
- ☐ **hormone blocker**: aminoglutethimide
- ☐ **oral contraceptives**
- ☐ **ulcer-healing drug**: sucralfate
- ☐ **vitamin K**: found in liver, salads and other green vegetables may reduce anticoagulation; avoid major changes in diet. Also vitamin K in some nutritional supplements for feeding by tube.

Unwanted effects

Likely Bleeding.
Less likely Skin rashes, hair loss, diarrhoea, abdominal pain, feeling or being sick, jaundice and other liver dysfunction, inflammation of the pancreas. You should see your doctor if any of these develop.

Contact your doctor immediately if you have signs of bleeding – for example bleeding gums, nosebleeds, heavy bleeding from cuts or wounds, abdominal pain, sudden lightheadedness, weakness, blood in urine, swelling of the ankles, feet or legs, purple toes.

Similar preparations

SINTHROME – Tablets
ACENOCOUMALONE (NICOUMALONE)

PHENINDIONE – Tablets

3

BREATHING PROBLEMS

Asthma
Chronic obstructive pulmonary disease
Allergies and hay fever
Coughs Colds

The lungs are the body's breathing machine. As you breathe air in through your nose or mouth, it passes down the back of the throat (*pharynx*), past the vocal cords (*larynx*) into the windpipe (*trachea*) and down into the lungs. Two lungs hang in the chest cavity above the heart. The windpipe branches into each lung through an airway called a *bronchus*. The bronchus divides into smaller and smaller air passages, the *bronchioles*, which in turn branch into air sacs (*alveoli*). The lungs resemble sponges made up of thousands and thousands of air sacs.

Each air sac is surrounded by a network of blood vessels. As air reaches the air sacs oxygen passes into red blood cells flowing through the blood vessels; carbon dioxide, waste gas that the body no longer needs, leaves the bloodstream and goes into the air sacs. As you breathe out, carbon dioxide is squeezed out of the lungs back into the surrounding air.

Asthma

Asthma is a long-term disturbance of the airways in the lungs. The cells of the airways become swollen. Plugs of phlegm or mucus are produced which sometimes block the air passages preventing the exchange of oxygen and carbon dioxide. The muscles of the bronchioles tighten, narrowing the airways. The inflamed airways become hyper-reactive: they are irritable and twitchy and narrow easily if they come into contact with any one of a number of trigger factors (page 155).

The main symptoms of asthma are wheezing, chest tightness, shortness of breath and coughing. Any one of these symptoms may indicate asthma, but your doctor will need to find out from you how and when chest problems occur and how long they last. Other conditions, such as bronchitis, have similar symptoms and must be distinguished from asthma. Symptoms are usually worst at night and first thing in the morning: they vary in severity and can even be life-threatening. Attacks may happen occasionally or you may live with regular symptoms. The bronchial airways usually recover from an attack and the narrowing reverses. If you have chronic asthma, the airways may stay inflamed, even if you have no symptoms or only mild ones occasionally and usually feel perfectly well. All grades of asthma need treatment.

WHAT CAUSES ASTHMA?

Even though asthma is a common condition, its cause is not completely understood. Asthma does run in families, often with other allergic conditions, such as hay fever and eczema, but it can affect people who have no family history of the condition or other allergic problems. Many factors can trigger an attack of asthma – you may find that any one of them or a combination sets off an attack, or that none of them does. Try to find out what makes you feel worse and tell your doctor. If you know that certain situations, such as a smoke-filled room, trigger an asthmatic attack, then you should obviously try to avoid them.

Allergies

Common triggers include: house dust which carries microscopic house dust mites; animals such as cats, dogs and birds; pollen; and fungal spores. When a susceptible person breathes in air full of house dust mites, for example, this may start an asthmatic attack. Occasionally, some foods and drinks such as fruits, milk, cheese, fizzy drinks, peanuts and alcohol, may trigger asthma. Airborne triggers are by far the most common cause.

FOOD ADDITIVES

Tartrazine – a dye that is often used to colour food, soft drinks and medicines – can trigger asthma. It can be identified on the label of packaged foods as E102, but it is not always obvious which medicines contain tartrazine. If you know you react to the dye, and you are not sure whether a medicine contains it, check with the pharmacist. Other similar dyes are E104 and E110. *Sodium metabisulphite* and its related compounds (E220–227) are preservatives commonly used in wines and beer and can also trigger asthma. The *benzoate* preservatives (E210–219) may also cause problems.

Illness

Colds, flu and viral infections can trigger an asthma attack, particularly in young children. Wheeziness and persistent coughing at night are common signs. About one in ten children has wheeziness that needs medical treatment at some time. Yet many wheezy babies with mild symptoms grow out of them as resistance to colds and coughs builds up by about the age of seven. In one study, eight out of ten children who wheezed in their first year no longer had asthma by the age of ten. *Atopic* children (those who had a tendency to develop other allergies) are more likely to have asthmatic symptoms when they are older.

Occupation

People in certain occupations may be exposed to the fumes or dusts of particular substances which can trigger asthma. When you leave work for a weekend or holiday, your symptoms improve, but on your return your condition worsens. People working in industries such as plastics, electronics and pharmaceutical manufacturing are likely to meet these *sensitising agents*. If you develop wheeziness or chest tightness during the time when you are at work (the symptoms may be worse at night), see your doctor. You may be able to get compensation if you are working with a recognised *sensitising agent* and your symptoms are clearly caused by it. Your asthma may clear up completely if you avoid working with a particular sensitising agent.

Smoke

For most people with asthma, symptoms are made worse by smoke, especially cigarette smoke. Children are particularly affected by smoke-filled rooms. You should avoid smoke and smoking.

HOW YOU CAN HELP YOURSELF

- ☐ Learn about asthma, the nature of the disease, its management and what triggers attacks. Complete avoidance of trigger factors may be difficult, but try to avoid things you know you are allergic to whenever you can. Allergy to the house dust mite is common and so it is helpful to vacuum regularly to reduce dust levels. In the bedroom, house dust mites can be reduced by not having a carpet or rugs; a mattress filled with man-made fibre and a washable mattress cover are also helpful.
- ☐ The National Asthma Campaign★ provides information and support, including a weekday helpline (9am – 5pm) and has set out an Asthma Charter of rights that you should expect if you have asthma.
- ☐ Asthma is a long-term, variable condition. Be prepared to visit your doctor regularly, even when your asthma is well-controlled, and not just when you are unwell.
- ☐ Know your medicines, both those that relieve and those that prevent attacks: asthma can be well controlled with medicines so that you can lead a full and active life. Use the medicine record sheet or a similar card to note the name of the medicine, how much to take and how often to take it each day, as well as other details. If you have an asthmatic schoolchild make sure the teacher understands that a reliever inhaler should be easily accessible. Never take more than the recommended dose or repeat the dosing more frequently. With an inhaler, ask your doctor up to how many inhalations you may take in 24 hours. If your usual dose appears not to be having its effect this often means your asthma has worsened and should be discussed with your doctor.
- ☐ Use a peak flow meter regularly (see box opposite) to monitor changes in your breathing. If you have an asthmatic attack, your peak flow reading is usually lower than usual.
- ☐ Learn to recognise the times when your asthma worsens and what you should do about it. Agree an asthma action plan with your doctor which should include deciding when to adjust your treatment. The written plan should also include when to call for help. Never be afraid to ask for urgent medical attention: uncontrolled asthma can be life-threatening.

Medicines

Beta blockers (for example **propranolol**) must not be taken by asthmatics because they can cause narrowing of the airways and provoke an asthma attack. If your doctor considers that it is absolutely essential for you to have a beta blocker, you should also have extra cover with a bronchodilator aerosol. Beta blocker eye drops for treating glaucoma (pages 403–9) should also be avoided. Aspirin and related medicines (non-steroidal anti-inflammatory drugs) can worsen asthma. If you are sensitive to aspirin, you may also react to ibuprofen, an over-the-counter NSAID. Paracetamol is the preferred pain-reliever for asthmatics.

Other causes

Emotion and stress can both start an asthmatic attack in someone who already has asthma, but cannot cause asthma. Going out suddenly into cold air can trigger asthma, as can a change in the weather or the different seasons. Many forms of exercise can provoke an attack.

HOW TO USE A PEAK FLOW METER

Peak expiratory flow rate or 'peak flow' is a measure of how quickly you can blow air out of your lungs. Your lung function depends on your age, height and sex and varies a great deal between people, even in those who have good lung function. If you have asthma, peak flow varies between morning and night as well as from day to day. Peak flow readings can help confirm the diagnosis of asthma, show you how good your lung function is, and help you and your doctor to assess both the severity of your asthma and the success of treatment.

If you have asthma the airways are narrowed and it is more difficult to blow air out. Your doctor or nurse may assess your peak flow at the surgery but you may also be asked to measure peak flow yourself for a couple of weeks at home and to keep a diary of measurements. Your doctor can prescribe a peak flow meter; with careful use it can last about three years.

To measure peak flow:

- ☐ stand or sit upright
- ☐ fit the mouthpiece (cardboard or plastic collar) around the neck of the meter
- ☐ make sure the marker or indicator is at the bottom of the scale
- ☐ check that your fingers are not over the scale
- ☐ take a good breath in and place your lips firmly around the mouthpiece
- ☐ blow out with a short, sharp blast (but not a cough)
- ☐ remove the meter from your mouth and take the reading
- ☐ note the reading, repeat the procedure twice more and record the best of the three readings.

Medicines for asthma

Asthma can be treated by using medicines regularly. Some relieve asthmatic symptoms (cough, chest tightness, wheezing and breathlessness) and are known as 'relievers'. The other type, 'preventers', prevent symptoms developing by reducing inflammation in the airways. Although there is no cure for asthma, symptoms can be controlled so well with medicines that you should not have any constraints on your life. With the help of your doctor and nurse you should draw up a written asthma action plan which aims to keep you free from the symptoms of asthma night and day. This will enable you to participate fully in physical activity, avoid emergency treatments or trips to hospital, and maintain your best possible peak flow (page 157). Each person will have different goals and you will need to balance these against the requirement to take medicines regularly to achieve optimum control of asthma.

Asthma treatments work on the inflamed cells of the air passages. When inhaled, small doses of medicine are very effective; much larger doses have to be used when medicine is given by mouth, because the drug reaches the lungs only after it has been absorbed into the body and distributed by the bloodstream. Getting the drug directly to where it is needed means not only that a smaller dose can be used but that unwanted effects are lessened. Medicines used simply to relieve symptoms – bronchodilators, also known as 'relievers' – also act more quickly when inhaled than when taken as tablets.

'STEPWISE' APPROACH TO TREATMENT

Guidance to health professionals on how to help people with long-term asthma suggests a 'stepwise' approach to treatment with the aim of abolishing symptoms speedily and optimising peak flow. Each step represents recommended treatment according to the current severity of the asthma symptoms, and you should start treatment at the level most likely to achieve control. The following guidance applies to adults and schoolchildren. The stepped approach and some of the same medicines are used for children less than five years old at appropriate doses, but referral to a specialist is more likely, depending on the severity of symptoms.

Step 1 For mild symptoms or occasional bouts of coughing, wheezing and breathlessness, you may need only a 'reliever' inhaler, such as one containing **salbutamol** or **terbutaline**. You should always keep an inhaler on hand so that any developing symptoms can be relieved speedily.

Step 2 If you find that you need to use your reliever inhaler more than once a day or have night-time symptoms, tell your doctor or nurse. At this stage you may start regular treatment with an inhaled 'preventer' medicine, usually a corticosteroid. A spacer (page 161) may help to get the drug into the lungs and will reduce the risk of throat infections and absorption of corticosteroid into the body. The daily dose of corticosteroid may vary depending on your symptoms and your peak flow meter readings. Alternative, but less effective, preventer therapies include inhaled **sodium cromoglicate** for adults or **nedocromil** for children, or by mouth a leukotriene receptor antagonist such as montelukast, or **theophylline,** which may be tried before a corticosteroid.

Step 3 If symptoms do not improve or control is inadequate, you should review how you use your medicines, inhaler technique and any possible trigger factors with your doctor or nurse. If control is still inadequate following this review then the dose of the inhaled corticosteroid may be increased for a trial period. More usually, a longer-acting bronchodilator, **salmeterol** (Serevent) or **formoterol** (eformoterol – Foradil; Oxis) can be added to corticosteroid treatment; this may avoid the need to increase the corticosteroid dosage, which remains an option after a thorough trial with the longer-acting bronchodilator. Inhalers combining a corticosteroid with either salmeterol or formoterol are now available. Like salbutamol, formoterol can be used for short-term symptom relief, but salmeterol must not be used for immediate relief of acute asthma attacks. You would continue to use your 'reliever' inhaler when required for immediate relief. Further treatment options, one of which may be added, include a leukotriene receptor antagonist, modified-release **theophylline** or other bronchodilator.

Step 4 If your asthma needs further control, the corticosteroid dosage can be increased still further. You will have your usual reliever inhaler as required, plus a longer-acting bronchodilator (either **salmeterol** or **formoterol**), plus in adults six-week trials in succession of one or more of a modified-release **theophylline** preparation, a leukotriene receptor antagonist, and other bronchodilators by mouth.

Step 5 At this stage you will have a reliever for immediate relief and a regular high-dose corticosteroid inhaler, plus one or more longer-acting bronchodilators as in step 4, plus **prednisolone**, a corticosteroid by mouth in a regular daily dose. Your doctor is also likely to refer you to an asthma specialist for a further opinion about your management. Courses of corticosteroid tablets may be necessary only from time to time when asthma symptoms worsen, but would be considered for longer periods if other treatments proved inadequate. The aim will be to use the lowest possible dose of corticosteroid to control symptoms. The risk of unwanted effects from long-term corticosteroids by mouth or three or four courses a year increases, and your doctor must monitor and treat you, for example for increases in blood pressure, the development of diabetes mellitus and brittle bones (osteoporosis), and must manage in children the possible effects of slowed growth and cataracts in the eye.

Stepping down Your doctor or nurse will want to review your treatment every three months. If you are aged 16 years or over, you should expect to be asked the following questions to assist in gauging how well your asthma is controlled:

In the last week/month (answer Yes or No):

- ☐ Have you had difficulty sleeping because of your asthma symptoms (including cough)?
- ☐ Have you had your usual asthma symptoms during the day (cough, wheeze, chest tightness or breathlessness)?
- ☐ Has your asthma interfered with your usual activities(e.g. housework, work, school etc.)?

You may be able to step down treatment gradually if your symptoms are well controlled. You should ask if this is possible if it is not mentioned at your review, as overtreatment can occur, for example if repeat prescriptions are continued for your regular asthma medicines without dose changes. Slow reduction of the inhaled corticosteroid dose is necessary because the condition can deteriorate at different rates in different people. The dose may be reduced by one quarter to one half if symptom control is good. Measuring your peak flow will be important during these periods and you should have a clear understanding of the signs that show your asthma is worsening:

- ☐ **night-time symptoms** – waking up with shortness of breath
- ☐ **morning symptoms lasting longer than usual**
- ☐ increased need for your reliever inhaler and symptoms not as well relieved
- ☐ **fall in peak flow** and an increasing variation between morning and evening readings.

Inhaler devices

Three main methods are available to deliver asthma treatment to the lungs by inhalation: using a pressurised metered-dose inhaler, a dry powder inhaler or via a nebuliser. A range of inhaler devices exist, so you should be able to find one that suits you and that you can manage easily. Your inhaler technique will need to be checked regularly and any difficulties identified.

Pressurised metered-dose inhalers

A pressurised metered-dose inhaler (aerosol) delivers a measured quantity of a drug carried by the aerosol propellant. Pressurised metered-dose inhalers may be operated by hand or breath-actuated. Each time the canister is pressed or you breathe from a breath-actuated device, a dose is released. You need careful instruction on how to use a metered dose inhaler manually; your technique should be checked before one is prescribed for you and then regularly at review. Even with correct use only about 10 to 20 per cent of the dose reaches the lungs; much of the drug catches on the back of the mouth and throat and is then swallowed. To use a metered dose inhaler, you have to press the canister and breathe in at the same time. Children, older people and those with arthritic hands may find this a problem. A breath-actuated device, such as an Autohaler or Easi-Breathe, fires a dose as you breathe in and this may be helpful for those who find metered-dose inhalers hard to use.

Spacer devices are used with pressurised metered-dose inhalers, either with a reliever or a preventer inhaler. There are two main types -- holding chambers and extension devices. **Holding chamber spacers**, such as the large-volume Volumatic or Nebuhaler, are helpful if you find it difficult to co-ordinate your breathing in at the same time as firing a dose. A face mask can be attached to the spacer, for example for a very young child. This type of spacer extends the gap between the inhaler and the mouth and slows the speed at which the propellant and drug travel to the back of the mouth. There is also more time for the propellant to start evaporating, leaving a higher proportion of the drug in the dose you inhale. Some people find the propellant causes irritation, and this may inhibit breathing in as fully as possible. You should inhale from the spacer as soon as possible after firing one puff into it, repeating the action until you have taken the prescribed dose, for example two puffs. Loading the spacer with several puffs at once before inhaling reduces the dose available to lungs. You can either take a slow, deep breath in or a series of smaller breaths – both ways are effective. Your spacer device should be replaced every 6–12 months. Many different spacers are now available and they vary widely, particularly in the dose of the drug they emit, so careful monitoring is needed if you have to change your type of device.

A metered-dose inhaler plus a spacer is as effective as any other hand-held inhaler, including dry powder devices. Some spacers are bulky to carry around, but a spacer is especially useful for people who have to use an inhaled corticosteroid, particularly in high doses, because it reduces the likelihood of thrush developing in the mouth and throat. With once- or twice-daily corticosteroid dosing, the spacer can be kept conveniently at home. For children aged under five years, both the reliever and the preventer inhaler should be given via a metered-dose inhaler plus spacer, with a facemask if necessary.

To maintain its performance, a spacer must be washed in warm water and detergent once a month (not weekly as manufacturers recommend) and without rinsing allowed to air dry. Wiping a spacer dry increases electrostatic activity and reduces the amount of drug delivered into the lungs. The mouthpiece should be wiped clean of detergent before use and the valve checked to see that it opens and closes with breathing.

Extension devices are smaller spacers that slow the aerosol down in the same way as holding chambers. They do not have a valve and still require good co-ordination.

Dry powder inhalers

There is no propellant with these inhaler devices: they rely on your efforts to breathe in the dry powder, which is then dispersed into small particles and the drug delivered to the lungs. You do not need to rely on co-ordinating the dose with your breathing, and some people find them easier to use than a metered-dose inhaler. Dry powder inhalers are unsuitable for children under six years old because they cannot breathe in reliably at the correct rate. Coughing may be a problem during the use of these inhalers. Around two-thirds of a dose may be deposited in the mouth and throat, and you should rinse your mouth with water routinely after inhaling from a dry powder device to minimise the development of thrush.

The Turbohaler device delivers the drug as pure drug powder which has no taste. The device is primed before each dose by holding it upright and twisting the base. A window on the device turns red when only a few doses remain. The Accuhaler device contains 60 doses in blisters on a foil strip. It has a dose counter that locks when the device is empty. Dry powder in capsules can be inhaled from a small device that breaks open the capsule containing the powdered drug, which may also contain sugar (lactose) to carry the drug (Spinhaler for use with Spincaps). The presence of lactose means that you can taste the dose, which some people prefer. You can get a whistle attachment for the Spincaps system that sounds when the dose has been taken properly. After each dose, a fresh capsule has to be loaded, which can be inconvenient, and the capsules may absorb moisture in humid climates. Diskhaler systems have several doses of dry powder packed on to a disk.

Nebulisers

A nebuliser converts a drug solution, when air or oxygen is forced through it, into an aerosol for inhalation through a mask or mouthpiece. It is used to deliver higher doses of asthma treatment to the lungs than is usual with other inhaler devices. Breathing does not need to be co-ordinated, so a nebuliser can be very useful for emergency treatment with a bronchodilator in an acute severe attack of asthma, particularly for adults and for young children who become too ill to use a metered-dose inhaler and large-volume spacer. Apart from emergency situations, a nebuliser for treating asthma would be used only after careful assessment and discussion with your doctor.

MEDICINES WHICH RELIEVE ASTHMA

Medicines that relax and open up the narrowed air passages (*bronchi*) are called *bronchodilators*, also known as 'relievers'. They relieve asthmatic symptoms of coughing, wheezing and breathlessness, but do not reduce inflammation. If you have mild asthma a bronchodilator may be all you need. It may also be added to other treatments and is used to treat an acute attack. There are two types of bronchodilator medicines – the adrenaline-like *beta$_2$-agonists* (or *beta-adrenoceptor stimulants*), and *theophylline* preparations. *Antimuscarinic bronchodilators* have been used to relieve asthmatic symptoms, but are mainly used now in chronic obstructive pulmonary disease (COPD), a term covering conditions such as chronic bronchitis and emphysema.

Beta$_2$-agonists

The body's chemicals act on receptor sites at the ends of nerves. Adrenaline and noradrenaline act on the beta$_1$- and beta$_2$-receptors to prepare you for activity ('flight or fight'). Among other effects, the airways open up, your heart beats faster and blood vessels dilate to allow blood to flow more easily around the body. Early bronchodilator treatments, such as ephedrine, mimicked adrenaline by working at both types of beta-receptor site. These *sympathomimetic* drugs relieved airway narrowing, but also affected the heart, sometimes adversely by disrupting its rate and rhythm. They should be avoided if possible. Drugs that mainly stimulate or enhance (agonist effect) the beta$_2$-receptors to relax the bronchioles, such as **salbutamol** and **terbutaline**, have much less of an effect on the heart. They may occasionally cause palpitations and fine tremor, usually of the hands, but when they are inhaled directly into the lungs they give fast relief and unwanted effects are rarely troublesome. Longer-acting beta$_2$-agonist bronchodilators **salmeterol** and **formoterol** are useful treatments to add by inhalation to corticosteroid therapy (see Step 3, page 159). They can be used for night-time or for exercise-induced asthma symptoms.

SALBUTAMOL

SALBUTAMOL – Inhaler, dry powder inhaler, tablets, liquid, nebuliser solution, injection
AIROMIR – Inhaler (CFC-free), breath-actuated Autohaler
ASMASAL CLICKHALER – Dry powder inhaler
CYCLOHALER Dry powder inhaler (Cyclocaps)
SALAMOL EASI-BREATHE Breath-actuated inhaler
VENTMAX SR Modified-release capsules
VENTODISKS – Dry powder inhaler (Diskhaler)
VENTOLIN – Dry powder inhaler (Accuhaler), liquid, nebuliser solution, injection
VENTOLIN EVOHALER – Inhaler (CFC-free)
VOLMAX – Modified-release tablets

Useful devices
Volumatic – Spacer device for use with inhalers. A face mask can be fitted to the spacer
Haleraid – For use with aerosol inhalers if your hands are too weak to press the canister (not NHS prescription)

Poor choice inhalers: combination preparations – ingredients better used separately (e.g. salbutamol should be used when needed, not regularly four times a day)

AEROCROM
SALBUTAMOL + SODIUM CROMOGLICATE

COMBIVENT
SALBUTAMOL + IPRATROPIUM

Salbutamol is a beta$_2$-agonist which opens up the airways in the lungs by relaxing the muscles around the bronchioles. It is used to relieve symptoms of asthma such as shortness of breath and wheezing. As a reliever, salbutamol acts quickly and the effect can last for up to four hours. Salbutamol may also be used in chronic obstructive pulmonary disease (COPD), a term covering conditions such as chronic bronchitis and emphysema. It is also useful for preventing exercise-induced asthma if taken about 20 minutes before exercise. Salbutamol is very effective when given by inhaler, rather than tablets, with few unwanted effects, although fine tremor of the hands may be noticeable. Modified-release tablets help lung function, but unwanted effects occur more commonly with this method.

Before you use this medicine

Tell your doctor if you are:
☐ pregnant – asthma must be well controlled. Inhalation of salbutamol means that very small doses can relieve asthma symptoms without high blood levels of the drug reaching the fetus. Salbutamol is sometimes used by injection in an attempt to prevent premature labour ☐ breast-feeding ☐ taking any other medicines, including vitamins and those bought over the counter.

Tell your doctor if you have or have had:
☐ high blood pressure ☐ an overactive thyroid ☐ diabetes ☐ heart disease ☐ irregular heartbeat ☐ an allergy to salbutamol or to other adrenaline-like drugs, such as the decongestants **pseudoephedrine** or **phenylpropanolamine**.

How to use this medicine

Inhaler Use one or two puffs of the inhaler device as directed and when symptoms require relief. If you need to use your inhaler regularly more than once a day to relieve symptoms, see your doctor. Your treatment may need to be stepped up to include a corticosteroid inhaler as a preventer. If you use a corticosteroid inhaler and a reliever bronchodilator inhaler, use the bronchodilator first. Allow about 15 minutes between inhaling the two medicines. Do not use a salbutamol inhaler more often or in a higher dose than that prescribed by your doctor. Contact your doctor or nurse if you do not feel better after taking your usual dose or your asthma worsens. Do not drive or do any other activities which require concentration until you know how you react to salbutamol.

Low blood levels of potassium may result from treatment with high doses of beta$_2$-agonists. If you take a beta$_2$-agonist with high doses of a corticosteroid, **theophylline** or a diuretic, blood levels of potassium may be further reduced; your doctor should monitor your blood levels of potassium.

Tablets Take one or two tablets three or four times a day. Modified-release tablets are longer-acting and need only be taken twice a day.

Over 65 If unwanted effects are troublesome you may need less than the adult dose, e.g. half the usual dose for the tablets.

Interactions with other medicines

Other adrenaline-like drugs enhance the effects of salbutamol, increasing the risk of unwanted effects.

Unwanted effects

Likely Fine tremor of the hands, headache, restlessness, anxiety, palpitations.
Less likely Muscle cramps, allergic reactions.

Contact your doctor if any of the likely symptoms are severe or if you have palpitations, muscle cramps or allergic reactions.

Similar preparations

BAMBEC – Tablets
BAMBUTEROL

BRICANYL – Inhaler, dry powder inhaler (Turbohaler), tablets, modified-release tablets, liquid, injection, nebuliser solution
TERBUTALINE

FORADIL – Dry powder inhaler
FORMOTEROL (EFORMOTEROL)

MONOVENT – Liquid
TERBUTALINE

OXIS – Dry powder inhaler (Turbohaler)
FORMOTEROL (EFORMOTEROL)

SEREVENT – Inhaler, dry powder inhaler (Accuhaler, Diskhaler)
SALMETEROL

Poor choice: Preparations of the following are less safe and more likely to cause unwanted effects
EPHEDRINE; ORCIPRENALINE (Alupent)

From a pharmacy
CAM – Liquid
EPHEDRINE

Theophylline preparations

Theophylline and related medicines have a direct relaxing effect on the muscles surrounding the air passages. They are bronchodilators that relieve the symptoms of asthma and can be added at steps 3–5 of the management scheme (page 159). The longer-acting modified-release preparations can be useful to control night-time symptoms and early-morning wheezing.

Theophylline has a narrow therapeutic range: the margin between helpful and harmful effects is small and blood tests may be needed to monitor levels in your body. There is also considerable variation between people's responses to the drug, particularly smokers and those with impaired liver function or heart failure in whom its effects are prolonged. Furthermore, theophylline interacts with a number of other drugs – its effects are either enhanced or reduced, so medicines containing it need to be used with your doctor's or pharmacist's guidance. It may be added to small doses of a $beta_2$-agonist to enhance the bronchodilator effect, but the risk of unwanted effects, including feeling sick, digestive disorders, effects on the heart rhythm, headache and sleeplessness, may increase.

Aminophylline, a more soluble form of theophylline, is used occasionally by injection to treat severe attacks of asthma.

THEOPHYLLINE

On prescription/from a pharmacy
NUELIN – Liquid, tablets, modified-release tablets
SLO-PHYLLIN – Modified-release capsules
UNIPHYLLIN CONTINUS – Modified-release tablets

Poor choice: From a pharmacy
Combination preparations – ingredients better used separately; also contain ephedrine, considered less safe (page 162)
FRANOL/FRANOL PLUS – Tablets
THEOPHYLLINE + EPHEDRINE
DO-DO Chesteze – Tablets
THEOPHYLLINE + EPHEDRINE + CAFFEINE

Theophylline is related to caffeine in tea and coffee and theobromine in chocolate. It relaxes the air passages in the lungs and stimulates breathing and the heart rate, but cannot be used for immediate relief of asthmatic symptoms. It is added to other asthma treatments only when further control of chronic symptoms is needed. A related preparation, aminophylline, may be used by injection to treat acute severe asthma. The margin between helpful and harmful effects is narrow. Blood tests are usually needed to monitor theophylline levels and are essential if aminophylline injection is added to existing treatment with theophylline taken by mouth.

Before you use this medicine

Tell your doctor if you are:
☐ a regular smoker ☐ a heavy drinker ☐ pregnant –- may cause irritability and breathing disturbance in the newborn ☐ breast-feeding –- may cause irritability

in infant (modified-release preparation preferred) □ taking any other medicines, including vitamins and those bought over the counter.

Tell your doctor if you have or have had:
□ liver disease □ irregular heartbeat □ peptic ulcer □ high blood pressure □ heart disease □ overactive thyroid □ prolonged fever □ epilepsy □ porphyria □ an allergy to caffeine or theobromine.

How to use this medicine

Tablets or liquid Take three or four times daily, after meals.
Modified-release preparations Take once or twice a day; swallow whole with plenty of water and do not chew or crush. The granules in the capsule preparation (Slo-Phyllin) can be removed and sprinkled on soft food such as yoghurt, which is useful for children. Do not change brands or dosage forms without checking with your doctor or pharmacist. If you leave hospital after your condition is stabilised with a particular brand, make sure you know the name of the theophylline preparation. Use a medicine record sheet to note details.

Do not use more often or in a higher dose than that prescribed by your doctor. Do not take several theophylline preparations together and always check with your doctor before using any theophylline-containing medicine, such as an over-the-counter product. Keep off charcoal-broiled foods and drinks containing caffeine, such as coffee, tea, chocolate, cocoa and colas. Alcohol and smoking may increase the need for theophylline, so discuss the dose with your doctor.

Do not stop taking this medicine suddenly without discussing treatment with your doctor. If you miss a dose, take it as soon as you remember, but skip it if it is almost time for your next dose. Do not take double the dose.

Over 65 You may need less than the normal adult dose.

Interactions with other medicines

Theophylline interacts with many medicines. Check with your doctor and pharmacist. Low blood levels of potassium may result from treatment combined with high doses of beta$_2$-agonists. If you take theophylline with a beta$_2$-agonist such as **salbutamol** or **terbutaline** in high doses, your doctor should monitor your blood levels of potassium and theophylline.

Theophylline's effects are enhanced by:
Antibacterials ciprofloxacin, norfloxacin, clarithromycin, erythromycin, isoniazid
Antidepressant fluvoxamine (avoid use together)
Antifungals fluconazole, ketoconazole
Antiplatelet drug ticlopidine
Calcium channel blockers diltiazem, verapamil and possibly other calcium channel blockers
Ulcer-healing cimetidine.

Theophylline's effects are reduced by:
Antidepressants St John's wort (avoid use together)
Antiepileptics carbamazepine, phenobarbital, primidone, phenytoin; also **theophylline** possibly reduces the effect of phenytoin
Antituberculosis medicine rifampicin
Antiviral ritonavir.

Unwanted effects

Likely Feeling or being sick, headache, digestive disorders.
Less likely Palpitations, irregular heartbeat, sleeplessness, diarrhoea. Contact your doctor if you feel unwell when taking a theophylline preparation. The margin between helpful and harmful effects is narrow and your doctor should monitor blood theophylline levels.

Similar preparations

On prescription/from a pharmacy
AMINOPHYLLINE – Tablets, injection (prescription-only)
PHYLLOCONTIN CONTINUS – Modified-release tablets
AMINOPHYLLINE

Combination preparations

Combination bronchodilator medicines are poor choices. These include Duovent, Franol, Franol Plus and Aerocrom. The ingredients are better taken as individual medicines (unless this is difficult for you); also the dose of each ingredient cannot be adjusted to suit different people.

MEDICINES WHICH PREVENT ASTHMA

Three main types of medicines can help to prevent asthmatic symptoms – corticosteroids, cromoglicate and related preparations, and leukotriene receptor antagonists.

Corticosteroids

Corticosteroids, sometimes called 'steroids', reduce both inflammation of the air passages and the production of extra fluid and mucus. They have been used to treat asthma for many years and are very effective. You may be concerned about having to take a corticosteroid because of the adverse effects of this group of medicines. However, inhaling a corticosteroid directly into the lungs is effective in very small doses and the drug has a local effect (like smoothing a cream directly on to a skin complaint), so that little of it is absorbed into the body. Unwanted effects are rarely a problem at low doses, but hoarseness and a fungal infection, thrush (candidiasis) can occur in the mouth or throat and particularly at higher doses. The corticosteroids used include **beclometasone**, **budesonide** and **fluticasone** –– all appear to be equally effective.

An inhaled corticosteroid is a very important treatment if you need to use an inhaled bronchodilator more than once a day, have night-time symptoms, a flare-up of symptoms or impaired lung function. The inhaled corticosteroid must be used regularly because it takes time to work (between three and seven days), and will not relieve sudden wheeziness or breathlessness. Conversely, corticosteroid treatment should not be stopped abruptly. The dose of corticosteroid must be tailored to you individually, sufficient to control your symptoms, and then stepped up or down as necessary. If you start **beclometasone** or **budesonide** (see Step 2, page 158) by metered-dose inhaler a typical dose might be 200 micrograms twice daily for adults and young people aged 16 years and over, and 100 micrograms twice daily for children. **Fluticasone** provides similar therapeutic activity to the other two drugs but at half the dosage for adults and children, that is 100 micrograms and 50 micrograms respectively. Some corticosteroid inhalers are available in high doses for those people who might otherwise have to take corticosteroid tablets. The risk of unwanted effects occurring throughout the body (*systemic*), such as adrenal suppression (page 333), increases for all three of the corticosteroids as the inhaled dose increases. Children are particularly at risk from adrenal suppression and slowed growth and need careful and regular checking. Fluticasone has been associated particularly with these risks, possibly because higher than recommended doses have been used in some cases. Occasionally, short courses of high-dose corticosteroid tablets may be necessary if symptoms increase and are not controlled by your usual medicines. High doses, in tablets, by injection or both, may be needed during a severe acute attack of asthma, which should be treated in hospital. Short courses of tablets rarely cause adverse effects, but the risk of systemic effects increases on long-term tablets or frequent courses.

One of the newer combination inhalers containing a corticosteroid and a long-acting bronchodilator – **fluticasone + salmeterol** (Seretide) or **budesonide + formoterol** (Symbicort) – may be useful if your asthma symptoms are stabilised with the fixed doses in these preparations. Both the corticosteroid and bronchodilator are used twice daily as single medicines, so that the combination is more logical than for some older products. A fixed-dose combination may help you to take both medicines regularly and reduce the number of different inhaler devices that you need, which means that you pay only one prescription charge for the combination. However, these fixed-dose combination products do not allow you to tailor the dose of each medicine to your symptoms, particularly the corticosteroid component, which should be stepped up or down according to symptom control.

BECLOMETASONE

BECLOMETASONE inhaler, dry powder inhaler, dry powder in capsules (Cyclohaler), nasal spray
AEROBEC – Breath-actuated inhaler, high-dose inhaler (Autohaler)
ASMABEC CLICKHALER – Dry powder inhaler, high-dose inhaler
BECLOFORTE – High-dose inhaler
BECODISKS – Dry powder inhaler (Diskhaler)
BECONASE (for allergic symptoms) – Nasal spray
BECOTIDE – Inhaler
BECLAZONE EASI-BREATHE – Inhaler, high-dose inhaler
QVAR – Inhaler, breath-actuated inhaler (Autohaler) (all CFC-free)

Useful devices
BABYHALER (not NHS)
VOLUMATIC – spacer

From a pharmacy
BECLOMETASONE e.g. Beclogen, Nasobec Hayfever, Pollenase Hayfever, Vivabec and stores' own brands, e.g. Boots Hayfever Relief
BECONASE ALLERGY

Beclometasone (beclomethasone) is a corticosteroid used for the prevention of asthma when a bronchodilator reliever does not fully control symptoms. In the lungs, it reduces inflammation of the air passages, as well as production of fluid and phlegm. On the skin it is used for severe inflammatory conditions such as eczema. Beclometasone nasal spray (on prescription or over the counter) helps the symptoms of an itchy, blocked nose in the hay fever season or due to perennial rhinitis. For maximum benefit beclometasone must be used regularly. Relief of symptoms may not begin for three to seven days after the start of treatment and may take four weeks to reach full effect. The drug is used locally in very small doses and there are few local unwanted effects. **Budesonide**, **fluticasone** and **mometasone** are similar.

Before you use this medicine

Tell your doctor if you are:
☐ pregnant or breast-feeding ☐ taking any other medicines, including vitamins and those bought over the counter.

Tell your doctor if you have or have had:
☐ tuberculosis of the lung ☐ viral, bacterial or fungal infections ☐ nasal disorders or surgery.

How to use this medicine

Inhaler Use regularly twice a day, in the morning and evening as directed. If your asthma symptoms are not controlled by lower-dose corticosteroid inhalers, using a high-dose inhaler may avoid the need to take a corticosteroid by mouth for long periods. If you are taking a regular dose of over 1,500 micrograms a day, some suppression of the body's adrenal function can occur (page 333). You should therefore carry a 'steroid card' and may need extra corticosteroid treatment (a short course of tablets) during periods of stress, such as an operation or an episode of infection. You may need to have a reserve supply of tablets.
Nasal spray Apply two puffs into each nostril in the morning and evening. When symptoms are controlled you may be able to reduce the dose to one puff twice a day.
Cream/ointment Apply thinly to the affected area twice daily. Beclometasone is a potent corticosteroid (for further information on the use of corticosteroid skin preparations see pages 432–5).

Do not stop taking this medicine suddenly without discussing treatment with your doctor. It may be possible to step down treatment but only with guidance from your doctor (see 'Stepwise approach to treatment', page 158). Do not use more often or in a higher dose than that prescribed by your doctor. If you miss a dose, take it as soon as you remember, but skip it if it is almost time for your next dose. Do not take double the dose.

Over 65 No special requirements.

Unwanted effects

Likely with inhaler Hoarseness or huskiness of the voice – if this persists you should tell your doctor.

An inhaled corticosteroid sometimes causes a sore throat due to a fungal infection (thrush) which can be treated with an antifungal drug. Rinsing your mouth out with water after inhalation can be helpful. Using a spacer with an aerosol inhaler helps the corticosteroid to reach the lungs and lessens fungal infections. If you use an aerosol inhaler and your daily corticosteroid dose is 1,000 micrograms or more, you should use a spacer. This reduces unwanted absorption of beclometasone into the body. Some absorption from the lungs can occur with **fluticasone** and also **budesonide**.

Likely with nasal spray Sometimes sneezing attacks immediately after using the aerosol, drying and crusting inside the nose and sometimes bleeding. This can be reduced by pointing the spray away from the nasal septum. You should ask the doctor or pharmacist to show you how to operate the nasal aerosol.

Similar preparations

▼ASMANEX – Dry powder inhaler (Twisthaler)
MOMETASONE

BETNESOL – Drops (for eye, ear or nose)
BETAMETHASONE

BUDESONIDE – Dry powder in capsules (Cyclohaler), nasal spray

▼EVOHALER – inhaler (CFC-free)
FLUTICASONE

FLIXONASE – Nasal spray, nasal drops
FLUTICASONE

FLIXOTIDE – Inhaler, dry powder inhaler (Accuhaler, Diskhaler), nebuliser solution
FLUTICASONE

NASOCORT – Nasal spray
TRIAMCINOLONE (also from a pharmacy)

NASONEX – Nasal spray
MOMETASONE

PULMICORT – Inhaler, dry powder inhaler (Turbohaler), nebuliser solution
BUDESONIDE

RHINOCORT AQUA – Nasal aerosol
BUDESONIDE

SERETIDE Inhaler, dry powder inhaler (Accuhaler, Diskhaler)
FLUTICASONE + SALMETEROL

SYMBICORT – Dry powder inhaler (Turbohaler)
BUDESONIDE + FORMOTEROL

SYNTARIS – Nasal spray
FLUNISOLIDE

VISTA-METHASONE – Drops (for the eye, ear or nose)
BETAMETHASONE

Poor choice: combination with a decongestant

DEXA-RHINASPRAY DUO – Nasal spray
DEXAMETHASONE + TRAMAZOLINE

Cromoglicate (cromoglycate) and related preparations

Sodium cromoglicate (Intal, Cromogen and Aerocrom) inhibits the release of body chemicals involved in allergic reactions. It also helps to prevent narrowing of the airways. It may be useful if asthma has an allergic basis, but does not help everyone. Sodium cromoglicate can only prevent an asthma attack and help exercise-induced asthma if inhaled half an hour beforehand. It is no use for relieving symptoms and acute attacks of asthma. Sodium cromoglicate is also used to prevent allergic nose and eye symptoms associated with hay fever (see below), and is taken by mouth occasionally for food allergy (Nalcrom). **Nedocromil** (Tilade) is similar to sodium cromoglicate for preventing asthma.

Leukotriene receptor antagonists

Montelukast (Singulair) and **zafirlukast** (Accolate) block the production of chemicals called leukotrienes in the airways, which are involved in the development of an asthma attack. They are taken by mouth and can be used alone or added to an inhaled corticosteroid when asthma symptoms need further control (Steps 3-5, page 159). The leukotriene receptor antagonists appear to have an additive effect with an inhaled corticosteroid, but taking one of these medicines with an inhaled corticosteroid does not necessarily allow you to reduce the dose of the corticosteroid. A leukotriene receptor antagonist can be used for exercise-induced asthma and may help if you have asthma and rhinitis. They are less effective in severe asthma and do not relieve acute asthma attacks. Montelukast tablets are available for adults and children and zafirlukast tablets for adults and children aged 12 and over.

Unwanted effects of leukotriene receptor antagonists include disturbances of the digestive system, headache, dry mouth and rarely allergic reactions (hypersensitivity). Chest infections can develop, particularly in older people. Montelukast can cause problems with sleep (insomnia, vivid dreams) and zafirlukast increases the risk of liver disorder. You should contact your doctor if you feel sick or are sick persistently, feel generally unwell or develop jaundice whilst taking zafirlukast. A rare syndrome or cluster of symptoms that appears together (the Churg-Strauss syndrome) is associated with the use of either of these medicines usually with corticosteroid tablets, following the reduction or withdrawal of corticosteroid treatment. You should contact your doctor if you develop skin rash, heart problems, tingling and numbness in the hands and feet and breathing problems worsen.

OTHER TREATMENTS

Antihistamines such as **ketotifen** (Zaditen) ought in theory to be helpful in treating asthma because of their anti-allergic action. In practice, antihistamines are disappointing in the treatment of asthma; they are poor choices and are not much used. Some people with asthma claim to benefit from the use of ionisers, acupuncture, homoeopathy and other forms of complementary treatment. The evidence is anecdotal and clinical trials have so far been disappointing. If you decide to try any of these treatments, you must continue to take any medicines prescribed by your doctor.

Chronic obstructive pulmonary disease

Chronic obstructive pulmonary disease (COPD) describes conditions such as chronic bronchitis, emphysema and small airways disease. Chronic bronchitis occurs when the cells lining the air passages produce excess mucus. This leads to long-term coughing, usually producing phlegm. Emphysema is the enlargement of the air sacs (*alveoli*) beyond the air passages. The walls of the air sacs break down, leading to breathlessness with or without a cough (page 182). These conditions, sometimes also called chronic obstructive airways or lung disease, were thought to be distinct and separate, but now research has shown that they occur together in people to a greater or lesser extent. Sometimes there is wheezing but the narrowing of the airways is not as reversible as with asthma. Some people may have mild chronic obstructive pulmonary disease with little more than cough and phlegm, but for others the condition is progressive and life-threatening. Chronic obstructive pulmonary disease is almost always the end result of years of cigarette smoking. Pollution and occupational hazards such as dusts or chemical fumes and hereditary factors may also contribute in a small way to the condition.

Cough and breathlessness are typical symptoms of chronic obstructive pulmonary disease, but your doctor or nurse may also ask you to blow out hard into a spirometer to measure your lung function. The measure, forced expiratory volume in one second (FEV_1) together with peak flow rates (page 157) measure the deterioration in the lungs and airflow limitations. The spirometer is also used to assess your response to an inhaled bronchodilator to which some people respond. Stopping smoking (page 156) is the most important factor in helping to reduce the rate of decline in lung function.

– HOW YOU CAN HELP YOURSELF –

- ☐ It is never too late to give up smoking – the condition of the lungs improves from the moment you stop.
- ☐ If you are overweight, lose weight. Carrying extra weight means that the heart and lungs have to work harder.
- ☐ Avoid smoky atmospheres and sudden changes of temperature; never go out in fog.
- ☐ Exercise within your capabilities. This will improve your general well-being.
- ☐ Always get chest infections treated promptly.

Medicines for chronic obstructive pulmonary disease

Medicines cannot halt the decline in lung function, but can help symptoms, such as breathlessness. Treatment involves bronchodilators, such as inhaled **salbutamol** and a longer-acting antimuscarinic bronchodilator, such as **ipratropium** (Atrovent). Depending on your symptoms, your doctor may suggest using a salbutamol inhaler when required and add ipratropium or similar inhaler if symptoms need further control. A combination inhaler of **salbutamol + ipratropium** (Combivent) may be useful only if you need regular bronchodilator treatment with both medicines. The usefulness of inhaled corticosteroids in chronic obstructive pulmonary disease is less certain. In people with advanced disease a corticosteroid such as **beclometasone**, inhaled or by mouth, may be given to reduce the frequency of exacerbations – a sustained worsening of symptoms that requires a change in your usual treatment.

Bronchial problems fluctuate and a worsening with increased amounts of phlegm which is green/yellow in colour or smelling may indicate infection and require treatment with an antibiotic, such as **amoxicillin** or **erythromycin**. Bronchodilator treatment may need to be increased, and your doctor may prescribe a short course of a corticosteroid by mouth.

Antimuscarinic bronchodilators

These block the nerve chemicals that control muscle contraction, which allows the air passages to open up. **Ipratropium** (Atrovent), **oxitropium** (Oxivent) and **tiotropium** (▼ Spiriva) are antimuscarinic drugs used by inhalation to relieve blocked airways, and are helpful for chronic obstructive pulmonary disease. Ipratropium by nebuliser may be added to beta$_2$-agonist treatment for acute severe or life-threatening asthma. Oxitropium is similar to ipratropium, whilst tiotropium is longer-acting and can be used once a day.

IPRATROPIUM

IPRATROPIUM – Nebuliser solution
ATROVENT – Inhalers, breath-actuated inhaler (Autohaler), dry powder inhaler (Aerocaps), nebuliser solution
RESPONTIN – Nebuliser solution
RINATEC – Nasal spray

Poor choice: combination product does not allow flexibility of dosage
DUOVENT
IPRATROPIUM + FENOTEROL

Ipratropium relieves tightened air passages by relaxing the muscles that form part of the bronchioles. It is used mainly to treat chronic bronchitis where airway obstruction is reversible. Ipratropium is used only by inhalation and little is absorbed into the body. It starts to act slowly, with the optimum effect occurring within half to one hour, and continues to work for three to six hours. The inhaler is used three to four times daily for long-term rather than rapid relief. Ipratropium nasal spray can help to dry a runny nose caused by perennial non-allergic rhinitis.

Before you use this medicine

Tell your doctor if you are:
☐ pregnant or breast-feeding ☐ taking any other medicines, including vitamins and those bought over the counter.

Tell your doctor if you have or have had:
☐ glaucoma ☐ prostate disorders ☐ bladder problems ☐ sensitivity to atropine or to soya lecithin, soya beans, peanuts. Both types of inhaler contain soya lecithin, but not the dry powder capsules.

How to use this medicine

Inhaler Use one or two puffs three or four times a day as directed. Your doctor will usually suggest a trial period of inhaled ipratropium with peak flow measurements (page 157) before prescribing a long-term course.
Nasal spray Use one or two puffs in the affected nostril up to four times a day. You may use a lower dose once symptoms are controlled.

For both preparations do not use more often or in a higher dose than that prescribed by your doctor. If you miss a dose, take it as soon as you remember, but skip it if it is almost time for the next dose. Do not take double the dose. Do not stop taking this medicine suddenly without discussing treatment with your doctor.

Over 65 You may be more sensitive to ipratropium than younger people.

Unwanted effects

Likely with inhaler Dry mouth, headache, feeling or being sick.
Likely with nasal spray Dry nose.
Less likely with inhaler Difficulty passing urine, constipation.
Less likely with nebulised solution Accidental contact with eyes may cause eye pain or discomfort, blurred vision, visual haloes or red eyes which are signs of acute closed-angle glaucoma. Contact your doctor immediately.
Less likely with nasal spray Stuffiness, irritation, burning sensation, bleeding.

If any unwanted effects are severe, discuss them with your doctor.

Similar preparations

OXIVENT – Inhaler, breath-actuated inhaler (Autohaler)
OXITROPIUM

▼SPIRIVA – Dry powder capsules for inhalation with Handihaler device
TIOTROPIUM

Allergies and hay fever

Allergy or *hypersensitivity* means that the body's immune system reacts excessively to an **allergen** – a harmless substance, usually a protein, which the immune system mistakes for an invading organism, such as a bacterium or a virus. When one of these foreign substances first gets into the body, white cells (*lymphocytes*) in the blood produce *antibodies*, which attach themselves to 'mast' cells, another type of white blood cell. When the same foreign substance enters the body for a second time it binds to the antibodies made on the first visit. This process causes the mast cells to release chemicals including histamine into the bloodstream. These chemicals help to destroy invading organisms and are an important defence mechanism in protecting the body from infection.

When the body responds to an allergen, the reaction is caused mainly by the effects of excess histamine, which acts at many places in the body on two types of cell receptor: H_1 and H_2. H_1-receptors are found in the skin, nose, blood vessels and airways; H_2-receptors are in the stomach lining, salivary and tear glands. *Antihistamines* block H_1-receptors to prevent the symptoms of allergic disorders. (H_2-receptor antagonists are used for healing peptic ulcers – page 66.) **Sodium cromoglicate** inhibits the release of chemicals from the mast cells. *Corticosteroids* reduce inflammation both internally and externally.

There are four common types of allergic disorder, ranging from anaphylactic reactions – type I hypersensitivity – to type IV – for example, contact dermatitis. The severity of an allergy can vary from person to person. Some people have mild symptoms occasionally while others may be severely affected, as in anaphylactic shock (see below). Many substances can cause more than one type of response in any person.

Hay fever

Typical symptoms of hay fever are runny nose and eyes, blocked nose, sneezing, itchy eyes, nose and palate and a tickle at the back of the throat. Hay fever (*seasonal allergic rhinitis*) is commonly caused by allergens in the air – tree and grass pollens, moulds, dust, animal feathers and hairs. Some people suffer from a runny, blocked nose all the year round. This is known as *perennial allergic rhinitis* and one of the common causes is the house dust mite. Not all perennial rhinitis is caused by allergens: *vasomotor rhinitis* appears to be a fault in the nervous control of the blood supply to the nose and results in a blocked and sometimes runny nose.

Skin allergies (urticaria)

A skin reaction can occur when something you eat disagrees with you: common allergens range from shellfish to strawberries to medicines such as aspirin. If your skin comes into contact with certain chemicals, such as household cleaners, soap powder, cosmetics or metals, these can cause rashes (*contact dermatitis*). Insect bites and stings also cause allergic reactions.

Asthma

Asthma can be triggered by exposure to allergens (page 174). Although the release of histamine plays a part in tightening the airways, other factors are involved in asthma and antihistamines are disappointing in the treatment of asthma symptoms.

Anaphylaxis

Anaphylaxis or anaphylactic shock is a rare and potentially fatal allergic response and needs emergency treatment. The signs are sudden, generalised itching and swelling around the mouth and throat, rapidly followed by breathing difficulties and extremely low blood pressure. Anaphylaxis can occur as a response to certain foods, such as eggs, shellfish and peanuts; to additives in foods and medicines; to some medicines, such as antibiotics, vaccines, arthritis medicines and hyposensitising preparations designed to treat allergies; and also to bee or wasp stings. The reaction is more likely to happen in someone who is already sensitive (*atopic*). The reaction may become increasingly severe with repeated exposure. If you have severe reactions (*hypersensitivity*) to something such as food or insect stings you should see your doctor to discuss the possibility of carrying an emergency supply of **adrenaline** (epinephrine) when you expect to be most at risk.

Medicines for allergies

Allergic symptoms such as hay fever may be treated locally with nose sprays or eye drops or systematically by medicines taken into the body. Treatment will depend on whether you are mildly affected throughout the season, for only a few days a year or suffer severe symptoms during the summer months.

LOCAL PREPARATIONS

Eye drops with an antihistamine and a decongestant (**antazoline** with **xylometazoline**; Otrivine-Antistin) may help allergic symptoms, but only for a short time. Nose drops and an eye preparation can be bought over the counter or your doctor may prescribe them for immediate symptom relief for a few days before medicines taken to prevent hay fever symptoms start to work.

Nasal symptoms alone are best treated with **sodium cromoglicate** or a corticosteroid (for example **beclometasone**) in the nose during the hay fever season. Either preparation must be used regularly to prevent symptoms. Starting treatment about a month before the hay fever season will 'prime' the nose to cope better.

SODIUM CROMOGLICATE

Inhaler, nebuliser solution, eye drops
CROMOGEN (for asthma) – Inhaler
HAY-CROM (for allergic symptoms) – Eye drops
INTAL (for asthma) – Inhaler (spacer devices Fisonair, Syncroner), dry powder inhaler (Spincaps), nebuliser solution
NALCROM (for food allergy) – Capsules
OPTICROM (for allergic symptoms) – Eye drops
RYNACROM (for allergic symptoms) – Nasal spray
VIVIDRIN (for allergic symptoms) – Eye drops, nasal spray

Poor choice: ingredients better used separately
AEROCROM
SODIUM CROMOGLICATE + SALBUTAMOL
RYNACROM COMPOUND
SODIUM CROMOGLICATE + XYLOMETAZOLINE

From a pharmacy
SODIUM CROMOGLICATE – Eye drops (e.g. Clariteyes, Opticrom Allergy, Vivicrom)
VIVIDRIN – Nasal spray
SODIUM CROMOGLICATE

Poor choice:
RYNACROM ALLERGY – Nasal spray
SODIUM CROMOGLICATE + XYLOMETAZOLINE

Sodium cromoglicate inhibits the release of body chemicals involved in allergic reaction. It also helps to prevent narrowing of the airways caused by exercise, cold air and chemicals. Sodium cromoglicate must be taken regularly and can only prevent symptoms, not provide instant relief. It may take from a few days up to six weeks to have an effect.

Before you use this medicine

Tell your doctor if you are:
☐ pregnant or breast-feeding ☐ taking any other medicines, including vitamins and those bought over the counter.

How to use this medicine

Inhaler Use two puffs of the aerosol inhaler or one capsule in the Spinhaler four to eight times a day.
Nasal spray Use one spray to each nostril four to six times daily.
Eye drops Apply one or two drops into each eye four times a day.
For food allergy (with dietary restriction) Take two capsules four times daily before meals. Children take a lower dose. Powder from the capsules can be dissolved in a little very hot water and then cold water added before drinking.

Storage and disposal Capsules containing powder must be kept in a cool, dry place to stop moisture getting in. Once opened, the eye drops may become contaminated with bacteria as you use them: throw any remaining drops away after four weeks.

Over 65 No special requirements.

Interactions with other medicines

Eye drops contain a preservative, benzalkonium chloride, and should not be used with soft contact lenses.

Unwanted effects

Likely with inhaler Throat irritation, cough.
Likely with nasal spray Irritation of the nose and sneezing, which usually lessens as you continue treatment.
Less likely with capsules Feeling sick, skin rashes, joint pain.
Less likely with inhaler The dry powder sometimes causes wheezing and breathlessness. If this happens, contact your doctor. Inhaling a beta$_2$-agonist a few minutes before sodium cromoglicate may help to overcome this.

Stop taking capsules if you develop a skin rash; see your doctor.

Similar preparations

RAPITIL (for allergic conjunctivitis) – Eye drops
NEDOCROMIL SODIUM

TILADE (for asthma) – Inhaler
NEDOCROMIL SODIUM

Corticosteroids

Corticosteroids (steroids) have a powerful anti-inflammatory effect. Nose sprays can help to control nasal symptoms of hay fever during the season. They should be started two or three weeks before the pollen season because their effect takes time to develop; they will not give immediate relief. They must be used regularly, usually twice daily. **Beclometasone** (Beconase), **betamethasone** (Betnesol, Vista-Methasone), **budesonide** (Rhinocort Aqua), **flunisolide** (Syntaris), **fluticasone** (Flixonase), **mometasone** (Nasonex) and **triamcinolone** (Nasacort) all have similar effects on symptoms – pages 167–170. Corticosteroids should not be used in the eye for hay fever symptoms.

ANTIHISTAMINES

If you have more widespread hay fever symptoms, such as itching of the mouth and ears as well as nose and eye symptoms, an antihistamine is usually helpful. An oral antihistamine can be used to treat symptoms throughout the season or an attack lasting a few days. Oral antihistamines are also used to treat allergic skin rashes, itchy skin (*pruritus*), insect bites and stings and drug allergies. Antihistamine creams or lotions applied to the skin to treat rashes, itchy skin or insect bites are marginally effective and may cause sensitivity reactions. The nasal sprays **azelastine** (Rhinolast) and **levocabastine** (Livostin) are also used for allergic rhinitis, but may cause irritation of the nasal membranes.

Widely advertised combination preparations of an antihistamine and a decongestant that are available over the counter should not be used to relieve hay fever symptoms because the decongestant is a *sympathomimetic*, a drug with adrenaline-like activity, which can cause serious unwanted effects (see 'Cold remedies', page 184).

Older sedating antihistamines

All of these have similar effects and there is no evidence that one preparation is better than another. People vary widely in their response to antihistamines, so you must find one that suits you. Most antihistamines work for a short time in the body and must be taken twice or even three or four times a day. Others, such as **promethazine**, are longer-acting and can be taken at night so that the effects last through the next day. Drowsiness (sedation) is the main unwanted effect; some of these older type antihistamines cause more drowsiness than others, but all do so to some extent. Performance is likely to be impaired, increasing the likelihood of work-related injuries or accidents when driving.

Other unwanted effects include dry mouth, blurred vision and inability to pass urine, which may be troublesome for some people. Antihistamines can be bought in a pharmacy – **chlorphenamine** (chlorpheniramine) and **brompheniramine** are effective and inexpensive. If you need to take an antihistamine for longer periods, such as throughout the hay fever season, your doctor can also prescribe them.

CHLORPHENAMINE

On prescription/from a pharmacy
CHLORPHENAMINE – Tablets, liquid, injection (prescription only)
PIRITON – Tablets, liquid

Not recommended
Over-the-counter preparations containing chlorphenamine with a decongestant:
CONTAC 400; DRISTAN; HAYMINE

Chlorphenamine is an antihistamine which reduces allergic symptoms such as swelling, inflammation, itchiness and runny nose and eyes. It is used to treat hay fever and other forms of rhinitis, nettle rash (*urticaria*), skin rashes caused by medicines or food, itchy skin (*pruritus*) and allergic swelling (*angioedema*). The injection, on prescription only, is used for acute allergies and as a supplementary medicine for the emergency treatment of anaphylactic shock.

Before you use this medicine

Tell your doctor if you are:
☐ pregnant or breast-feeding ☐ taking any other medicines, especially a tricyclic antidepressant, a monoamine-oxidase inhibitor antidepressant or the anti-epileptic phenytoin, and including vitamins and those bought over the counter.

Tell your doctor if you have or have had:
☐ asthma ☐ glaucoma ☐ difficulty passing urine ☐ enlarged prostate ☐ liver disease ☐ epilepsy ☐ kidney disease.

How to use this medicine

Take the tablets or syrup three or four times a day. The syrup can be given to young children, but at lower than the adult dose.

Until you know how you react to chlorphenamine, do not drive, operate machinery or do other activities that require alertness. Avoid alcohol as chlorphenamine enhances its effects.

If you miss a dose, take it as soon as you remember, but skip it if it is almost time for your next dose. Do not take double the dose.

Over 65 Less than the usual adult dose may be necessary. Older people are more sensitive to the unwanted effects. These include confusion, short-term memory problems and impaired attention as well as antimuscarinic effects – dry mouth, blurred vision, difficulty passing urine (especially for a man with an enlarged prostate gland), worsening of glaucoma, and sexual difficulties.

Interactions with other medicines

Sedatives and anti-anxiety drugs enhance the effects of chlorphenamine. **Antimuscarinic drugs**, such as the tricyclic antidepressants **amitriptyline** and **imipramine**, and **monoamine-oxidase inhibitors** (pages 206–7) increase the antimuscarinic effects of chlorphenamine (see **Over 65**). **Phenytoin** (an anti-epileptic) may build up to toxic levels.

Unwanted effects

Likely Drowsiness.
Less likely Headache, inability to concentrate, gastrointestinal disturbances (feeling or being sick, diarrhoea), dizziness, anti-muscarinic effects (see **Over 65**), **in high doses:** over-excitement in children and older people.

If any of the less likely effects occur and are severe, contact your doctor.

Similar preparations

On prescription/from a pharmacy

DIMOTANE – Tablets, liquid
BROMPHENIRAMINE

PERIACTIN – Tablets
CYPROHEPTADINE

PHENERGAN – Tablets, liquid, injection (prescription only)
PROMETHAZINE

TAVEGIL – Tablets, liquid
CLEMASTINE

Prescription-only

ATARAX – Tablets
HYDROXYZINE

UCERAX – Tablets (not NHS), liquid
HYDROXYZINE

VALLERGAN – Tablets, liquid
ALIMEMAZINE

Newer non-sedating antihistamines

These cause much less drowsiness than the older ones – a major advantage – but although drowsiness is rare your ability to drive a car or operate machinery may be affected. Alcohol intake should be kept low. **Loratadine**, **cetirizine** (Zirtek), **fexofenadine** (Telfast) **desloratadine** (▼Neoclarityn), **levocetirizine** (▼Xyzal) and **mizolastine** (Mizollen) are equally effective. Desloratadine and levocetirizine are very similar (*isomers*) to loratadine and cetirizine respectively but are no more effective. Fexofenadine is a metabolite of terfenadine, but is not associated with irregular heart beats. Fexofenadine, mizolastine, levocetirizine and terfenadine must be prescribed.

Antihistamines and irregular heart beats

Terfenadine is an effective antihistamine but it can cause irregular heart beats which can be hazardous, particularly when the blood levels of the drug increase, for example through drug interactions, in liver disease or with low levels of body potassium. If you have existing heart irregularities, then you must not take terfenadine on its own or with medicines that also affect heart rhythm. You must not take more than the recommended dose and must avoid taking it at the same time as grapefruit juice or any of the following medicines because the combination increases the risk of hazardous heart beats: **Antibiotics erythromycin**, **clarithromycin** and similar preparations, **antifungals**, **antiarrhythmics**, **antipsychotics**, **antimalarials** (**quinine**), **antivirals**, **antidepressants**, **diuretics**, the **beta blocker sotalol**, **bicalutamide** (Casodex) and **pentamidine** (Pentacarinat).

The potential to affect heart beats does not occur with all antihistamines. Other antihistamines which may also be associated with heart rhythm disturbances include **alimemazine**, **hydroxyzine**, **promethazine** and **mizolastine**.

Many antihistamines such as **acrivastine**, **cetirizine** and **loratadine** can be bought in smaller pack sizes from a pharmacy.

LORATADINE

On prescription

LORATADINE – Tablets

CLARITYN – Liquid
LORATADINE

Loratadine reduces allergic symptoms such as swelling, inflammation, itchiness and runny nose and eyes. It is taken by mouth and is used to treat allergic rhinitis, such as hay fever, and nettle rash (urticaria). It causes much less drowsiness than the older antihistamines, although sedation may occur and can affect driving and other skilled tasks.

Before you use this medicine

Tell a doctor or pharmacist if you are:
□ pregnant or breast-feeding (avoid) □ taking any other medicines including vitamins and those bought over the counter.

Tell your doctor if you have or have had:
□ a previous reaction to loratadine.

How to use this medicine

Take the tablets with water once a day. Do not exceed the recommended dose. Do not drive or do other activities that require alertness until you know how you react to loratadine. The effects of loratadine are not increased with small amounts of alcohol, but avoid large quantities. If you miss a dose, take it as soon as you remember, but skip it if it is almost time for your next dose. Do not take double the dose.

Over 65 No special requirements.

Interactions with other medicines

Unlikely to be a problem, but **caution with:** the antibiotic **erythromycin**, **antifungals ketoconazole** and **fluconazole**, **quinidine**, **fluoxetine**, **cimetidine**.

Unwanted effects

Less likely Headache, feeling sick, fatigue.
Rare Drowsiness, fainting and/or palpitations, hair loss, allergic reactions, liver changes.

Stop taking loratadine and contact your doctor if you experience any of the rare symptoms.

Similar preparations

On prescription

CETIRIZINE – Tablets

MISTAMINE – Tablets
MIZOLASTINE

MIZOLLEN – Tablets
MIZOLASTINE

▼ NEOCLARITYN – Tablets, liquid
DESLORATADINE

TELFAST – Tablets
FEXOFENADINE

ZIRTEK – Liquid
CETIRIZINE

XYZAL – Tablets
LEVOCETIRIZINE

From a pharmacy

BENADRYL ALLERGY RELIEF – Capsules
ACRIVASTINE

BENADRYL ONE A DAY – Tablets
CETIRIZINE

PIRITEZE ALLERGY – Tablets
CETIRIZINE

ZIRTEK ALLERGY RELIEF – Tablets (not NHS)
CETIRIZINE

MEDICINES FOR SEVERE HAY FEVER

When hay fever symptoms are severe and likely to disrupt an important occasion (such as taking an exam), a short course of a corticosteroid taken by mouth, such as **prednisolone**, or by injection (**methylprednisolone** or **triamcinolone**) may be considered by your doctor.

Hyposensitisation (also known as desensitisation or immunotherapy) may help a few people with severe symptoms that cannot be controlled by other medicines. Anaphylaxis, an acute and severe allergic reaction to the desensitising vaccine, can occur. Patients with asthma appear to be particularly sensitive. Treatment should be carried out only where there are adequate facilities for resuscitation and patients should remain under medical observation for at least one hour after the injection. For adults with severe reactions to bee or wasp stings a course of venom injections may help.

Cough

The lungs clean themselves constantly so that breathing continues efficiently. Cells lining the air passages produce mucus which traps foreign substances such as smoke, chemicals or invading organisms (bacteria or viruses). Coughing helps to remove unwanted material from the lungs. A cough is therefore a natural function with a purpose, especially a productive cough which brings up phlegm (*sputum*). A dry, irritating cough that does not bring up phlegm, or a non-productive cough that may also keep you awake at night, can be a nuisance. Coughing is controlled by a signal from the brain, so a dry cough can sometimes be relieved by a medicine which reduces the cough reflex.

Coughing may be a temporary nuisance or it may indicate that there is a more serious disorder of the lungs. You should consult your doctor if:

- ☐ you cough up green or yellow mucus or if it is foul-smelling
- ☐ you have a high temperature lasting a few days
- ☐ coughing or breathing in causes sharp chest pain
- ☐ you wheeze or have shortness or breath
- ☐ mucus contains blood
- ☐ a cough continues for longer than ten days.

A cough can be a symptom of a long-term condition such as asthma (pages 144–5), or it can signify chronic obstructive pulmonary disease (pages 171–2) or an acute inflammation of the air passages. *Acute bronchitis* is usually a viral infection, causing cough, yellow or green sputum and fever. The infection is self-limiting and will not respond to an antibiotic. Treatment consists of rest and drinking plenty of fluids.

Cough medicines

MUCOLYTICS

These contain enzymes which make mucus less sticky so that it should be easier to cough up. They may help people with chronic obstructive pulmonary disease and are prescribed as **carbocisteine** (Mucodyne) or

mecysteine (methylcysteine) (Visclair – also from a pharmacy). Drinking extra fluids, inhaling steam and postural drainage are also useful for thinning the mucus or sputum if you have chronic bronchitis.

EXPECTORANTS

A productive cough is the body's way of clearing debris from the lungs and it helps you to recover from a self-limiting condition such as a cold or flu. Expectorants are taken with the aim of thinning mucus in the lungs so that phlegm is coughed up more easily. Most expectorants are claimed to act by irritating the lining of the stomach. This causes a reflex stimulation of the nerves to the air passages in the lungs which encourages the production of mucus. This effect occurs only at high doses which would normally make you ill with nausea and vomiting. Cough medicines containing expectorants such as **ammonium chloride** and **ipecacuanha** have only small ineffective doses. Furthermore, there is no evidence that any ingredient of a cough medicine can act as an expectorant. Expectorants are of no more value than a placebo.

SOOTHING COUGH MEDICINES

These contain syrup or **glycerol** (glycerine) and may help an irritating dry cough. Your doctor can prescribe Simple Linctus BP or you can buy it cheaply over the counter. Simple Linctus Paediatric BP is particularly useful for young children, but it contains large quantities of sugar which can damage teeth; a sugar-free version is available. Similar remedies, such as glycerol, lemon and honey in hot water, can easily be prepared at home.

COUGH SUPPRESSANTS

These may reduce troublesome symptoms if you are kept awake at night or if your cough is interfering with normal activities. A cough suppressant does not shorten the course of colds, coughs and other respiratory infections. People with acute or chronic bronchitis should not take a cough suppressant because it does not help with the removal of phlegm. A cough suppressant reduces breathing control, which could be dangerous if you have asthma or chronic bronchitis.

Pholcodine, **codeine** and **dextromethorphan** are used to suppress cough but they all tend to cause constipation. Codeine and dextromethorphan are equally effective, but dextromethorphan causes fewer unwanted effects. Doctors cannot prescribe dextromethorphan on the NHS, but it is an ingredient of various preparations that can be bought at a pharmacy. Pholcodine Linctus BP may be helpful and is inexpensive. Cough suppressants should not usually be given to children, especially those under one year old.

COMPOUND COUGH MEDICINES

These are not at all helpful in the treatment of respiratory infections and lung conditions and cannot be prescribed on the NHS. As with most combination preparations the ingredients are often present in too low a dose for them to be effective. Many compound cough remedies are a therapeutic nonsense, with some of the ingredients acting in the opposite way to others. Manufacturers may claim that these remedies have a dual action of suppressing a cough and drying up mucus. This is unhelpful: if you have a productive cough with extra phlegm you need to remove it from your lungs by coughing, not drying it up. If the desire to cough (the cough reflex) is suppressed by another ingredient, phlegm remains on the lungs.

Other cough preparations have an unnecessary number of ingredients with similar actions. Some cough medicines contain an antihistamine which will also have a drying effect on phlegm and therefore will not help you to cough it up from your lungs. For people with chronic obstructive pulmonary disease an antihistamine may prevent the waste gas, carbon dioxide, leaving the lungs.

Colds

The common cold is a viral infection of the nose, throat and upper airways (upper respiratory tract). The mucous membranes become swollen and inflamed, resulting in a blocked and runny nose. Other symptoms include sneezing, sore throat, cough, mild fever and a general aching feeling.

There are a number of different cold viruses and having one cold does not give you immunity from the other viruses. A cold is spread to others by breathing out or sneezing. Colds are also spread by hands and it is a good idea to wash your hands frequently if you have a cold to prevent the virus spreading. A cold is self-limiting: it can be cured only by time. The illness has to run its course – anything from four to fourteen days. An antibiotic works against bacteria but not against viruses. Sometimes a secondary bacterial infection may develop, such as sinusitis or an ear infection, and your doctor may then prescribe an antibiotic.

Other more serious illnesses may appear similar to a cold; you should contact your doctor if you have a high fever (above 101°F; 38.3°C) with shaking chills and you are coughing up thick phlegm, or if you have a sharp chest pain when you cough or breathe deeply.

Cold remedies

No medicine can prevent or cure a cold, but many remedies are sold for the relief of symptoms. Combination preparations – cocktails of aspirin or paracetamol with decongestants, antihistamines and expectorants – cannot be recommended and should be avoided. They cause unwanted effects and do not alter the course of the cold. A nasal decongestant, aspirin or paracetamol and a single-ingredient cough syrup should be all that is needed.

NASAL DECONGESTANTS

When you have a cold the inability to breathe through your nose is uncomfortable and can aggravate a sore throat. A nasal decongestant may lessen swelling and stuffiness in the nose. **Ephedrine** nose drops 0.5 per cent, one or two drops in each nostril, are the mildest and can give relief for several hours. Nose drop preparations containing **xylometazoline** (Otrivine – not NHS), **phenylephrine** or **oxymetazoline** (not NHS: Afrazine; Sudafed; Vicks Sinex) are effective but stronger. They relieve swelling by constricting the blood vessels in the nose, but this effect can wear off, resulting in further swelling and stuffiness (rebound congestion) after a few days' use. This congestion is caused by the nose drops, not the cold.

PAIN RELIEF

Aspirin or **paracetamol** can help fever and the general aching feeling. It is important not to take more than the correct dose of paracetamol: two tablets four times a day, and no more than eight tablets in 24 hours (equivalent to 4g of paracetamol in 24 hours). If you have bought an over-the-counter cold remedy containing either aspirin or paracetamol, do not take additional aspirin or paracetamol. Unbranded aspirin or paracetamol tablets are good value compared with branded products. You should not take aspirin if you have or have had a peptic ulcer.

COUGH MEDICINES

You will not need a medicine if you have a productive cough. Steam inhalations and drinking plenty of warm liquids will help to thin mucus so that it is easier to cough up from the lungs. If a dry, irritating, non-productive cough prevents you sleeping, use a single-ingredient cough suppressant such as **pholcodine**.

HOW YOU CAN HELP YOURSELF

- ☐ Time and rest are the best healers of a common cold. If you are prone to heavy colds you may need a day in bed, but otherwise early nights are helpful.
- ☐ Drink plenty of fluids – at least eight to ten glasses a day.
- ☐ Fever is the body's way of dealing with infection, but paracetamol may help to ease aches and pains.
- ☐ Gently blow a blocked nose. Inhaling steam can ease congestion. Menthol and Eucalyptus inhalation added to a bowl of hot (not boiling) water may encourage you to inhale but does not cure the cold.
- ☐ A sore throat may be eased by sucking a boiled sweet or anything to promote saliva flow. Antiseptic lozenges sometimes cause irritation and sensitivity in the mouth and there is no evidence that these preparations are any more beneficial than a sweet.
- ☐ Gargling with warm salt water may also ease a sore throat. There is no evidence that antiseptic gargles are any more effective.
- ☐ A home-made drink of lemon juice, honey and warm water is also soothing.
- ☐ Avoid smoking.

DECONGESTANTS

The decongestant drugs used locally in the nose are also ingredients in cold and cough remedies. When taken by mouth not only do these drugs constrict blood vessels in the nose, but they also tighten blood vessels throughout the rest of the body, causing a rise in blood pressure and an increase in heart rate. Decongestants are *sympathomimetic* drugs which mimic the effects of adrenaline. They are potentially hazardous for people with high blood pressure, heart disease (angina or coronary thrombosis), and over-active thyroid (*hyperthyroidism*). Decongestants also enhance the effects of the antidepressant drugs monoamine-oxidase inhibitors and cause a dangerous rise in blood pressure if the two are used together. You should avoid preparations containing **ephedrine**, **pseudoephedrine**, **phenylephrine** or **phenylpropanolamine (PPA)**. These decongestants should be used with caution if you have glaucoma, prostatic enlargement or diabetes as they can aggravate these conditions. The Committee on Safety of Medicines (CSM) has reviewed evidence of a possible link between PPA and haemorrhagic stroke (page 144) but concluded that the association is weak. Some of the evidence came from the USA where the drug is used at higher doses and for other purposes. The CSM has therefore advised that people should take no more than 100mg a day, the maximum daily dose of PPA.

Other unwanted effects include headache, giddiness, nervousness, anxiety, palpitations, restlessness and sleeplessness. Although taking a decongestant by mouth does not cause rebound congestion in the nose, the risk of other unwanted effects is too much to make them worthwhile treatments. Preparations containing decongestants cannot be recommended. They are also combined with antihistamines in many over-the-counter cold remedies, which may cause drowsiness and affect your ability to make decisions, drive or operate machinery.

WHAT THE LABELS REALLY MEAN

What the packet may say	What it means	One or more of these drugs will be on the label	Notes	Non-drug alternative
'Aches, pain and fever'	Pain reliever	aspirin, paracetamol, ibuprofen, codeine	Relieves aches and pains, reduces fever	Stoicism is the only real alternative to using a pain reliever, or you could try a hot water bottle
'To dry up a runny nose' or 'to help you sleep'	antihistamine	diphenhydramine, promethazine, brompheniramine, chlorphenamine, triprolidine, doxylamine	Not proven to be useful in colds. Can cause drowsiness	Just let the runny nose run its course. If it's sore, use petroleum jelly to soothe skin
'For a stuffy nose'	decongestant	*Sprays/drops:* phenylephrine, oxymetazoline, xylometazoline *Tablets/capsules/liquid:* phenylephrine, phenylpropanolamine, ephedrine, pseudoephedrine	Preferable in spray or drop form, but beware rebound congestion	Try inhaling hot water vapour with aromatic oils if you like
'For a chesty cough'	expectorant	ammonium chloride, guaifenesin, ipecacuanha, squill	Not recommended – efficacy doubtful	Let the cough run its course. Keep your fluid intake up. Steam inhalation may help
'For a dry or tickly cough'	suppressant	dextromethorphan, pholcodine, codeine	Use sparingly if your sleep or work is being disturbed by your cough	Use sweets to soothe your throat. Menthol or camphor can help soothe a tickle

4

MIND AND NERVES

Sleeping and anxiety problems   Depression
Psychotic illnesses   Sickness and dizziness
Pain   Migraine   Epilepsy
Parkinson's disease and parkinsonism

The brain resembles a telephone junction box, with ten billion nerve cells receiving electrical and chemical impulses from all over the body. Part of the brain works out how to respond to these impulses, checking with the memory to help it decide on the action the body should take, and another part controls body action. As signals come to the brain and are interpreted, the responses are sent through nerves to trigger the muscles into action. Nerve cells (*neurons*) are grouped together to form the main path that takes messages to and from the brain – the spinal cord. The spinal cord runs most of the length of the back from the bottom of the brain, inside, and protected by, the backbones. The brain and the spinal cord form the central nervous system.

Nerves that branch off from the central nervous system to the rest of the body form the peripheral nervous system. Nerves from one part of this system run to the skin and muscles while another part in the head connects the brain to the sense organs – eyes, ears, nose and taste buds.

The *autonomic* nervous system works 'automatically', to regulate the heart and circulation, breathing, digestion, the processes for removing waste from the body and the *endocrine glands*. The autonomic system works in harmony with the endocrine glands which release hormones, chemical messengers to regulate certain organs and body functions. The autonomic nervous system has two parts – the *sympathetic* and *parasympathetic* nervous systems – which work in a 'push–pull' way.

The sympathetic system stimulates a particular organ to make it work harder; the parasympathetic system dampens or inhibits activity, opposing the sympathetic system. Daily body functions such as food digestion and passing urine are mostly controlled by the parasympathetic system. The sympathetic system controls body functions during exercise and emotion; for example, when you are angry or frightened it makes the heart beat faster, widens the airways in the lungs, enlarges the pupils of the eyes and diverts blood flow from the intestines and skin to the muscles.

How nerves send messages

Nerve messages travel to and from the brain in rapid bursts by electrical means. The minerals sodium, potassium and calcium in association with chloride are present everywhere in the body as tiny electrically charged particles (*ions*), so the inside of the nerve cell has a slight negative charge while the fluid outside is positively charged. As the nerve message approaches, the nerve cell membrane alters to change the electrical balance within the cell, allowing the transmission of the message. As the message flows on from one end of the nerve cell to the other, the balance is restored to the resting state. The whole process takes about one thousandth of a second.

The nerve cells do not actually touch each other: the message must pass across a gap (*synapse*). To bridge this gap the cell releases a chemical or *neurotransmitter* which binds on to receptor sites of nearby cells. The message is relayed by the neurotransmitter to the next cell which in turn sends the message to another nerve cell or causes activity in a muscle or organ.

The neurotransmitters in the sympathetic system are the hormones adrenaline and noradrenaline. The activity of the sympathetic system is increased by the release of adrenaline and noradrenaline from the central part of the adrenal gland (*medulla*). These body chemicals act on alpha- and beta-receptors in the tissues. There are several types of beta-receptors, the main ones being $beta_1$ in heart muscle and $beta_2$ in smooth muscle, such as that found around the airways. Drugs that promote the release of adrenaline or noradrenaline or mimic their effects are known as *adrenergic drugs*, *adrenoceptor stimulants* or *sympathomimetics*. Drugs that oppose the sympathetic nervous system are blocking drugs, such as *beta-adrenoceptor blocking drugs* (beta blockers), *adrenergic neuron blocking drugs* or *alpha-adrenoceptor blocking drugs* (alpha blockers).

The nerves that carry messages in the parasympathetic system are *cholinergic* nerves; the chemical nerve transmitter is *acetylcholine*. The actions of acetylcholine can be increased or decreased by other chemicals or drugs. Drugs that stimulate the parasympathetic system and increase acetylcholine activity are called *cholinergic* medicines. Drugs that reduce the action of acetylcholine and the parasympathetic system are *anticholinergic* or *antimuscarinic* medicines, for example **atropine** and **hyoscine**.

The way the neurotransmitters adrenaline, noradrenaline and acetylcholine act has been known for many years and drugs to increase or oppose their effects have been developed. More recently, other neurotransmitters and their receptors – in particular dopamine and serotonin – have been discovered. Drugs that affect serotonin, for example, include the antimigraine drug **sumatriptan** (Imigran) and the selective serotonin re-uptake inhibitors (SSRIs) such as **fluoxetine** (Prozac).

Sleeping and anxiety problems

SLEEPING PROBLEMS

Insomnia, or the feeling of being awake for long periods at night, is common: about one person in five suffers from it, although it affects women more often than men. People sleep for variable amounts of time – from three to ten hours – at night, with an average of seven to eight hours. The amount of sleep that each person needs varies: babies sleep a great deal; elderly people need less than the average. Many people suffer from sleeplessness or insomnia occasionally, but persistent lack of sleep can be a problem which needs sorting out. You will need to tell your doctor whether you have difficulty in getting to sleep, or whether you wake during the night or wake too early in the morning. Causes include stress and anxiety; depression; medical problems such as pain, indigestion, cough or itching; the need to pass urine; menopausal symptoms such as hot flushes and sweating; noise; and drinking tea or coffee too late in the evening. Knowing the cause of a sleeping problem is important, particularly where there is an underlying medical condition, such as pain or depression, which can be treated.

A short-term sleeping problem may be related to an emotional problem and will clear up once the problem is resolved. One or two nights of broken sleep caused by noise, shift work or travel (for example 'jet lag') do not usually lead to disruption in your life, but longer periods may do so. Taking medicine for a short time may help but a long-term sleeping problem can rarely be solved by taking a sleeping tablet routinely.

HOW YOU CAN HELP YOURSELF

- ☐ Avoid daytime napping or going to bed too early.
- ☐ Do not be determined that you must have a fixed number of hours sleep a night.
- ☐ Make sure that environmental factors such as light, heat and noise are right for you. A quiet, dark room with some ventilation promotes restful sleep.
- ☐ Avoid drinking stimulants such as tea, coffee or cola before bedtime; some people find that caffeine prevents sleep for six hours or more.
- ☐ Avoid over-the-counter medicines containing caffeine and decongestant preparations containing phenylpropanolamine. Asthma preparations containing theophylline or aminophylline are also stimulants.
- ☐ Avoid alcohol late at night.
- ☐ Make sure you establish a good bedtime routine. Have a light, bland snack or milky drink and a warm, relaxing bath.
- ☐ Exciting television programmes and loud noisy music before you go to bed can interfere with sleep; reading a dull book and having sex both help sleep.
- ☐ If you really cannot sleep it is often better to get up and do something pleasant than to lie feeling frustrated.

ANXIETY

Anxiety is a mixture of emotional and physical symptoms, such as fear, nervousness, tension and sometimes overwhelming panic; physical signs include tense muscles, headaches, rapid heartbeat or palpitations, breathlessness, sweating, shaking and lightheadedness. The physical symptoms occur because of increased stimulation of the sympathetic nervous system and the release of adrenaline and noradrenaline. The balance of certain other chemicals in the brain may also be disturbed.

Stress is one of the commonest causes of anxiety. A degree of stress is important in your life to act as a springboard for action or a change of circumstances. Events such as the death of your spouse or a close friend, marriage problems, divorce, poor housing or losing your job cause a great deal of stress; if it becomes too much, symptoms of anxiety may set in. Other psychological factors are important, such as your ability to cope and your self-esteem.

Anxiety symptoms are now understood as a natural psychological reaction to social and physical problems. The best treatment is likely to be counselling in the form of explanation, reassurance and encouragement by your doctor or another suitably trained professional, such as a clinical psychologist or community psychiatric nurse or social worker.

– HOW YOU CAN HELP YOURSELF –

- ☐ Discuss your problems with someone; confiding in a friend, your partner or a relative may help to identify causes of anxiety and potential solutions as well as lessening the burden.
- ☐ Express your thoughts: try to find out what makes you anxious and make a list of your problems.
- ☐ Get plenty of rest and sleep if you can.
- ☐ Regular exercise can be very important and help to release tension; swimming is especially beneficial, particularly for older people.
- ☐ Yoga or relaxation classes can relieve tension; assertiveness training may also help.
- ☐ Eat sensibly at regular intervals; avoid drinking stimulants such as tea, coffee or cola and avoid medicines containing caffeine, phenylpropanolamine, theophylline or aminophylline.
- ☐ Join a self-help group: ask your doctor or local Patient Advice and Liaison Services (PALS)* for addresses and phone numbers. There are groups for supporting the bereaved and ethnic and other minorities as well as groups for psychological disorders.

Medicines for sleep and anxiety problems

Medicines to treat anxiety and sleeping problems are discussed together because most anti-anxiety medicines will induce sleep when given in higher doses at night and most sleeping tablets will dampen anxiety when given in lower doses during the day. For example, the benzodiazepine **diazepam** (which was known as Valium) can be used both as a tranquilliser and as a sleeping tablet, although it is more commonly used to relieve anxiety. However, a sleeping tablet should be used only when lack of sleep markedly affects your life, work or the family, and when other approaches or treatments have failed.

Anti-anxiety medicines (tranquillisers or *anxiolytics*) and sleeping tablets (sedatives or *hypnotics*) have been widely used since the 1960s when benzodiazepines became available. They appeared to have fewer unwanted effects than **barbiturates**, which are now rarely used for their calming and sedative effects, but see 'Benzodiazepine use', below. The adverse effects of barbiturates include a tendency to cause 'hangover effects' the next day and toxicity in overdose. Barbiturates also cause problems of dependence. Some barbiturates are still useful: for example **phenobarbital** (phenobarbitone), which is used for the treatment of epilepsy.

Children should never be given an anti-anxiety medicine or a hypnotic unless your doctor feels there is a strong reason, such as night terrors.

BENZODIAZEPINES

If the balance of body chemicals is disrupted in some way, you may experience changes to your mental or physical well-being. *Gamma-aminobutyric acid* (GABA) reduces the flow of electrical impulses across nerve cells in the part of the brain where emotion is controlled. The main action of a benzodiazepine is to increase the effect of GABA, further reducing the electrical flows across cells, and so reducing feelings of anxiety and agitation and slowing mental activity. Benzodiazepines relax muscles and are particularly helpful for reducing muscle spasm, for example after sports injuries. They also have an anticonvulsant action and some are used to treat epilepsy.

Benzodiazepine use

Doctors are likely to want to try non-drug management at first, but if a benzodiazepine appears to be appropriate then its use should be limited to the lowest possible dose for the shortest possible time. Tranquillisers and sleeping tablets must not be used indiscriminately and should be given only for short courses. They should never be given on repeat prescription without the doctor seeing the patient. The reason is that tolerance of and dependence on the effects of benzodiazepines can occur. Tolerance means that the medicine becomes less effective even though you continue to take the same dose, and it can develop after 3 to 14 days of continuous use.

Taking a benzodiazepine can become habit-forming and dependence develops. Physical dependence means the regular use of a substance which when stopped, especially abruptly, causes the person to develop physical symptoms of withdrawal. With benzodiazepines these include sweating, nervousness, inability to sleep, broken sleep with vivid dreams or nightmares, loss of appetite and body weight, tremor and disturbed vision. These symptoms are similar to the original complaint and may encourage further prescribing of the same benzodiazepine. Psychological dependence, when you feel that you cannot do without the medicine, often accompanies the physical problems.

When you stop taking a sleeping tablet you should expect disturbed sleep for a few nights before a normal sleep routine is re-established, but withdrawing a benzodiazepine after long-term use should be done with the help of your doctor by gradually reducing the dose over a period of time, so that withdrawal symptoms will be lessened if not eliminated. It may be helpful to keep a written record of your dose reduction schedule. Withdrawal may take months to achieve but it is better to go slowly rather than too quickly. You may have to be prepared for the withdrawal process to go on for a year or more. Joining a self-help group, where you can share your experiences and get support, may be helpful (see box, page 191).

The National Service Framework for Mental Health asks doctors to review benzodiazepine prescribing regularly. The Committee on Safety of Medicines (CSM) now advises doctors that:

- ☐ benzodiazepines should be prescribed only for the short-term relief (2–4 weeks only) of anxiety that is severe, disabling or subjecting the individual to unacceptable distress
- ☐ it is inappropriate and unsuitable to use a benzodiazepine to treat short-term 'mild' anxiety
- ☐ a benzodiazepine should be used to treat sleeplessness only when it is severe, disabling or subjecting the individual to extreme distress.

All benzodiazepines should be avoided for the treatment of anxiety and sleeplessness whenever possible. A benzodiazepine is not recommended for loss or bereavement, for example, because it can inhibit the period of adjustment. Other strategies can help with life events, such as family illness, bereavement, unemployment or feelings of social isolation and personal inadequacies. These problems need to be recognised, talked about and relieved without the use of medicines where possible. Your doctor may be able to put you in contact with other professionals, such as a clinical psychologist or a counsellor. Always ask your doctor what alternatives there are to drug treatment. If you have to take a tranquilliser or hypnotic make sure it is for a short time only. Note down how you feel at the start of treatment and how you progress from day to day during the treatment.

Unwanted effects

Benzodiazepines have fewer unwanted effects than barbiturates and are less dangerous in overdose. Common unwanted effects include unsteadiness and drowsiness and the elderly are particularly vulnerable to them. Benzodiazepines can also cause confusion, memory loss, slurred speech, hostility and aggression. Dependence and withdrawal symptoms are recognised unwanted effects of benzodiazepines. Dependence can develop, particularly in people who are prone to alcohol or drug misuse and also in those with marked personality disorders.

Confusion and poor co-ordination can result in falls and fractures, especially of the hips in older people. Sleeping tablets and tranquillisers impair judgement and increase reaction time, so the ability to drive or operate machinery is affected. The daytime drowsiness or hangover effects of sleeping tablets may also impair driving on the following day. The effects are increased by alcohol and by other tranquillisers or hypnotics.

In older people the adverse effects of a benzodiazepine may be attributed to old age rather than the effects of the medicine itself. The onset of impaired intelligence with memory loss, confusion or loss of co-ordination in a young person is likely to be attributed to the drug. The same symptoms in an older person, especially if they develop more slowly, are often dismissed with the remark, 'You must expect these things at your age.' However, an older person cannot clear a drug from the body (particularly through the liver and kidneys) as rapidly as a young person and is more sensitive to adverse effects of drugs.

Drug-induced impaired thinking and learning disability is one of the most reversible or treatable forms of mental illness. It is a by-product of the increased use of potent medicines during the last 40 years. Stopping a drug with your doctor's guidance can often be better treatment than continuing with a medicine, but it should be done gradually.

A benzodiazepine usually reduces feelings of agitation and restlessness, but in some people it has the opposite effect. There have been some reports of increased hostility and aggression with effects ranging from talkativeness and excitement to aggressive and antisocial acts. US research has shown that, like alcohol, diazepam increases aggressive behaviour. Both benzodiazepines and alcohol depress central nervous system activity and in some people this releases certain patterns of behaviour which would normally be controlled. Some people experience increased anxiety, delusions and hallucinations.

Choice of benzodiazepines

Twelve benzodiazepine medicines are marketed, some as tranquillisers (anxiolytics) and some as hypnotics. This is a bewildering array, particularly because all of these drugs can both tranquillise and promote sleep depending on the dose taken. Calling some anti-anxiety drugs and others hypnotics has more to do with marketing than with pharmacology. However, the benzodiazepines do differ in one important respect and that is how quickly or slowly they are cleared from the body.

Longer-acting benzodiazepines, including **diazepam**, **loprazolam** and **nitrazepam**, have a prolonged action in the body and may cause residual or hangover effects, so that drowsiness persists. The effects of a longer-acting benzodiazepine accumulate so that a steady state of anxiety control and side effects such as drowsiness is reached in the body. Many benzodiazepines break down into one or more chemicals (*metabolites*) in the body and these may have further tranquillising or hypnotic effects.

Shorter-acting benzodiazepines, such as **lorazepam** and **oxazepam**, pass through the body more quickly and therefore produce little hangover effect. However, they can cause more withdrawal problems, particularly if they are taken every day and then stopped abruptly. If you have taken a short-acting benzodiazepine for a prolonged period, your doctor may transfer you to a longer-acting one, usually diazepam, to lessen the impact of withdrawal symptoms.

A short-acting benzodiazepine used as a hypnotic, such as **temazepam**, causes little drowsiness the next day, although this can vary between people. Taking a hypnotic intermittently, for example every third or fourth night for a short period of time at the lowest possible dose, should avoid dependence and also withdrawal problems. Diazepam at low dose (2mg) up to three times a day can be appropriate for the short-term relief of severe anxiety. A benzodiazepine may also be used in conjunction with or following an antidepressant for alleviating panic disorders at the start of treatment.

Since the Selected List was introduced (page 18), certain benzodiazepines used for sleep and anxiety problems can no longer be paid for by the NHS. Also, prescribing by brand names is disallowed, so doctors must prescribe the benzodiazepines by generic name.

DIAZEPAM

DIAZEPAM – Tablets, liquid, injection, rectal solution, suppositories

Diazepam is a long-acting benzodiazepine used for relieving severe disabling anxiety. It has a depressant effect on the part of the brain controlling emotion. Treatment should be for no more than two to four weeks. Diazepam is also used as a muscle relaxant, for relieving epileptic fits, to help withdrawal symptoms for people with acute alcohol poisoning and sometimes as premedication before operations or uncomfortable diagnostic procedures. Like all benzodiazepines, diazepam can cause tolerance, dependence and withdrawal symptoms.

Before you use this medicine

Tell your doctor if you are:
☐ pregnant or breast-feeding – avoid diazepam ☐ taking any other medicines, including vitamins and those bought over the counter.

Tell your doctor if you have or have had:
☐ liver or kidney problems ☐ mental health problems or depression ☐ brief periods of not breathing during sleep (sleep apnoea) ☐ lung disease or breathing problems ☐ alcohol or drug dependence ☐ myasthenia gravis ☐ porphyria.

Do not use if you have:
☐ severe breathing problems or acute lung disease ☐ severe mental health problems such as schizophrenia ☐ severe liver disease ☐ muscle weakness.

How to use this medicine

Take the tablet according to the schedule agreed with your doctor. Ask your doctor to limit the prescription, for example up to seven days of treatment, and do not obtain further supplies of diazepam on a repeat prescription. It is important to see your doctor and for you both to evaluate how you feel after the course of treatment.

Do not drive a car or do other activities that require alertness until you know how you react to diazepam. Diazepam may cause drowsiness, impair judgement and increase reaction time. People who take a benzodiazepine are more likely to have traffic accidents. Do not take alcohol, as it increases the effects of diazepam. Do not stop taking this medicine suddenly if treatment lasts more than seven days; ask your doctor for a dosage reduction schedule that will allow you to stop gradually and prevent withdrawal symptoms. If you miss a dose, take it as soon as you remember but if it is nearly time for your next dose skip it. Do not take double the dose or more than the prescribed dose.

Over 65 Older people and those who are seriously ill or debilitated, for example with severe kidney or liver impairment, need only half the standard adult dose or even less.

Interactions with other medicines

Always check with your doctor or pharmacist if you can take diazepam with another medicine. All drugs that have a sedative or tranquillising effect on the central nervous system will increase the effect of diazepam. The antibacterial **rifampicin** may speed up the breakdown of diazepam (making it less effective), while **cimetidine**, and possibly **omeprazole** and **esomeprazole**, may inhibit the breakdown of diazepam (increasing its duration in the body).

Unwanted effects

Likely Drowsiness, dizziness, lightheadedness, confusion, clumsiness, unsteadiness or falling, forgetfulness, dependence.
Rare Headache, digestive disorders, rashes, blurred vision, low blood pressure, dry mouth, increased thirst or unusual mouth watering, difficulty passing urine, blood disorders, jaundice, unusual excitability, hallucinations, changes in libido, aggression.
Dependence and withdrawal symptoms – page 193.

The unwanted effects of drowsiness and dizziness may fade as treatment continues or a lower dose may help. If you experience any of the rare effects contact your doctor. Stop taking diazepam if you develop a skin rash, reducing the dose gradually.

Similar preparations

Prescribed (generically) for anxiety – brands not on NHS
CHLORDIAZEPOXIDE (LIBRIUM) – Capsules, tablets
LORAZEPAM – Tablets, injection
OXAZEPAM – Tablets

Prescribed (generically) for sleeping problems – brands not on NHS
LOPRAZOLAM – Tablets
LORMETAZEPAM – Tablets
NITRAZEPAM – Tablets, liquid
TEMAZEPAM – Tablets, liquid

Not available on NHS prescription in any form
For anxiety:
ALPRAZOLAM (XANAX); **CLOBAZAM*** (FRISIUM); **CLORAZEPATE** (TRANXENE)
For sleeping problems:
FLUNITRAZEPAM (ROHYPNOL); **FLURAZEPAM** (DALMANE)

* **CLOBAZAM** may be prescribed for epilepsy under the Selected List Scheme (SLS) – page 18.

• *OTHER HYPNOTICS* •

Newer preparations, **zopiclone** (Zimovane), **zolpidem** (Stilnoct) and **zaleplon** (Sonata) (known collectively as the 'Z drugs'), are not benzodiazepines, although they act at the same places on the nerve cell as a benzodiazepine and they are similarly effective. These hypnotics are for short-term use only (no more than 28 days for zopiclone or zolpidem;

only 14 days for zaleplon), and like benzodiazepines intermittent use may be a reasonable strategy. They are short-acting but have little or no advantage over a benzodiazepine such as temazepam. Like benzodiazepines, these hypnotics have the potential to cause withdrawal symptoms and rebound insomnia, where sleeplessness recurs which may be worse than before, leading to dependence. Zaleplon is very short-acting and a second dose should not be taken during the same night. As with all other hypnotics, they can cause dizziness, lightheadedness and poor co-ordination. Drowsiness may continue into the next day and you should avoid driving if you are affected by treatment.

Clomethiazole (chlormethiazole) (Heminevrin) may be useful for short-term use for older people with severe insomnia. It is available in capsules and in liquid form. Younger people with alcohol problems are sometimes prescribed it for a very short time to ameliorate alcohol withdrawal symptoms.

Older hypnotics – **chloral hydrate** (Welldorm) and a derivative **triclofos** – predate benzodiazepines and were used widely. They are limited by their unwanted effects which include giddiness, vertigo and hangover effects. Chloral hydrate causes digestive system upsets, for example feeling or being sick, abdominal distension and flatulence. They are no longer recommended.

Diphenhydramine (Dreemon; Nightcalm; Nytol; Panadol Night) and **promethazine** (Phenergan Nightime; Sominex) are old antihistamines with marked sedative effects, now marketed as 'sleep aids' and sold in pharmacies. They act in the body for a long time and can cause confusion and day-time sedation, particularly in older people. These types of preparation should only be used short-term and are not recommended for children. You should always let any health professional know that you also take an over-the-counter medicine.

Alcohol cannot be recommended because it disturbs sleep later in the night. It has a diuretic (water-removing) action and causes thirst. Heavy long-term use disturbs sleep and causes insomnia.

OTHER MEDICINES FOR ANXIETY

Buspirone (Buspar) is not related to the benzodiazepines and it has no muscle relaxant, hypnotic or anti-epileptic effects. Buspirone can be used for the short-term relief of anxiety, but its effects may not be felt for up to two weeks after starting treatment. It does not help to relieve benzodiazepine withdrawal symptoms, and a benzodiazepine should be withdrawn gradually before buspirone is started. Buspirone may cause dizziness, lightheadedness, nervousness, headache, nausea, excitement and rarely rapid heart beat, palpitations, chest pain, drowsiness, confusion, seizures, dry mouth, fatigue and sweating. You should not drive a car or perform skilled tasks until you know how you react to buspirone. The potential for buspirone to cause dependence seems to be low.

A beta blocker such as **propranolol** or **metoprolol** may be helpful if you are troubled by the physical symptoms of anxiety, such as sweating, palpitations and shaking, but it will not affect your emotions such as worry, tension and fear. Nevertheless if a beta blocker helps to control the physical symptoms, then the emotional symptoms may be relieved. Beta blockers are not suitable for asthmatics. **Meprobamate** is less effective than a benzodiazepine, more hazardous in overdose and can cause dependence. It is no longer recommended.

Depression

Depression is the most common mental disorder, affecting many thousands of people – as many as one in five at some stage during their lifetime. The exact nature of the illness is poorly understood but it appears to be a blend of biochemical and psychological factors, often coupled with adverse life experiences. Sad moods usually pass with time and need no medical treatment, but when the feeling does not fade it may lead to loss of interest in working or living. Sufferers may experience low self-esteem, a feeling of hopelessness, loss of appetite for food and sex and disturbed sleep. Depression may be masked by anxiety or by physical symptoms such as backache, headaches, dizziness, chest pains or weight loss. In severe depression someone may consider taking his or her own life.

Social factors or events such as bereavement, someone losing their job or divorce can trigger depression. Feeling physically low because of a debilitating illness or the aftermath of a virus infection or continuous, nagging pain can cause depression, which is sometimes worse than the physical condition itself. People may suffer depression after childbirth, during the menopause or at a mid-life crisis. Some drugs can cause depression, for example methyldopa, the blood pressure-lowering drug. If a depressive episode begins after the start of treatment with a new medicine, ask your doctor whether the drug could be causing the depression.

Depressive episodes may alternate with periods when you feel perfectly well (*unipolar depression*) or with periods of over-activity and with normal mood (*bipolar* or *manic depression*; page 218). Depression occurs in episodes and a bout may last for a few weeks or months or more – for example, a chronic low depressive mood lasting for more than two years is known as *dysthymia* or minor depression. Depression is classified as minor or major and then by degrees as mild, moderate or severe depending on the severity of symptoms, particularly for research purposes in clinical trials. Researchers need to gauge the effectiveness of treatments and use a variety of rating scales to assess the degree of depression and response to antidepressants and to placebo.

In assessing depression your doctor may ask you whether, during the past month, you have often been bothered by feeling down, depressed or hopeless and whether you have often been bothered by having little interest or pleasure in doing things. If you answer 'no' to both questions depression is unlikely; if 'yes' to either question then depression is possible, but further discussion between you and your doctor will be needed to explore the issues. You may recover spontaneously, particularly if symptoms are mild and you can carry on with your daily routine, but treatment with medicines and/or counselling may be needed and can help moderate to severe major depressive illness. Major depression is characterised by depressive symptoms that become pronounced and start to interfere with normal functioning. It may not be easy to help yourself when you are depressed, but some tips are given in the box below.

HOW YOU CAN HELP YOURSELF

These suggestions are also useful for anyone trying to help a depressed friend or relative.

- ☐ Share your sadness with a friend or neighbour. Try not to bottle your feelings up.
- ☐ Keep a record of the pleasant things that happen to you and discuss these with someone, too. If you have no one to talk to, find out if there is a counselling service near to you or available by telephone. The Samaritans*, a 24-hour listening and befriending service, has local branches throughout Britain – see your telephone directory or ask the operator (dial 100). Organisations such as the Fellowship of Depressives Anonymous* and the British Association for Counselling and Psychotherapy* have lists of self-help groups and counsellors.
- ☐ Do not try to overcome depression with large amounts of alcohol. Alcohol depresses brain and nervous activity and may make you even further depressed.
- ☐ Eat properly and try to take regular exercise – this could be as simple as a daily walk.
- ☐ Try to rest and sleep if possible: have a quiet time before bedtime, perhaps a warm bath to try and relax; avoid caffeine-containing drinks.
- ☐ If your depression seems to be lasting, see your doctor.

Antidepressants

Treatment with an antidepressant medicine can help to moderate severe lingering depression. Drug treatment will not cure the underlying cause but may help you to function more normally again. A period of drug treatment may lift you sufficiently from melancholic thoughts and low self-esteem to allow you to get on with life. You may not begin to feel the beneficial effects of some medicines for 10–14 days, with full effects taking four to six weeks to develop. Treatment is usually needed for at least four to six months after the acute symptoms of depressive illness have faded. Older people may need 12 months of treatment, and some people may need to continue treatment for a number of years to prevent a relapse. Your doctor should withdraw treatment very gradually over a period of six to eight weeks to prevent a recurrence of symptoms and will need to see you for another three or four weeks once you have stopped your medicine altogether.

Many of the clinical trials for antidepressants have been conducted with hospital patients who have major depression, i.e. their lives are disrupted by symptoms. Studies that demonstrate the effectiveness of antidepressants in people with mild depressive symptoms in the community are lacking, particularly for long-term treatment. Yet many antidepressants are prescribed by general practitioners to ameliorate troubling symptoms – there were over 22 million prescriptions for antidepressants in England in 2000, an increase from nine million in 1991. An immediate prescription from your GP may not be needed, but your doctor must balance this against concerns if symptoms worsen or become life-threatening. You should expect a supportive approach from your general practice, a period of 'watchful waiting' and time to discuss problems. Many people prefer supportive treatments such as counselling, which can help to relieve depressive symptoms and refocus thoughts and behaviour, and these therapies are becoming more accessible.

Depression is thought to be caused by a decrease in brain chemicals called neurotransmitters, such as noradrenaline and serotonin (also called 5-hydroxytryptamine). In depression the brain cells release less of the neurotransmitters to excite neighbouring cells and stimulate activity. Antidepressants increase the amount of neurotransmitters outside brain cells, which prolongs their stimulatory effect on the brain.

Choice of antidepressant

Two types of antidepressant are mainly used: the *tricyclics*, of which **amitriptyline** is a good example, and the *selective serotonin re-uptake inhibitors* (SSRIs) such as **fluoxetine**. Both types of antidepressant are effective and there is no significant difference in efficacy between these classes. The tricyclic antidepressants increase brain levels of both noradrenaline and serotonin whereas the SSRIs increase serotonin and hardly affect noradrenaline. These differences in action between the classes account for the different profiles of unwanted effects.

The choice of antidepressant depends on each person's requirements, such as other co-existing conditions and current medicines, suicide risk and whether they have responded before to a particular type of antidepressant. The older tricyclic antidepressants (except **lofepramine**) can be sedating and affect heart rhythm in overdose, whereas the SSRIs are safer in overdose. Only one class of of antidepressant is used at a time; they are generally not prescribed in combination. All antidepressants can cause withdrawal reactions if stopped suddenly, but the SSRIs are associated with a specific set of symptoms, which are a problem for some people (page 204).

Other newer antidepressants include medicines that act mainly by increasing noradrenaline levels in the brain such as **reboxetine** (Edronax), while **mirtazepine** (Zispin) and **venlafaxine** (Efexor) increase both noradrenaline and serotonin selectively. Their unwanted effect profile may be better than the tricyclics, but there is less experience of their use than with the tricyclics and SSRIs and so they are likely to be reserved as second-line antidepressants. **Flupentixol** (Fluanxol) is an older medicine used for short-term treatment of depression. The older *monoamine oxidase inhibitors (MAOIs)* such as **phenelzine** increase the levels of neurotransmitters in the brain by blocking the enzyme which breaks them down.

They can be tried after tricyclics, SSRIs or other antidepressants, and are usually started by a hospital specialist.

The herbal remedy St John's wort, extracted from the plant Hypericum perforatum, can be used for depression, but evidence of efficacy and safety are lacking for long-term treatment beyond six to eight weeks. It is not licensed as a medicine in the UK and the active constituents have not been precisely identified. St John's wort enhances the unwanted effects of SSRIs and they should not be taken together.

TRICYCLIC ANTIDEPRESSANTS

The tricyclic and related antidepressants, so-called because of their chemical structure, are well established, relatively safe and effective at normal doses. Some of the medicines have a more sedative effect and are helpful if you have sleeping difficulties because the single daily dose can be taken at night; these include **amitriptyline**, **dosulepin** (dothiepin) and **doxepin**. Other medicines are less sedative, for example **imipramine** and **lofepramine**, and may help if you feel lethargic.

When starting treatment with a tricyclic antidepressant, your doctor should increase the dose gradually as this will minimise the impact of unwanted effects. This has to be balanced against the need to obtain a full treatment effect as early as possible. All may cause unwanted effects such as dry mouth, blurred vision, constipation and difficulty passing urine as well as dizziness (from postural hypotension) and heart problems (except for **lofepramine** and **trazodone**). Some unwanted effects may fade as you continue treatment; older people are more sensitive to them. Overdosage can cause severe heart problems that need emergency treatment.

AMITRIPTYLINE

AMITRIPTYLINE – Tablets, liquid

Poor choice
Combination preparations – ingredients better used separately:
TRIPTAFEN/TRIPTAFEN M – Tablets
AMITRIPTYLINE + PERPHENAZINE

Amitriptyline is a tricyclic antidepressant which lifts mood, increases activity and improves appetite. It has a sedative effect and because it acts in the body for a long time, it can be taken at night as a single dose. Amitriptyline improves sleep once treatment has started but it may take two to four weeks before you feel the full antidepressive effect.

It may also be used to help children over seven years old with bed-wetting problems, for no longer than three months. Other, unofficial uses of amitriptyline include its use in low dosage (25–50mg) to reduce nerve irritation (neuropathic pain), which may develop with back pain, after shingles, with phantom limb pain or in terminal illness. Unwanted effects can be troublesome, especially in older people. Amitriptyline should be used with care in people with heart disease because it may cause hazardous irregular heart rhythms and heart block.

Before you use this medicine

Tell your doctor if you are:
□ pregnant – safety of amitriptyline not established □ breast-feeding □ taking any other medicines, including vitamins and those bought over the counter.

Tell your doctor if you have or have had:
□ heart disease, especially irregular heart rhythms, heart failure □ epilepsy or seizures □ liver disease □ thyroid disease □ psychoses □ angle-closure glaucoma □ prostate disorders □ urinary retention.

Do not take if you have or have had:
□ a recent heart attack □ heart block □ mania □ porphyria □ severe liver disease.

How to use this medicine

Take the tablet with water at night or in divided doses during the day. The effective dose range is 125–200mg, but your doctor may prescribe a lower dose to minimise unwanted effects. Increasing the dose gradually at intervals also helps.

Do not drive or do other activities that require alertness until you know how you react to amitriptyline. You may feel dizzy or faint when you get up from sitting or lying down, especially during the first few days of treatment. Get up slowly and stay beside the chair or bed until you are sure you are not dizzy. Avoid alcohol because it increases the sedative effects of amitriptyline.

Do not stop taking this medicine suddenly. Your doctor will give you a schedule to reduce the dose gradually if you are on long-term treatment, to prevent a recurrence of your symptoms. If you miss a dose, take it as soon as you remember. For example, if you have forgotten your night-time dose, take it the next morning if drowsiness is not a problem. Otherwise, skip it and take your next dose as usual. Do not take double doses.

Over 65 You should have a third to half the normal adult dose. Unwanted effects may be troublesome, especially antimuscarinic effects of dry mouth, blurred vision, drowsiness, constipation and difficulty passing urine, and also mental effects such as confusion, short-term memory problems, disorientation.

Interactions with other medicines

Amitriptyline interacts with many other medicines. Do not take other medicines without checking with your doctor or pharmacist. These are some important ones:

Analgesics Tramadol increases risk of nervous system unwanted effects, e.g. confusion, hallucinations. Opioids increase sedation.

Adrenaline and adrenaline-like drugs (sympathomimetics) result in high blood pressure and irregular heart rhythms.

Anaesthetics Amitriptyline may need to be stopped before you have a general anaesthetic. Always tell your doctor or dentist that you take this drug.

Antiarrhythmics Increased risk of abnormal heart rhythms. Avoid with **amiodarone**.

Antiepileptics and tricyclic antidepressants antagonise each other's effects.

Antihistamines increase some unwanted effects such as drowsiness and dry mouth.

Antihypertensives Blood pressure-lowering effect enhanced.

Antiobesity sibutramine Increases risk of central nervous system effects.

Other antidepressants Monoamine-oxidase inhibitors (MAOIs) cause excitation of the central nervous system, restlessness, high blood pressure and other signs of overactivity. They must not be taken for at least 14 days before or after another antidepressant. SSRIs such as **fluoxetine** increase blood levels of some tricyclic antidepressants.

A number of drugs increase the risk of abnormal heart rhythms with amitriptyline, including the antibacterial **moxifloxacin**, the antihistamine **terfenadine**, **antipsychotics**, **pimozide**, **thioridazine**.

Unwanted effects

Likely Drowsiness, dizziness, fainting, dry mouth, stuffy nose, blurred vision, difficulty passing urine, feeling sick, constipation, fluid retention, weight gain.
Less likely Irregular heart rhythms, palpitations, sweating, tremor, rashes, disorientation, confusion, sexual dysfunction, breast enlargement, discharge from nipples, movement disorders, hypersensitivity reactions including nettle rash, photosensitivity.
Rare Jaundice.

Unwanted effects may be noticed before the antidepressive effects are felt, although they usually fade as treatment continues and if the dose is increased slowly; dry mouth may persist. If unwanted effects are troublesome discuss with your doctor. If you have irregular heart rhythms and severe dizziness or fainting, stop taking amitriptyline and call your doctor.

Similar preparations

ALLEGRON – Tablets
NORTRIPTYLINE

ANAFRANIL – Capsules
CLOMIPRAMINE

ASENDIS – Tablets
AMOXAPINE

CLOMIPRAMINE – Capsules

DOSULEPIN (DOTHIEPIN) – Capsules, tablets

GAMANIL – Tablets
LOFEPRAMINE

IMIPRAMINE – Tablets

LOFEPRAMINE – Tablets, liquid

PROTHIADEN – Capsules, tablets
DOSULEPIN (DOTHIEPIN)

SINEQUAN – Capsules
DOXEPIN

SURMONTIL – Capsules, tablets
TRIMIPRAMINE

TOFRANIL – Tablets
IMIPRAMINE

TRAZODONE – Capsules, tablets

Poor choice
ANAFRANIL SR – Modified-release tablets
CLOMIPRAMINE

Combination preparations – ingredients better used separately
MOTIVAL – Tablets
NORTRIPTYLINE + FLUPHENAZINE

Related preparations
LUDIOMIL – Tablets
MAPROTILINE

MIANSERIN – Tablets

MOLIPAXIN – Capsules, tablets, liquid
TRAZODONE

Combinations in one preparation of an anti-anxiety drug with an antidepressant, such as **perphenazine** with **amitriptyline**, are not recommended. An anti-anxiety medicine is taken for a short time only, while antidepressant treatment may continue for several months or more. The doses of the individual drugs cannot be adjusted in a combination preparation.

• *SELECTIVE SEROTONIN RE-UPTAKE INHIBITORS* •

Fluoxetine (Prozac), **fluvoxamine** (Faverin), **sertraline** (Lustral), **paroxetine** (Seroxat), **citalopram** (Cipramil) and related medicine **escitalopram** (▼Cipralex) are selective serotonin re-uptake inhibitors (SSRIs), which increase body levels of the neurotransmitter serotonin. In general, these newer antidepressants are no more effective than the older tricyclic type and may be less effective than them in major depression. Unwanted effects of SSRIs include digestive system problems, feeling or being sick, indigestion, abdominal pain, diarrhoea or constipation, loss of appetite and weight loss, difficulty sleeping and headache. Lowering the dose may ease those symptoms. Although SSRIs cause less drowsiness, dry mouth or blurred vision than the tricyclics, these symptoms can still occur and your ability to drive may be affected. SSRIs have less effect on the heart and appear safer than tricyclics if you have ischaemic heart disease, or take an overdose.

In some people the SSRIs are associated with psychiatric and neurological reactions at the start of therapy. These problems include hallucinations, mania, anxiety, confusion, restlessness, agitation, depersonalisation, panic attacks, nervousness, seizures and movement disorders. These symptoms of mental turmoil have been linked allegedly in some to self-harm, harm to others and even suicide in a number of high-profile legal cases and in the media. The Committee on Safety of Medicines (CSM) has reviewed the issue of whether SSRIs are linked directly to suicidal behaviour since reports started in the early 1990s. In December 2001 following further assessment, the CSM concluded that there was insufficient evidence to confirm a link, although an effect in a small number of high-risk people could not be ruled out. You and your partner or carer need to be aware that these unwanted effects are a possibility with any of the SSRIs, particularly at the start of therapy. If bizarre reactions develop, contact your doctor urgently.

The market for SSRIs, already large for the treatment of depression, has been expanded further by manufacturers gaining authorisation for new uses such as social phobia, generalised anxiety disorder and panic disorder. Some doctors have prescribed them for children and adolescents, for whom these medicines are generally not recommended. Their use for depressive illness in children and young people under 18 years is not licensed. Some evidence supports the use of fluoxetine in this age group, but good-quality information is lacking for other SSRIs (sertraline, citalopram, escitalopram, paroxetine and fluvoxamine). The CSM has now advised doctors that, apart from fluoxetine, SSRIs should not be used for treating depression in people aged under 18 years. There are concerns that many psychological problems are being medicalised and that SSRIs have been oversold. They are not effective in all people and in some clinical trials for depression were only ten per cent better than placebo.

FLUOXETINE

FLUOXETINE – Capsules PROZAC – Capsules, liquid

Fluoxetine is a selective serotonin re-uptake inhibitor (SSRI) antidepressant. Low amounts of body chemicals for triggering brain activity (noradrenaline and serotonin) are thought to cause depression. Fluoxetine prevents reabsorption of serotonin so that an increased amount is available to stimulate brain cells. Fluoxetine hardly affects noradrenaline levels. Like all antidepressants it may take up to four weeks before you feel the depression starting to respond. It acts in the body for a long time (page 36) and also breaks down to a metabolite (page 36) with a long action. The advantages are that a single dose can be given once a day and that when stopping fluoxetine, the drug effect wears off slowly.

Fluoxetine is also used for obsessive-compulsive disorder and bulimia nervosa (the eating disorder).

Before you use this medicine

Tell your doctor if you are:

☐ pregnant – fluoxetine can be taken during pregnancy but caution during late pregnancy ☐ breast-feeding – avoid if possible ☐ taking any other medicines, including vitamins and those bought over the counter.

Tell your doctor if you have or have had:

☐ heart disease ☐ liver disease ☐ kidney disease (avoid if kidney problems are severe) ☐ epilepsy ☐ diabetes mellitus ☐ mania ☐ angle-closure glaucoma ☐ bleeding disorders (especially from the intestines).

Do not take an MAOI for at least five weeks after stopping fluoxetine.

How to use this medicine

Depression Take the capsule(s) once a day in the morning, usually 20mg at first, but the dose can be increased by your doctor. Do not drive or do other activities that require alertness until you know how you react to fluoxetine. Do not stop taking fluoxetine or any other SSRI antidepressant abruptly. Your doctor should give you a schedule to withdraw gradually from treatment. If you miss a dose, take it as soon as you remember, but skip it if it is almost time for your next dose. Do not take double the dose.

Over 65 The dose is one to three capsules a day.

Interactions with other medicines

The SSRIs interact with a number of other medicines; the important ones are given here.

Other antidepressants The effects of MAOIs, some tricyclics and St John's wort are increased – avoid use together.

Analgesics Tramadol Increased risk of nervous system unwanted effects; NSAIDs and **aspirin** increase risk of bleeding.

Anticoagulants (**warfarin** and **acenocoumarol**) Effects enhanced, dosage adjustments may be needed.

Antiepileptics SSRIs lower the threshold for when seizures may occur. Fluoxetine increases **phenytoin** and **carbamazepine** blood levels and increases the risk of toxicity.

Antihistamines Terfenadine Increased risk of irregular heart rhythms – avoid use together.
Antipsychotics Fluoxetine increases the effects of **clozapine**, **haloperidol**, **sertindole**, **risperidone** and **zotepine** and therefore the risk of toxicity.
Selegiline Risk of high blood pressure and nervous system toxicity – selegiline should not be started until five weeks after stopping fluoxetine; avoid starting fluoxetine for two weeks after stopping selegiline.
Other drugs: Lithium, sibutramine (for obesity) Increased risk of toxicity.
Sumatriptan Risk of nervous system toxicity – avoid use together.

Unwanted effects

Likely Feeling or being sick, diarrhoea or constipation, loss of appetite, weight loss (may affect blood sugar level), headache, nervousness, sleeplessness, dry mouth, dizziness, blurred vision, anxiety.
Less likely Confusion, low blood pressure, drowsiness, blood disorders, gastrointestinal bleeding (especially in older people), sexual dysfunction, vaginal bleeding on stopping treatment, violent behaviour, mania and movement disorders.

At low doses unwanted effects are mild. If violent, manic behaviour develops at the start of therapy, contact your doctor urgently. Rarely, a hypersensitivity reaction with facial swelling, rash (urticaria), itching, joint and muscle pains and sometimes anaphylaxis can occur. If you develop a rash, this may be a warning of a pending hypersensitivity reaction – stop taking fluoxetine and contact your doctor.

Similar preparations

CIPRAMIL – Tablets
CITALOPRAM

▼CIPRALEX – Tablets
ESCITALOPRAM

CITALOPRAM – Tablets

EDRONAX
REBOXETINE

ESCITALOPRAM – Tablets

FAVERIN – Tablets
FLUVOXAMINE

FLUVOXAMINE – Tablets

LUSTRAL – Tablets
SERTRALINE

MIRTAZAPINE – Liquid

PAROXETINE – Tablets

SEROXAT – Tablets, liquid
PAROXETINE

ZISPIN – Tablets
MIRTAZAPINE

MONOAMINE-OXIDASE INHIBITORS (MAOIs)

Monoamine oxidase inhibitors (MAOIs) have been in use for about 40 years, but their unwanted effects and interactions with other medicines, certain foods, beer and wine limit their usefulness. They increase neurotransmitter levels in the brain (serotonin, dopamine and noradrenaline) by blocking enzymes (monoamine oxidase A and B) which normally break them down. MAOIs may be tried after other antidepressants, but no antidepressant should be given for at least 14 days before or after treatment with an MAOI because of the risk of toxic effects. An MAOI should not be started for five weeks after a course of **fluoxetine** or two weeks after **paroxetine** or **sertraline**. Of the MAOIs, **phenelzine** (Nardil) and **isocarboxazid** are preferred, because they are safer than **tranylcypromine**.

Combining a tricyclic antidepressant with an MAOI is no more effective than either drug used alone and can be hazardous. Tranylcypromine with **clomipramine** (Anafranil) is a particularly unsafe combination. You should always carry a treatment card with you reminding you of interactions with medicines, including cough and cold remedies, food and alcohol.

Moclobemide (Manerix) has a more selective and reversible action than MAOIs and prevents the enzyme monoamine oxidase A from breaking down brain neurotransmitters. It may have fewer unwanted effects and less risk of dietary and drug interactions than standard MAOIs.

STOPPING TREATMENT

Unlike benzodiazepines and other tranquillisers, treatment with an antidepressant medicine does not generally cause dependence. The medical definition of dependence is that people only become dependent if they develop tolerance to a drug, sometimes with a desire to increase the dose, suffer unpleasant symptoms when they stop using it and crave for the drug when they cannot have it. A cluster of symptoms, a 'discontinuation syndrome' can occur following antidepressant withdrawal, rather than a true dependence, although for some it may seem like a form of dependence, because the effects can be so severe.

Such withdrawal symptoms can occur after stopping regular antidepressant treatment suddenly, particularly with the SSRI **paroxetine** (Seroxat) but also with tricyclic and monoamine-oxidase inhibitor antidepressants, and with **venlafaxine** (Efexor). Symptoms begin within 24 to 72 hours after suddenly stopping the treatment and include headaches, feeling and being sick, dizziness and lethargy. Other symptoms are sleeplessness, vivid dreams, anxiety, panic attacks, 'pins and needles', shock-like sensations, balance problems, tremor and sweating. About one in five people experience SSRI withdrawal effects and difficulties on stopping treatment. In some, symptoms are so severe that normal functioning is impossible and the dose may need to be increased before attempting a slow withdrawal. Your doctor will give you a schedule to withdraw treatment gradually over a period of six to eight weeks following a standard course of six to eight months of treatment. After courses lasting less than eight weeks, treatment can generally be withdrawn in one to two weeks. Many symptoms are mild and short-lasting and if your doctor has explained what is likely to happen, this can help you to deal with any symptoms.

ELECTROCONVULSIVE THERAPY

Electroconvulsive therapy (ECT) may help severe acute depressive illness, particularly if someone has hallucinations, delusions, a risk of suicide and is not eating or drinking properly. It may also be used for a person with a prolonged or severe episode of mania or for catatonia, characterised by abnormal movement or posture, and occasionally to treat schizophrenia. ECT is used to achieve rapid and short-term improvement of severe symptoms after other treatments have been thoroughly tried.

ECT is usually effective and has few adverse effects, although heart rate and blood pressure and short- and long-term memory may be affected. ECT may not be suitable for children and old people or during pregnancy. You are given a general anaesthetic and a small current of electricity is passed through the brain, producing a mild convulsion. Recovery may take a few weeks. The need for valid consent before ECT treatment with the involvement of a carer or patient advocate is recommended.

Psychotic illnesses

Psychoses – mental disorders such as schizophrenia, paranoia symptoms, mania and depression – are serious illnesses. Thoughts and behaviour are disturbed in some cases for only a short time, but in others the disorders may be permanent.

Schizophrenia is an illness in which thought processes become fragmented: you lose touch with reality, often seeing or hearing things which are not really there (hallucinating) and believing things that are not true (suffering delusions). Paranoid delusions are common, for example the belief that everyone is against you. You may hear or talk to imaginary (mainly negative) voices, and try to protect yourself from people who you believe want to harm you. These symptoms are known collectively as 'positive' symptoms. You may also experience severe mood problems, such as depression, apathy, loss of emotion and difficulties relating to people – so-called 'negative' symptoms.

About one person in a hundred is at risk of developing schizophrenia, regardless of culture, social class or sex. It is most common in young people, especially between the ages of 15 and 45. The illness can run in families and if one of your parents has schizophrenia the risk of your developing it increases to about one in eight. Theories that family interaction causes schizophrenia are now rejected, although if you have had schizophrenic symptoms the tendency to relapse can be affected by family relationships and attitudes. A combination of factors seems to be the most likely explanation for schizophrenia and these include genetic make-up, upbringing and environment, psychological factors and your vulnerability to stressful life events.

FAMILY THERAPY

If a schizophrenic's family is supportive, tolerant and keep the emotional temperature low, the person is far less likely to have a relapse than if they are critical or emotionally demanding. Of the people who return from hospital to a 'high-emotion' home, 53 per cent have a relapse during the following year. For those who return to a 'low-emotion' home, the figure is only 23 per cent.

Family therapy sessions help people adjust to the idea that their son, daughter or spouse is unlikely to regain the same levels of achievement and emotional strength that they had before they were ill. This adjustment in itself can improve the sufferer's chances.

Manic depression (bipolar disorder) is a mental illness in which changes in mood are greatly exaggerated. In a mentally healthy person, your mood or state of mind may alter slightly from day to day depending on events. With manic depression episodes of deep depression may alternate, sometimes rapidly, with periods of normal moods and periods of elation or overactivity (*mania*). Manic episodes occur less frequently than depressive symptoms and range in intensity from milder symptoms (*hypomania* as in bipolar II disorder) to severe mania with psychotic features (bipolar I disorder) which may require hospital admission. The intensity, presentation and frequency of these episodes vary in people. It is a distressing and disabling disorder in which sufferers may attempt suicide. Treatment aims to prevent recurrences and suicidal acts. Lithium is the most effective long-term treatment for manic depression (page 218), but other medicines are used, including antiepileptics and antipsychotics.

Other mental illnesses include acute states of confusion, dementia and behaviour and personality disorders. *Dementia* is a deterioration in brain function leading to impairment of intellect, memory and personality, but without impairment of consciousness. There are various causes of dementia, for example degeneration in brain function (e.g. Alzheimer's disease) or blockage of blood vessels usually following mini strokes (*vascular dementia*) or as a result of some other disease (e.g. low thyroid levels or infection which can be treatable). Alzheimer's disease accounts for about 60 per cent of dementias, vascular dementia for around 25 per cent and other types of dementias for 10 to 15 per cent. Dementia is common in old age; it is often progressive and sometimes associated with disruptive behaviour, for example agitation and aggression. Antipsychotics, often in low doses, have been widely used unofficially to control the behaviour of elderly people with dementia, although they should be reserved for people whose disturbances are causing severe problems.

The new medicines for **Alzheimer's disease – donepezil** (Aricept), **rivastigmine** (Exelon), **galantamine** (▼Reminyl) and **memantine** (▼Ebixa) – are not necessarily helpful for behavioural and psychological problems, although they slow the rate of cognitive decline.

The exact cause of psychoses is not known but it may be a blend of a number of factors including stress, heredity and brain injury. What is known is that parts of the brain become oversensitive to the brain chemical *dopamine.* This chemical is a neurotransmitter carrying messages between brain cells. In mental illness the brain cells release too much dopamine, resulting in mental overactivity. This process is thought to produce abnormal thoughts and behaviour. There may also be an imbalance in the electrical messages between the left and right sides of the brain.

Temporary psychotic symptoms can occur with drug or alcohol misuse. The abuse of mind-altering drugs such as cocaine, cannabis and amphetamines can cause hallucinations and psychosis. If mental symptoms, such as hallucinations, develop in older people the medicines they take or have just started should be examined. Certain prescription medicines, such as antiparkinsonian drugs, analgesics, the heart drug digoxin, beta blockers, sedatives and anti-anxiety drugs, can cause psychotic signs.

The government, recognising the need to improve services to people with mental health problems, has published a National Service Framework for mental health, as well as a separate framework for problems in older people. Standards that the NHS and Social Services should deliver include combating discrimination against those with mental health problems, providing timely access to services and effective treatments and having a written care plan. It will take time to turn mental health services around, but opportunities exist for you to become involved in influencing the shape of local services by linking into the Expert Patient Programme* or the Preparing Professionals for Partnership with the Public* (4Ps) initiative. The National Institute for Clinical Excellence (NICE)* has also looked at the choice of antipsychotic medicines.

– HOW YOU CAN HELP YOURSELF –

Friends and relatives of a person suffering from a psychotic illness should encourage the following actions.

- ☐ Seek advice, support and professional help.
- ☐ Become actively involved with your treatment and discuss the pros and cons of treatment with your doctor and other members of the healthcare team.
- ☐ Take exercise or be active for a part of each day.
- ☐ Take care with what you eat and try to limit weight gain. Some believe that fish oils and nutritional supplements play a role in better mental health.
- ☐ Balance life between seeing people and being alone.
- ☐ Join a local help group; depending on your condition contact Rethink* (previously the National Schizophrenia Fellowship), the Schizophrenia Association of Great Britain* or the Manic Depression Fellowship*. Sane* and the National Association for Mental Health (MIND)* offer general advice on mental health issues.

Antipsychotic medicines

Antipsychotic medicines (*neuroleptics*; also misleadingly called major tranquillisers) can help to relieve psychotic symptoms, but they are not cures for mental illness. Drug treatment can improve the quality of life for a mentally ill person and may prevent relapse after the illness first becomes apparent. Someone with acute schizophrenia – a dramatic crisis lasting days or weeks – generally responds to treatment better than someone who has developed the illness gradually and has chronic (long-term) symptoms. Chronic schizophrenia is usually a slow and often permanent deterioration in mental health. Although an antipsychotic medicine may be less effective in someone who is apathetic and withdrawn, drug treatment sometimes appears to have an enlivening influence. You should discuss the relative benefits of medication and potential unwanted effects with your doctor and involve an advocate or carer where possible. Making an advanced directive, that is, written instructions with the healthcare team about future treatment – for example during an acute schizophrenic episode when you may be unable to respond – can be helpful. In addition to taking an antipsychotic, support for other medical, emotional and social needs should be available.

Antipsychotic medicines act by interfering with the flow of nerve signals within the brain. They block dopamine receptors, areas on the cell wall where dopamine locks on to the cell to produce its effect; some newer medicines also affect serotonin receptors. Antipsychotic drugs should not be used to treat mild cases of anxiety or depression. Two main groups of antipsychotic medicines exist – the older 'typical' antipsychotics, such as **chlorpromazine** and a similar drug **haloperidol**, and the newer or 'atypical' antipsychotics, such as **risperidone** or **olanzapine**.

Choice of antipsychotic medicine

The choice of antipsychotic depends on a person's response to the drug, how well symptoms improve and how unwanted effects are tolerated. Of the older medicines, **chlorpromazine** acts widely, not just on dopamine receptors to bring about therapeutic effects, but also on other receptors to cause unwanted effects, for example dry mouth, blurred vision and constipation (antimuscarinic receptors), dizziness and faintness when changing position suddenly (adrenergic receptors) and drowsiness (histamine receptors). Other typical antipsychotics act at the same sites to varying degrees, for example **haloperidol** is less sedating than chlorpromazine and has less antimuscarinic and dizziness effects.

All antipsychotics can cause unwanted effects but the types of effect and their significance varies between different people. The atypical antipsychotics, such as **risperidone**, are so-called because they are less likely to cause unwanted extrapyramidal effects (see below). NICE recommends that an antipsychotic from this group should be considered if someone is newly diagnosed with schizophrenia. If you relapse on treatment with a typical antipsychotic or find the unwanted effects intolerable then a newer medicine should be tried. The typical antipsychotics remain useful and unwanted effects may not be a problem, particularly at low dosage, so you do not need to change treatment unless there are problems. The lowest possible dose of any antipsychotic should be used, but sometimes higher than licensed doses are tried. Your doctor should limit the period when you are on a higher than usual dosage, monitor you for signs of unwanted effects and review the need for high-dose treatment regularly.

Unwanted effects

Extrapyramidal symptoms of antipsychotics cause the most trouble. They cannot be predicted and depend on the dose, the type of drug and how susceptible you are to it. The extrapyramidal system is a network of nerve pathways running from the brain to the spinal cord, which controls and co-ordinates movement in skeletal muscles, including posture. If the extrapyramidal system is damaged or degenerates, your voluntary control over muscle movements decreases and involuntary movements, such as jerks and tremors, develop. This happens in Parkinson's disease, a degenerative problem, and as unwanted effects of some medicines, for example some of the antipsychotics. Antipsychotic drugs can cause several types of extrapyramidal disorders.

- ☐ **Parkinsonian symptoms** (or parkinsonism) – difficulty speaking or swallowing, loss of balance, mask-like face, muscle spasms, stiffness of the arms or legs, trembling or shaking.
- ☐ **Dystonia** – jaw clenching and other abnormal face, neck and body movements, unusual eye movements with eyeballs becoming fixed in one position.
- ☐ **Akathisia** – restlessness, inability to sit or stand still.
- ☐ **Tardive dyskinesia** – lip smacking, chewing movements, puffing of cheeks, rapid darting tongue movements, uncontrolled movements of arms or legs.

Parkinsonian effects and akathisia may come on gradually within the first months of treatment but can be suppressed with an anti-parkinsonian medicine, such as **orphenadrine** or **trihexyphenidyl** (benzhexol) (pages 256–8). Alternatively, a change of antipsychotic medicine may be needed. Dystonia may appear after only a few doses but can also be treated with an antiparkinsonian drug. Parkinsonian disorders disappear slowly when the drug is withdrawn, although akathisia and dystonia disappear more rapidly.

Tardive dyskinesia occurs fairly frequently, especially in older people, on long-term treatment (over one year) and at high doses. However, it can occur occasionally at low dosage after a short period of treatment. If you experience spontaneous or uncontrolled movements of the face, tongue, arms or legs, contact your doctor as soon as possible. It may be irreversible and result in immobility and difficulty with chewing and swallowing. Prompt detection of this unwanted effect may prevent an irreversible problem developing. Contact your doctor if you are concerned; the dose of your medicine may need to be lowered or the drug changed.

Other unwanted effects that can occur variously with new and old antipsychotics include low blood pressure, which can result in falls and accidents, and interference with the body's temperature regulation which may result in low or high body temperature in older people, especially during very cold or hot weather. These effects can be lessened by reducing the dose, and other effects such as sedation can wear off with time. Antimuscarinic effects can cause confusion, short-term memory problems and other mental impairment as well as dry mouth, constipation, difficulty passing urine, blurred vision, worsening of glaucoma, sexual problems and decreased sweating. Antipsychotics can also affect the threshold at which seizures can occur. Weight gain is also a problem. The body chemical prolactin, a hormone produced by the pituitary gland, influences breast development and the production of milk for breast feeding. Antipsychotics stimulate overproduction of this hormone leading to breast enlargement (*gynaecomastia*), breast milk production (*galactorrhoea*) and sexual dysfunction. Sexual problems include loss of sex drive, difficulty in achieving orgasm, and in women irregular periods. Some antipsychotics, for example **thioridazine** (Melleril) or **sertindole** (▼Serdolect), affect heart rhythm and are reserved as second-line drugs, treatments that will be supervised only by a specialist. *Neuroleptic malignant syndrome* is a very rare but potentially fatal adverse effect, which can occur early in treatment with any type of antipsychotic, where the body temperature increases, muscular rigidity and fluctuating consciousness occur and body systems such as blood pressure become unstable.

PHENOTHIAZINES

Chlorpromazine is a well-known member of a group of drugs called the phenothiazines; **haloperidol** is a butyrophenone which has similar properties. These sorts of drugs are similar in effect but differ in their main actions and unwanted effects, and people have different responses to them. Your doctor will need to find the right medicine at the lowest effective dose to suit you. Taking two antipsychotic medicines is not recommended; it does not produce twice the effect or lessen unwanted effects. An acutely disturbed person needs a higher dose of medicine at first but the dose can be reduced when symptoms are controlled. Do not alter the dose or stop treatment yourself because the illness may relapse. Your doctor will give you a schedule to withdraw treatment gradually if this seems appropriate. Some phenothiazines have other uses – for example, haloperidol or **levomepromazine** prevent feeling or being sick in patients with advanced cancer.

Phenothiazines and similar medicines may be taken by mouth but they are also given by injection or long-acting depot injection, for example **flupentixol** (Depixol) or **fluphenazine** (Modecate). If you are having regular treatment, your doctor may suggest a depot injection which is given deep into a muscle at intervals of one to four weeks and releases the drug slowly into the body, so you don't have to remember to take tablets every day.

CHLORPROMAZINE

CHLORPROMAZINE – Tablets, liquid, injection, suppositories
LARGACTIL – Tablets, liquid, injection

Chlorpromazine is a phenothiazine used for treating schizophrenia and other mental illnesses, especially paranoid symptoms. It is used as a short-term measure to quieten disturbed patients. Chlorpromazine calms and sedates without impairing consciousness, but should not be regarded as a straightforward tranquilliser for use in non-psychotic people. Chlorpromazine acts in many different ways, blocking the actions of a range of body chemicals, dopamine, serotonin, histamine (H_1), acetylcholine and adrenaline/noradrenaline alpha receptors (page 189). Although its main use and those of related medicines is in psychiatry, the phenothiazines are useful for controlling nausea and vomiting (page 224). Chlorpromazine is used in terminal illness to help increase the effects of other pain relievers and also to blunt response to pain. It can help intractable hiccup.

Chlorpromazine dosage varies depending on its use. When high dosage is required the dose should be increased gradually.

Before you use this medicine

Tell your doctor if you are:
☐ pregnant or breast-feeding ☐ taking any other medicines, including vitamins and those bought over the counter.

Tell your doctor if you have or have had:
☐ heart or circulation problems e.g. heart failure ☐ severe breathing problems ☐ Parkinson's disease ☐ epilepsy or seizures ☐ underactive thyroid gland ☐ glaucoma ☐ enlarged prostate or difficulty urinating ☐ poor liver function ☐ poor kidney function ☐ myasthenia gravis ☐ blood disorders e.g. agranulocytosis ☐ hypersensitivity to chlorpromazine.

How to use this medicine

Take the tablet with food or a full glass of water three times a day. Chlorpromazine can cause a skin rash (contact dermatitis); tablets should not be crushed and liquids must be handled with care. It can also cause a dry mouth; drink extra fluids to prevent dryness.

You may feel dizzy, especially when you get up from sitting or lying down. Get up slowly and stand beside the chair or bed until you are sure you are not dizzy. Do not drive or do other activities that require alertness until you know how you react to chlorpromazine. Avoid alcohol as it increases the effects of chlorpromazine.

Do not stop taking chlorpromazine suddenly – even if you feel well. Always discuss your treatment with the doctor who will give you a schedule to reduce the dose gradually if treatment can be stopped. If you miss a dose, take it as soon as you remember but skip it if it is almost time for your next dose. Do not take double doses.

Over 65 You should have a third to half the adult dose: older people are more susceptible to unwanted effects. You should take particular care in very hot or very cold weather because chlorpromazine affects the body's regulation of temperature. You or a relative should find out why you are being prescribed a phenothiazine. Doctors should give serious consideration to prescribing these drugs to people aged over 70 because of the many possible adverse effects.

Interactions with other medicines

Chlorpromazine interacts with many other medicines. Do not take other medicines without checking with your doctor or pharmacist. These are some important ones.
General anaesthetics increase the blood pressure-lowering effect of chlorpromazine. If you have to have surgery tell your doctor or dentist that you take this medicine.
Anti-anxiety and sleep-inducing drugs increase drowsiness with chlorpromazine; depressed breathing.
Antidepressants, **tricyclics** increase the antimuscarinic unwanted effects of chlorpromazine, such as dry mouth, blurred vision, difficulty in passing urine and constipation.
Antiepilectics Increased risk of agranulocytosis, a blood disorder.
Lithium Increased risk of extrapyramidal effects.
Sibutramine Increased risk of nervous system toxicity.
Ulcer-healing **cimetidine** may enhance the effects of chlorpromazine.

A number of types of medicine interact with chlorpromazine and related drugs to increase the risk of abnormal heart rhythms. These include: **antiarrhythmic drugs**, **antibacterials** e.g. **moxifloxacin**, **tricyclic antidepressants**, **antihistamine terfenadine**, other antipsychotics, **beta-blockers**, **diuretics**, **antivirals for HIV**.

Unwanted effects

Likely Drowsiness, lethargy, antimuscarinic effects including dry mouth (see above), dizziness, fainting, sleeplessness, agitation, weight gain, fewer periods, extrapyramidal symptoms (see below), headache, menstrual irregularities, discharge from nipple, sexual difficulties, impotence.

Less likely Jaundice, irregular heart rhythm, blood disorders indicated by fever and sore throat, abnormal bleeding or bruising, skin rash (contact dermatitis); with high dosage sensitivity to sunlight – avoid exposure, eye changes, nasal stuffiness, upset in body temperature regulation, breast enlargement, seizures, neuroleptic malignant syndrome.

Contact your doctor if you feel unwell on chlorpromazine but especially if you develop these extrapyramidal symptoms:

Parkinsonian symptoms Difficulty speaking or swallowing, loss of balance, mask-like face; muscle spasms; stiffness of arms and legs; trembling and shaking.

Dystonia Muscular spasms of face, neck, shoulders and body; facial distortions and grimacing; unusual eye movements when eyeballs become fixed in one position.

Akathisia Restlessness, inability to sit or stand still, pacing up and down.

Tardive dyskinesia Lip smacking, chewing movements, puffing of cheeks, darting tongue movements, uncontrolled movements of arms and legs.

Similar preparations

BENQUIL – Tablets
BENPERIDOL

CLOPIXOL – Tablets, depot injection
ZUCLOPENTHIXOL

DEPIXOL – Tablets, depot injection
FLUPENTIXOL

DOLMATIL – Tablets
SULPIRIDE

DOZIC – Liquid
HALOPERIDOL

FENTAZIN – Tablets
PERPHENAZINE

HALDOL – Tablets, liquid, injection, depot injection
HALOPERIDOL

HALOPERIDOL – Tablets

ORAP – Tablets
PIMOZIDE

*MELLERIL – Tablets, liquid
THIORIDAZINE

MODITEN – Tablets, depot injection (Modecate)
FLUPHENAZINE

NEULACTIL – Tablets, liquid
PERICYAZINE

NOZINAN – Tablets, injection
LEVOMEPROMAZINE (METHOTRIMEPRAZINE)

PIPORTIL DEPOT – Depot injection
PIPOTIAZINE

PROCHLORPERAZINE – Tablets

PROMAZINE – Tablets, liquid (*not recommended for use by mouth as antipsychotic*)

SERENACE – Capsules, tablets, liquid, injection
HALOPERIDOL

STELAZINE – Tablets, modified-release capsules, liquid
TRIFLUOPERAZINE

STEMETIL – Tablets, liquid, granules, injection, suppositories
PROCHLORPERAZINE

SULPIRIDE – Tablets

SULPITIL – Tablets
SULPIRIDE

SULPOR – Liquid
SULPIRIDE + SERTINDOLE

***THIORIDAZINE** – Tablets, liquid

TRIFLUOPERAZINE – Tablets, liquid

* Under specialist supervision only

NEWER ATYPICAL ANTIPSYCHOTIC MEDICINES

'Atypical antipsychotics' include **amisulpride** (Solian), **olanzapine** (Zyprexa), **quetiapine** (Seroquel), **risperidone** (Risperdal) and **zotepine** (Zoleptil). **Sertindole** (▼Serdolect) and **clozapine** (Clozaril) cause potentially life-threatening conditions very occasionally and therefore their use is restricted.

Atypical antipsychotics are not necessarily more effective than older established drugs, but are generally easier to tolerate because they cause fewer unwanted (e.g. antimuscarinic and parkinsonian) effects and have less effect on prolactin (see unwanted effects above). They can cause dizziness, especially at the start of treatment; you may faint after standing up too quickly (postural hypotension). Several of these newer medicines increase weight and olanzapine and clozapine also affect blood sugar adversely, which can trigger diabetes. None of the newer antipsychotics is more effective than the others, but the range of unwanted effects varies.

Clozapine (Clozaril) is an effective antipsychotic, but occasionally (the risk is less than 1 in 100) it can cause a serious blood disorder (*agranulocytosis*) of a type of white blood cells (granulocytes), and so is used only with strict monitoring – the Clozaril Patient Monitoring Service – in those who do not respond to, or cannot take, other antipsychotics. Clozapine can exacerbate heart and circulatory disease, as it causes inflammation of the heart muscle and weakening of the heart contractions leading to poorer circulation. Your doctor must check your health, particularly your heart, before you start clozapine and must monitor you very carefully during the first two months of therapy. If you develop heart problems while taking clozapine, your doctor will stop the treatment; you must not take clozapine again. Clozapine also has antimuscarinic unwanted effects, such as constipation. These effects are increased if clozapine is taken with other drugs with similar unwanted effects, such as tricyclic antidepressants.

RISPERIDONE

RISPERDAL – Tablets, dispersible tablets, liquid, ▼depot injection

Risperidone is an atypical antipsychotic used for schizophrenia, both sudden (acute) and longer-term (chronic) episodes where you experience hallucinations, confusion, delusions, paranoia, emotional and social withdrawal. It acts by blocking dopamine and serotonin receptors, but also blocks alpha- and histamine- receptors, which causes unwanted effects such as dizziness and faintness at the start of treatment and also weight gain. Risperidone causes less extrapyramidal symptoms than the older antipsychotics, although these can become a problem at high doses (over 10mg a day).

Before you use this medicine

Tell your doctor if you are:

☐ pregnant ☐ breast-feeding – avoid ☐ taking any other medicines, including vitamins and those bought over the counter.

Tell your doctor if you have or have had:
☐ heart or circulation problems ☐ Parkinson's disease ☐ epilepsy or seizures ☐ poor liver or kidney function.

Do not take if you have phenylketonuria
☐ Risperidone dispersible tablets (Risperdal Quicklet) contain the artificial sweetener aspartame and must not be taken if you have phenylketonuria.

How to use this medicine

Risperidone dosage should be increased slowly at first to avoid low blood pressure that results when you move position suddenly (postural hypotension). Take the tablet with food or a full glass of water twice a day for the first and second days, and thereafter either as a single dose once or twice a day. Your doctor may recommend a slower increase, if necessary. Six different tablet strengths are available, ranging from 500 micrograms (0.5mg) to 6mg. The total daily dose is usually between 4–6mg and for older people and those with liver or kidney problems 2–4mg; take no more than a total of 16mg a day. A dispersible preparation that dissolves in the mouth (Risperdal Quicklet) does not need to be taken with water. A long-acting depot injection given every two weeks is also available. When starting treatment with the injection, tablets are continued for up to three weeks while the injection takes effect. The injection is not recommended for people under 18 years.

You may feel dizzy, especially when you get up from sitting or lying down at the start of treatment. Get up slowly and stand beside the chair or bed until you are sure you are not dizzy. This effect should fade with time. Do not drive or do other activities that require alertness until you know how you react to risperidone. Avoid alcohol as it increases the effects of risperidone.

Do not stop taking risperidone suddenly, even if you feel well. Always discuss your treatment with the doctor, who will give you a schedule to reduce the dose gradually if treatment can be stopped. If you miss a dose, take it as soon as you remember but skip it if it is almost time for your next dose. Do not take double doses.

Over 65 and those with poor liver or kidney function You should have a quarter of the adult dose. Risperidone by mouth is not recommended if you are under 15 years of age.

Interactions with other medicines

Antiepileptics Opposing effects, seizure threshold lowered; **carbamazepine** decreases the amount of risperidone in the body and therefore its effectiveness.
General anaesthetics increase the blood pressure-lowering effect of risperidone. If you have to have surgery, tell your doctor or dentist that you take this medicine.
Antidepressant fluoxetine increases blood levels of risperidone and therefore the amount in the body.

Unwanted effects

Likely Sleeplessness, agitation, anxiety, headache.
Less likely Drowsiness, lethargy, dizziness, impaired concentration, constipation, blurred vision, weight gain, feeling or being sick, dyspepsia, abdominal pain, sexual dysfunction, fluid retention, fewer periods, breast milk production (galactorrhoea) and breast enlargement (gynaecomastia), runny or stuffy nose, urinary problems, hypersensitivity reactions, extrapyramidal symptoms at high dosage, blood disorders, stroke.

Rarely seizures, low blood sodium, low blood pressure, abnormal body temperature.

Contact your doctor if you feel unwell on risperidone and especially if you develop extrapyramidal symptoms.

Similar preparations

*CLOZARIL – Tablets
CLOZAPINE

▼SERDOLECT – Tablets
SERTINDOLE

*SEROQUEL – Tablets
QUETIAPINE

*SOLIAN – Tablets, liquid
AMISULPRIDE

*ZOLEPTIL – Tablets
ZOTEPINE

*ZYPREXA – Tablets, dispersible tablets, injection
OLANZAPINE

* Under specialist supervision only

LITHIUM AND OTHER MEDICINES FOR MANIA

Lithium as a salt, lithium carbonate or citrate, is used for the prevention and treatment of acute mania, for preventing the recurrence of manic depression (bipolar depression) and also for depressive mood swings or recurrent depression. A benzodiazepine and/or an antipsychotic medicine may be given at first to relieve immediate manic symptoms when lithium treatment is started because it can take up to two to three weeks to work.

Although lithium's effect in controlling mania was discovered in the late 1940s, the link between its effect in the body and how it helps manic symptoms is not clear. Nevertheless it is an effective treatment, although the level between its therapeutic and adverse effects is narrow (the level is measured as serum concentration. Serum is the clear fluid that separates from blood when it clots). It is important that you have the same brand of lithium preparation once you have started therapy because of possible variations between products, although no one product is preferred over another.

Other medicines, particularly antiepileptics, are being increasingly used as 'mood stabilisers'. **Carbamazepine** (Tegretol) may be useful for preventing manic depression if lithium does not help. It can help where manic-depressive illness cycles rapidly, for example four or more episodes a year. **Valproic acid** (Depakote) is specially licensed for use in manic episodes associated with bipolar disorder, but other antiepileptics (pages 250–2) such as **sodium valproate**, **gabapentin** and **lamotrigine** are sometimes used unofficially. The advantage of antiepileptics is that they have fewer unwanted effects than lithium. The antipsychotics **olanzapine** (Zyprexa) and **quetiapine** (Seroquel) are licensed for the treatment of moderate to severe episodes of mania, but others such as **risperidone** may be used unofficially. They may be used additionally with lithium or valproic acid. Non-drug treatment such as psychotherapy and cognitive behavioural therapy can be helpful additions to treatment with medicines.

LITHIUM

Lithium carbonate: tablets, modified-release tablets
CAMCOLIT LITHONATE
LISKONUM PRIADEL

Lithium citrate: liquid
LI-LIQUID PRIADEL

Lithium is used for preventing and treating mania, manic depression, recurrent depression and aggressive behaviour or intentional self-harm. It lessens the intensity and frequency of mood swings. The decision to start treatment with lithium has to be carefully considered because there is a narrow range between a helpful and a harmful dose. Treatment is usually started by a hospital specialist and blood levels of the drug must be measured frequently at the start of therapy and then regularly at three-monthly intervals so that the dose can be tailored to your needs. Treatment may be for a period of up to five years, or even longer. Lithium can cause serious adverse effects, which you should know about, and medical help must be sought immediately if they occur.

Before you use this medicine

Tell your doctor if you are:
☐ pregnant – do not become pregnant without talking to your doctor because lithium can affect the fetus ☐ breast-feeding – you must not breastfeed whilst on lithium ☐ on a low-salt diet ☐ taking any other medicines, including vitamins and those bought over the counter.

Tell your doctor if you have or have had:
☐ heart or circulation problems ☐ kidney disease ☐ Addison's disease (page 327) ☐ myasthenia gravis ☐ under- or overactive thyroid – thyroid function should be measured every 6–12 months.

Your doctor should check your heart, kidney and thyroid function before you start lithium treatment.

How to use this medicine

Take the tablet with plenty of water as a single daily dose, either in the morning or at bedtime, once treatment has been stabilised. At the start of lithium therapy you may take it in divided doses as directed by your doctor. Swallow each tablet whole, especially modified-release tablets. Try to take the dose at the same time each day. Liquid preparations of lithium are usually taken twice a day. It may take up to two or three weeks before you can tell whether the drug is working.

Different preparations vary in how much lithium reaches the blood. Never accept a different preparation from the one you have, unless your doctor specifically prescribes it. Ask the pharmacist to give you a treatment card with information about lithium and space to note the brand name, or use the medicine record sheet at the back of this book. If you change preparation, blood levels need to be re-measured.

Lithium blood levels are affected by the amount of sodium in your body. Be especially careful to keep your salt and fluid intake constant. Avoid dieting and discuss any plans you have for dieting with your doctor. Drink more fluids during hot weather or illness such as diarrhoea. Alcohol can enhance the sedative effects of lithium.

Do not drive or do other activities that require alertness until you know how you react to lithium.

Do not stop taking this medicine suddenly as your condition may worsen. Your doctor will give you a schedule to reduce the dose of lithium gradually. If you miss a dose, take it as soon as you remember, but skip it if it is less than eight hours until your next scheduled dose. Do not take double doses.

Monitoring treatment

See your doctor regularly to make sure lithium is working. You will need regular three-monthly blood tests, exactly 12 hours after your last dose, and a check to see that you are not developing unwanted effects. You will also need regular tests for thyroid function (every 6–12 months) and kidney function.

If you have an illness such as an infection, diarrhoea or vomiting or where you sweat profusely, you should have a lower dose or temporarily stop lithium treatment. Around one third of people taking lithium may pass more urine than usual. This should return to normal when you stop lithium. If you have lithium therapy for a long time, permanent changes can occur and function can be impaired.

Over 65 You need less than the normal adult dose; older people are more sensitive to the effects of lithium.

Interactions with other medicines

Lithium interacts with many other medicines. Do not take other medicines, including those bought over the counter, without checking with your doctor or pharmacist.

Some medicines reduce the usual pattern of lithium leaving the body so blood levels of lithium increase, and therefore the risk of toxicity. Dosage should be adjusted or combinations avoided:

Analgesic anti-inflammatory drugs Aspirin and NSAIDs e.g. ibuprofen, diclofenac, indometacin, mefenamic acid, naproxen, rofecoxib and others.

Blood pressure-lowering drugs: ACE inhibitors, angiotensin II receptor antagonists

Diuretics, especially thiazide diuretics – avoid.

Other medicines increase the risk of unwanted effects variously:

Antidepressants Citalopram, fluoxetine, fluvoxamine, paroxetine and **sertraline** Increased risk of nervous system effects e.g. drowsiness, tremor, giddiness, blurred vision.

Antipsychotics Clozapine, **haloperidol**, **phenothiazines** Increased risk of extrapyramidal effects and possibly nerve damage; **sulpiride** increased risk of unwanted extrapyramidal effects; **amisulpride**, **sertindole** and **thioridazine** increased risk of abnormal heart rhythms

Methyldopa for lowering blood pressure may cause nerve damage such as numbness or weakness.

Unwanted effects

Likely at the start of treatment, but should fade as treatment stabilises: feeling sick, dizziness, muscle weakness, dazed feeling.

Likely to remain Thirst, fine hand tremor, needing to urinate more often.

Less likely weight gain, fluid retention in the legs (may respond to dose reduction).

If you develop any the following symptoms of toxicity, stop taking lithium and contact your doctor immediately:

Early signs Diarrhoea, feeling or being sick, loss of appetite, muscle weakness, drowsiness, slurred speech, trembling.
Late signs Blurred vision, giddiness, clumsiness, lack of co-ordination, confusion, coarse tremor, trembling.

Sickness and dizziness

Feeling sick (nausea) and being sick (vomiting) are common symptoms of a variety of disorders. Vomiting is one of the ways that the body gets rid of harmful substances, as in the case of food poisoning, but it may also be a sign of disease. Causes of sickness include gastroenteritis, bacterial and viral infections, hormonal changes during pregnancy, diabetes, motion sickness, migraine, cancer chemotherapy, Ménière's disease, vertigo and unwanted effects of medicines.

Vomiting is a reflex action in response to stimulation of the *vomiting centre* in the brain. The vomiting centre can receive signals from the stomach and intestines, from the inner ear and from the brain. Another part of the brain, the *chemoreceptor trigger zone*, which is thought to be sensitive to foreign substances in the blood, can also stimulate the vomiting centre. Medicines to prevent or control sickness seem to suppress the stimulus to vomit. Treatment of vomiting depends on its cause.

Giddiness is described clinically as vertigo – a condition in which you feel that either you or the room is spinning. You may lose balance and feel or be sick. The inner ear controls balance and responds to changes in bodily movements and if it is damaged through illness, such as infection, your balance may be affected. Sudden attacks of vertigo, associated with hearing loss and noises in the ear (*tinnitus*), occur in a wide variety of disorders of the inner ear. When there appears to be no direct cause of the condition, the disorder is known as Ménière's disease.

A dizzy feeling (a swimming, lightheaded feeling) can also be caused by anxiety, lack of food when blood-sugar is low and overbreathing (*hyperventilation*). If you stand up or lift your head up quickly when your blood pressure is low, you may feel dizzy or faint (*postural hypotension*).

Medicines for sickness and dizziness

The choice of medicine depends on the cause of sickness. Sometimes a medicine is unnecessary because the body may be reacting to an infection, such as food poisoning. Taking a medicine to stop sickness (an anti-emetic) can delay the removal of bacteria and toxins from the body. An anti-emetic may mask diagnosis of a medicine's unwanted effect, when lowering the dose or stopping the drug would be better treatment.

MOTION SICKNESS

The most effective drug for preventing motion or travel sickness on short journeys is **hyoscine** (related to **atropine**). It should be taken about half

HOW YOU CAN HELP YOURSELF

- ☐ If you have vomited, drink fluids to replace those lost from the body. The rehydration solution of glucose and salt used for diarrhoea is ideal (pages 74–5). If vomiting occurs over a few days, for example as a result of gastroenteritis, rehydration is important and food should be avoided until vomiting has stopped. Re-introduce food gradually.
- ☐ If you are prone to travel sickness, find a medicine that suits you to take before you travel. Avoid overindulging in food and drink before the journey; find a good position on an aeroplane, stay on deck on a boat and look out of the window in a car. Avoid reading in the car – children are particularly liable to feel sick doing this. Take something to drink and/or suck, such as bottled water and some glucose sweets.
- ☐ If you are sick during pregnancy, eat a little food before you get up in the morning and take small amounts frequently throughout the day.
- ☐ Eat meals regularly if lack of food makes you dizzy; carry glucose sweets as a standby.
- ☐ If you feel dizzy after resting, get up slowly from sitting or lying down and stay beside the chair or bed until you are sure you are not dizzy. If you have been lying down, hang your legs over the side of the bed for a few minutes then get up slowly.

Contact your doctor:

- ☐ if you have severe vomiting for 24 hours
- ☐ if you have taken a medicine for sickness and it is not having any effect after two days
- ☐ if a young child has diarrhoea and vomiting with a temperature
- ☐ if you are vomiting and feeling very ill
- ☐ if you vomit after a head injury.

an hour before travelling and is effective for around four hours. You can take another dose after six to eight hours, but no more than three doses in 24 hours. Remedies to prevent travel sickness, such as Kwells (hyoscine hydrobromide 0.3mg), can be bought from a pharmacy. Children under the age of three years should not take a hyoscine-containing preparation, but older children can take a lower dose than adults – Joy-Rides or Kwells Junior, for example. Unwanted effects include drowsiness, dry mouth, blurred vision and difficulty passing urine which may be particularly troublesome in older people. Hyoscine can cause troublesome visual disturbances; you should avoid activities such as driving until vision has recovered. You should not take hyoscine if you have glaucoma.

Hyoscine can also be applied to the skin as a plaster (Scopoderm), which for longer protection, for instance on sailing voyages, may be more convenient than taking tablets. Plasters are not recommended for children under ten years of age. Unwanted effects are similar to the tablets. Doctors can prescribe the plasters but you cannot buy them over the counter.

Antihistamines such as **cinnarizine** (Cinazière, Stugeron), **cyclizine** (Valoid), **meclozine** (Sea-Legs) and **promethazine** (Phenergan; Avomine) are slightly less effective than hyoscine, but unwanted effects are fewer. Drowsiness can be a problem with antihistamines; cinnarizine and cyclizine are less sedating while promethazine causes greater drowsiness than the others. Alcohol and other medicines that affect the brain, such as tranquillisers and antidepressants, should not be taken with hyoscine or an antihistamine. Both hyoscine and antihistamines commonly cause drowsiness and interfere with your ability to drive or operate machinery. Alcohol increases this effect.

VERTIGO

Giddiness and sickness associated with Ménière's disease and middle-ear disorders, such as labyrinthitis, may sometimes be helped by hyoscine, an antihistamine or a phenothiazine (for example **prochlorperazine** – Stemetil). **Betahistine** (Serc) and **cinnarizine** have been used specifically for Ménière's disease. Cinnarizine has no advantage over other antihistamines or a phenothiazine. Betahistine is specifically used for Ménière's disease and may be helpful at a starting dose of 16mg three times daily. In acute attacks of vomiting, cyclizine or prochlorperazine may be given by injection or by suppository.

Non-drug management such as vestibular rehabilitation exercises (e.g. Cawthorne Cooksey) can also be helpful. If you have severe vertigo for more than six weeks, accompanied by hearing loss or dizziness and neurological problems, then your doctor may consider referral to a specialist. Surgery is sometimes tried, but its use is controversial.

Vague symptoms of dizziness which often afflict older people need investigation rather than long-term treatment with prochlorperazine. Many medicines cause dizziness as an unwanted effect, for example the heart drug digoxin and diuretics, and altering the dose of these can stop the dizziness. Prochlorperazine can cause extrapyramidal effects (pages 211–12) especially in older people and when treatment is prolonged.

VOMITING DURING PREGNANCY

It is quite usual to feel sick or to be sick during the first three months of pregnancy at any time of the day, not just in the morning. This gradually fades, usually by 16 weeks, and does not need drug treatment. Occasionally vomiting may be severe and your doctor may prescribe an antihistamine such as **promethazine** or **cyclizine**; there is no evidence that they can harm the fetus.

Prochlorperazine or **metoclopramide** are alternatives but there is less evidence for their use in pregnancy. You should always see your doctor if you think that you need something to help with sickness. Non-drug management includes eating small meals regularly and avoiding any trigger points, such as certain smells or stress. Keep rehydrated by drinking plenty of fluids. If vomiting is severe and continues (for example with *hyperemesis gravidarum*), you may need to see a specialist and be rehydrated in hospital.

UNDERLYING DISORDERS

Some medicines, such as opioid analgesics, general anaesthetics and anticancer drugs, some diseases, terminal illness and radiotherapy can cause nausea and vomiting. A phenothiazine, such as **chlorpromazine**, **haloperidol** or **levomepromazine** (methotrimeprazine) in low dose is recommended for preventing and treating this sort of sickness.

Metoclopramide is another anti-emetic which acts on the gut as well as on the brain to stop vomiting. Like the phenothiazines, metoclopramide may cause extrapyramidal effects, usually uncontrolled movement of the neck, face, tongue and eyes (*dystonia*), especially in children and young people. It is therefore given to people under 20 only when vomiting is severe.

Domperidone is similar to metoclopramide but is less likely to cause drowsiness and dystonia and can be used in younger people, for example for sickness with emergency hormonal contraception. Domperidone is useful in Parkinson's disease to control sickness associated with certain medicines such as levodopa.

Nabilone, a synthetic medicine derived from cannabis that helps to relieve sickness caused by anticancer drugs, is used when other anti-emetics have not worked.

Ondansetron (Zofran) is a type of anti-emetic that helps to prevent nausea and vomiting induced by anticancer medicines. This class of drug affects the neurotransmitter 5-hydroxytryptamine (5-HT) by blocking $5HT_3$ receptors, specifically in the small intestine and in the brain where this appears to trigger nausea and vomiting. Ondansetron and similar medicines **granisetron** (Kytril) and **tropisetron** (Navoban) block these stimuli. They can be given by injection, suppository or by mouth before the start of chemotherapy or radiotherapy. They are also used for sickness following surgery. Unwanted effects include headache and constipation or diarrhoea, rash and occasionally hypersensitivity.

METOCLOPRAMIDE

METOCLOPRAMIDE – Tablets, liquid, injection
MAXOLON – Tablets, liquid, injection

Antimigraine preparations

MIGRAMAX – Powder
METOCLOPRAMIDE + ASPIRIN

PARAMAX – Tablets, soluble powder
METOCLOPRAMIDE + PARACETAMOL

Poor choice
Modified-release preparations:
GASTROBID CONTINUS; MAXOLON SR

Metoclopramide is used in adults to relieve nausea and vomiting caused by digestive, liver and biliary disorders and occasionally with anticancer treatment. It blocks dopamine receptors in the intestines and in the vomiting centre in the brain. Metoclopramide may also help non-ulcer dyspepsia and oesophageal reflux because it acts on the gut, speeding the stomach contents along the intestines. Metoclopramide's anti-emetic and stomach-emptying effect also helps in migraine attacks, although absorption of low doses taken by mouth is variable. Metoclopramide in modified-release preparations is absorbed too slowly to help with nausea and vomiting. Metoclopramide is also used after operations to restore gastric activity and in some diagnostic procedures.

Before you use this medicine

Tell your doctor if you are:
☐ pregnant – may be used for sickness ☐ breast-feeding – avoid ☐ taking any other medicines, including vitamins and those bought over the counter.

Tell your doctor if you have or have had:
☐ liver or kidney disease ☐ porphyria ☐ phaeochromocytoma (a tumour causing high blood pressure) ☐ epilepsy ☐ obstruction, bleeding or perforation of the gut.

How to use this medicine

Take the 10mg tablet three times a day. Tablets should not be used for children under 15, but a liquid preparation can be used – this must be measured accurately to get the exact dose for the weight of the child. People weighing less than 60kg should have half the usual dose.

Do not drive or do other activities that require alertness until you know how you react to metoclopramide. Avoid alcohol because it works against metoclopramide's actions and enhances drowsiness.

If you miss a dose, take it as soon as you remember. If the next dose is due within two hours, take the missed dose immediately and skip the next one.

Under 20 Only used for severe, intractable sickness following radiotherapy or anticancer treatment, or in selected hospital procedures.

Over 65 Usually you need less than the normal adult dose. Prolonged treatment has caused extrapyramidal effects. Your doctor should review treatment regularly.

Interactions with other medicines

Metoclopramide can interact with any other medicine that has a sedative effect on the central nervous system, such as tranquillisers.

Hyoscine and atropine-like drugs, opioid pain relievers decrease metoclopramide's effect on the stomach and gut.

Unwanted effects

Unlikely Extrapyramidal symptoms (pages 211–12) such as uncontrolled movements of the face or eyes (dystonia – in children and young adults it is **likely**) and tardive dyskinesia (after prolonged treatment, mainly affecting elderly people).
Rarely Drowsiness, restlessness, diarrhoea, confusion, depression, leaking from breasts, breast enlargement in men.

Metoclopramide causes few problems in adults. If extrapyramidal symptoms develop in people under 20 or over 65 (usually within 36 hours of starting treatment), stop metoclopramide and contact your doctor immediately. Effects usually disappear within 24 hours.

Similar preparations

BUCCASTEM – Tablets (dissolve in the mouth)
PROCHLORPERAZINE

DOMPERIDONE – Tablets
MOTILIUM – Tablets, liquid, suppositories
DOMPERIDONE

PROCHLORPERAZINE – Tablets

STEMETIL and other phenothiazine preparations: pages 213–15

From a pharmacy
DOMPERIDONE – Tablets (for relief of stomach discomfort after eating, such as fullness, bloating and heartburn)

MOTILIUM 10 – Tablets
DOMPERIDONE

Pain

Pain is a symptom not a disease. It is an unpleasant sensory and emotional experience associated with actual or likely damage to the body. You learn the nature of pain from early childhood, for example when falling over as a toddler and cutting a knee. When the body is hurt, nerve endings detect the damage and relay impulses to the brain via the central nervous system. Your brain registers pain and the need to act to avoid further damage. This is known as *nociceptive pain*. Pain may be short-lived (*acute*), intermittent or become a long-term problem (*chronic*), defined as pain that persists after the time when healing would be expected to have finished. The severity of pain varies according to the cause or your condition, for example pain from an accident, post-operatively or pain from malignant or non-malignant disease. The intensity with which pain is felt also varies from person to person, so the amount of pain relief needed for any problem varies. However, pain is not always associated with damage to the body; there may be one or more other psychological, social or behavioural causes.

You and your doctor or dentist should try to discover the underlying cause of pain. Understanding what causes your pain can help you cope with it: when you see a cut finger and know how it happened, you attend to the physical damage first and then cope mentally with the sensation of pain afterwards, but it is much harder to understand pain from within the body, whether it is backache or a symptom of a disease. Anxiety, lack of sleep and depression lessen your tolerance of pain. If pain becomes a worry or a nagging fear then you must see your doctor.

Treating the underlying cause generally relieves pain, so a pain-relieving medicine (*analgesic*) may not always be needed; treatment with another type of medicine or other pain-relief technique may be better. Your doctor may prescribe a combination of medicines, one to relieve the underlying cause and one to tackle pain. Other medicines (e.g. **amitriptyline**, some antiepileptic drugs such as **carbamazepine**) are *adjuvants*, enhancing pain relief from analgesics by various mechanisms such as altering the emotional response to pain. They are useful for *neuropathic pain*, which is pain resulting from damage to or dysfunction in the nervous system. This type of pain can be intermittent and you may experience a variety of shooting, stabbing, stinging or electric shock-like sensations. Sometimes numbness or tingling can occur, or burning sensations (*dysaesthesia*) or pain caused by normally harmless stimuli, such as stroking the skin of the affected area (*allodynia*). Examples of neuropathic pain include trigeminal neuralgia (*tic douloureux*), a severe shooting pain across one side of the face, and pain after shingles (*post-herpetic neuralgia*) in which chronic burning and shooting pain can occur with allodynia. Neuropathic pain appears to arise from slowed or blocked electrical messages from damaged nerve cells; other specific causes include diabetes mellitus, deficient diets and excessive alcohol consumption. Sometimes no obvious cause can be found and this can be distressing.

You are the authority on the degree to which you experience pain and how it affects daily living. You need to convey these experiences, but doctors can also assess pain by using a variety of measures, such as patient questionnaires, rating scales and the visual analogue scale where you mark

– HOW YOU CAN HELP YOURSELF –

Short-lived or acute pain:

- ☐ Use simple local treatments where relevant – ice packs or cold compresses for sports injuries.
- ☐ Rest if possible to help the injured part relax.
- ☐ Exercise gently and within the capability of the damaged part to strengthen the injured muscles and tissue.
- ☐ Keep a small supply of pain-relief medicines in the house, one for adult use and one for children. Do not use more than the recommended dose.
- ☐ If you are still in pain and simple remedies have not helped after 48 hours, see your doctor.

Long-term or chronic and severe pain:

- ☐ Work with your doctor to try to establish the cause of pain, describing accurately where the pain is and how severe you think it is.
- ☐ You are the authority on your pain and only you can feel it; do not be afraid to ask for pain relief. Suffering pain after an operation, however minor, is unnecessary and may slow your recovery.
- ☐ If you have continuous pain you should have regular doses of a pain-relieving medicine to prevent pain breaking through.
- ☐ Your doctor may be able to refer you to a pain-relief clinic if you have severe intractable pain.
- ☐ Rehabilitation is important with physiotherapy or other therapists, including complementary therapies.
- ☐ Useful organisations include the Pain Society* (for healthcare professionals but which has some information for the public) and BackCare* for healthier backs.

on a line scale of 0 to 100 how your pain is at the moment. Analgesia can help with the management of pain, but a combination of approaches is likely to give better results. Therapies can be complementary or alternatives to analgesics and include physiotherapy; rest and heat (massaging a pulled muscle, for example) or cold (for burns); graduated exercise, retraining and strengthening; acupuncture; transcutaneous electrical nerve stimulation (TENS); manipulation or chiropractic; meditation; and hypnosis. The aim should be for the best possible rehabilitation with a reduction in distress, disability and pain.

Analgesics

There are two main types of pain-relieving medicine: *non-opioid analgesics* such as **paracetamol** and **aspirin**, and *opioid analgesics* (*narcotics*) such as **morphine**. Non-opioid medicines are helpful for headaches and muscular pain, stopping the transmission of pain stimuli in nerve endings at the site of pain. Non-steroidal anti-inflammatory drugs (NSAIDs), for example **ibuprofen** and **diclofenac**, are non-opioid medicines and are widely used for pain relief.

Opioid analgesics are used for moderate to severe pain. They act directly on the brain, altering your perception of pain. A simple, non-opioid analgesic may be tried first (Step 1) before you move up the 'analgesic ladder' to using a non-steroidal anti-inflammatory drug or a codeine-based medicine (Step 2) and then finally to morphine or a related medicine (Step 3) plus, if necessary, a non-opioid. An adjuvant can be taken at any stage to enhance analgesia. Pain relief should be started at the step most appropriate to your level of pain and can be stepped up or down according to your needs. If you have continuous pain, you will need regular analgesia but if pain is intermittent then you can take an analgesic when required.

NON-OPIOID ANALGESICS

Paracetamol is the analgesic of choice for mild to moderate pain, for example headache, backache, toothache, rheumatic and muscle pains. Doctors commonly recommend it and a range of paracetamol preparations can be bought over the counter in tablet, capsule, powder sachet and liquid form. How paracetamol works in the body is unclear, but it appears to act centrally on the brain by blocking the body chemicals (*prostaglandins*) that contribute to pain and swelling. Unlike aspirin and NSAIDs, paracetamol has little effect on prostaglandins elsewhere in the body. This means that it does not reduce inflammation which contributes to some pain, for example in rheumatoid arthritis or sports injuries. Paracetamol does not irritate the stomach and intestines, which is a risk with aspirin and NSAIDs. It acts for a short time in the body and must be taken up to four times a day to achieve consistent pain relief. Paracetamol is particularly suitable for children with minor illnesses and for reducing fever. It can be taken during pregnancy or when breast feeding and is the preferred analgesic for older people who are more susceptible to the unwanted effects of NSAIDs (page 236). Unwanted effects of paracetamol are rare at recommended dosages, but it can cause skin rashes and allergic reactions and occasionally blood disorders. In overdose paracetamol is harmful (see below).

Aspirin is useful for relieving headache, sore throat, muscular pains and period pains, provided you can tolerate its irritant effect on the stomach. It brings the body temperature down and reduces inflammation. Aspirin blocks the effect of prostaglandins, which are released when tissue is damaged. Taken regularly, aspirin can relieve the pain and swelling in rheumatoid arthritis, although NSAIDs are usually preferred. Aspirin is increasingly used for its antiplatelet effect in thinning blood after a heart attack or stroke, or if you are at high risk of having a coronary event (page 94).

Aspirin can cause indigestion, irritate the stomach lining and sometimes cause ulceration and bleeding. These unwanted effects arise probably through aspirin's direct action on the gut lining and the blocking effect on the prostaglandins. Taking aspirin, particularly as the dispersible form in water after food, helps to reduce these effects. Dispersible aspirin is absorbed more quickly into the bloodstream from the digestive system and pain relief is faster, but dispersible aspirin does not protect the stomach completely. Enteric-coated aspirin tablets, designed to release aspirin in the small intestine, are specially formulated to overcome aspirin's unwanted effects, but even these formulations do not do so completely. Bleeding from the gut can still occur and there appears to be little difference between plain and enteric-coated tablets in this respect, particularly at the lower doses used for blood thinning. Enteric-coated tablets take time to work, and may be helpful for relieving long-lasting pain, for example taken regularly at night, but are not suitable for immediate pain relief, say for a headache.

Toxic effects of aspirin and paracetamol

Although aspirin and paracetamol are found in ordinary, everyday medicines used for the relief of minor aches and pains, both can be toxic if more than the recommended dose is taken. Always check the label of compound preparations, such as cold remedies and analgesics, or ask the pharmacist about the contents of prescription medicines. Never take more than one type of pain- or cold-relief preparation at any one time and always follow the instructions on how much to take and how often. Plain aspirin or paracetamol sold generically give the clearest indication of the ingredients and dosage of the preparation.

You should take no more than 12 aspirin tablets of 300mg strength a day, at intervals of at least four hours. If you need to use aspirin for more than a few days, you should see your doctor for a review. Regular use of even lower doses of aspirin may cause stomach upsets and bleeding; the higher the dose, the higher the risk of bleeding. You should take no more than eight paracetamol tablets of 500mg strength a day, two tablets per dose at intervals of at least four hours. If you need to take eight tablets of paracetamol every day for more than a few days, again see your doctor for a review.

An overdose of aspirin or paracetamol needs immediate and urgent medical attention. Signs of too high a dose of aspirin include noises or ringing in the ears (*tinnitus*), deafness, overbreathing, high body temperature and sweating, thirst, stomach pain and vomiting, and an upset in the body's acid-base (alkaline) balance. Both aspirin and paracetamol can also cause kidney damage. Signs of too high a dose of paracetamol are not very obvious, but there may be some nausea and vomiting at first. An overdose of paracetamol causes severe liver damage, which may be fatal unless you have immediate treatment in hospital. Damage occurs because the body chemicals in the liver (enzymes) that break paracetamol down become saturated and cannot continue to work effectively. A by-product then develops that reacts with cell proteins, which causes the death of liver and kidney cells. With normal doses and frequency of dosing the enzymes can cope with paracetamol. In overdose, liver damage can be prevented by giving another chemical, either **acetylcysteine** by injection or **methionine** by mouth, to increase the break down of paracetamol by liver cells.

Pack sizes

The amount of paracetamol or aspirin that you can buy in a single pack is now restricted (page 9). Pack sizes of capsules and tablets containing aspirin or paracetamol (including combinations of these with codeine) on sale from pharmacies are restricted to a maximum of 32 capsules/tablets. The restriction includes dispersible, but excludes effervescent tablets. Pharmacists can sell up to 100 capsules/tablets (in multiples of 32) in certain circumstances, for example for someone who needs regular treatment with any of these preparations; this is at the pharmacist's discretion. The maximum pack size that can be bought from non-pharmacy outlets is 16 tablets/capsules. Low-dose aspirin tablets (75mg) can now be bought from pharmacies in packs of 100 tablets for preventing blood clots after heart attacks or stroke.

PARACETAMOL

Over the counter/on prescription
PARACETAMOL – Tablets, soluble tablets, liquid, suppositories

PARADOTE – Tablets (methionine protects the liver from overdose)
PARACETAMOL + METHIONINE

CO-METHIAMOL 100/500
METHIONINE + PARACETAMOL

Poor choice
Combination pain-relief preparations – ingredients better used separately:

Over the counter/on prescription
CO-CODAMOL 8/500 – Tablets (Low dose of opioid)
CODEINE 8mg + PARACETAMOL 500mg

On prescription
CO-CODAMOL 15/500 – Tablets
CODEINE 15mg + PARACETAMOL 500MG
(CODIPAR)

CO-CODAMOL 30/500 – Tablets, capsules, soluble powder sachets
CODEINE 30mg + PARACETAMOL 500mg
(KAPAKE; SOLPADOL; TYLEX)

CO-CODAMOL 60/500 – Soluble powder sachets
CODEINE 60mg + PARACETAMOL 500mg
(KAPAKE)

CO-DYDRAMOL 10/500 – Tablets
DIHYDROCODEINE 10mg + PARACETAMOL 500mg

CO-PROXAMOL 32.5/325 – Low dose of both drugs
DEXTROPROPOXYPHENE 32.5mg + PARACETAMOL 325mg
(DISTALGESIC; COSALGESIC – not NHS)

DIHYDROCODEINE 20mg + PARACETAMOL 500mg – Tablets
(REMEDEINE)

DIHYDROCODEINE 30mg + PARACETAMOL 500mg – Tablets
(REMEDEINE FORTE)

From a pharmacy
PARAMOL (not NHS)
DIHYDROCODEINE 7.46mg + PARACETAMOL 500mg

Antimigraine preparations
On prescription
PARAMAX – Tablets, soluble powder
PARACETAMOL + METOCLOPRAMIDE

Poor choice
Over the counter/on prescription
MIGRALEVE (lose dose of antihistamine and CODEINE)
MIDRID (low dose of PARACETAMOL, with adrenaline-like drug of unproven value)

Paracetamol relieves mild to moderate pain in many situations such as headache and backache, and it reduces fever by lowering raised body temperature. When taken by mouth it is rapidly absorbed into the body and will be effective within 30 minutes. Paracetamol can be used by people of all ages and is suitable for children for relieving fever and pain, such as toothache. However, unlike aspirin and NSAIDs, it has only a mild anti-inflammatory effect and does not reduce joint swelling effectively. As it does not cause stomach irritation, people with a stomach ulcer can take paracetamol and it is a good pain-reliever for older people. People allergic to aspirin can usually take paracetamol. Paracetamol is a safe and effective analgesic provided the dosage instructions are followed carefully. In overdose, a medical emergency, it can cause fatal liver and kidney damage.

Before you use this medicine

Tell your doctor if you are:
☐ pregnant or breast-feeding ☐ taking any other medicines, including vitamins and those bought over the counter.

Tell your doctor if you have or have had:
☐ severe liver or kidney disease ☐ alcohol dependence.

How to use this medicine

Take two tablets, or follow dosage instructions for other preparations, every 4–6 hours if needed. Do not take more often than every four hours. Do not take more than eight tablets or four doses in 24 hours (this is equivalent to 4g of paracetamol in 24 hours). Children older than three months may be given paracetamol. Babies who are immunised at two months can have paracetamol if fever develops after vaccination. Your doctor or nurse will recommend this, but otherwise do not give it to babies under three months of age.

If you are a moderate to heavy regular drinker, routine use of paracetamol carries a risk of liver damage and so a lower dose or less frequent dosing should be used.

If you are treating yourself with paracetamol, contact your doctor if you have a fever that lasts for more than three days or if your symptoms do not improve.

Over 65 Paracetamol is a suitable analgesic for self-treatment. As you get older paracetamol remains in the body for longer, which is increased with liver and/or kidney impairment, so that you may need less than the normal adult dose.

Interactions with other medicines

Paracetamol interacts with few medicines, but check with your doctor or pharmacist that it does not interact with any medicine you are already taking.

Anticoagulants The dose of **warfarin** may need adjusting if paracetamol is taken regularly for prolonged periods because of a risk of bleeding.

Antimigraine metoclopramide and **domperidone** accelerate the absorption of paracetamol, an advantage in treating migraine attacks

Unwanted effects

Less likely Skin rash, blood disorders, acute pancreatitis.

Unwanted effects are rare when paracetamol is taken as recommended. **Immediate medical attention must be sought if you suspect an overdose**, whether by design or accident. Overdosage leads to feeling or being sick and then liver damage after 1–2 days. Treatment within 12 hours of the overdose can prevent liver damage. Families with an unstable teenager or a depressed person in the house may wish to buy **co-methiamol, methionine + paracetamol** (Paradote) to have as the analgesic in the medicine cupboard instead of other aspirin or paracetamol products. Methionine helps to prevent liver damage caused by an overdose of paracetamol. The co-methiamol combination should not be taken together with a monoamine oxidase inhibitor antidepressant (page 206). Co-methiamol is not recommended for children under 12 years, because it has not been tested in this age group.

COMBINED ANALGESIC PREPARATIONS

Many preparations combine aspirin or paracetamol with one of the weaker opioid analgesics such as **codeine** (page 238). When pain is inadequately controlled with aspirin or paracetamol alone, it seems logical to combine one or other with a stronger analgesic, particularly as they work in different ways. Yet there is little evidence that combined analgesics are more effective than either drug given alone. The doses of the two analgesics are fixed in a combined preparation and the dose of the opioid analgesic is often too small to be felt, or each drug acts in the body for a different length of time.

Combinations of **dextropropoxyphene** with **paracetamol (co-proxamol)** or with aspirin cannot be recommended because they provide little more analgesia than either paracetamol or aspirin alone. In co-proxamol the amount of both dextropropoxyphene and paracetamol is lower per tablet than if either drug was given alone. A dose of two co-proxamol tablets provides less paracetamol (650mg) than paracetamol alone at the recommended dose of two tablets (1,000mg). Combined analgesics at lower dose might mean fewer unwanted effects.

Dextropropoxyphene, a milder opioid analgesic than codeine, still causes depressed breathing even when combined with paracetamol, which can complicate the treatment of overdose. Codeine's unwanted effects, principally constipation, can still occur at low dosage. Taking separate analgesics in appropriate doses provides more flexibility for you to tailor the use of each medicine, for example if your pain level fluctuates.

Preparations containing paracetamol with higher doses of opioids (page 238), for example with **dihydrocodeine** (Remedeine), or with codeine (Kapake, Solpadol, Tylex) may be more effective, particularly once pain is controlled, but it is questionable whether the paracetamol component is still needed. Again, taking each drug individually allows better flexibility in managing pain relief. These combination analgesics are not recommended for children.

Some pain-relief preparations contain other ingredients such as caffeine, an antihistamine or a muscle relaxant. However, such ingredients add nothing to the pain-relieving properties of an analgesic. Caffeine may aggravate the gastric irritation caused by aspirin. High doses or stopping caffeine may cause headaches.

The names of combination analgesics, both generic and brand, do not reveal the ingredients of the preparations. This information has to be carefully looked for on the label of products bought over the counter or in the patient information leaflet for prescribed analgesics. Packs and leaflets now declare 'contains paracetamol' and warn the consumer to seek advice even if he/she does not feel unwell in the event of an overdose. Always check the ingredients of a pain-relief product with the pharmacist. *Acetylsalicylic acid* is another name for aspirin which you may come across, and all salicylates are similar to aspirin. If you take a combination analgesic you should not take any other type of pain-relief product with it, unless under medical guidance. It is usually best to find a single-ingredient preparation that suits you for occasional pain relief and stick to the product. If pain relief is inadequate with paracetamol or aspirin, discuss other methods of pain relief with your doctor.

ASPIRIN IS NOT FOR CHILDREN

Aspirin should not be given to children under 16 for treating minor illnesses nor taken during breastfeeding. A rare but potentially fatal illness involving the brain and liver (Reye's syndrome) has been linked to aspirin usage in children, particularly those with a viral infection. Aspirin may occasionally be used to treat children with juvenile rheumatoid arthritis (Still's disease) or Kawasaki syndrome (a rare acute illness from which most children recover completely) under the guidance of a specialist. Paracetamol is an effective alternative treatment for relieving the pain and fever of minor complaints for young people under 16.

ASPIRIN

On prescription/over the counter for pain relief
ASPIRIN – Tablets, dispersible (soluble) tablets, enteric-coated tablets, suppositories

CAPRIN – Enteric-coated tablets

NU-SEALS ASPIRIN – Enteric-coated tablets

Some branded pain-relievers contain aspirin (see table pages 236–7): check the ingredients and the dose

Antimigraine preparation on prescription
MIGRAMAX – Powder sachets
ASPIRIN + METOCLOPRAMIDE

Poor choice
Combination preparations – ingredients better used separately (on prescription)
ASPAV (**ASPIRIN + PAPAVERETUM**); **CO-CODAPRIN 8/400** (each tablet: **CODEINE PHOSPHATE 8mg + ASPIRIN 400mg**) – also from a pharmacy
LOW DOSE ASPIRIN (75mg)

On prescription/over the counter for blood thinning (antiplatelet)
ASPIRIN – Dispersible tablets, enteric-coated tablets

Branded enteric-coated tablets:
ANGETTES 75
NU-SEALS
CAPRIN

Aspirin (*acetylsalicyclic acid*) is a non-opioid analgesic for headache, migraine, toothache, muscular injuries and period pains. Aspirin also helps the symptoms of cold and influenza. It blocks the effects of prostaglandins, which are released when body tissue is injured. Aspirin reduces a raised temperature and inflammation. Aspirin is also used in low doses (75–150mg) to prevent blood clots after heart attacks or strokes and may be useful for preventing heart attacks in people at serious risk (e.g. those who have angina, peripheral vascular disease). Irritation of the stomach is the main unwanted effect; enteric-coated preparations only partially reduce aspirin's effects on the stomach. Aspirin should not be given to children aged under 16 except under medical guidance, or taken during breastfeeding, because a rare, but often fatal, disorder – Reye's syndrome – has been linked to its use.

Before you use this medicine

Tell your doctor if you are:
☐ pregnant – avoid aspirin for pain relief, particularly in the last few weeks of pregnancy unless low dose prescribed under medical guidance ☐ breast-feeding – avoid aspirin ☐ taking any other medicines, including vitamins and those bought over the counter.

Tell your doctor if you have or have had:
☐ asthma ☐ allergies ☐ nasal polyps ☐ a previous reaction to aspirin or a non-steroidal anti-inflammatory drug such as ibuprofen ☐ blood-clotting disorders ☐ kidney or liver disease – avoid aspirin if severe ☐ anaemia ☐ dehydration ☐ glucose 6-phosphate dehydrogenase (G6PD) deficiency.

Do not take if you have or have had:
☐ a stomach or duodenal ulcer ☐ haemophilia ☐ gout.

Do not give to a child or adolescent, particularly with a fever or viral infection (see box, page 233).

How to use this medicine

Take one to three tablets every four or more hours if needed, with milk or water at or just after meals. Do not take aspirin more often than every four hours. If you are treating yourself do not take regular doses of aspirin for more than two days without contacting your doctor. If you are taking a high dose of aspirin for long periods, see your doctor for regular checks. Avoid alcohol because it increases the risk of gastric or intestinal bleeding.

If you are going to have surgery, regular treatment with aspirin should be stopped about five days beforehand. Aspirin interferes with your ability to stop bleeding.

Storage Keep aspirin tablets in a cool dry place. Do not use if the tablets smell of vinegar, look mottled or are crumbling. Renew stocks of aspirin for household use once a year.

Over 65 You can take the normal adult dose.

Interactions with other medicines

Aspirin interacts with several other medicines. Do not take other medicines without checking with your doctor or pharmacist. These are the important interactions:
Anticoagulants e.g. warfarin Increased risk of bleeding due to antiplatelet effect.
NSAIDs Increased risk of stomach irritation; aspirin's protective effects on the heart may be opposed by regular use of ibuprofen and other NSAIDs.
Methotrexate (anticancer and antirheumatic drug) Increased risk of methotrexate toxicity.
Sulphinpyrazone for gout Uric acid-lowering effect reduced by aspirin, which must not be used for gout.

Unwanted effects

Likely Heartburn, indigestion, feeling or being sick, stomach pain, abnormal weakness.
Less likely Gastrointestinal bleeding; hypersensitivity reactions: skin rash, itching, wheezing, chest tightness, trouble breathing.

Unwanted effects are generally mild and infrequent but indigestion, stomach irritation and bleeding can occur at any dosage. Vomiting bloody or coffee ground-like matter or black, tarry stools are signs of serious gastrointestinal bleeding and you should contact your doctor. Some people are hypersensitive to the effects of aspirin: if a skin rash develops or you have wheezing or difficulty breathing, stop taking aspirin and contact your doctor immediately. For treatment of overdose symptoms see above.

Similar preparations

BENORAL – Tablets, granules, liquid
BENORILATE (BENORYLATE)

This is a derivative of aspirin and paracetamol, occasionally used to relieve pain and swelling in arthritic conditions. If you take benorilate it is very important **not** to take other aspirin- or paracetamol-containing preparations with it.

Other non-opioid analgesics

Non-steroidal anti-inflammatory drugs (NSAIDs) (page 379) such as **ibuprofen**, **diclofenac** and others are mainly used to relieve the pain and inflammation of arthritic diseases, but they are also useful pain-relievers for a variety of conditions, for example period pains or sports injuries. NSAIDs also lower raised body temperature (*antipyretic*). They are useful for long-term conditions, for example bone pain where bones have tumour deposits in them. They are used for relieving pain after surgery and may reduce the need for opioid analgesics.

NSAIDs are related to aspirin and, like aspirin, they can be irritant to the stomach and duodenum. Protection with one of the ulcer-healing medicines, such as **ranitidine** or **omeprazole**, can lessen NSAID gastric effects. Newer NSAIDs (COX II inhibitors) such as **meloxicam** and **rofecoxib** are no more effective than the traditional NSAIDs, but the risk of serious irritant effects, such as bleeding and ulceration in the upper gut, is less. However, this advantage appears to be lost if you also take low-dose aspirin regularly to protect the heart. Diclofenac is used by injection or suppository to relieve the acute and excruciating pain of renal colic.

WHAT'S IN PAIN-RELIEVERS?

Analgesic ingredients of branded pain-relievers sold over the counter and in pharmacies.

Aspirin

ALKA-XS GO
ANADIN
ANADIN EXTRA SOLUBLE
ASKIT
ASPRO CLEAR
BEECHAMS POWDERS
CAPRIN
DISPRIN
DISPRIN DIRECT
MRS CULLEN'S HEADACHE POWDERS
PHENSIC

Paracetamol

ALVEDON
ANADIN PARACETAMOL
BEECHAMS POWDER CAPSULES
CALPOL
CALPOL SIX PLUS
DE WITT'S
DISPROL
DOAN'S BACKACHE PILLS
FENNINGS
GALPAMOL
HEDEX
HEDEX EXTRA
INFADROPS
MEDINOL
MANDANOL
OBIMOL
PANADOL
PANADOL ACTIFAST
PANADOL EXTRA
PARACETS
PARADOTE (with methionine)
RESOLVE
RESOLVE EXTRA

Ibuprofen

ADVIL
ANADIN IBUPROFEN
ANADIN ULTRA
CALPROFEN
CUPROFEN
GALPROFEN
HEDEX IBUPROFEN
IBUFEM

LIBROFEM	NUROFEN MELTLETS
MANDAFEN	NUROFEN MIGRAINE PAIN
MANORFEN	NUROFEN RECOVERY
MIGRAFEN	OBIFEN
NUROFEN	ORBIFEN
NUROFEN FOR CHILDREN	RELCOFEN
Aspirin + paracetamol	
ANADIN EXTRA	DISPRIN EXTRA
ANADIN EXTRA SOLUBLE	NURSE SYKES
Aspirin + codeine	
CODIS 500	
Paracetamol + codeine	
FEMINAX	SOLPADEINE
PAINEX	SOLPADEINE MAX
PANADOL ULTRA	ULTRAMOL
PARACODOL	VEGANIN
PARAMOL (dihydrocodeine)	
with antihistamine:	
DOZOL	PANADOL NIGHT
MEDISED	PROPAIN
MIGRALEVE	SYNDOL
Ibuprofen + codeine:	
NUROFEN PLUS	SOLPAFLEX

OPIOID ANALGESICS

Morphine and related drugs are extracted from the head of the opium poppy. The opioids, also called narcotic analgesics, relieve moderate to severe pain, for example pain after surgery and the pain of terminal illnesses such as cancer. An opioid may be considered for severe enduring pain of non-cancer origin, such as chronic pancreatitis or osteoporotic vertebral collapse. Pain relief would usually be managed by a specialist, for example in a pain clinic. They act directly on the areas of the brain where pain is perceived. They also block the flow of pain signals.

Morphine is the most valuable opioid analgesic for relieving severe pain and is the standard against which other opioids are compared. In addition to relieving pain morphine also causes euphoria, a sense of well-being, and mental detachment. Sixteen other opioid analgesics are available including **diamorphine** (heroin), **fentanyl**, **hydromorphone**, **oxycodone**, and **pethidine**. Opioid analgesics all have similar actions and effects, although they differ in when and for how long they work and whether they can be taken by mouth or by another method such as injection or patches. Syringe drivers – devices for giving medicines by continuous infusion under the skin (subcutaneous) – can be useful if someone is very ill and cannot take or tolerate medicines by mouth or by injection into muscles. A range of medicines can be added to the driver and doses adjusted, allowing symptoms to be well controlled. For example, to control nausea and vomiting, unwanted effects of morphine that usually fade within four or five days of treatment, an antinauseant such as **haloperidol** or **meto-**

clopramide can be added to the driver. Pain relief should be given regularly, not on an 'as required' basis when pain recurs.

Some opioids have specific uses and are less used for pain relief – for example **methadone** and **buprenorphine** are used in the management of opioid dependence.

The opioids have similar unwanted effects, although these may vary in intensity, the most common being nausea and vomiting, drowsiness and constipation. Unwanted effects that occur with higher doses include depressed breathing and low blood pressure. People vary in their response to opioids and to their unwanted effects. Constipation is almost universal with an opioid, and laxatives, for example both a softener (e.g. **lactulose**) and a stimulant (e.g. **senna**), should be started at the same as the analgesic. Drowsiness may affect the performance of skilled tasks, such as driving, and the effects of alcohol are enhanced.

High doses of morphine or any other opioid analgesic lead to breathing difficulties, narrowing of the pupil to pinpoint size, and even coma. **Naloxone**, a drug that blocks the effects of morphine, can be given by injection to reverse morphine poisoning.

The use of opioid analgesics has to be strictly controlled because of their tendency to cause dependence (addiction). But when morphine or related medicines are used medically for the control of severe pain the risk of dependence is small.

Tramadol (e.g. Tramake, Zamadol, Zydol and modified-release preparations) is a newer analgesic used for moderate to severe pain relief. It is claimed to act partly as an opioid but by also enhancing the effects of the body chemicals serotonin and noradrenaline (pages 188–9). Tramadol may not cause constipation as much as opioid analgesics, but it is associated with dependence and withdrawal symptoms. It can worsen epilepsy and lower the seizure threshold, particularly when taken in high doses or with an antidepressant medicine. Tramadol also causes wheezing and can worsen asthma.

Weaker opioid analgesics

Dihydrocodeine and **codeine** are used to relieve mild to moderate pain. Codeine and dihydrocodeine (DF118 Forte, DHC Continus) in higher doses are useful for relieving more severe pain, but both cause constipation (page 84).

MORPHINE

MORPHINE – Liquid, injection, suppositories
MORCAP SR – Modified-release capsules
MST CONTINUS – Modified-release tablets, granules
MXL – Modified-release capsules
ORAMORPH – Liquid
SEVREDOL – Tablets
ZOMORPH – Modified-release capsules

With anti-emetic
CYCLIMORPH – Injection
MORPHINE + CYCLIZINE

Morphine – the main active ingredient of opium – is an opioid analgesic used to relieve severe pain caused by surgery, heart attack or injury and is most valuable in controlling pain in terminal illnesses such as cancer. Morphine acts on the brain and alters your perception of pain. It makes you drowsy, light-headed and less anxious. Tolerance (when the dose needs to be increased to produce the same effect) and dependence may occur, but short courses of morphine do not usually cause dependence and the drug can be stopped or gradually withdrawn without problems.

Before you use this medicine

Tell your doctor if you are:
☐ pregnant – morphine is not usually prescribed ☐ breast-feeding – usual doses are unlikely to affect the baby, but discuss with your doctor ☐ taking any other medicines, including vitamins and those bought over the counter.

Tell your doctor if you have or have had:
☐ heart and circulatory disorders, including low blood pressure ☐ asthma, breathing problems or lung disease (chronic obstructive pulmonary disease) ☐ kidney or liver disease – reduce dose or avoid ☐ enlarged prostate ☐ low levels of thyroid hormones ☐ opioid dependence – severe withdrawal reactions can occur if morphine withdrawn abruptly.

Morphine should not be used if you have:
☐ acute depressed breathing ☐ raised pressure in the brain or head injury ☐ seizures ☐ biliary colic – pain caused by obstruction of the gall bladder or bile duct ☐ acute alcoholism and risk of paralytic ileus, where the intestinal muscle is paralysed and gut contents cannot pass through. ☐ phaeochromocytoma (a tumour causing high blood pressure).

How to use this medicine

Take the tablet or liquid or use suppositories regularly every four hours for serious constant pain. Modified-release tablets or capsules should be taken every 12 or 24 hours according to your doctor's instructions.

You may feel dizzy or faint when you get up from sitting or lying down, especially during the first few days of treatment. Get up slowly and stay beside the chair or bed until you are sure you are not dizzy. Do not drive or do other activities that require alertness until you know how you react to morphine. Avoid alcohol as it will make you more drowsy.

If you miss a dose take it as soon as possible, but skip it if it is almost time for the next dose. Do not take double the dose. If you have been taking morphine for more than a few weeks, do not stop taking it suddenly. Ask your doctor to give you a schedule to reduce the dose gradually. If you take morphine for a short period you can stop the drug as soon as you no longer need pain relief.

Over 65 The dose of morphine varies from person to person but you may need less than the standard adult dose, especially if you have poor liver or kidney function.

Interactions with other medicines

Morphine will enhance the sedative effects of all drugs acting on the brain such as **tranquillisers**, **antidepressants**, **sleep-inducing drugs**, **antihistamines** and **antipsychotics**.

Antidepressants, especially monoamine-oxidase inhibitors (MAOIs), affect the brain, causing either excitation or depression with high blood pressure or low blood pressure. Avoid use together and for two weeks after stopping an MAOI.

Unwanted effects

Likely Feeling or being sick, drowsiness, dizziness, confusion, lightheadedness, constipation.
Less likely Breathing difficulties, sudden drop in blood pressure, dry mouth, difficulty passing urine, colic of the bile duct or kidneys, sweating, palpitations, abnormal heart rhythms, headache, facial flushing, hallucinations, hypothermia, mood changes, dependence, pin-point pupils, decreased sexual desire or potency, skin rashes, itching.

Feeling or being sick initially and constipation are common unwanted effects which may be alleviated with other medicines. Call the doctor immediately if someone has slow and troubled breathing, severe drowsiness or loss of consciousness.

Similar preparations

ACTIQ – Lozenges
FENTANYL

DIAMORPHINE (HEROIN) – Tablets, injection

DICONAL – Tablets (with anti-emetic)
DIPIPANONE + CYCLIZINE

DUROGESIC – Patches
FENTANYL

MEPTID – Tablets, injection
MEPTAZINOL

METHADONE – Liquid, tablets, injection

NUBAIN – Injection
NALBUPHINE

OXYCONTIN – Modified-release tablets
OXYCODONE

OXYNORM – Capsules, liquid
OXYCODONE

PALLADONE – Capsules, modified-release capsules
HYDROMORPHONE

PAMERGAN P100 – Injection
PETHIDINE + PROMETHAZINE (not recommended)

PAPAVERETUM – Injection

PENTAZOCINE – Capsules, tablets, injection, suppositories (not recommended as can cause hallucinations)

PETHIDINE – Tablets, injection

PHYSEPTONE – Tablets, injection
METHADONE

TEMGESIC – Tablets (for placing under the tongue), injection
BUPRENORPHINE

▼TRANSTEC – Patches
BUPRENORPHINE

Migraine

Migraine is a recurring severe headache, usually affecting the front of the head on only one side, although both sides may be painful. Before the pain begins you may have warning signs (*aura*) when you see flashing lights, bright or coloured lines or even lose sight temporarily; you may experience 'pins and needles' in the arms or legs; occasionally speech may be affected. These symptoms disappear as the headache develops, and as it comes on you may feel or be sick, lose your appetite and want to avoid light or some sounds or smells. About one person in three has aura before a migraine attack. Most people have migraine without aura, but all types of migraine, with or without aura, can be very painful and debilitating.

At least one in ten adults in Britain has migraine attacks, yet the exact cause of these severe headaches is unknown. Migraine may be caused by the action of neurotransmitters, such as *5-hydroxytryptamine (serotonin)*, on blood vessels surrounding the brain and scalp. The blood vessels surrounding the brain may tighten, triggering the warning signs, followed by blood vessels in the scalp temporarily widening and swelling, causing the severe throbbing headache. The headache may last for several hours, or even days, usually between 4 and 72 hours. A number of factors or 'triggers', which should be avoided whenever possible, are known to set off migraine, including:

- ☐ physical factors – exercise, too much or too little sleep, hormonal changes before a period, pains in the head, neck, teeth, eyes and sinuses
- ☐ psychological factors – stress, shock, anxiety and worry
- ☐ nutritional factors – chocolate, alcohol, fish and cheese or hunger due to missed meals
- ☐ medical factors – the oral contraceptive pill
- ☐ environmental factors – loud noises, strong smells and bright lights.

Most migraine sufferers have their first attack before the age of 30. Some people have only two or three attacks during a lifetime, but others may have one or two a week. Women are two to three times more likely to have migraine attacks than men. This may be associated with hormonal changes during the menstrual cycle. Attacks may start during puberty and continue until or after the menopause. It is unusual to have the first one after the age

– HOW YOU CAN HELP YOURSELF –

- ☐ Identify your trigger factors so that you can avoid them whenever possible.
- ☐ Keep a diary and note any likely triggers; after an attack jot down: the time you got out of bed that day; the time the attack started and how long it lasted; any medicines you took, the dose and time taken; the way your migraine developed; food and drink; work and social activities; your mood; any unusual events or news; extra travel or exercise; the stage of your menstrual cycle.
- ☐ Always keep a supply of medicine such as aspirin or paracetamol immediately to hand; note what works as pain relief. Take an analgesic at the first signs of a migraine, before the headache develops.
- ☐ Rest or lie down. Many sufferers have to lie in a quiet, darkened room until the attack is over; others may be able to carry on working, but should still rest after an attack.
- ☐ See your doctor if your migraine attacks change in severity or frequency; severe headaches can be caused by other conditions such as high blood pressure.
- ☐ Alternative or complementary therapies can also be helpful.
- ☐ Find out about migraine. Migraine Action Association* and the Migraine Trust* can help.

of 40, but not unknown. Migraine attacks can suddenly stop at any time and generally become less frequent and less severe with age. Headaches have other causes and your doctor should question you carefully about the nature and severity of your headache to exclude other possibilities such as a brain lesion, haemorrhage, or temporal (giant cell) arteritis.

There is some evidence that migraine runs in families, but there is no typical sufferer. Children can also have migraine attacks: around three or four out of every hundred are likely to be sick and have severe stomach cramps and headache – but migraine is very rare in children under the age of five.

Cluster headache

Cluster headache is a very severe headache occurring usually on one side of the head. It does not usually respond to standard analgesia. This type of headache mainly affects men and is quite distinct from migraine. Headaches occur daily and last from half an hour to two hours in clusters of 4–16 weeks or longer periods. The pain is aching, boring or stabbing and often occurs at night an hour or so after sleep. It may recur in the daytime and often at the same time – it is sometimes called 'alarm-clock headache'. **Sumatriptan** injection is the most helpful treatment, or oxygen gas can help to abort an attack. Other medicines are used unofficially such as **verapamil** (calcium channel blocker – page 141) or **lithium** (antidepressant – page 218) to prevent attacks if they are frequent or last over three weeks. **Ergotamine** may be used, but not for prolonged periods, or **methysergide**, but only if other treatments are ineffective (see below).

Medication-overuse headache

Some people get a chronic headache for which they take analgesics every day. Chronic headache can sometimes be due to underlying depression, or can be caused by some medicines (for example, headache is an unwanted effect of **nifedipine**). Sometimes chronic headache may result from headache treatments themselves (paracetamol or aspirin, either alone or in combination with codeine or caffeine): initial relief of pain by the treatment is followed by rebound headache, which can lead to people taking pain-relief medication every day. This type of headache is called medication-overuse headache and affects up to 1 in 20 people.

If you treat a headache with more than about 12 doses of analgesic in a week, or on more than three to four days a week, you could risk getting analgesic-induced headache. Headaches usually improve when the analgesic is stopped, although symptoms may worsen temporarily. Medication-overuse headache is not usually a problem for people who need to take regular analgesics, for instance for severe arthritis pain.

Medicines for migraine

There are medicines for treating an acute attack, but if you get frequent migraine attacks you may need a preventive drug. Resting in a quiet, dark room is an important part of treatment and judicious use of complementary therapies can also be helpful. Migraine cannot be cured, but it is possible to control the condition, particularly if you find a treatment that lessens your symptoms. The aims of migraine treatment include reducing the frequency of attacks, the intensity of symptoms and the duration of headache with a medicine that produces the least unwanted effects.

ACUTE MIGRAINE ATTACK

Many people manage their migraine headaches by buying a simple pain-reliever over the counter. A migraine that responds to an analgesic such as **paracetamol**, **ibuprofen** or **aspirin** (not for children under 16) should be taken as soon as you notice warning signs or other features of an imminent attack. The digestive system slows down during a migraine attack so that aspirin or paracetamol may not be absorbed in time to be effective. A dispersible (soluble) or effervescent pain-relief preparation can help to overcome this and act more quickly than conventional preparations. Combined preparations of aspirin or paracetamol with another analgesic or an antihistamine (for example Migraleve) are no more effective than an analgesic used on its own.

The anti-emetic **metoclopramide** or **domperidone** is used to speed up stomach emptying and the absorption of the analgesic. A single dose can be taken as soon as symptoms start and before the analgesic. Alternatively, your doctor can prescribe one of the combination preparations of aspirin or paracetamol with metoclopramide (MigraMax; Paramax) in dispersible form, or paracetamol with domperidone tablets (Domperamol). Metoclopramide is not suitable for everyone, either taken on its own or in combination with an analgesic. Young people aged under 20 years are more susceptible to the unwanted extrapyramidal effects that are a risk with metoclopramide treatment (page 224). Metoclopramide must be avoided in this age group. Domperidone by mouth or by rectum as a suppository is an alternative antiemetic, although not licensed for children, except for managing sickness in cancer treatment.

An NSAID is also suitable for managing a migraine attack. Some are specifically licensed for treating migraine, including **ibuprofen**, **diclofenac potassium** (Voltarol Rapid), **naproxen** (Synflex), **flurbiprofen** (Froben) and **tolfenamic acid** (Clotam), although other NSAIDs may be as satisfactory. Some preparations are available as dispersible or soluble tablets or in suppository form, which can be helpful if you are unable to stop vomiting. You can buy some of these NSAIDs over the counter, but others will need a prescription. Paracetamol or ibuprofen are suitable for children and adolescents.

Some doctors recommend a stepped approach to antimigraine treatment, advising trials of a simple analgesic at first (in adequate dosage, e.g. 900mg aspirin), then a NSAID before considering one of the 'triptan' class (see below). Alternatively if your symptoms are severe and disabling, your doctor could consider a triptan from the outset.

'Triptan' class drugs

As the body's neurotransmitter 5-hydroxytryptamine (serotonin) plays a role in migraine headache, the search for better migraine treatments led to the development of 5-HT_1 receptor agonists – otherwise known as the triptans. They act on receptors in the brain's blood vessels to enhance the tightening (constriction) effect which in turn reduces the width and swelling of the blood vessels during a migraine attack. The original triptan, **sumatriptan** (Imigran), relieves migraine attacks or cluster headache. It can be taken in tablet form, or given by injection just under the skin or as a nasal spray (both are useful if vomiting is a problem).

Other triptans similar to sumatriptan have been developed – **almotriptan** (▼Almogran), **eletriptan** (▼Relpax), **frovatriptan** (▼Migard), **naratriptan** (Naramig), **rizatriptan** (Maxalt) and **zolmitriptan** (Zomig). All the triptans are available in tablet form; **rizatriptan** (Maxalt Melt) and **zolmitriptan** (Zomig Rapimelt) can also be dissolved under the tongue for a rapid effect.

People vary in how they respond to one of the triptans and so you should be able to try one or two to find which one suits you. Studies have shown that headache improves in 30 to 40 per cent of people within one hour of taking a triptan, and that this increases to 50 to 70 per cent after two hours. For many sufferers a triptan has dramatically reduced the time taken to recover from a migraine, allowing a speedier resumption of daily activities.

Not everyone can take a triptan, and you should not use one if you have had a heart attack or stroke, or have any of the following – ischaemic heart disease, peripheral vascular disease, severe liver impairment, uncontrolled or severe high blood pressure or transient ischaemic attacks. There is little experience of triptan use in people aged over 65 years and in general they have not been tested for use in children or adolescents under 18 years. Sumatriptan nasal spray is the exception as it can now be used for younger people aged 12 to 17 years. A triptan should be used on its own and not combined with other treatments for acute migraine.

Ergotamine, a derivative of ergot – a mould that grows on rye – is rarely used nowadays and only if you do not respond to other treatments. It relieves migraine headache by narrowing the blood vessels in the scalp, but does not improve visual and other warning signs and may make vomiting worse. It is used in short courses only; maximum recommended doses and length of treatment must not be exceeded.

SUMATRIPTAN

IMIGRAN – Tablets, injection, nasal spray

Sumatriptan is used for relieving attacks of migraine with or without aura. The injection can also be used for treating cluster headache. Sumatriptan should not be used for preventing migraine or cluster headache. It is chemically similar to the body's neurotransmitter 5-hydroxytryptamine and acts at 5-HT_1 receptors. Sumatriptan appears to prevent the widening of certain blood vessels, which is thought to cause migraine. The injection and nasal spray begin to act after 10–15 minutes, the tablets within 30 minutes.

Before you use this medicine

Tell your doctor if you are:

☐ pregnant – there is limited experience of the effects of sumatriptan on the fetus ☐ breast-feeding – sumatriptan passes into breast milk; stop breastfeeding for 24 hours after use ☐ taking any other medicines, including vitamins and those bought over the counter.

Tell your doctor if you have or have had:
☐ ischaemic heart disease ☐ angina (Prinzmetal's variety) ☐ peripheral vascular disease ☐ severe or uncontrolled high blood pressure ☐ heart attack ☐ stroke ☐ transient ischaemic attacks ☐ severe liver impairment.

Do not use if you:
are taking an MAOI antidepressant or one of the SSRI antidepressants that affects 5-HT receptors – **citalopram**, **fluvoxamine**, **fluoxetine**, **sertraline**, **paroxetine, ergotamine** or **methysergide**.

How to use this medicine

Tablets Swallow one tablet whole with water. If this dose gives some relief but the migraine returns, take another tablet two hours or more after the first. Take no more than three tablets in 24 hours. If the first tablet gives no relief there is no point in taking a second dose for the same attack.
Injection Sumatriptan is injected just under the skin, usually the outside of the thigh, as early as possible in an attack. Detailed instructions are provided in the pack. The recommended dose is one injection, but a further dose may be used if necessary one hour or more after the first dose. The maximum dose is two injections in 24 hours.
Nasal spray The recommended dose is one puff of the spray into one nostril. A further dose may be used if necessary two hours or more after the first dose. The maximum dose is two puffs in 24 hours.

Do not drive or do other activities that require alertness until you know how you react to sumatriptan – drowsiness may occur as a result of the migraine or sumatriptan. Avoid alcohol in a migraine attack. Sumatriptan does not appear to interact with alcohol.

Over 65 Experience with sumatriptan in people over 65 is limited.

Interactions with other medicines

Antidepressants MAOIs, SSRIs and **St John's wort** Increased risk of nervous system toxicity – avoid using with sumatriptan and for two weeks after an MAOI.
Ergotamine or **ergometrine** and sumatriptan should not be used together as they add to each other's effects on the nervous system.

Unwanted effects

These are mostly mild to moderate and pass off.
Likely Slight but fleeting pain at the injection site; nasal irritation and taste disturbance with nasal spray; sensations of tingling, heat, heaviness, pressure or tightness in any part of the body (especially the chest), flushing, dizziness, weakness, drowsiness.
Less likely Feeling or being sick, initial increase in blood pressure which wears off, irregular heart rhythms, palpitations, low blood pressure.
Rarely Visual disturbances, seizures, colitis, Raynaud's phenomenon, hypersensitivity reactions.

Similar preparations

▼ALMOGRAN – Tablets
ALMOTRIPTAN

MAXALT – Tablets, wafers (for dissolving under the tongue)
RIZATRIPTAN

▼MIGARD – Tablets
FROVATRIPTAN

NARAMIG – Tablets
NARATRIPTAN

▼RELPAX – Tablets
ELETRIPTAN

ZOMIG – Tablets, tablets (for dissolving under the tongue), ▼nasal spray
ZOLMITRIPTAN

PREVENTING MIGRAINE

If you have migraine attacks often you should try to find out what factors might provoke them. For example, some women taking the combined oral contraceptive 'pill' may find migraine gets worse. If you have migraine with visual disturbances or if your attack worsens when you start the oral contraceptive, you should change to another form of contraception. However, some women experience fewer migraine attacks when they start oral contraception.

If you have more than two attacks a month that are disabling then taking a medicine to prevent migraine may be helpful. A beta blocker may be used twice or three times a day, or a longer-acting preparation taken once a day. **Propranolol** is most commonly used, but **metoprolol**, **nadolol** and **timolol** are also available. Treatment with a beta blocker is limited by interactions, for example it should not be taken with ergotamine and by people with certain medical conditions in which a beta blocker must not be used (pages 106–7).

Pizotifen (Sanomigran) is an antihistamine and a 5-HT blocker which gives some protection against both types of migraine (with and without warning signs) and cluster headache. It may cause drowsiness but can be given as a single dose at night to lessen this problem. It may also cause weight gain, dry mouth and occasionally nausea and dizziness.

Occasionally **sodium valproate**, a tricyclic antidepressant (e.g. **amitriptyline**) or the antihistamine **cyproheptadine** may be helpful. **Methysergide** (Deseril) is effective at preventing migraine but has unpleasant unwanted effects and is given only under hospital supervision. **Clonidine** (Dixarit) is less effective than other medicines for preventing migraine and is not recommended.

Epilepsy

Epilepsy is a common condition of the nervous system which affects around 400,000 people in the UK. An epileptic seizure (fit or convulsion are older terms) occurs when the normal co-ordinated electrical activity of the brain's nerve cells is disrupted. The chaotic discharge of electrical activity usually results in loss of control over muscle and body movements and/or perceptual changes in the mind. The tendency to have repeated seizures, even if a long interval separates them, is known as epilepsy.

Epilepsy can start at any time of life but is mostly diagnosed before the age of 20 and after 60 years. Types of epilepsy and seizures are classified to help with diagnosis and treatment. If you have epilepsy, the same type of seizure usually recurs, but some people experience different types of seizures at different times.

Antiepileptic medicines can control seizures and symptoms in about four out of five people, and nine years after diagnosis around three quarters of people can expect to have had no seizures in the previous three years. Some people can stop medication without recurrence of seizures. Neurosurgery (*temporal lobectomy*) can be helpful in selected cases.

Having one isolated epileptic seizure does not mean you have a tendency to epilepsy. Each person has a different threshold above which a seizure may occur and the threshold varies from time to time, depending on the stimulus or provocation. For most people that threshold is never reached, but for someone with a low threshold or tolerance to abnormal electrical activity in the brain, any of a number of stimuli may trigger seizures.

Diagnosis Your account and that of any witness are important to help the doctor determine what has happened during a seizure. Other conditions can sometimes resemble epileptic seizures, for example collapse during a heart problem. Investigations can include an *electroencephalogram* (EEG) to assess the brain's electrical activity. This can occasionally help to establish whether or not you have epilepsy, but is particularly helpful in deciding what type of epilepsy may be occurring. Sometimes an EEG may be normal in between seizures in someone with epilepsy and abnormal in a person who has not had a seizure. A brain scan may also be performed to look for anomalies, for example a lesion that may be contributing to seizures, but it is not a diagnostic test in itself. Blood tests, for example to measure calcium levels, may also help to determine the cause of seizures.

Causes Epilepsy may start as a result of injury to the brain caused by infection, stroke or an accident. An underlying brain condition or damage is sometimes present at birth, which is a common cause of childhood epilepsy. In older people epilepsy can occur as a result of damage through a stroke or in Alzheimer's disease and in other rare degenerative diseases. Seizures can also occur as a result of upset in the body's metabolic control, for example with low blood sugar, low sodium or calcium levels or in liver failure. Seizures sometimes occur with acute (one-off) excessive alcohol intake or as a result of drug toxicity. Long-term abuse of alcohol may result in seizures which may continue even if you stop drinking. In some people generalized seizures may be genetically linked but in others no obvious cause can be identified. However, there may be any number of factors or triggers that precipitate, but are not the cause of, a seizure and these vary from person to person. Common examples include lack of sleep, lack of food, menstruation, flashing bright lights (*photosensitivity*) and repetitive patterns on a floor or wall. Seizures may occur in young children with a high temperature and these are known as *febrile convulsions*. Epilepsy is generally not inherited, but a history of epilepsy in both parents' families does increase the likelihood of a tendency to epilepsy. A low seizure threshold appears to run in some families, but for most people with epilepsy, the chance of your child developing it is very small.

HOW YOU CAN HELP YOURSELF

- ☐ Keep a diary record of your attacks and the circumstances in which they occur – this information will be very helpful to your doctor.
- ☐ If you take an antiepileptic medicine, take it regularly. It may take you and your doctor some months to establish the best treatment plan. Keep a note of unwanted effects and discuss them with the doctor.
- ☐ Wear an identification bracelet or carry a card with details of your medicines.
- ☐ Get information and advice – there are over 20 organisations concerned with epilepsy to choose from, such as the National Society for Epilepsy* or Epilepsy Action*. Epilepsy Bereaved* provides information on sudden unexpected death in epilepsy.
- ☐ If there are trigger factors that precipitate your seizures, try to avoid them. Keep a record of events leading up to attacks – the trigger factors may become apparent.
- ☐ Lead as healthy and independent a life as possible, eating, exercising and sleeping regularly. You can safely participate in most activities except climbing and underwater diving.
- ☐ Avoid alcohol: small amounts (1–2 units) are acceptable, but generally can interfere with your medicine or may start an attack.
- ☐ If you drive, you must inform the DVLA (Driver and Vehicle Licensing Agency) of your epilepsy. Generally you are allowed to drive a car, but not heavy goods or public service vehicles, if you have had a seizure-free period of one year or if you have only had attacks while asleep over a three-year period.

TYPES OF SEIZURE

Types of seizure are classified broadly into *generalised seizures*, where abnormal electrical activity is widespread in the brain, and *partial seizures*, where abnormal activity is localised and starts in a particular area of the brain. Some types of seizure are as follows.

Tonic-clonic (*grand mal*) seizures are generalised seizures characterised by electrical disturbance across the whole brain. As the tonic phase begins you may have a warning sensation or aura, such as flashing lights, a smell or taste, before the body becomes rigid and you suddenly lose consciousness. The chest muscles contract, forcing air through the larynx and causing an involuntary grunt or cry. Sometimes you lose bladder or faecal control or bite your tongue. The clonic phase starts with a generalised seizure and foaming at the mouth. Limbs jerk as muscles contract and relax uncontrollably in a rhythmic way. The seizure usually lasts for only a few minutes and afterwards you may have a headache and feel dazed and exhausted. A prolonged attack as seizures follow each other without stopping is called *status epilepticus* and is a medical emergency.

Absence (*petit mal*) seizures commonly occur in children and may be mistaken for daydreaming. An absence attack is brief and lasts only a second or two. The child loses consciousness for a moment and appears to go pale and blank, stares and may flutter the eyelids. Sometimes body movements occur, such as dropping the head forwards.

Partial (*focal*) seizures occur in one part of the brain only, although they may sometimes become generalised (secondarily generalised seizures). Partial seizures vary from person to person. They may start with muscle contractions or unusual sensations at one point of the body such as the mouth, a finger or a toe and then spread without your losing consciousness. You may experience loss of speech, confusion and involuntary movements, and may not remember what has happened.

HOW TO HELP

Tonic-clonic seizures

Note the time as soon as a seizure begins and clear a space around the person having the seizure. Cushion the head and loosen clothes; remove glasses, false teeth (if this is easily done) and any sharp objects in the vicinity. Do not move the person having the seizure (unless in a dangerous place, e.g. in a road) or force anything between his or her teeth. Do not try to rouse the person or to make him or her drink anything.

As soon as the seizure begins to settle, turn the person on one side to keep the airways open. As the person begins to recover, offer reassurance and talk quietly until full recovery.

Seek urgent medical assistance if the seizure lasts longer than five minutes or if one seizure follows another without the person regaining consciousness (status epilepticus).

Partial seizures

These seizures do not require medical attention. The person having the seizure may wander around with a blank expression and should be accompanied to make sure he or she is safe. Do not interfere or attempt to stop the seizure, but talk calmly after the seizure to provide reassurance.

Febrile convulsions

Some children have a seizure only when they develop a high temperature. A febrile convulsion is a seizure that occurs in a child aged between three months and five years with a fever, but without any evident underlying cause. As a parent you may be very frightened by your child having a febrile convulsion, but most seizures are brief and there is no lasting problem. You can take some measures to help. Place the child on his or her side to keep the airway open. There is no need to intervene unless the convulsions last longer than 15 minutes. Seek medical help if the convulsions last longer than 15 minutes or if your child is under 18 months.

Reduce the child's temperature by removing clothing, sponging with tepid water and gentle fanning. Paracetamol elixir for children may help to reduce the fever.

If your child has a tendency to have febrile convulsions, your doctor may teach you how to use rectal diazepam solution in an emergency.

IMPROVING OUTCOMES IN EPILEPSY

People with epilepsy are two to three times more at risk of premature death then the general population and sadly around 1,000 people die every year as a result of their epileptic seizures, probably because of a heart attack or breathing difficulties during or following the seizure. In about half the death is unexpected, known as sudden unexpected death in epilepsy (SUDEP). Many of these people are young or have uncontrolled epilepsy, learning disability, seizures during sleep, or problems remembering to take their medication.

Following a national audit which evaluated the care received by people before they had died from an epilepsy-related death, the Department of Health has started to take action to inform local health communities about how to improve epilepsy services. The National Service Framework for Long-term Conditions will include standards of care for epilepsy and a ten-year implementation programme starting in 2005. National Institute for Clinical Excellence guidance will be available soon for a range of antiepileptic medicines suitable for children and adults to address 'post-code' prescribing, where access to health services, neurologists specialising in epilepsy care, and medicines can be a lottery. Clinical guidelines for health professionals will recommend best practice in the diagnosis, management and treatment of epilepsy.

Antiepileptic medicines

Your doctor will look for any underlying disorder that might cause seizures and try to identify any trigger factors. You should be referred to a specialist for further investigation as epilepsy is not always easy to diagnose with certainty. Treatment with an antiepileptic medicine will not usually be started after just one seizure, but this decision should be made by you and the specialist after weighing the pros and cons. If you have recurrent seizures, an antiepileptic medicine can prevent attacks, allow you to lead a normal life with few restraints, and reduce the risk of brain damage which may occur with frequent, uncontrolled seizures. Antiepileptics act on the brain to increase the seizure threshold and to prevent the spread of abnormal electrical activity in the brain. The choice of medicine depends on the type of epilepsy, also on your age, whether you take medication for other conditions, your response to treatment and any unwanted effects. Most people are treated with one medicine (*monotherapy*), but it may take time to establish which drug suits you best. Treatment is started with a low dose and gradually increased until seizures are controlled or unwanted effects develop. You may need to have blood tests with some of the medicines to help to establish the dosage. A second medicine should only be added if seizures continue; some people seem to need more than one drug and occasionally three antiepileptics may be needed. Taking two or three antiepileptics is not always beneficial because the drugs may interact and cause more unwanted effects. When you are settled on medication, your doctor should review your treatment once a year.

Medicines recommended for use in generalised (tonic-clonic) seizures include **sodium valproate** (Epilim) or **lamotrigine** (Lamictal). Sodium valproate can also be used for other forms of epilepsy. Occasionally it affects the liver, so tests for liver function may be necessary before and once in a while during treatment. Lamotrigine can be used on its own or added to another antiepileptic drug. Unwanted effects include headache, tiredness, feeling sick, dizziness, drowsiness and insomnia. Rash is quite common, especially in children, and occasionally a severe allergic, hypersensitivity reaction with rash, fever, and 'flu-like' symptoms develops, usually within the first month of starting treatment. Blood disorders (e.g. aplastic anaemia) also occur very rarely; watch out for signs (bruising and infection). If either the hypersensitivity reaction or signs of blood disorder occur, contact your doctor immediately.

For partial seizures and where they have spread across the brain (secondarily generalised), treatment includes **carbamazepine** (Tegretol) or related medicine **oxcarbazepine** (▼Trileptal), sodium valproate or lamotrigine. Absence seizures can be treated with either **ethosuximide** (Zarontin, Emeside) or sodium valproate. Blood disorders can occur rarely with ethosuximide treatment and you or your carer need to recognise the symptoms – fever, sore throat, mouth ulcers, bruising or bleeding. If these develop you should contact your doctor urgently.

Phenytoin (Epanutin), an older antiepileptic, is effective in both types of seizures and has been widely used but the range between an effective dose and one which causes adverse effects is narrow. Blood levels of the drug may have to be measured to help with dosage adjustment and because of these practical difficulties, it is less likely to be used for people newly diagnosed as epileptic. Carbamazepine has a wider therapeutic range and fewer unwanted effects than phenytoin. Most of carbamazepine's unwanted effects, such as blurred vision, dizziness and unsteadiness, are dose-related. If the dose is effective, but unwanted effects remain a nuisance your doctor may alter the time when you take carbamazepine or recommend a modified-release preparation to overcome this problem. **Phenobarbital** (phenobarbitone) and the related **primidone** (Mysoline), both older antiepileptics, remain in use, usually under specialist supervision. Benzodiazepines **clonazepam** or **clobazam** are sometimes used, but their effectiveness may wane with long-term use. They remain useful for status epilepticus (page 253).

Newer antiepileptics have extended treatment choice recently. Several medicines are used as 'add on' treatment – for example **gabapentin** (Neurontin), **levetiracetam** (▼Keppra), **tiagabine** (Gabitril) and **topiramate** (Topamax) for partial seizures; topiramate is also used for generalised seizures. Topiramate can also be used on its own if you have recently been diagnosed with epilepsy; it is suitable for children from the age of six years. Common unwanted effects of topiramate include sleepiness, dizziness, lack of co-ordination of movement (ataxia) and also eye problems through raised intraocular pressure, which can occur within one month of starting treatment. As with all antiepileptic therapy, careful monitoring is needed, especially at the start of treatment. If you notice changes to your vision, contact your doctor immediately. **Vigabatrin** (Sabril) is now used only when all other appropriate antiepileptic medicines, either singly or in combination, have not been satisfactory. Visual field defects can occur in about one third of patients taking vigabatrin. These defects may not be noticeable in some, but in others may be severe and potentially disabling. The Committee on Safety of Medicines (CSM) warns that visual field loss may be irreversible even after vigabatrin has been stopped. Vigabatrin should be used only under specialist supervision, with appropriate assessments of vision followed by regular six-monthly screening.

Treatment aims to keep you seizure-free and if you have a period of two years without a seizure, you may want to discuss the possibility of stopping medication with your specialist and GP. A shared care plan should be agreed. Your doctor may consider withdrawing treatment very gradually over at least six months, depending on the antiepileptic. Whether it will be possible to withdraw treatment depends on your age and when epilepsy started, how many and what type of attacks you have had, for example seizures whilst on medication and over what period, how many antiepileptic medicines you take and whether you want to drive. If you take several antiepileptics, only one medicine should be withdrawn at a time. There is no guarantee that seizures will not recur and the likelihood of this happening is greatest during withdrawal and the following six months after withdrawal has been completed. Driving, and other situations in which a seizure could be dangerous, should be avoided during this period.

Pregnancy and breast-feeding

Around 3 per cent of births in general result in a baby with a major birth defect. In women with epilepsy the risk of congenital abnormalities, such as cleft lip and palate, increases to around 7 per cent if you take one antiepileptic drug and 15 per cent if you take two or more medicines. Some combinations of three antiepileptics can increase the risk to 50 per cent. Genetic and other factors may contribute, but drug treatment may be responsible for the excess of abnormalities. Research also suggests that some antiepileptics taken during pregnancy may have an effect on the child's subsequent development. No antiepileptic drug is completely free from the risk of causing abnormalities. So these risks of continuing medication during pregnancy must be carefully weighed with the risks of having seizures if you stop taking antiepileptics. Ideally you want to be on one medicine at the lowest dose that controls seizures. Your management during pregnancy needs careful discussion of the various options, preferably with a specialist before conception. Any changes to medication should ideally be completed before conception.

Women taking antiepileptics, especially sodium valproate, carbamazepine and phenytoin, during the first three months of pregnancy are at increased risk of having a baby with spina bifida. More is known about the effects of the older antiepileptics during pregnancy because of experience in use. Women of child-bearing age are often excluded from drug trials but a UK epilepsy and pregnancy register shows that 95 per cent of babies born to women with epilepsy show no major birth defects. You will need to take a daily folic acid 5mg supplement before becoming pregnant, as soon as you stop contraception, and for 12 weeks after conception, whether or not you continue an antiepileptic. Careful monitoring during the first three months of pregnancy and throughout will be essential. During the week before delivery you should take vitamin K to prevent bleeding in the baby.

Breast-feeding is possible with most antiepileptic medicines taken in normal dosage, except for barbiturates, which can cause drowsiness (such as phenobarbital), ethosuximide (the manufacturer advises against use), and some of the newer antiepileptics – check with your doctor.

Status epilepticus

Status epilepticus is a medical emergency and is treated with diazepam, clonazepam or lorazepam, given intravenously. These benzodiazepines, of which lorazepam is preferred because of its longer action, must be used cautiously because they can cause breathing difficulties. Diazepam can also be given by rectal solution. Alternatively, midazolam (also a benzodiazepine) can be applied to the inside of the mouth, between the teeth and gums (buccal route) or inserted up the nose. If seizures recur or fail to respond to treatment after half an hour, other drugs that may be used include phenytoin, fosphenytoin and phenobarbital.

SODIUM VALPROATE

SODIUM VALPROATE – Tablets, liquid
EPILIM – Tablets, crushable tablets, modified-release tablets, liquid, injection
CONVULEX – Capsules
VALPROIC ACID

Sodium valproate is an antiepileptic which stabilises a person's seizure threshold and prevents the spread of abnormal electrical activity across the brain. Is it used for all forms of epilepsy, especially generalised tonic-clonic seizures. Valproic acid is also used for the acute manic phase in bipolar disorder and sodium valproate is sometimes used unofficially for treating other conditions (page 218).

Before you use this medicine

Tell your doctor if you are:
□ pregnant or considering pregnancy – risk of abnormalities increases with antiepileptics (see above); the risk may be higher with sodium valproate compared to some other drugs. Sodium valproate should not be started during pregnancy without specialist medical advice □ breast-feeding – acceptable at normal dosage □ taking any other medicines, including vitamins and others bought over the counter. Women need to take a daily folic acid tablet 5mg for three months before and during the first three months of pregnancy.

Tell your doctor if you have or have had:
□ liver disease or someone in your family has had severe liver impairment □ kidney impairment □ diabetes – sodium valproate may give a false positive urine test □ systemic lupus erythematosus □ porphyria.

How to use this medicine

You should take the tablets or liquid twice a day, preferably after food in the morning and evening. The modified-release tablets can be taken once or twice daily. A sugar-free liquid is available. It may be important to the control of your epilepsy to have the same make of medicine, including generic medicines, each time you get a prescription. Discuss this with your doctor and pharmacist.

Eat plenty of fresh, green vegetables because folic acid deficiency may occur with long-term treatment. You will need to take additional folic acid before becoming pregnant and during the first 12 weeks of pregnancy (see above).

Do not drive or do other activities that require alertness until you know how you react to sodium valproate. You may not be allowed to drive a car at all.

Do not stop taking this medicine suddenly as seizures may recur. Discuss the possibility of stopping treatment with your doctor. You will need a gradual reduction of dosage over a period of time. Do not withdraw treatment without medical guidance. If you miss a dose take it as soon as you remember.

Over 65 Dosage should be adjusted to control seizures. With poor kidney function, the dose may need to be lower.

Before you start treatment with sodium valproate, and during the first six months of treatment, your liver function must be assessed to ensure no undue risk of bleeding. Blood tests to check your liver function and blood clotting function may also be needed periodically, e.g. before surgery. Liver function usually settles as treatment continues, but toxicity can develop very occasionally (see below).

Interactions with other medicines

Interactions of antiepileptic medicines with each other, when used together, and with other medicines can be complex and not entirely predictable. Check with your doctor and pharmacist about which combinations are suitable.

Effects of sodium valproate on other medicines:

Antidepressants, including MAOIs, antipsychotics and benzodiazepines – effects enhanced.

Antiepileptics carbamazepine, **lamotrigine**, **phenytoin**, **phenobarbital**, **primidone** Increased risk of adverse effects – lower doses may be needed.

Anticoagulants Warfarin and related drugs – possibly increased anticoagulant effect. Blood tests to monitor clotting time (INR) are needed.

Effects of other medicines on sodium valproate:

Antiepileptics carbamazepine, **phenytoin**, **phenobarbital** decrease blood valproic acid levels – adjust dosages.

Antimalarials chloroquine and **mefloquine** lower seizure threshold; mefloquine antagonises sodium valproate's effects.

Other medicines Aspirin, **cimetidine**, **erythromycin** may increase valproic acid blood levels. Lipid-lowering **colestyramine** may decrease absorption of sodium valproate.

Unwanted effects

Likely Stomach upsets, feeling sick, increased appetite and weight gain, temporary hair loss (regrowth may be more curly than before).

Less likely Tremor, unsteadiness, fluid retention, sedation, increased alertness, aggression, irregular periods, severe stomach pain, blood disorders, skin rash, hearing loss. High levels of ammonia can occur in the body but this usually fades with time. If this causes sickness, unsteady gait and clouding of consciousness, contact your doctor.

Rare Serious liver, blood or pancreas toxicity.

You or a carer should tell your doctor immediately if you develop a sudden illness, especially if it is within the first six months of treatment and particularly if you are repeatedly sick, or feel sick, have extreme tiredness, abdominal pain, lose your appetite, your skin becomes yellowish (jaundice) or your epilepsy worsens. Children are most at risk of liver and pancreas toxicity. Blood disorders can also occur – symptoms include spontaneous bruising or bleeding. Drug treatment needs to be carefully withdrawn under medical guidance.

Similar preparations

CARBAMAZEPINE – Tablets

CLOBAZAM – Tablets

CLONAZEPAM – Tablets, injection
RIVOTRIL

EMESIDE – Capsules, liquid
ETHOSUXIMIDE

EPANUTIN – Tablets, chewable tablets, liquid
PHENYTOIN

GABAPENTIN – Capsules

GABITRIL – Tablets
TIAGABINE

▼KEPPRA – Tablets
LEVETIRACETAM

LAMICTAL – Tablets, dispersible tablets
LAMOTRIGINE

NEURONTIN – Capsules, tablets
GABAPENTIN

PHENOBARBITAL – Tablets, liquid, injection

PHENYTOIN – Capsules, tablets

SABRIL - Tablets, dispersible powder
VIGABATRIN

TEGRETOL – Tablets, chewable tablets, modified-release tablets, liquid, suppositories
CARBAMAZEPINE

TERIL RETARD – Modified-release tablets
CARBAMAZEPINE

TIMONIL RETARD – Modified-release tablets
CARBAMAZEPINE

TOPAMAX – Tablets, capsules (contents can be sprinkled on to soft food)
TOPIRAMATE

▼TRILEPTAL – Tablets, liquid
OXCARBAZEPINE

ZARONTIN – Capsules, liquid
ETHOSUXIMIDE

Parkinson's disease and parkinsonism

Parkinson's disease, described by a London doctor James Parkinson in 1817, is a degenerative condition of the nervous system in which voluntary movement is disturbed. The most noticeable features of the disease are slowness of movement (*bradykinesia*), tremor – shaking and a rhythmic rolling movement in the fingers – difficulty starting to walk and stopping once walking, stiffness and muscle rigidity. Tremor is often first noticed by others. Other signs include the face becoming blank and mask-like and the voice soft and monotonous. Other symptoms include heartburn, difficulty swallowing, constipation, urinary difficulties and weight loss. Sweating increases and the skin becomes greasy. Handwriting becomes small and spidery and may tail off at the end of the line. The disease may be more prominent on one side of the body. People with the disease may have one or more of the symptoms and in different proportions. Sadly, the condition is progressive and some sufferers are eventually disabled by it. However, for many people medical treatment can dampen symptoms for many years, allowing them to lead full lives.

Nerve cells in part of the brain responsible for controlling movement, the *basal ganglia*, lose supplies of the body chemical **dopamine**.

Dopamine and another body chemical, **acetylcholine**, are neurotransmitters, which help to relay messages along the nerves which control movement. The control of movement is finely balanced between sets of nerves which respond to one of the two chemicals. When dopamine supplies are reduced, an imbalance between the two chemical transmitter systems, *cholinergic* and *dopaminergic*, occurs in the brain. The resulting imbalance means that the basal ganglia are unable to modify the nerve messages to the muscles, which leads to rigid joints, slow movements and tremor.

The exact cause of Parkinson's disease is unknown, nor why dopamine loss occurs. It seems likely that a combination of factors plays a role including environmental, genetics and viruses. It is rare in people aged under 40 years. The rate at which the disease progresses varies considerably.

Parkinsonian symptoms (*parkinsonism*) or movement disorders can be caused by a drug treatment; for example by antipsychotic medicines such as chlorpromazine (pages 213–15). These are drug-induced extrapyramidal symptoms, unwanted effects which usually improve when the dose is reduced or the drug is stopped. Other causes of parkinsonism include brain damage and narrowed blood vessels in the brain.

– HOW YOU CAN HELP YOURSELF –

- ☐ In the early stages of Parkinson's disease, often before drug treatment is needed, regular moderate exercise may help.
- ☐ Learn what your capabilities and energy levels are; plan your day around your best times.
- ☐ Find out whether other treatments would help, such as physiotherapy, speech therapy or occupational therapy.
- ☐ Find out about equipment which could help you to get around or you could use at home, such as special utensils and hand rails in the bathroom and toilet. The Disabled Living Foundation* produces information and has a centre where equipment can be tried out. The local branch of the British Red Cross Society may also be able to help with equipment – see the Phone Book for your nearest branch.
- ☐ Get advice on shoes and clothing which are easy to put on and take off.
- ☐ Get more information from the Parkinson's Disease Society*.

Medicines for Parkinson's disease

Treatment is not usually started until symptoms become troublesome and start to disrupt daily living. Medicines can help to relieve the symptoms of Parkinson's disease, but cannot halt the degeneration of brain cells or permanently restore the chemical imbalance; areas of research include gene therapy (page 41) and stem cell transplantation. Surgery can provide temporary relief for severe tremor and dyskinesia in some instances, but drug treatment continues to be the mainstay for managing Parkinson's disease.

Medicines boost dopamine levels in the brain and include levodopa and dopamine receptor agonists (dopamine agonists) such as **bromocriptine** and related drugs, or **pramipexole** or **ropinirole**. **Entacapone**, **apomorphine** and occasionally **amantadine** are also used. Antimuscarinic medicines were used in Parkinson's disease to reduce acetylcholine action, but are mainly used now to relieve drug-induced parkinsonian symptoms.

MEDICINES BOOSTING DOPAMINE ACTIVITY

Levodopa is the most commonly used medicine; it is the chemical which brain cells convert into dopamine. Dopamine itself is not effective as a medicine because it is not absorbed very well from the digestive system, nor can it pass from the bloodstream into the brain, where it is needed. Levodopa replenishes dopamine in the brain and in particular helps to improve difficulty in starting movement, slow walking and rigidity. However, a large proportion of the drug is broken down in the body before it ever reaches the brain. To overcome this levodopa is always given with **carbidopa** or **benserazide**, drugs that block the breakdown of levodopa in the body, but do not themselves enter the brain. Levodopa therapy without either drug is not recommended.

Levodopa can produce a range of unwanted effects such as feeling or being sick and a sudden drop in blood pressure, sleeplessness, vivid dreams and changes to the mental state, including hallucinations. If nausea and vomiting are problematic, **domperidone** (Motilium) can help (page 224). As it is given with carbidopa or benserazide, levodopa can be given in much smaller doses so that adverse effects are minimised. The combination of carbidopa + levodopa has the generic name of **co-careldopa** (Sinemet) while benserazide + levodopa is known as **co-beneldopa** (Madopar).

Levodopa treatment is started at a low dose and gradually increased until a satisfactory response occurs. High doses do not always increase the benefit, and risk causing unwanted effects. There is evidence that high doses of levodopa cause its advantages to wear off faster.

SWITCHING ON AND OFF

As time goes on you may start to experience fluctuations or swings between mobility and immobility – a kind of 'on-off' phenomenon. 'On' periods are the relatively normal times when the medicines are working. 'Off' periods are times when you are immobile, stiff, rigid, tremulous and sometimes in pain. Your voice may be slurred or inaudible, and you may perspire profusely. You also have 'over-stimulated' periods due to excess stimulation by the medicines. When this happens, you have no control over your body: you writhe and make involuntary movements.

Swings between these extremes may occur with little or no warning and sometimes frequently throughout the day – as if the 'mains' switch is repeatedly being thrown. It can be alarming for you and your carer. Contact the Parkinson's Disease Society* for support.

During the first 6–18 months of levodopa treatment you may slowly improve, perhaps for up to two years. After that time the benefit from levodopa treatment wanes because the disease progresses, and possibly because drug levels in the brain fluctuate. Former disabilities may return insidiously, new ones appear and unwanted effects of levodopa may increase. This long-term levodopa syndrome includes abnormal involuntary movements, 'end-of-dose' deterioration – when effective treatment is limited to three or four hours – and the 'on-off' phenomenon (see box, page 257). Falls are common and there may also be changes to the mental state, such as hallucinations, confusion and psychotic behaviour. Sometimes drug treatment causes these changes but dementia may also be part of the underlying disorder in later stages. Depression and anxiety are also common in Parkinson's disease. To preserve levodopa's usefulness, specialists may start you on a dopamine agonist first (see below) and add levodopa later.

LEVODOPA

MADOPAR – Capsules, dispersible (soluble) tablets, modified-release capsules
CO-BENELDOPA

SINEMET – Tablets, modified-release tablets
CO-CARELDOPA

▼STALEVO – Tablets
LEVODOPA + CARBIDOPA + ENTACAPONE

Poor choice
LEVODOPA – Tablets

Levodopa is the chemical the body converts to dopamine, the neurotransmitter that is lacking in the brain of someone with Parkinson's disease. Levodopa is an effective antiparkinsonian drug, but higher and higher doses have to be given to maintain an effect. Unwanted effects such as abnormal movements, nausea and vomiting then become a problem. Carbidopa and benserazide stop levodopa being converted into dopamine in the body, thereby increasing the amount of levodopa available to the brain for conversion into dopamine: the combination preparations, co-careldopa and co-beneldopa, enable a lower dose of levodopa to be given. Unwanted effects are also reduced. The dose is increased slowly to achieve a balance between mobility and unwanted effects.

Before you use this medicine

Tell your doctor if you are:
□ pregnant – not recommended – or breast-feeding □ taking any other medicines, including vitamins and those bought over the counter.

Tell your doctor if you have or have had:
□ lung disease or bronchial asthma □ heart or circulation problems □ diabetes □ overactive thyroid gland □ closed-angle glaucoma – levodopa must not be used. Use with caution in open-angle glaucoma □ peptic ulcer □ history of skin cancer – may re-activate cancer □ kidney or liver disease □ psychiatric illness – avoid if severe □ osteomalacia – weakening of the bones due to lack of vitamin D.

How to use this medicine

Take the tablet or capsule with or after meals to minimise stomach upsets. The constituents of protein (amino acids) can reduce levodopa's absorption at meal-times. Later as the disease progresses preparations should be given before meals to enhance absorption.

Dosage has to be tailored to each person. Your doctor will start you with a low dose, gradually increasing the dosage to balance improvement and unwanted effects. A modified-release preparation may help to reduce night-time loss of movement (akinesia). A faster-acting dispersible preparation may help in the morning to allow you to dress. You may feel dizzy or faint when you get up from sitting or lying down, especially during the first few days of treatment. Get up slowly and stay beside the chair or bed until you are sure you are not dizzy. Do not drive or do other activities that require alertness until you know how you react to levodopa. Daytime sleepiness and sudden onset of sleep can occur with levodopa and other dopamine agonists. You should not drive or operate machinery until these effects have stopped recurring. Alcohol increases levodopa's effect on driving.

Do not stop taking this medicine suddenly as this will lead to a return of the disease symptoms. Discuss any problems with the medicine with your doctor. If you miss a dose, take it as soon as you remember; but delay or omit the next dose. Do not take double the dose.

Over 65 Levodopa is used mainly in older people. You may be more susceptible to unwanted effects, especially a sudden drop in blood pressure when getting up from sitting or lying down. Modified-release preparations help to reduce unwanted effects and sudden surges of the drug released from standard preparations.

Interactions with other medicines

Anaesthetics e.g. halothane increase risk of irregular heart rhythm.
Antidepressants – Monoamine-oxidase inhibitors produce a dangerous rise in blood pressure with levodopa. An MAOI must be stopped at least two weeks before levodopa is started. An SSRI antidepressant can be given with levodopa. The antiparkinsonian drug **selegiline** (similar to the MAOIs) can be given with levodopa preparations, although low blood pressure may be a problem.
Bupropion for smoking cessation increases the risk of levodopa's unwanted effects.
Antipsychotics should be avoided in people with suspected Parkinson's disease.

Unwanted effects

Likely Abnormal body movements, feeling or being sick, loss of appetite, sleep-lessness, agitation, nervousness, sudden drop in blood pressure (postural hypotension), palpitations and irregular heart rhythm.
Less likely Mood changes, aggressive behaviour, depression, drowsiness, headache, unusual tiredness or weakness, hypersensitivity, flushing, sweating, gastrointestinal bleeding, duodenal ulcer, taste disturbance.

Reddish discoloration of urine and and other body fluids such as sweat may occur but is nothing to worry about. Discuss how you feel and all levodopa's unwanted effects that you notice with your doctor. Muscle twitching, prolonged and uncon-trolled contraction of an eyelid muscle can indicate a possible dose reduction.

Similar preparations

APO-go – Injection
APOMORPHINE

BROMOCRIPTINE – Tablets

CABASER – Tablets
CABERGOLINE

CELANCE – Tablets
PERGOLIDE

COMTESS – Tablets
ENTACAPONE

ELDEPRYL – Tablets, liquid
SELEGILINE

LISURIDE – Tablets

▼MIRAPEXIN – Tablets
PRAMIPEXOLE

PARLODEL – Tablets, capsules
BROMOCRIPTINE

REQUIP – Tablets
ROPINIROLE

SELEGILINE – Tablets

SYMMETREL – Capsules, liquid
AMANTADINE

ZELAPAR – Tablets (dissolvable in mouth)
SELEGILINE

Dopamine agonists act by directly stimulating surviving dopamine receptors in the brain. Although the approach may vary, dopamine agonists are increasingly being used before a levodopa combination, particularly in people aged less than 70 years, to preserve levodopa treatment for the later stages of the disease. Dopamine agonists are slightly less effective than levodopa, but have fewer late unwanted abnormal movements (dyskinesia). The original dopamine agonists, **bromocriptine** (Parlodel) and **lisuride**, are less used as similar, newer drugs have fewer unwanted effects. These include **cabergoline** (Cabaser), **pergolide** (Celance), **ropinirole** (Requip) and **pramipexole** (▼Mirapexin).

Unwanted effects such as feeling or being sick can be a problem initially although these fade with time. The anti-emetic **domperidone** is helpful. Also at the start of treatment low blood pressure may be a problem, and you should avoid activities such as driving until you know how you react to dopamine agonist treatment. Very rare, serious reactions can develop during treatment with bromocriptine or one of the related medicines (cabergoline, lisuride, pergolide) including tissue overgrowth in some organs such as the lungs. The CSM has advised doctors that people should have blood tests and a chest X-ray before starting treatment and certainly if long-term treatment is intended. Careful monitoring is required.

Apomorphine can help some people with unpredictable 'off' periods with levodopa treatment. It starts to work within 5–10 minutes and acts for about one hour.

Apomorphine has to be given by injection under the skin (subcutaneously) – you can be taught the injection technique once you have been stabilised on treatment or you can have a continuous infusion pump. Specialist supervision in hospital is usual, especially at the start of treatment to adjust the dose and also because apomorphine causes nausea and vomiting. Domperidone is essential to control these predictable unwanted effects, started two days before apomorphine treatment begins and continued for at least three days afterwards. Apomorphine, in much lower doses than for Parkinson's disease, is also used for erectile dysfunction.

All the dopamine agonists can cause psychiatric problems such as hallucinations, confusion and paranoia. Relatives and helpers should note any mood changes, aggressive behaviour or even mild disturbances, and discuss them with the doctor.

All dopamine-enhancing drugs, including levodopa, apomorphine and dopamine agonists, are associated with sudden sleep attacks, falling asleep suddenly without warning and waking up a few minutes later, and also sleep episodes – waves of sleepiness lasting about one hour. Driving or operating machinery can be very dangerous until you know how you react to one of these medicines; driving accidents have occurred.

Other medicines Entacapone (Comtess) is a catechol-O-methyl-transferase (COMT) inhibitor drug used in addition to co-beneldopa or co-careldopa to reduce 'end of dose' deterioration. Levodopa is broken down in the body by the COMT enzyme when other routes are blocked by carbidopa or benzerazide. **Entacapone** enhances the effect of levodopa, allowing reduction in the dose of levodopa. A new combination of levodopa, carbidopa and entacapone (▼Stalevo) in one tablet reduces the number of different medications that you may need to take in a day.

Selegiline (Eldepryl; Zelapar) is used in severe parkinsonism with levodopa to reduce 'end-of-dose' deterioration. It is a monoamine-oxidase-B inhibitor which prevents the breakdown of dopamine in the brain. The dietary restrictions needed with monoamine-oxidase-A antidepressants (page 206) are not necessary.

Amantadine (Symmetrel) has modest antiparkinsonian effects and may help if you have not responded to levodopa. It may help mild slowness of movement (bradykinesia), rigidity and tremor, but tolerance to its effects occurs. Amantadine treatment should be withdrawn gradually.

DRUG-INDUCED PARKINSONIAN SYMPTOMS

Antimuscarinic medicines dampen cholinergic activity in the brain, which allows a better balance between the dopaminergic and cholinergic systems. They were the mainstay for relieving symptoms of Parkinson's disease before levodopa was introduced in the late 1960s. Their effects are modest (they help muscle rigidity and tremor) and so they are no longer used routinely for Parkinson's disease except for reducing excessive salivation, which causes dribbling and drooling.

Antimuscarinic medicines lessen some of the extrapyramidal symptoms of drug-induced parkinsonism that can occur, for example with phenothiazines or other antipsychotic medicines (pages 212–13). An antimuscarinic drug should not be taken routinely with an antipsychotic as a preventative just in case parkinsonism develops. Antimuscarinic medicines do not help tardive dyskinesia (page 212) and may worsen this condition. There are no important differences between the antimuscarinic medicines, but some people appear to tolerate one preparation better than another. Commonly used medicines include **orphenadrine** (Disipal; Biorphen) and **trihexyphenidyl** (benzhexol) (Broflex), **benzatropine**, **procyclidine** (Kemadrin; Arpicolin) and **biperiden** (Akineton). Doses may be taken before meals if dry mouth is a problem, or after food if the particular drug upsets the stomach. Apart from the common antimuscarinic unwanted effects of constipation, difficulty in passing urine and visual disturbances, these drugs can impair memory and cause nightmares and confusion, especially if someone has dementia.

5

INFECTIONS

Bacterial infections Cystitis
Fungal infections Viruses
Protozoa Worms

Micro-organisms, creatures too small to be seen with the naked eye, are all around us and some of them, given the right conditions, can cause disease. There are four main groups of disease-causing micro-organisms: *bacteria*, *viruses*, *fungi* and *protozoa*, and medicines used to combat them are called *antimicrobials*. Very few of the organisms in these groups are harmful. Many live side by side with humans without generating disease. Some bacteria and fungi co-exist happily with people, living on skin or other areas of the body, such as the bowel, and stop harmful organisms getting a hold. The body's immune system protects you from constant invasion by harmful organisms, commonly known as germs.

In the body, germs are usually killed before they multiply to large numbers and cause disease. Blood contains various types of white cells responsible for killing germs, which are carried to the site of infection. It also produces antibodies specific to the invading organism. Antibodies and special white cells remain in the bloodstream so that the next time the organism enters the body, they recognise it and disarm it. This process builds up the body's immunity, but white blood cells are sometimes overwhelmed by an invading germ or the immune system may be destroyed (as in AIDS), allowing a disease to take hold. Symptoms of infection can be confined to one part of the body, such as the bladder and urine or the lungs, or extended throughout the body, as in the case of chicken pox or septicaemia.

Disease is also caused by other organisms or parasites which depend for part of their life cycle on an animal or human host, and sometimes both. Examples include worms (*helminths*) such as tapeworm, and malaria, scabies and lice.

The body's defences

The body is under constant attack from organisms but it is reasonably well defended. Invading organisms enter the body by several routes:

- **Nose** As you breathe in through your nose you take in micro-organisms. The inside of the nose is lined with a layer of cells (*membrane*) covered in very fine projections (*cilia*). Mucus produced by the nasal membranes traps germs and foreign particles. The cilia move the foreign bodies along the membranes to the throat where they are swallowed; alternatively they may be sneezed out.

- ☐ **Mouth** Micro-organisms enter the body when you breathe in through your mouth and in food and drink. Stomach juices contain hydrochloric acid and kill many germs that can cause gastroenteritis.
- ☐ **Eyes** When you sleep or blink the eyes are cleaned by liquid from the tear glands; tears can kill some germs.
- ☐ **Skin** is a natural barrier to micro-organisms. However, they can enter through cuts, scratches and when the skin is pierced by a disease-carrying insect such as a mosquito. Bacteria causing boils and acne can enter through hair follicles.
- ☐ **Vagina and urinary tract** The vagina is naturally acidic, which kills many germs. Urine washes bacteria out of the bladder and urethra.

HOW INFECTION IS SPREAD

Infection is illness or disease that is spread from person to person. Infection results when, for instance, a virus entering the nose attacks and damages some of the cilia, allowing the organism to get into your body. Once you are infected with the organism the virus is carried on drops of liquid in your breath to another person (droplet infection).

Micro-organisms can also transfer from one person to another on direct physical contact. For example, the cold virus can be passed on with a handshake. The cold-sore virus *herpes* can be transferred by direct contact or from sharing the same article, such as a toothbrush, with someone with an active cold sore. Some diseases can be passed from one person to another through sexual intercourse. Genital contact also allows pubic lice to transfer from an infected person to another.

Many types of food are ideal breeding grounds for micro-organisms, particularly bacteria. Water can carry infections, especially where there is no clean water supply or sewage system. For example, cholera is passed on this way.

Flies, fleas and mosquitoes are among the animals that pass on disease. They convey the infecting organism from one host to another. For example, malaria is caused by species of the protozoon *Plasmodium*, which depends on a female mosquito for part of its life-cycle and a human for the other part. The mosquito passes on the protozoon in saliva when it bites a human. Other blood-sucking animals such as fleas transmit disease. Bubonic plague is carried from rats to humans by fleas. Flies acquire germs on their feet, for example from dirty places such as rubbish dumps, which they pass on to food.

A doctor is required to notify the local authority when a patient is suspected of having any disease from a list of 30 which have implications for public health. Examples of notifiable diseases include cholera, food poisoning, viral hepatitis, measles, mumps and meningitis. Immunisation against diseases which have the potential to cause long-term damage and disability if you do not have the vaccine – for example poliomyelitis – has improved individual and public health immeasurably.

– HOW YOU CAN HELP YOURSELF –

Many infections cannot be avoided but you can cut down the risk.

- ☐ Always wash hands after going to the toilet or changing a nappy and immediately before eating.
- ☐ Store food at recommended temperatures and take note of 'Use by' or 'Best before' dates. Keep raw and cooked food covered and on separate shelves.
- ☐ Prepare food hygienically: wash your hands before preparing a meal.
- ☐ Cook food thoroughly, especially ready-prepared meals.
- ☐ Avoid passing colds on – do not go to work if the cold is heavy; wash your hands after blowing your nose.
- ☐ Do not share towels, toothbrushes, swimwear or underwear.
- ☐ Use a condom for sex, to prevent the transmission of diseases such as gonorrhoea, syphilis, genital warts, herpes, chlamydia and AIDS.

Bacterial infections

Infections are common even though the body's defences and the immune system are protective. A healthy body can often control and overcome infections naturally with time. It is only when the defence systems break down or harmful micro-organisms overwhelm you that treatment may be needed. The most frequently infected parts of the body are the respiratory system, the digestive system, the skin, and the bladder and urinary tract.

Bacteria multiply very rapidly – every 20 to 30 minutes – and may release poisons (toxins) that damage body cells. You may have a high temperature and feel unwell. Bacteria may stay at one site in the body or spread throughout the body in the bloodstream. Bacteria are classified according to their shape – *cocci* are spherical, *bacilli* rod-shaped and *spirochaetes* are spiral-shaped – and also by whether or not they are stained by a dye (Gram's stain). If they take up the stain, bacteria are classified as Gram-positive; if not, they are Gram-negative.

Some antibiotics can be less effective against Gram-negative bacteria because their cell walls tend to be more complex and more able to resist antibiotic action. Examples of bacteria that can cause infection include Gram positive *Staphylococcus* (e.g. skin infections), *Streptococcus* (e.g. septic infections) and *Pneumococcus* (e.g. pneumonia); and Gram negative *Escherichia coli* (e.g bladder infections) and Salmonella (e.g. gut infections such as typhoid). Bacteria are also classified by whether they require oxygen to grow (*aerobic*) or whether they can live without it (*anaerobic*).

Antibacterial medicines

A *bactericidal* drug kills the invading organism by interfering with either the bacterial cell wall or the cell contents; a *bacteriostatic* drug stops the multiplication of bacteria. Both types of antibacterial drugs are also known as *antibiotics*. An antibiotic is usually given to treat an infection, but may also be given to prevent one. For example, if you have an artificial heart valve and need to have routine surgery, you will be given antibiotic cover before you have the operation.

Each year around half the British population visits the doctor for the treatment of infections. If it seems appropriate your doctor may prescribe an antibacterial medicine and may also advise some simple pain relief and rest. Your doctor may be able to diagnose the type of bacteria involved from the symptoms of your illness, for example with a bladder infection, or may make 'a considered guess'. Sometimes the bacterium will need to be identified in a laboratory in order to select the appropriate antibiotic for your illness. In practice this is difficult because laboratory testing takes time, so the doctor may decide to prescribe a *broad-spectrum* antibiotic – one that affects a wide range of bacterial species – while waiting for the results of tests. Treatment may be switched to another antibiotic in light of the laboratory results and local policies. Sometimes no specific organism can be identified in apparent infections, for example an upset stomach (gastroenteritis).

Micro-organisms which have not previously grown and caused infection are constantly being discovered, particularly viruses. Over 30 infectious diseases have become important since the early 1970s, for example severe acute respiratory distress syndrome (SARS). Examples of antibacterial medicines and infections for which they may be used are shown in the table overleaf.

Many infections, particularly of the throat and other parts of the upper respiratory tract, are caused by viruses and not by bacteria. An antibacterial drug is not effective against a virus. Even if a bacterium is responsible for the infection, it is now known that antibiotics offer little benefit in minor infections, for example for acute bronchitis or sinusitis, if your underlying health is good. When considering whether or not to prescribe an antibiotic the doctor has to consider your resistance to infection, the severity of your illness and the likelihood of another or secondary infection developing subsequently, where the infection is and the likely organism(s) causing the problem. Other important factors are your age, ethnic origin and history of allergies, the state of your kidney and liver function and, if you are a woman, whether you are pregnant, breast-feeding or taking an oral contraceptive. Don't expect your doctor to give you an antibiotic automatically: you may not need one. Your doctor may suggest a period of watchful waiting or suggest delaying a prescription for an antibiotic to see whether your illness improves with time. These strategies aim to conserve the usefulness of antibiotics for use when they are essential. If you do need an antibiotic, don't stop taking it until the course is complete, even if you feel better. Failing to complete the course, for instance to treat tuberculosis, may mean that you don't get better properly. It also encourages bacterial resistance. Don't be tempted to take the few tablets left over from a previous prescription for a new problem without talking to your doctor, and don't give your antibiotics to anyone else in the family or your friends.

Common infections and examples of antibacterial treatment (by mouth except where indicated)

Infection	Antibacterial medicine
Gastroenteritis	Usually self-limiting – medicine not needed
Salmonella	Ciprofloxacin or trimethoprim
Chronic bronchitis flare-up	Amoxicillin, tetracycline or erythromycin
Pneumonia (uncomplicated community-acquired)	Amoxicillin or erythromycin
Meningitis	Initial treatment by injection: benzylpenicillin or cefotaxime if tolerated, or if these have caused anaphylaxis previously, chloramphenicol
Cystitis	Trimethoprim or amoxicillin, or a cephalosporin or nitrofurantoin
Inflammation of the kidneys (acute pyelonephritis)	Cefadroxil (or other cephalosporin) or norfloxacin (or other quinolone)
Chlamydia	Doxycycline or azithromycin
Sinusitis (with discharge and lasting at least 7 days)	Amoxicillin, doxycycline or erythromycin
Middle ear infection (if not resolved after 72 hours, or start antibacterial treatment earlier if symptoms worsen)	Amoxicillin or erythromycin
Throat infections (bacterial)	Phenoxymethylpenicillin for ten days, or erythromycin or a cephalosporin
Impetigo (widespread)	Flucloxacillin or erythromycin
Cellulitis	Phenoxymethylpenicillin or flucloxacillin
Animal bites	Co-amoxiclav

UNWANTED EFFECTS

Most antibiotics prescribed by your GP are unlikely to cause many serious unwanted effects. Common unwanted effects include feeling sick (nausea) and diarrhoea, often caused by the increased growth of other micro-organisms not killed by the antibiotic (*superinfection*). The other main unwanted effect is allergic reaction to the antibiotic, arising from breakdown products of the antibiotic that combine with the body's proteins and cause an immune response. These hypersensitivity reactions range from skin rashes to acute anaphylactic shock. Most antibiotics are either broken down in the liver or leave the body via the kidneys. If you have reduced liver or kidney function you are more liable to unwanted effects, especially if you are over 65.

Allergy

Rashes and fever occur commonly, not always at the start of treatment. A delayed reaction (*serum sickness*) may sometimes occur after stopping the medicine. Symptoms include itchy rash, joint pains, fever and swollen lymph nodes (part of the body's immune system). The most serious unwanted effect, especially of the **penicillin** group, is severe allergic reaction (*anaphylaxis*), which affects around one person in 5,000 and is very occasionally fatal. If you are allergic to penicillin, you will be allergic to all the medicines in the penicillin group. **Cephalosporin** antibiotics are similar to the penicillins, and about ten per cent of patients who are sensitive to penicillin will also react to a cephalosporin. You must always tell your doctor, particularly one you have not consulted before, if you have had a severe reaction to an antibiotic – keep a note of its name on the medicine record sheet. It is important to distinguish between true allergy, including anaphylaxis, and the expected unwanted effects, such as feeling sick or having diarrhoea.

Interaction with oral contraceptives

The effectiveness of the oral contraceptive may be reduced. **Rifampicin** and the antifungal drug **griseofulvin** (and possibly other antifungal medicines taken by mouth) reduce the activity of all oral contraceptives, and additional precautions are needed if you are taking either drug. Diarrhoea caused by an antibiotic may disrupt the absorption of an oral contraceptive, and broad-spectrum antibiotics such as **ampicillin** and **doxycycline** may reduce the effectiveness of the combined oral contraceptive by decreasing the amount of oestrogen available in the body. Women should follow the advice for a missed pill (page 358), or use another contraceptive measure.

Upsetting the body's flora

Sometimes antibiotic treatment may upset the natural balance of micro-organisms living in or on your body, thus affecting the organisms which co-exist with the body, without causing harm – especially if you have a long course of treatment. For example, antibiotics can kill off the bacteria that check the growth of *Candida albicans*, a yeast which normally lives in or on the body without harming you. If the yeast, a member of the fungus family, grows unchecked, it also causes infection (superinfection), with symptoms of soreness and irritation (thrush) in the mouth, throat, gullet and vagina.

Pseudomembranous colitis

Antibiotic treatment occasionally leads to the overgrowth of one type of bacterium (*Clostridium difficile*) which is not killed by the antibiotic. These bacteria release a toxin that causes *pseudomembranous colitis*, unremitting diarrhoea which can be fatal, especially in elderly people. This complication can occur with cephalosporins, penicillins and **erythromycin**, but is most common with **clindamycin**, an antibiotic reserved for serious infections. If you develop unremitting diarrhoea while taking an antibiotic, stop treatment immediately and contact your doctor.

BACTERIAL RESISTANCE

Bacteria live life at a pace: they are born, mature and multiply in the space of a few hours and can change and adapt to a new environment. Bacteria develop ways to avoid the effects of antibiotics, for example by adapting their growth and reproductive cycles or by producing an enzyme to neutralise the antibiotic. Not all bacteria causing an infection are necessarily killed during a course of antibiotic treatment and the ones that survive eventually become the dominant strain by a process of natural selection. Their resistance becomes inherent and can spread, but this is not the only route that bacteria take to overcome antibiotic treatment. Bacteria acquire resistance by permanently building it into their genes (*mutation*) or by receiving genetic material already resistant to a range of antibiotics from other bacteria (*gene transfer*).

When penicillin was first introduced it was a powerful killer of *Staphylococcus aureus*, a bacterium capable of causing infections from impetigo to life-threatening pneumonia following influenza, and blood poisoning (septicaemia). After 20 years of treatment, penicillin was no longer effective against almost all strains of staphylococcus because the bacteria had developed an enzyme to counter the effects of penicillin. A new antibiotic, **methicillin**, was developed and was successful at first. Gradually methicillin-resistant strains developed to produce a 'super staph', known as *methicillin-resistant Staphylococcus aureus* (MRSA), which is resistant virtually to all antibiotics. This 'superbug' emerged in hospitals but has spread to the community – for example to nursing homes – as patients, and their bacteria, moved between these locations. Infections have become more difficult to treat, prolonging the length and severity of illness. Even with the development of new antibiotics, often more toxic alternatives to older medicines, bacteria continue to find ways to become resistant to treatment. Exposure to antibiotics is therefore the key factor to bacteria developing resistance. Reducing inappropriate use is essential if antibiotics are to remain effective therapies in the future.

Antibiotics must be used only when they are really needed. Diagnostic tools and sensitivity testing to find out which antibiotic will be most effective against a particular bacterium are important, but a lack of these tools have contributed to the overuse of antibiotics, as have demanding patients. If you have an established bacterial infection, other than a minor self-limiting one, the benefits of using an antibiotic to treat it far outweigh the risks of not taking the antibiotic. However, using an antibiotic to treat a viral infection, such as a cold or cough, is a misuse of an antibiotic because antibiotics act against bacteria and will not help infections caused by viruses. If you take an antibiotic, it may make you more susceptible to further bacterial infection.

GROUPS OF ANTIBIOTICS

Many antibiotics have been developed from substances produced naturally by moulds and fungi. Penicillin was the first antibiotic developed from a mould, *Penicillium notatum*, some years after Alexander Fleming noticed that the mould, which had accidentally contaminated some culture dishes, inhibited the growth of bacteria. There are now many different types of penicillin, some capable of eliminating a wide range of bacteria, while others have a more specific action. Over the years many more antibacterial drugs have been discovered and developed. Most are produced synthetically in the laboratory, and the search for new antibiotics in the attempt to counteract bacterial resistance continues.

Antibacterial medicines are classified into several groups. The main ones are featured in drug profiles: **penicillins**, **cephalosporins**, **tetracyclines**, **erythromycin**, **sulphonamides** and **trimethoprim**, **quinolones** and **metronidazole**.

AMOXICILLIN

AMOXICILLIN – Capsules, soluble powder, liquid, injection
AMOXIL – Capsules, liquid, soluble powder, injection

Co-amoxiclav
AUGMENTIN – Tablets, soluble tablets, liquid, injection
CO-AMOXICLAV – Tablets, liquid
AMOXICILLIN + CLAVULANIC ACID

The addition of clavulanic acid makes amoxicillin effective against more infections.

Amoxicillin (amoxycillin) is bactericidal. It interferes with the bacterial cell wall, which allows water to enter the cell until bursting point. A member of the penicillin group, it is used for treating a wide range of bacterial infections of the ear, chest and bladder, and also for the sexually transmitted disease, gonorrhoea.

Amoxicillin can be used during pregnancy for bladder infections. It is normally taken three times a day (less often at higher doses) for treating dental abscesses and urinary tract or middle ear infections. It is also used to prevent bacterial growth developing inside the heart (infective endocarditis) in people who are at risk of such infection, for example those who have artificial heart valves, valve disease or heart inflammation (for example as a result of rheumatic heart disease) and who then require dental or other surgical procedures.

Amoxicillin is similar to an older pencillin, ampicillin, but is better absorbed and can be taken with food. A blotchy skin rash is a common unwanted effect, but this is not necessarily an allergic reaction. Rash almost always occurs if amoxicillin is given to people with glandular fever. These penicillins should not be used for treating a sore throat until the cause is known.

Before you use this medicine

Tell your doctor if you are:
☐ pregnant or breast-feeding – amoxicillin can be used ☐ taking any other medicines, including vitamins and those bought over the counter.

Tell your doctor if you have or have had:
☐ a rash, hypersensitivity or allergy to a penicillin or cephalosporin antibiotic ☐ glandular fever ☐ severe kidney impairment.

How to use this medicine

Take the capsules regularly three times a day or the powder as prescribed.

Liquid preparations should be shaken thoroughly before use. You can take amoxicillin with or after food if necessary.

Always take all the amoxicillin prescribed for you, even if you feel better before the prescription is finished. If you stop too soon, your symptoms may come back. If you miss a dose, take it as soon as you remember, but skip it if it is almost time for your next dose. Do not take double the dose. Dose reduction may be needed if kidney function is severely impaired. Small amounts of alcohol should not be a problem. Amoxicillin and alcohol do not interact, but an infection means that your body needs rest and recuperation.

Liquid preparations should be stored in a refrigerator, but not frozen.

Over 65 No special requirements except caution with co-amoxiclav (see below).

Interactions with other medicines

Combined oral contraceptives may not be as effective and there may be breakthrough bleeding, e.g. with ampicillin, which can reduce the amount of oestrogen available to the body. Discuss this with your doctor.

Unwanted effects

Likely Loose stools, diarrhoea, skin rashes (hives or itching).
Less likely Feeling or being sick, sore mouth and tongue from superinfection, e.g. with Candida.
Rarely Severe hypersensitivity or allergic reaction.

Unwanted effects are usually mild. Rashes are more likely with long or repeated courses or because of underlying medical conditions (e.g. chronic lymphocytic leukaemia). If you develop a severe rash or unremitting diarrhoea contact your doctor. If you have a severe allergic reaction (wheezing, swollen mouth and tongue, itching), stop taking amoxicillin and call your doctor immediately.

Co-amoxiclav Liver toxicity (cholestatic jaundice) may occur during, or shortly after, treatment with co-amoxiclav. This is more likely in men and in people above the age of 65. If jaundice develops it is usually self-limiting and very rarely fatal. Amoxicillin is preferred, but when co-amoxiclav is needed it should not be taken for longer than 14 days.

Similar preparations

AMPICILLIN – Capsules, liquid

CO-FLUAMPICIL – Capsules
AMPICILLIN + FLUCLOXACILLIN

MAGNAPEN – Capsules, liquid, injection
CO-FLUAMPICIL

PENBRITIN – Capsules, injection
AMPICILLIN

Narrower range, but useful preparations: **BENZYLPENICILLIN** injection (Crystapen); **PHENOXYMETHYLPENICILLIN** (PENICILLIN V); **FLUCLOXACILLIN** (FLOXAPEN)

CEFALEXIN

CEFALEXIN – Capsules, tablets, liquid KEFLEX – Capsules, tablets, liquid
CEPOREX – Capsules, tablets, liquid

Cefalexin (cephalexin) is a broad-spectrum cephalosporin antibiotic. Cephalosporins are related to penicillins and, like them, they are bactericidal. They have a similar range of action that may be used for pneumonia, meningitis, septicaemia, biliary tract infection and urinary tract infections, although this varies for individual cephalosporins. Some cephalosporins are only available as an injection and are used mostly in hospital; others such as cefalexin or cefaclor can only be taken by mouth. About one person in ten who is sensitive to penicillin will also react to a cephalosporin.

Cefalexin is useful for treating bladder infections that have not responded to other drugs; it can be used during pregnancy. It may also be used for skin and infected wounds or deep cuts, and middle ear or respiratory infections, although other antibiotics are generally preferred as first-line treatments, because cephalosporins are prone to cause resistance.

Before you use this medicine

Tell your doctor if you are:
☐ pregnant or breast-feeding – cefalexin can be used ☐ taking any other medicines, including vitamins and those bought over the counter.

Tell your doctor if you have had:
☐ an allergic reaction or hypersensitivity to a cephalosporin or a penicillin.

How to use this medicine

Take the tablet or capsule every six hours (or you may be able to take a higher dose every eight hours). Shake liquid preparations thoroughly before use. You can take cefalexin before or with food.

Always take all the cefalexin prescribed for you, even if you feel better before the prescription is finished. If you stop too soon, your symptoms may recur. If you miss a dose, take it as soon as you remember, but skip it if it is almost time for your next dose. Do not take double the dose. Dose reduction may be needed if kidney function is severely impaired. Small amounts of alcohol should not be a problem. Cefalexin and alcohol do not interact but an infection means that your body needs rest and recuperation.

Liquid preparations should be stored in a refrigerator, but not frozen.

Over 65 No special requirements.

Interactions with other medicines

No significant interactions, but always check with your doctor or pharmacist if you take cefalexin with other medicines.

Unwanted effects

Likely Mild diarrhoea.
Less likely Feeling or being sick, indigestion and abdominal pain, superinfection e.g. with Candida, sore mouth or tongue, itching in the genital or rectal area, fever, rashes.

Rarely Severe allergic or hypersensitivity reactions, including skin reactions, Stevens-Johnson syndrome, toxic epidermal necrolysis; pseudomembranous colitis at high doses, blood disorders.

Unwanted effects are usually mild and fade as you continue treatment. If you develop a severe rash or unremitting diarrhoea contact your doctor. If you have a severe allergic reaction (wheezing, swollen mouth and tongue, itching) stop taking cefalexin and call your doctor immediately.

Similar preparations

BAXAN – Capsules, liquid
CEFADROXIL

CEFACLOR – Capsules, liquid

CEFRADINE – Capsules

▼CEFZIL – Tablets, liquid
CEFPROZIL

DISTACLOR – Capsules, liquid, modified-release tablets
CEFACLOR

ORELOX – Tablets, liquid
CEFPODOXIME

SUPRAX – Tablets, liquid
CEFIXIME

VELOSEF – Capsules, liquid, injection
CEFRADINE (CEPHRADINE)

ZINNAT – Tablets, liquid, powder
CEFUROXIME

TETRACYCLINE

TETRACYCLINE – Tablets
TOPICYCLINE – Skin lotion for acne

Poor choice combination preparation
DETECLO – Tablets
TETRACYCLINE + CHLORTETRACYCLINE + DEMECLOCYCLINE

The tetracyclines are bacteriostatic broad-spectrum antibiotics which have been widely used, although increasing bacterial resistance has now limited their effectiveness. They are used for the long-term treatment of acne – either by mouth, for example minocycline, or applied directly on to the skin, for example tetracycline. Tetracyclines are also especially useful for treating *Chlamydia* infections, such as inflammation of the urinary tract (*urethritis*), pelvic inflammatory disease, certain types of respiratory disease, Lyme disease (a bacterial infection caused by *Borrelia burgdorferi* and transmitted by the bite of a tick associated with deer) and sometimes skin infections or pneumonia. There is little to choose between the tetracyclines in terms of effectiveness; **doxycycline** and **minocycline** may be used when kidney function is poor. Doxycycline is also used for preventing malaria and unofficially for treating rosacea, an acne-like skin condition.

Like other members of the class, tetracycline may cause stomach upsets and overgrowth of the fungus *Candida*. Tetracycline combines with calcium in the body and is laid down in growing bones and teeth of unborn babies and young children. This causes yellow-brown staining not just of the milk teeth, but also of the permanent teeth. **Tetracycline should not be given to pregnant or breast-feeding women and children under the age of 12 or to those with severe impairment of kidney function.**

Before you use this medicine

Tell your doctor if you are:
☐ pregnant or breast-feeding – tetracycline must be avoided ☐ taking any other medicines, including vitamins and those bought over the counter.

Tell your doctor if you have or have had:
☐ poor liver or kidney function ☐ allergic reaction or hypersensitivity to a tetracycline antibiotic.

Do not use tetracycline:
☐ if you are pregnant ☐ for children under 12 years ☐ if you have severe kidney disease ☐ if you have systemic lupus erythematosus or myasthenia gravis – tetracycline exacerbates these conditions.

How to use this medicine

By mouth Take the dose every six hours with a full glass of water while sitting or standing to avoid the antibiotic irritating the gullet, one hour before meals or two hours afterwards. Avoid taking milk, dairy products and any other medicine, especially antacids, calcium and iron preparations, for an hour before or two hours after tetracycline as they reduce absorption. Although hard water contains some calcium, it seems unlikely to affect the absorption of tetracycline significantly. The absorption of doxycycline and minocycline is not affected significantly by food and they can be taken at meal times.

On the skin for acne Apply to clean skin twice daily. Other local preparations are used for skin and eye infections.

Always take all the tetracycline prescribed for you, even if you feel better before the prescription is finished. If you stop too soon, your symptoms may come back. If you miss a dose, take it as soon as you remember, but skip it if it is almost time for your next dose. Small amounts of alcohol should not be a problem. Tetracycline and alcohol do not interact, but an infection means that your body needs rest and recuperation.

If you have poor kidney function a tetracycline antibiotic can damage the kidneys further. Doxycycline and minocycline are less harmful to the kidneys. If you have severe kidney disease you should not take tetracycline. If you have liver disease you may need a lower dose of tetracycline.

Over 65 As kidney and liver function decreases with age, tetracycline should be used with care.

Interactions with other medicines

Acitretin for acne. Avoid use with tetracycline.
Bismuth chelate, calcium, antacids (containing aluminium/magnesium) and dairy products may reduce the absorption and therefore the effectiveness of tetracyclines.
Iron and zinc salts reduce tetracycline absorption and vice versa.
Combined oral contraceptives may not be as effective and there may be breakthrough bleeding; tetracycline can reduce the amount of oestrogen available to the body. Discuss this with your doctor.
Oral anticoagulants such as **warfarin** Tetracycline may increase the risk of bleeding.

Unwanted effects

Likely Feeling or being sick, diarrhoea.
Less likely Increased sensitivity to the sun (increased sunburn), sore mouth or

tongue or itching in the genital or rectal area due to candidal overgrowth, difficulty swallowing and gullet irritation, liver toxicity.
Rarely Severe allergic or hypersensitivity reactions, blood disorders, antibiotic-associated colitis; headache and visual disturbances may indicate raised pressure within the brain.

Contact your doctor if diarrhoea or stomach upsets are severe. Stop taking tetracycline and contact your doctor if you have a skin reaction or severe itching and soreness.

Unwanted effects of minocycline, which is commonly used for acne, include dizziness and vertigo (more common in women), and skin coloration (pigmentation), which is sometimes irreversible on stopping treatment. Rarely other effects include sensitivity to sunlight, systemic lupus erythematosus, and lung problems – shortness of breath, cough and fever (reversible on stopping treatment).

Similar preparations

DALACIN T – Skin lotion for acne
CLINDAMYCIN

DOXYCYCLINE – Capsules

LEDERMYCIN – Capsules
DEMECLOCYCLINE

MINOCIN – Tablets, modified-release capsules
MINOCYCLINE

MINOCYCLINE – Capsules, tablets

OXYTETRACYCLINE – Tablets

TETRALYSAL 300 – Capsules
LYMECYCLINE

VIBRAMYCIN – Capsules, soluble tablets
DOXYCYLINE

ZINACLIN – Gel for acne
CLINDAMYCIN

ERYTHROMYCIN

ERYTHROMYCIN – Tablets, capsules, liquid, injection
ERYMAX – Capsules
ERYTHROCIN – Tablets
ERYTHROPED – Liquid
ERYTHROPED A – Tablets
STIEMYCIN – Skin lotion for acne
ZINERYT – Skin lotion for acne

Erythromycin is used in a similar way to penicillin, although it does not affect an identical range of bacteria. It is widely used and people who are allergic to penicillins or who must avoid tetracycline can usually take erythromycin safely. Erythromycin is used for treating middle-ear, throat and chest infections in children, legionnaires' disease, sinusitis, pneumonia, and intestinal infections caused by Campylobacter bacteria. It is also used for treating genital infections caused by sexually transmitted diseases, such as syphilis or gonorrhoea. Erythromycin may also be given to prevent the spread of whooping cough or diphtheria. It can also be used for the long-term treatment of acne and skin infections either by mouth or applied directly to the skin.

Three other related medicines have similar uses to erythromycin but also have some specific uses. For example, **clarithromycin** is used in combination with other antimicrobials and an ulcer-healing drug to eradicate *Helicobacter pylori*, a bacterium associated with peptic ulcer disease. **Azithromycin** can be used as an alternative, but unofficial treatment of Lyme disease (page 272). A new erythromycin derivative, **telithromycin** (▼Ketek), can be used for community-acquired pneumonia, chest infections, sinusitis and as an alternative to penicillin in severe (streptococcal) throat infections. These erythromycin relatives are taken once or twice daily.

Before you use this medicine

Tell your doctor if you are:
□ pregnant or breast-feeding □ taking any other medicines, including vitamins and those bought over the counter.

Tell your doctor if you have or have had:
□ an allergic reaction or hypersensitivity to erythromycin □ liver disease or poor kidney function □ myasthenia gravis – erythromycin may exacerbate this condition.

Do not use erythromycin:
□ if you are taking the antihistamine **terfenadine** or the antipsychotics **pimozide** or **sertindole**.

How to use this medicine

By mouth Take the tablet or capsule every six hours, that is four times daily, with a full glass of water, before or with meals. Higher doses can be taken twice daily. For the long-term treatment of acne you may take erythromycin twice or three times a day, reducing to once a day, depending on the response. Liquid preparations are suitable for children; the dose is usually four times daily. Shake liquid thoroughly before use.
On the skin for acne Apply to clean skin twice daily.
Always take all the erythromycin prescribed for you, even if you feel better before the prescription is finished. If you stop too soon, your symptoms may come back. If you miss a dose, take it as soon as you remember, but skip it if it is almost time for your next dose.

Small amounts of alcohol should not be a problem. Erythromycin and alcohol do not interact but an infection means that your body needs rest and recuperation.

Liquid preparations should be stored in a refrigerator, but not frozen.

Over 65 No special requirements.

Interactions with other medicines

Erythromycin is broken down in the liver and can alter the effectiveness or safety of a number of medicines. Interactions with erythromycin 'relatives' can vary and are not always the same as with erythromycin. Check with your doctor or pharmacist for specific interactions if you are about to start a course of erythromycin or a similar preparation and already take another medicine, including any bought over the counter such as **St John's wort**, which reduces the effectiveness of telithromycin.

Erythromycin and similar preparations can increase the blood levels of some medicines that affect heart rhythm, an unwanted effect. This in turn increases the potential of these medicines to trigger irregular heart rhythms (ventricular arrhythmias) which can be fatal. The following medicines must not be taken with erythromycin and similar preparations:
Antihistamine terfenadine
Antipsychotics pimozide, sertindole, amisulpride
Disopyramide, amiodarone – medicines for irregular heart rhythms.

Erythromycin and similar preparations can increase blood levels of the following medicines, increasing the risk of their toxicity:

Antiepileptics carbamazepine, sodium valproate
Antipsychotics clozapine, quetiapine
Antianxiety medicines midazolam, zopiclone, buspirone
Antiasthma theophylline
Antimigraine eletriptan
Blood pressure-lowering felodipine
Irregular heart rhythms: digoxin
Immunosuppressants ciclosporin, tacrolimus.

Erythromycin and similar preparations should be avoided with the following:
Antibacterial rifabutin
Antidepressant reboxetine
Antimalarial artemether with lumefantrine
Antimigraine ergotamine
Incontinence: tolterodine
Lipid-regulating simvastatin, atorvastatin, rosuvastatin Blood levels decreased
Oral anticoagulants such as **warfarin** Erythromycin increases the risk of bleeding
Vasodilator cilostazol.

Unwanted effects

Likely Feeling or being sick, abdominal pain, diarrhoea.
Less likely Allergic reactions, reversible deafness after high doses, itching, jaundice, skin rashes.
Rare Chest pain, irregular heart rhythms, severe skin rashes – Stevens-Johnson syndrome or toxic epidermal necrolysis.

Erythromycin is a valuable alternative to penicillin and a useful antibiotic for community-acquired pneumonia. Some infections must be treated with a high dose. At the start of treatment you may feel or be sick with erythromycin, particularly with higher doses, but this should wear off as you continue with the course. Contact your doctor if you are very sick while taking erythromycin: a lower dose or a change of antibiotic may avoid this. **Clarithromycin** and **azithromycin** cause less stomach upset. Deafness is reversible on stopping treatment and is usually associated with doses over 4 grams a day. Erythromycin taken for longer than 14 days may occasionally cause jaundice, which clears up on stopping treatment.

Similar preparations

▼KETEK – Tablets
TELITHROMYCIN

KLARICID – Tablets, liquid, granules, injection
CLARITHROMYCIN

ZITHROMAX – Capsules, tablets, liquid
AZITHROMYCIN

SULPHONAMIDES AND TRIMETHOPRIM

The sulphonamides are bacteriostatic antibacterials which originated from the dye industry in the 1930s. **Sulphanilamide**, from the red dye *prontosil rubra*, was the first to be found to have antibacterial activity. The sulphonamides have been widely used for many years, but with increasing bacterial resistance to their effects they are seldom used today and have been replaced by more active and less toxic antibiotics.

Co-trimoxazole is a combination of **trimethoprim** and the sulphonamide **sulfamethoxazole** (sulphamethoxazole). Like all sulphonamides, sulfamethoxazole causes unwanted effects, some severe, such as blood disorders (e.g. bone marrow depression, agranulocytosis) and the Stevens-Johnson syndrome – a condition of the skin and mucous membranes with swelling, blistering and ulcers, which is sometimes fatal. There have been reports of deaths in people over the age of 65 treated with co-trimoxazole and also with trimethoprim. Co-trimoxazole (Septrin) should be used only when there is no alternative. It is now used mainly for treating *Pneumocystis carinii* pneumonia, which can occur when your immune system is impaired, for instance with HIV infection, also for toxoplasmosis – a protozoal infection acquired from undercooked meat or from cat faeces – and the lung infection nocardiasis, which also occurs when the immune system is deficient.

Trimethoprim on its own is used for bladder and chest infections, prostatitis, and serious gastrointestinal infections such as salmonella. Unwanted effects are less frequent and less severe than with co-trimoxazole. Bacterial resistance to trimethoprim is also increasing.

TRIMETHOPRIM

TRIMETHOPRIM – Tablets
MONOTRIM – Liquid
TRIMOPAN – Liquid

Trimethoprim is an antibacterial drug used for treating and preventing bladder (urinary tract) infections, chest infections such as a flare-up in chronic bronchitis, prostate infections and sometimes salmonella infections. It is also a component of co-trimoxazole, the use of which is now restricted to treating serious or unusual infections because of the risk of rare, life-threatening adverse effects.

Before you use this medicine

Tell your doctor if you are:

□ pregnant – trimethoprim must be avoided (teratogenic risk, page 49) □ breast-feeding – a short course of trimethoprim can be taken □ taking any other medicines, including vitamins and those bought over the counter.

Tell your doctor if you have or have had:

□ hypersensitivity to trimethoprim □ folic acid deficiency or any other blood disorder □ severe kidney or liver disease.

How to use this medicine

Take one tablet every 12 hours, twice daily. You may be able to take the dose once a day (usually at night) if it is to prevent recurrent bladder or kidney infections. Liquid preparations are available for children. The usual length of a course of trimethoprim is seven to ten days, but a three-day course is often adequate for simple bladder infections. Trimethoprim can be taken with food and this may help if the drug irritates your stomach. Small amounts of alcohol should not be a problem. Trimethoprim and alcohol do not interact, but an infection means that your body needs rest and recuperation.

Always take all the trimethoprim prescribed for you, even if you feel better before the prescription is finished. If you stop too soon, your symptoms may come back. If you miss a dose, take it as soon as you remember. If you are taking trimethoprim twice a day, take the dose you missed and wait about six hours before taking the next dose. For once-a-day trimethoprim, take the dose you missed and wait about 12 hours before the next one.

Over 65 You may be more susceptible to unwanted effects, such as blood disorders, particularly if you are lacking in folic acid. You may need less than the usual dose, particularly if kidney function is impaired.

Interactions with other medicines

Antimalarials Pyrimethamine in Fansidar – increased risk of low folic acid levels.
Anticancer azathioprine, **mercaptopurine** Increased risk of blood disorders; with **methotrexate** increased risk of low folic acid levels.
Oral anticoagulants such as **warfarin** Possible increased risk of bleeding.
Ciclosporin Increased risk of adverse effects on the kidneys.

Unwanted effects

Likely Feeling or being sick, rashes and itching.
Rarely Blood disorders, Stevens-Johnson syndrome, severe skin reactions, photosensitivity and allergic reactions, anaphylaxis, aseptic meningitis.

Trimethoprim causes few unwanted effects. If stomach upsets or skin reactions are severe, contact your doctor. On long-term treatment you need to recognise signs of blood disorders such as fever, sore throat, rash, mouth ulcers, reddish-purplish skin spots, bruising or bleeding. If these develop, contact your doctor immediately.

Similar preparations

CO-TRIMOXAZOLE – Tablets, liquid, injection

SEPTRIN – Tablets, liquid, injection
CO-TRIMOXAZOLE

SULFADIAZINE – Tablets, injection

CIPROFLOXACIN

CIPROFLOXACIN – Tablets
CIPROXIN – Tablets, liquid, injection

CILOXAN – Eye drops

Ciprofloxacin is an antimicrobial of the quinolone group, a relative of an older drug, nalidixic acid. It is active against a wide range of bacteria and the micro-organism Chlamydia, which causes pelvic inflammatory disease and urethritis, and is used for certain chest infections – for example in cystic fibrosis, and infections of the urinary tract and digestive system. Ciprofloxacin is also used for treating septicaemia and gonorrhoea if the bacteria are sensitive to its effects. It is used with other antibiotics to combat anthrax, if exposure to the disease is confirmed or suspected. Ciprofloxacin is used unofficially (unlicensed) to prevent the spread of meningitis during an outbreak. The eye drops are used for treating corneal ulcers. The quinolones are best reserved for treating particular bacterial infections as resistance to their effectiveness is emerging with common bacteria such as *Staphylococcus aureus*.

Before you use this medicine

Tell your doctor if you are:
☐ pregnant or breast-feeding – not recommended ☐ taking any other medicines, including vitamins and those bought over the counter.

Tell your doctor if you have or have had:
☐ hypersensitivity to ciprofloxacin or other quinolones – do not use these antibiotics ☐ poor kidney function ☐ excessive alkalinity of the urine – ciprofloxacin can cause crystal formation ☐ epilepsy or other central nervous system disorders – ciprofloxacin may exacerbate these conditions ☐ myasthenia gravis – ciprofloxacin may exacerbate ☐ deficiency of the enzyme glucose-6-phosphate dehydrogenase ☐ tendonitis, e.g. Achilles tendon damage – do not take ciprofloxacin.

Ciprofloxacin is not recommended for children or growing teenagers, except where the benefit outweighs the risk – for example for exacerbations of cystic fibrosis, inhalation anthrax and as a single dose for preventing the spread of meningitis. Studies have shown damage to weight-bearing joints in animals and this is a potential risk in humans.

How to use this medicine

Take the tablets, usually twice daily, with a glassful of water. Ciprofloxacin is absorbed more rapidly if it is taken on an empty stomach. Avoid taking ciprofloxacin at the same time as dairy products, those with a high calcium content or indigestion remedies, because they affect its absorption. A normal diet with small amounts of calcium will not affect ciprofloxacin's absorption significantly. Drink plenty of fluids during treatment with ciprofloxacin to avoid crystals forming in the urine.

Ciprofloxacin may impair driving and the performance of skilled tasks. Do not drive or do other activities that require alertness until you know how you react to ciprofloxacin. Avoid alcohol because it enhances these effects. Always take all the ciprofloxacin prescribed for you, even if you feel better before the prescription is finished. If you stop too soon, your symptoms may come back. If you miss a dose, take it as soon as you remember, but skip it if it is almost time for your next dose.

Ciprofloxacin is generally well tolerated, but can cause a range of potential, rare unwanted effects, including tendon damage, exacerbation of mind and nerve problems, and skin rashes such as photosensitivity. Whilst taking ciprofloxacin, you should avoid excessive exposure to sunlight as this can trigger skin reactions.

Over 65 No dose reduction needed unless kidney function is moderately impaired, when half the normal dose is needed. Older people are more prone to tendon damage with ciprofloxacin and other quinolones (see below).

Interactions with other medicines

The quinolones can interact with a range of medicines; check with your doctor or pharmacist because these can vary depending on the quinolone. The most significant ones for ciprofloxacin are listed here.
Theophylline for asthma – ciprofloxacin prolongs and increases the blood levels of theophylline, causing toxicity. If you have to use the two drugs together, your doctor should reduce the dose of theophylline. Blood tests to measure the level of theophylline may be necessary. Possible increased risk of seizures.
Anticoagulants such as **warfarin** The risk of bleeding is increased.

Non-steroidal-anti-inflammatory drugs (NSAIDs) Possible increased risk of seizures.
Ciclosporin Increased risk of kidney toxicity. Monitoring required.
Indigestion remedies, iron tablets and supplements containing iron and zinc Reduce absorption of ciprofloxacin. Allow four hours between taking ciprofloxacin and these preparations.
Methotrexate Ciproflxacin may increase methotrexate blood levels and increase the risk of toxicity. Monitoring required.

Unwanted effects

Likely Feeling or being sick, diarrhoea, indigestion, abdominal pain, headache, restlessness, sleep disorders, dizziness, rash, itching.
Less likely Tremor, confusion, convulsions, depression, hallucinations, blurred vision, loss of appetite, pins and needles, sensitivity to sunlight (photosensitivity), hypersensitivity including hives, muscle and joint pain, swollen throat, anaphylaxis.
Rarely Stevens-Johnson syndrome, toxic epidermal necrolysis, blood disorders, jaundice, pseudomembranous colitis.

Ciprofloxacin and other quinolones can rarely cause tendon inflammation and damage (including rupture), especially in older people and in those also taking corticosteroids. Tendon rupture may occur within 48 hours of starting quinolone treatment. At the first sign of pain or inflammation in the tendons, you should stop taking ciprofloxacin and contact your doctor.

Stop taking ciprofloxacin or other quinolone and contact your doctor if any unwanted effects (psychiatric, neurological or hypersensitivity, including severe rash) occur.

Similar preparations

▼AVELOX – Tablets
MOXIFLOXACIN

EXOCIN – Eye drops
OFLOXACIN

MICTRAL – Soluble granules
NALIDIXIC ACID

NEGRAM – Tablets, liquid
NALIDIXIC ACID

NORFLOXACIN – Tablets

OFLOXACIN – Tablets

TARIVID – Tablets, injection
OFLOXACIN

TAVANIC – Tablets, injection
LEVOFLOXACIN

URIBEN – Liquid
NALIDIXIC ACID

UTINOR – Tablets
NORFLOXACIN

Cystitis

Cystitis is inflammation of the bladder, usually involving painful passing of urine, caused by infection. The kidneys or bloodstream may be infected by the infection spreading upwards from the bladder. You may pass urine frequently or uncontrollably and sometimes urine is blood-stained. The tube leading down from the bladder to outside the body (the urethra) usually becomes inflamed first, causing urination to sting. The bladder may also be inflamed, causing a dull ache in the lower part of the abdomen. Sometimes the kidneys are involved, which you feel as a dull backache. You may have a fever. Bacterial infection of the kidney is known as acute pyelonephritis; rarely this infection can lead to kidney damage.

Bacteria are responsible for around half the cases of cystitis. They live harmlessly in the bowel and around the anus, but they can spread to the urethra and bladder where they can cause infection and inflammation by attaching themselves to the tissues lining the inside of the bladder. Factors that contribute to colonisation include the use of antibiotics by mouth for other infections, leading to upset in the body's bacterial balance, dryness and shrinkage of the vagina in older age, use of a diaphragm and jelly for contraception, and previous bladder infections, which may be difficult to eliminate completely. Sexual intercourse and catheterisation (the introduction of a flexible tube to drain the urine) facilitate bacterial transfer. The openings of the urethra and anus are closer together in a woman than in a man and the urethra is shorter – it is therefore easier for bacteria to contaminate the urethra and reach the bladder in a woman. Men are also protected by fluid from the prostate gland, which has bactericidal properties.

Cystitis is therefore much more common in women than men. When it occurs in men, especially those who are middle-aged or older, there is frequently an underlying disorder, such as enlargement of the prostate (benign prostatic hyperplasia) or a tumour in the prostate or bladder. A low flow rate of urine and infrequent and incomplete emptying of the bladder predispose to infection.

Children who get cystitis should see a doctor. Cystitis is more difficult to spot in children under two years old because the symptoms – loss of appetite, being sick, diarrhoea, drowsiness and fever – are similar to other

– HOW YOU CAN HELP YOURSELF –

- ☐ Drink at least three to four pints of liquid a day – more if the weather is hot. This helps to flush out bacteria. Cranberry juice is helpful.
- ☐ If you find you get cystitis after drinking coffee, tea or alcohol try diluting them – or avoid them altogether.
- ☐ Pass urine when you need to. Holding on can encourage an attack of cystitis.
- ☐ After passing urine count to 20 and then see if any more will come, but don‘t strain.
- ☐ If you are a woman who gets cystitis after sexual intercourse, it will help to pass water and wash your genitals and anus before and after sex. A man can also help by washing his penis before and after intercourse. Women who suffer from soreness and bruising may find it helps to use a lubricating jelly during intercourse.
- ☐ Wash your genital area morning and night; and always wipe the anus from front to back. This helps to prevent any of the bacteria from the genitals or anus reaching the urethra and causing infection.
- ☐ Avoid using bubble bath or bath gels if you find they irritate your skin. Do not use perfumed soap, deodorants, talcum powder or antiseptics on the genital area.
- ☐ Avoid wearing tight trousers or nylon pants or tights. They can create a warm moist environment which helps bacteria to breed. Cotton pants allow the skin to breathe.

childhood conditions. It can make older children wet the bed. Cystitis in children is usually a sign that there is something wrong with the kidneys and may lead to permanent kidney damage.

Vaginal candidiasis and other sexually transmitted diseases such as Chlamydia can also produce cystitis-like symptoms. If cystitis keeps coming back, you must see your doctor.

Medicines for cystitis

Self-treatment can be helpful to alleviate pain and discomfort in simple cystitis. Preparations available from a pharmacy include **sodium citrate** as a powder to make into a liquid (Canesten Oasis; Cymalon; Cystemme; Cystocalm) and **potassium citrate** as a liquid (Potassium Citrate Mixture BP), as effervescent tablets (Effercitrate) or as granules (Cystopurin). Drink plenty of water to flush the bacteria out of the bladder. Cranberry or blueberry juice helps to prevent bacteria attaching themselves to the bladder. You should see your doctor if cystitis continues for more than two days or you have recurrent attacks. If you have blood in your urine, a temperature, backache or you are pregnant, you should see your doctor at once, without trying self-help remedies. Blood in the urine usually means that bacteria are attacking the lining of the urethra.

Your doctor or nurse will usually prescribe an antibiotic, such as **trimethoprim**, **amoxicillin**, a **cephalosporin** or **nitrofurantoin** (Furadantin, Macrodantin, Macrobid) for up to seven days. Shorter courses of amoxicillin or trimethoprim may be appropriate. Nitrofurantoin is a synthetic antimicrobial, first used in the 1960s. It is effective, but unwanted effects, particularly feeling or being sick, limit its use. Newer formulations (Macrodantin or Macrobid) reduce the likelihood of unwanted reactions. Other unwanted effects of nitrofurantoin include loss of appetite, diarrhoea, allergic reactions (rashes, urticaria), changes to the lungs, and nerve damage in the fingers and toes. This last effect may occur if you take nitrofurantoin and have severe kidney impairment. Other medicines that are sometimes used for uncomplicated urinary tract infections include **ampicillin** and **nalidixic acid**. However, increasing bacterial resistance is a drawback to the use of most of these medicines. A urine sample may be needed so that the bacteria can be identified and the choice of antibiotic checked in the laboratory if the first one does not work. A reagent strip or dipstick dipped into the urine can indicate whether infection is present or not. This is a quick way to check for infection so you can start treatment before the laboratory results are ready. After treatment of the initial infection, some people need to take a low dose of antibacterial long-term to prevent a recurrence, particularly with repeated infections and significant kidney damage; trimethoprim or nitrofurantoin are used.

Fungal infections

There are around 100,000 different kinds of fungi in the world, growing on all kinds of plants and animals, and their derivatives. They are prolific and many are able to live either as parasites or to co-exist happily with their host, depending on the food supply and local conditions. One of the common fungi associated with humans is *Candida albicans*, a simple yeast. *Aspergillus* is another fungus that can cause allergies or infections. Some fungal infections involve the skin and other parts of the body, such as ringworm (*Tinea*) infections of the scalp, nails and skin.

CANDIDA ALBICANS

Candida lives on the skin and in the mouth, the gut and the vagina without causing any harm until its living conditions are changed. Taking an antibiotic by mouth changes the composition of micro-organisms in the digestive system, killing harmless bacteria that keep Candida under control and allowing it to proliferate unchecked. Fungal infection often begins when the body's resistance is lowered in some way. An antibiotic is taken when the body is already under attack by bacteria. Other conditions such as pregnancy, and illnesses such as diabetes, cancer or AIDS alter the body's natural resistance and immunity to infection, and allow the fungus to flourish. The oral contraceptive or prolonged treatment with a corticosteroid may also predispose the body to candidal infection.

Symptoms of candidal infection are patchy white spots (thrush), usually in the mouth or vagina. The mouth is a common site of infection and in babies it may be hard to distinguish Candida from milk curds. Older people who wear dentures are also at high risk of fungal mouth infections. A baby's nappy rash may become infected with Candida. In women the vulva and vagina are common sites of infection and also the skin under the breasts and other areas of skin folds. Nipple infection can occur if you are breast-feeding. In uncircumcised men, the area under the foreskin is liable to candidal infection. Candidal infection can also occur in the absence of other predisposing factors described above.

TINEA

Tinea species commonly cause fungal infections of the scalp (*Tinea capitis*), the nail (*Tinea unguium*), the body (*Tinea corporis*), the feet (athlete's foot – *Tinea pedis*) and in the groin area (*Tinea cruris*). These ringworm infections can be passed from human to human, from animal to human and from soil to human.

Antifungal medicines

Fungal infections generally need treatment because they rarely clear up alone. Most antifungal drugs affect the cell wall of the fungus, allowing the cell contents to leak out; the cell then dies. Severe fungal infections within the body (*systemic infections*) may need treatment with an antifungal by injection into the veins, for example with **amphotericin** or **flucytosine**, usually in hospital. Aspergillosis and the rarer *cryptococcal* and *histoplasmosis* infections can be challenging to treat. Systemic fungal infections may need weeks of treatment, especially if the immune system is damaged (*immunocompromised*).

The choice of antifungal by mouth includes **ketoconazole** (Nizoral), **fluconazole** (Diflucan), **itraconazole** (Sporanox) or **voriconazole**

(▼Vfend). Antifungal medicines which are taken by mouth can interact with a range of other medicines, but when used locally interactions are not usually a problem. **Miconazole** gel (Daktarin), even when used locally, is absorbed into the body and interacts with some medicines.

Fungal infections, particularly candidiasis, occur commonly in the mouth, on the skin, in the external part of the ear, the vagina, and rarely in the bladder and eye. Antifungal medicines are used directly on the infection, that is applied locally.

CANDIDIASIS

Candidal skin infections are treated locally with an imidazole cream, spray or powder such as miconazole, or another antifungal such as **nystatin**. In the mouth, lozenges or pastilles of **amphotericin** (Fungilin) or nystatin (Nystan) are used. These medicines are not absorbed into the body. Babies can be treated with amphotericin or nystatin suspension or miconazole gel. Treatment should continue for 48 hours after the infection appears to have cleared.

Vaginal and vulval infections are treated with pessaries and cream (pages 286–8). Nystatin has been widely used, but must be used for up to a fortnight and stains clothing yellow. The imidazole antifungal preparations such as miconazole or clotrimazole can be used for up to 14 days, but are also effective in shorter courses as a single dose or a three-day course, which are more convenient. Medicines in this class are equally effective. The triazole antifungal drugs – fluconazole or itraconazole – are taken by mouth to treat various fungal infections, including vaginal candidiasis. Recurrent vaginal candidiasis may need treating with one of these oral drugs, which cannot be used during pregnancy.

Recurrent infection is common if the course of treatment is not completed, but may also be due to underlying causes, such as long-term antibiotic treatment (page 268) or diabetes mellitus (pages 301–4). Your doctor may need to take swabs for culture. Ideally your partner should wear a condom during sexual intercourse, but note that antifungal creams and pessaries can damage rubber condoms and diaphragms.

MICONAZOLE

On prescription
DAKTARIN – Mouth gel, cream (also from a pharmacy)
GYNO-DAKTARIN – Pessaries, intravaginal cream, combination pack (pessaries + cream), single high-dose vaginal capsule (also from a pharmacy)

With a corticosteroid
DAKTACORT – Skin preparations for eczema
DAKTACORT HC (from a pharmacy)
MICONAZOLE + HYDROCORTISONE

Available over the counter (not NHS)
DAKTARIN Dual Action – Cream, dusting powder, spray for fungal skin infections

Miconazole is a broad-spectrum imidazole antifungal drug which acts against yeasts such as Candida. Miconazole gel is used for treating and preventing fungal infections of the mouth, throat and gut. It can be used on the skin to treat Candida infections such as nappy rash, or relieve irritation of the vulva (*vulvitis*) or the penis. Pessaries and creams are available for use in the vagina, and there is also a high-dose pessary for use as a single-dose treatment. Miconazole can be absorbed into the body from the gel or vaginal preparations, despite local use, and so interactions with other medicines remain important.

Before you use this medicine

Tell your doctor if you are:
□ pregnant or breast-feeding □ taking any other medicines, including vitamins and those bought over the counter.

Tell your doctor if you have or have had:
□ hypersensitivity to miconazole □ poor liver function □ porphyria.

Avoid miconazole in these situations.

How to use this medicine

Gel Take the dose four times a day after meals for ten days or for up to two days after the symptoms have cleared. For mouth and throat infections, keep the gel in the mouth for as long as possible before swallowing. For local use in the mouth, the gel can be put directly on to the affected areas with a clean finger.
Skin Apply to the affected area, rub in gently.
Vagina Insert the cream or pessaries at night high into the vagina. Pessaries and creams may damage the rubber of diaphragms and condoms.

Always take or use all the miconazole prescribed for you, even if you feel better before the prescription is finished. If you stop too soon, your symptoms may come back. If you miss a dose, take or use it as soon as you remember, but skip it if it is almost time for the next dose.

Over 65 No special requirements.

Interactions with other medicines

Miconazole (and other antifungals, although these need to be checked specifically with your doctor or pharmacist) should not be used with medicines that affect the heart rhythm, including **quinidine** (anti-arrhythmic), **terfenadine**, **mizolastine** (**antihistamines**), **pimozide** and **sertindole** (**antipsychotics**).
Midazolam by mouth (**benzodiazepine**) – increased risk of irregular heart rhythms. Blood levels increased by miconazole – avoid use together:
Anticoagulants such as **warfarin** Effect enhanced by miconazole.
Antidiabetic oral hypoglycaemics e.g. **glibenclamide**, **tolbutamide** – blood levels increased by miconazole, increasing the risk of hypoglycaemia.
Antiepileptic phenytoin Effect enhanced by miconazole, increasing the risk of toxicity.
Immunosuppressants ciclosporin, **sirolimus** Blood levels increased by miconazole, increasing the risk of toxicity.
Lipid-lowering simvastatin Increased risk of muscle weakness (myopathy) with miconazole – avoid use together.

Unwanted effects

Less likely Feeling or being sick, diarrhoea (on long-term treatment).

Rarely Allergic reactions, hepatitis.
With skin and vaginal preparations Irritation, occasionally local sensitivity reaction – if this occurs, discontinue treatment and contact your doctor.

Similar preparations

CANESTEN – Skin and vaginal preparations (from pharmacies)
CLOTRIMAZOLE

CANESTEN HC – Skin cream (from pharmacies)
CLOTRIMAZOLE + HYDROCORTISONE

CANESTEN ORAL – for vaginal candidiasis
FLUCONAZOLE

CLOTRIMAZOLE – Skin cream, pessaries

DIFLUCAN – Capsules, liquid, injection
FLUCONAZOLE

DIFLUCAN ONE – for vaginal candidiasis (from pharmacies)
FLUCONAZOLE

ECOSTATIN – Skin and vaginal preparations (from pharmacies)
ECONAZOLE

EXELDERM – Skin cream (from pharmacies)
SULCONAZOLE

FLUCONAZOLE – Capsules, injection

GYNO-PEVARYL – Vaginal preparations (from pharmacies)
ECONAZOLE

LOMEXIN – Pessaries
FENTICONAZOLE

NIZORAL – Tablets, skin cream (not NHS), shampoo (also from pharmacies)
KETOCONAZOLE

NYSTAN – skin, vaginal and mouth preparations
NYSTATIN

NYSTATIN – Mouth preparations

PEVARYL – Cream (from pharmacies)
ECONAZOLE

SPORANOX – Capsules, liquid, injection
ITRACONAZOLE

TROSYL – Nail solution
TIOCONAZOLE

• *VAGINAL CANDIDIASIS* •

Antifungal creams and pessaries for vaginal use and preparations for use on the skin can now be bought from pharmacies, under the supervision of a pharmacist. This is an important advance for women in whom vaginal candidiasis is a common condition. Almost half of all women will have at least one attack during their lifetime.

Symptoms of vaginal candidiasis include soreness, itching and sometimes swelling of the vagina and vulva. A curd-like whitish discharge with little or no smell may be noticed. You may also experience a burning sensation at the opening to the vagina and sexual intercourse may be uncomfortable. It is a good idea for your partner to use a condom but antifungal creams and pessaries can damage rubber condoms and diaphragms. Your partner may need to use a skin cream on the penis as the infection can be transmitted during intercourse.

Once you recognise the signs of vaginal candidiasis with confidence, you may decide to treat yourself with a specially formulated vaginal cream or pessary. If however, you are a first-time sufferer and have not treated yourself before, always seek help and advice from your doctor. See your doctor if:

☐ you are under 16 or over 60
☐ you have had more than two attacks in the last six months

- ☐ you are pregnant
- ☐ you have pain and discomfort on passing urine – it is sometimes difficult to tell whether you have a bladder or vaginal problem
- ☐ you have a temperature or chills
- ☐ you feel sick or have diarrhoea
- ☐ you have a history of sexually transmitted disease
- ☐ you have a foul-smelling or blood-stained discharge
- ☐ you have ulcers, sores or blisters.

VAGINAL ANTIFUNGALS FROM A PHARMACY

Name	*Form*	*Pack size*
CLOTRIMAZOLE	Pessary Skin cream	1 20g, 50g
CANESTEN PREPARATIONS **CLOTRIMAZOLE**	Pessary Vaginal cream Skin cream	1; 3; 6 5g with applicator 20g
CANESTEN COMBI	Pessary + Skin cream	1 + 10g
DIFLUCAN ONE **FLUCONAZOLE**	Capsule	1
ECOSTATIN **ECONAZOLE**	Pessary Skin cream	1 15g; 30g
GYNO-PEVARYL **ECONAZOLE**	Pessary Skin cream	1;3 15g; 30g
GYNO-PEVARYL COMBI PACK	Pessaries + Skin cream	3 + 15g

The imidazole antifungal medicines – **clotrimazole**, **econazole**, **fenticonazole** and **miconazole** – appear to be equally effective against candidal infections. The products have been prescribed by doctors for many years, so their effectiveness and safety are well established. A single overnight application of vaginal cream or a pessary, also called a vaginal capsule or a soft pessary, seems to be as good as longer courses of treatment and is more convenient. The imidazole preparations are well tolerated, but very occasionally they can cause irritation and skin preparations can cause a mild local burning. Very rarely they cause sensitisation and treatment may need to be stopped. The antifungal drug **fluconazole** is available from a pharmacy as a single-capsule treatment for taking by mouth as Diflucan One or Canesten Oral, but is expensive.

Each antifungal product should contain comprehensive instructions and information. Follow the directions carefully. Larger pack sizes can be bought for three, six or seven nights' treatment. Small sizes of the skin cream, for twice- or three-times daily use, can be bought for just less than the prescription charge. Some products (Canesten 1 and Canestan Once) are advertised direct to the public, for example in women's magazines.

Symptoms should ease or clear up within three days of a course of treatment with a single-dose pessary or vaginal cream. If you still have symptoms after seven days you should see your doctor. It is unwise to repeat the course if the treatment fails to relieve symptoms.

Other treatments, such as live yogurt inserted into the vagina, are of unproven value. A teaspoon of sodium bicarbonate to half a litre (one pint) of warm water may soothe the vulva and surrounding skin, but should not be used as a vaginal douche because this upsets the normal balance of the vagina. After going to the toilet, wipe from front to back away from the vagina because infection can be transferred from the bowel. Your doctor may suggest a course of an oral antifungal if it seems likely that the gut is acting as a reservoir of infection or you have an underlying condition that predisposes to candidal infection. See also 'How you can help yourself', below.

– HOW YOU CAN HELP YOURSELF –

- ☐ Cleanliness is essential and it is important to keep potential areas of infection dry and cool. Take care with drying skin folds and creases and use a light dusting of a non-perfumed talcum powder to absorb remaining moisture.
- ☐ Avoid using perfumed soaps and irritant bath additives.
- ☐ Avoid tight-fitting clothes such as jeans or tights.
- ☐ Wear natural fabrics, rather than nylon, next to your skin to allow it to breathe.
- ☐ Wash clothes in non-biological powder and rinse thoroughly.
- ☐ Do not share towels, swimwear, underwear or toothbrushes. Candida and other infections can spread this way.
- ☐ Use a condom for sex if your partner has or has recently had Candida infection.
- ☐ If you wear dentures, keep them and your mouth clean. Watch out for the slightest sign of infection, such as redness and soreness at the corners of the mouth, which should be treated.
- ☐ Change babies' nappies regularly and clean the nappy area well with warm water. Dry thoroughly and leave the area exposed to the air whenever practical. Avoid tight-fitting plastic pants.
- ☐ Sterilise teats and bottles before putting them into the baby's mouth and avoid putting sugary solutions in bottles.

TINEA

Mild ringworm infections, for example athlete's foot (*Tinea pedis*) – scaling and itching between the toes – can be treated locally with ointment, cream or powder. **Terbinafine** (Lamisil) cream, applied once or twice daily for a week, is the most effective antifungal treatment for athlete's foot. Other products include **tolnaftate** (Tinaderm; Mycil) and the **undecenoates** (Mycota). The *imidazole* antifungal skin preparations, such as **clotrimazole**, **econazole**, **sulconazole** and **miconazole**, are also used and reduce the risk of spreading the infection. You can buy these preparations over the counter. **Amorolfine** cream (Loceryl) can be used once a day for skin infections such as Tinea. Treatment lasts for three to six weeks and should be continued for up to five days after the infection has cleared. Older preparations that are less effective or less easy to use include salicylic acid-containing preparations such as **Phytex**, **Monphytol** and **compound benzoic acid** ointment (Whitfield's ointment), a sticky ointment which is less cosmetically acceptable. More severe and widespread ringworm infections of the nails and scalp usually need treatment by mouth with an antifungal drug.

The **scalp infection** (*Tinea capitis*) is increasing in developed countries and is more common in children, particularly black African children. It has a variable appearance and can be difficult to diagnose. Scalp ringworm must be treated with an antifungal by mouth, such as **griseofulvin** (Grisovin), and local application of antifungal to the scalp may reduce the risk of it spreading.

Nail infections, especially on toenails, are difficult to treat locally and may also need treatment by mouth as well. Treatment may have to be continued for weeks or months. Griseofulvin has been widely used, but treatment is not always successful and it can cause unwanted effects. Itraconazole in particular or fluconazole by mouth are effective for nails and have largely replaced griseofulvin for this. Itraconazole can be taken daily for three months or intermittently as 'pulse' therapy twice daily for seven days, with two or three repeated courses after 21-day intervals. Terbinafine by mouth is also helpful for nail infections. It is generally well tolerated. The dose should be reduced if kidney function is impaired and the drug stopped if liver function deteriorates or jaundice develops. Amorolfine is also available as an antifungal lacquer for painting on infected nails, but it is not clear whether the drug is effective without additional treatment by mouth. The product is applied once or twice a week for six months (fingernails) or up to 12 months (toenails). Nail varnish or artificial nails should be avoided during treatment. Antifungals taken by mouth should be avoided during pregnancy.

TERBINAFINE

LAMISIL – Tablets, cream

Terbinafine is used for treating fungal infections of the skin and nails and also Tinea infections of the body, groin and scalp. Treatment needs to continue for between two weeks and three months, depending on the site of infection, or for six months or longer with some nail infections. Although terbinafine is not licensed officially for children, they can take it under medical advice, for example for *Tinea capitis*.

Before you use this medicine

Tell your doctor if you are:

☐ pregnant ☐ breast-feeding – do not take terbinafine ☐ taking any other medicines, including vitamins and those bought over the counter.

Tell your doctor if you have or have had:
☐ liver disease – avoid terbinafine ☐ impaired kidney function ☐ hypersensitivity to terbinafine ☐ psoriasis – risk of exacerbation.

How to use this medicine

Take one tablet daily – usually for up to six weeks for skin infections, or up to three months or longer for nail infections (sometimes six months or longer for toenail infections). The cream should be applied once or twice a day.

Always take all the terbinafine prescribed for you, or use the cream for as long as recommended, even if the infection appears to have cleared up. If you stop too soon, your symptoms may come back. You should continue the treatment for at least two weeks after all the signs of infection have disappeared.

Reservoirs of infection may remain in clothing, footwear and bedding, so general measures of care and hygiene are important. Pets can carry infection, too.

If you miss a dose, take it as soon as you remember. If it is nearly time for your next dose, skip the missed dose and take the next one as usual.

Over 65 No special dose requirements, unless kidney function is impaired when half the dose is needed. Avoid terbinafine if liver function is poor.

Interactions with other medicines

Antibacterial rifampicin reduces blood levels of terbinafine.
Cimetidine increases blood levels of terbinafine.
Oral contraceptives Occasional reports of breakthrough bleeding.

Unwanted effects

Likely
Tablets Abdominal discomfort, headache, loss of appetite, feeling sick, diarrhoea.
Cream Redness, itching or stinging.
Less likely Numbness, dizziness, tiredness, aching joints or muscles, temporary taste disturbance or taste loss, skin rash.
Rare Severe skin reactions, liver toxicity, blood disorders.

Stop taking terbinafine and contact your doctor if a skin rash develops and gets progressively worse, if symptoms of liver damage develop (itching, loss of appetite, feeling or being sick, tiredness, stomach pain or dark-coloured urine) or if blood disorders develop (fever, sore throat, rash, mouth ulcers, reddish-purple skin spots, bruising or bleeding).

Viruses

Viruses are much smaller than bacteria and depend on living cells for their survival. A virus penetrates a cell and then uses the cell's DNA (basic cell matter which carries genetic codes) to multiply and spread to other cells. As new viruses are released the body's cell dies and the viruses go on to infect other cells. There are many different types of virus, from the common cold and influenza to German measles and other childhood infections such as chicken pox, measles and mumps. Infections of the throat, lungs and digestive system are often caused by viruses. Individual viral infections cause a variety of symptoms with differing degrees of severity; for example, some strains of the influenza virus may produce severe symptoms and cause an epidemic. The human immune deficiency virus (HIV), the cause of the acquired immune deficiency syndrome (AIDS) is an epidemic in many countries such as Africa and a major cause of death worldwide.

Antiviral medicines

Treatment of viral infections with specific antiviral medicines is difficult because the virus gets right into, and sometimes becomes a permanent part of, the body's cells. The ideal antiviral drug should kill the virus within the cell or prevent it from multiplying without harming the human cell. Antibiotics are of no use in the treatment of viral infections. Many viral infections clear up spontaneously as the body's immune system overcomes them. Symptoms of infection can be eased with bed rest and a medicine for pain relief and lowering temperature. Some viral illnesses, such as polio, German measles (*rubella*) or measles, can cause lasting damage but developments in immunisation against these diseases over the last 30 to 50 years have reduced their significance in developed countries. However, if no effective vaccine exists for a particular virus, a viral infection can have serious consequences, particularly if your immune system is weakened or compromised.

More antiviral drugs are being developed and treatments are available for *herpes simplex* (cold sores and genital herpes), *herpes zoster* (chicken pox and shingles), HIV, cytomegalovirus (a herpes virus that is important if you are immunocompromised), chronic hepatitis, bronchiolitis in babies (respiratory syncytial virus) and influenza. The medicines sometimes have unpleasant and toxic unwanted effects, particularly where combinations of medicines have to be taken regularly for HIV, but other antiviral treatments, such as **aciclovir** (acyclovir – Zovirax), are well tolerated. Treatment success can be variable and resistance to antiviral medicines has started to occur, including the spread of drug-resistant viruses into communities.

Immunisation remains a very effective way of combating viral infections and their complications, for example pneumonia, which can develop following influenza (flu) in older people or those with long-term conditions such as asthma or diabetes. Two new antiviral medicines, **zanamivir** (Relenza) and **oseltamivir** (▼Tamiflu) are available to treat flu. Either zanamivir or oseltamivir should be taken within the first 48 hours of flu symptoms developing. This helps to stop the virus from spreading in the body and should allow the immune system to overcome the infection. These 'antiflu' medicines appear to reduce the infection by a day or a day and half, two at most, and so benefit is rather limited. Oseltamivir can also be used to prevent flu during a local outbreak, if you are at high risk, providing it is taken within 48 hours of exposure to someone with flu. Both medicines have to be prescribed by your doctor.

Aciclovir was the first selective antiviral medicine to be developed. It halts the herpes virus in its reproductive phase and stops it multiplying, but does not rid the body of the virus. Treatment must be started at the first sign of infection – for example, within 48 hours of the appearance of a shingles rash. Herpes can cause pain and discomfort in whatever part of the body it affects. In people with a weakened immune system, chicken pox and shingles are life-threatening diseases; aciclovir can be life-saving and is usually given by injection in hospital. Aciclovir is also given by mouth to prevent herpes infections and to prevent recurrences of infections.

Shingles is an infection caused by the chicken pox virus (*herpes zoster*). After you have had chicken pox, the virus lies in the nerves of the body inactive for many years. Sometimes the virus will suddenly become active and spread down the nerve, causing a painful, itchy rash in the area of the nerve. Occasionally a nerve of the face and eye is affected; chicken pox blisters may develop on the cornea. Aciclovir lessens the complications of herpes zoster in the eye. Shingles can be very painful and the pain can continue after the rash has gone (*post-herpetic neuralgia*). Aciclovir by mouth helps to shorten the length of time of pain during the illness and reduces the duration of post-herpetic neuralgia. Adequate pain relief will be needed if post-herpetic neuralgia is troublesome. A skin cream (Axsain) containing capsaicin – a derivative of the capsicum pepper – has analgesic properties and may help relieve the pain of severe post-herpetic neuralgia once the skin has healed. It can be applied locally to the affected area up to four times a day, but cannot be used on broken or irritated skin. Other antiviral medicines for treating shingles, **famciclovir** (Famvir) and **valaciclovir** (Valtrex), are as effective as aciclovir in reducing post-herpetic pain, but need only be taken three times a day compared with a five-times-daily dosage for aciclovir.

Chicken pox Aciclovir is also used to lessen the impact of chicken pox in adults and young people who are otherwise healthy but have not had the disease in childhood. Aciclovir is not usually given to younger children with chicken pox because the disease is milder.

Cold sores and genital herpes (*herpes simplex*) can be treated with aciclovir cream applied to the affected areas, but it should not be used inside the mouth, in the vagina or in the eye. The cream is available from pharmacies for the treatment of cold sores (see below). An eye ointment is used for herpes simplex of the eye. Aciclovir tablets may be needed for acute herpes simplex infections of the genital area. If this is a first occurrence your doctor may refer you to hospital to get an accurate diagnosis and to exclude other sexually transmitted infections. Aciclovir tablets should be started within the first five days of infection and should reduce the severity of recurrences. Pain relief by mouth and local application of an anaesthetic gel or ointment for up to seven days may be needed. Other measures include increasing fluid intake to help with passing urine, bathing in salt water and applying Vaseline to the affected area.

ACICLOVIR

On prescription
ACICLOVIR – Tablets, dispersible tablets, cream, injection
ZOVIRAX – Tablets, liquid, cream, eye ointment, injection

From a pharmacy, for cold sores
ZOVIRAX COLD SORE TREATMENT, BOOTS AVERT, CLEARSORE, SOOTHELIP, VIRASORB

Aciclovir is an antiviral drug. It is active against herpes simplex and herpes zoster viruses. It prevents the viruses from multiplying or replicating themselves but does not rid the body of them. Treatment is effective only if it is started at the onset of the infection. Aciclovir is used to treat shingles (caused by the chicken pox virus, herpes zoster) and herpes simplex infections of the skin, lips, genital area or the eye.

Before you use this medicine

Tell your doctor if you are:
☐ pregnant – aciclovir tablets not known to be harmful, but specialist advice is needed for genital herpes (simplex) – or breast-feeding ☐ taking any other medicines, including vitamins and those bought over the counter.

Tell you doctor if you have or have had:
☐ reduced kidney function.

Do not use the cream if:
☐ you are hypersensitive to aciclovir or to propylene glycol.

How to use this medicine

Tablets To treat infection, swallow the tablets whole with water, five times a day, usually for five days for herpes simplex infections, or seven days for herpes zoster infection. Dispersible tablets can be added to a quarter of a glass of water, or swallowed whole with a little water. Tablets should be taken after meals. Drink plenty of fluids during a course of tablets.

Aciclovir tablets can also be used to suppress recurrent herpes simplex infections and to prevent infection in people with an impaired immune system (e.g. someone who has had a bone marrow transplant).

Cream For cold sores, start using the cream at the first sign of an attack. Apply five times a day (every four hours) for five days. A small tube of aciclovir cream can be bought from a pharmacy for less than the prescription charge.

Eye ointment Apply a 1cm ribbon of the eye ointment inside the lower eyelid five times a day and continue for at least three days after complete healing.

Over 65 No special dose requirements.

Interactions with other medicines

No significant interactions with aciclovir tablets.

Unwanted effects

Tablets
Likely Skin rash which usually disappears after treatment, feeling or being sick, diarrhoea, abdominal pain.
Less likely Headache, dizziness, tiredness, confusion, hallucinations.
Rarely Anaphylaxis, swollen throat, shortness of breath, hepatitis, jaundice.

Cream
Likely Temporary stinging or burning.
Less likely Mild drying or flaking of the skin, itching or redness.
Rare Contact dermatitis.

Eye ointment
Less likely Mild stinging, irritation, inflammation.

Similar preparations

FAMVIR – Tablets
FAMCICLOVIR

VALTREX – Tablets
VALACICLOVIR

VECTAVIR – Cream (cold sores)
PENCICLOVIR

Protozoa

Protozoa are microscopic single-celled organisms. They are abundant creatures, mostly found in soil and water, and some can exist for years in cyst form, resistant to temperature and climatic changes. Some can be passed to humans through contaminated food or water. Protozoal diseases can also be spread by sexual contact and through insect bites or by other animal carriers. Diseases caused by protozoans include *amoebic dysentery* (a severe bowel infection), *trichomoniasis* (predominantly a vaginal infection), *giardiasis* (a bowel infection), *cryptosporidiosis* (which causes severe diarrhoea) and *malaria*. Protozoal infections are sometimes difficult to cure and must always be treated promptly. The antimicrobial drug **metronidazole** is used for treating amoebic dysentery, trichomonal infections and giardiasis. In addition metronidazole combats a wide range of anaerobic bacterial infections (for example dental infections), a severe form of diarrhoea as a result of antibiotic treatment (*pseudomembranous colitis*), and is also used in combination treatment to eradicate Helicobacter pylori, which causes duodenal ulceration.

METRONIDAZOLE

METRONIDAZOLE – Tablets, liquid, injection
FLAGYL – Tablets, liquid, injection, suppositories

Skin preparations for acne rosacea
METROGEL – Gel
METROSA – Gel
NORITATE – Cream
ROZEX – Cream, gel
ZYOMET – Gel

Skin preparations for malodorous tumours and skin ulcers
ANABACT – Gel
METROTOP – Gel

Metronidazole is an antimicrobial drug active against a variety of bacterial infections, particularly anaerobic bacteria, and protozoa. It is used for treating protozoal diseases including some vaginal infections (e.g. Trichomonas, Gardnerella), amoebic dysentery and giardiasis. It is also used to treat or prevent infections following surgery and is effective in treating pseudomembranous colitis. Metronidazole is used with other antibiotics in ulcer-healing treatments to eradicate Helicobacter pylori (page 72). Infections of the gums and other dental infections succumb to metronidazole treatment and it is also used on the skin for infected tumours, leg ulcers, pressure sores and rosacea (a facial infection).

Before you use this medicine

Tell your doctor if you are:
☐ pregnant or breast-feeding ☐ taking any other medicines, including vitamins and those bought over the counter.

Tell your doctor if you have or have had:
☐ severe liver disease – dose reduction ☐ hypersensitivity to metronidazole ☐ a central nervous system disorder, e.g. epilepsy ☐ blood disorders.

How to use this medicine

Swallow the tablets whole with water, generally three times daily during or after meals. Treatment usually lasts for five to ten days. The liquid should be taken at least one hour before a meal.

Always take all the metronidazole prescribed for you, even if you feel better before the prescription is finished. If you stop too soon, your symptoms may come back. A course of metronidazole should not last more than ten days, but if it does your doctor should monitor your treatment. If you miss a dose take it as soon as you remember, but if your next dose is due within two hours, take it and skip the next dose.

Skin preparations For acne rosacea the gel or cream should be applied once or twice daily to the face for at least two months. Metronidazole will usually be applied by a nurse as part of treatment for skin ulcers or malodorous tumours. Skin ulcers and pressure sores may also be treated with metronidazole by mouth.

Avoid alcohol. Metronidazole with alcohol may cause headache, stomach cramps, nausea, vomiting, flushing.

Over 65 No special dose requirements.

Interactions with other medicines

Oral anticoagulants such as **warfarin** Blood-thinning effects may be increased.
Antiepileptic drugs Metronidazole increases blood levels of **phenytoin** and risk of phenytoin toxicity. **Phenobarbital** reduces the blood levels of metronidazole and therefore its effectiveness.

Unwanted effects

Likely Feeling or being sick, digestive disorders, unpleasant taste in mouth, furred tongue, rashes.
Less likely Drowsiness, headache, dizziness, unsteadiness, itching, swollen face, throat and tongue. Metronidazole may darken your urine.
Rarely Anaphylaxis.

Serious adverse effects rarely occur with standard courses of treatment. During prolonged or intensive treatment, numbness or tingling of the hands and feet, seizures and blood disorders have been reported. If you feel unwell while taking metronidazole, contact your doctor.

Similar preparations

FASIGYN – Tablets
TINIDAZOLE

MALARIA

The most important and serious protozoal infection is malaria, which is transmitted to humans by the female mosquito. Four types of malaria parasite affect humans. *Plasmodium falciparum* causes the most serious infection. Benign malaria, a less severe form of the disease, is usually caused by *Plasmodium vivax*, but other species *P. ovale* and *P. malariae* may be involved. Infection can occur with more than one species at any one time. Malaria symptoms include aching joints, soaring temperatures, shivering, vomiting, headache, malaise and delirium. In extreme cases, malaria can lead to coma and death. Each year there are approximately 2,000 cases of malaria imported into Britain, and a number of deaths – usually from falciparum malaria. Throughout the world over three million people are infected every year and 1–2 million die, mostly children.

There are medicines for preventing malaria as well as for treating it. **Quinine** and **chloroquine** (Avloclor, Nivaquine) have been used for many years for both treatment and prevention, but resistance to them has developed. Chloroquine is no longer used for treatment and quinine is not suitable for preventing malaria. A number of other medicines are now used, sometimes sequentially or in combination, or as separate treatment. Treatment of malaria may require specialist advice, particularly if someone is seriously ill.

Treatment

Quinine, **mefloquine** (Lariam), **proguanil + atovaquone** (Malarone) or **artemether + lumefantrine** (▼Riamet) can be taken by mouth for falciparum malaria, but in serious illness quinine is given by injection. A course of quinine may be followed by a combination medicine, **pyrimethamine + sulfadoxine** (Fansidar), in a single dose, or if resistant to Fansidar by **doxycycline** for at least seven days.

If you are pregnant, falciparum malaria is particularly dangerous, especially during the last three months. Quinine can be given safely. Doxycycline should be avoided because it can discolour teeth. Malarone, mefloquine and Fansidar are also best avoided.

Benign malaria is usually treated effectively with chloroquine. This form of malaria can occur many months after the initial infection and can recur for years afterwards. Sometimes another antimalarial, **primaquine**, is needed after initial treatment with chloroquine to destroy the parasites that linger in the liver. Chloroquine may be taken during pregnancy, but primaquine treatment should be delayed until after the baby is born. Children tolerate the same antimalarials as adults but dosages depend on the child's body weight.

Prevention

Malaria is a life-threatening disease and the following notes may be helpful in planning trips to areas in the world where malaria is rife.

- ☐ Everyone visiting a malarious area is at risk of infection, whether or not medicines have been taken to prevent the disease. Using a medicine to prevent malaria is a part of a strategy that must also include reducing bites from mosquitoes that carry the parasite. Taking an antimalarial does not provide total protection.

- ☐ The disease may develop after you return from a visit abroad, and any illness that occurs within one year, but particularly within three months of your return, may be malaria. You must see your doctor for advice and mention that you have been exposed to malaria even if you have taken antimalarials exactly as directed.
- ☐ People who have been resistant to malaria in the past but then live in Britain for long periods will lose this resistance.
- ☐ Areas in the world that were once free from malaria may no longer be so and it is essential to check with your doctor or pharmacist for the latest information on which antimalarials are appropriate before travelling. You can also get advice from the Malaria Reference Laboratory* and the Medical Advisory Service for Travellers Abroad (MASTA)*.
- ☐ Prolonged travel increases the risk of contracting malaria, and preventive measures remain essential. Antimalarials for preventing malaria are not available on the NHS and so you will need to purchase them from a pharmacy, either directly or with a doctor's private prescription.
- ☐ Some people are at higher risk of severe malaria than others. If you are pregnant, malaria can be life-threatening and it is wise to avoid travel to malarious areas unless essential. If your immune system is compromised, for example through illness or from taking medicines such as anti-cancer medicines or a corticosteroid by mouth, then you will also be at increased risk. Discuss any concerns with your doctor before making arrangements to travel.
- ☐ The malaria mosquito bites between dusk and dawn, but mostly at night. Personal protection against mosquito bites, including the use of mosquito nets impregnated with an insecticide, insect repellents and adequate clothing to cover as much of the body as possible, is also essential.

MEDICINES FOR PREVENTING MALARIA

The choice of medicine depends on the risk of exposure to malaria – that is, the countries you intend to visit, the patterns of resistance in those areas, the effectiveness and potential unwanted effects of antimalarials and your state of health. The medicines used for prevention change because of changing patterns of resistance and it is important to check that you have the most up-to-date information before you travel.

Prevention with antimalarials should be started preferably one week before travel so that therapeutic levels of the medicine are circulating in the bloodstream by the time you reach the malarious area. For mefloquine, treatment should begin two to three weeks before travel, but for Malarone you can start one or two days before travel. Antimalarials should be taken at the same time each day or on the same day each week.

Antimalarials can cause unwanted effects and these may develop before travel; if they are troublesome ask your doctor for advice.

Antimalarials must be continued for at least four weeks (seven days for Malarone) after you have returned from a malarious area to counter any infection contracted on the last day of exposure. You should take the full course of antimalarial on your return, otherwise you are at increased risk of malaria.

Medicines currently used include one of the following:

- ☐ a combination of chloroquine once weekly and proguanil (Paludrine) daily
- ☐ mefloquine once weekly
- ☐ doxycycline once daily
- ☐ Malarone once daily
- ☐ chloroquine once weekly
- ☐ proguanil once daily.

Unwanted effects of Malarone include feeling or being sick, diarrhoea, abdominal pain, mouth ulcers, loss of appetite and fever. Chloroquine or proguanil is sometimes used singly in low risk areas.

Mefloquine is effective as a weekly dose in areas where there is a high risk of falciparum malaria resistant to chloroquine. It is an effective antimalarial, but unfortunately adverse effects can occur – the majority do so at the start of a course, usually by the third dose. If you start mefloquine two or three weeks before travel this allows you to see how you tolerate the drug.

Mefloquine should not be used for prevention if you have or have had epilepsy, psychiatric problems, abnormal heart conduction problems, or severe liver problems. Mefloquine should be avoided in pregnancy, although it could be used for travel in chloroquine-resistant areas. No evidence of harm has been revealed where mefloquine has been taken during pregnancy. Mefloquine is not recommended during breastfeeding, although the risk to the baby is minimal. It is not recommended for babies under three months old.

Around one in five people is likely to experience unwanted effects, and because mefloquine acts in the body for a long time, reactions to it may persist for several weeks after the last dose. The list of reported effects is now long, and the patient information leaflet should be consulted for the full list. Any concerns, particularly about neuropsychiatric problems, should be discussed with your doctor.

Likely unwanted effects include feeling or being sick, dizziness or vertigo, loss of balance, headache, drowsiness, loose stools or diarrhoea and abdominal pain, and sleep disorders, including sleeplessness and abnormal dreams.

Less likely, but more serious problems include **psychiatric disorders** such as anxiety, depression, mood changes, confusion, hallucinations, panic attacks, restlessness, forgetfulness, psychosis, paranoia, emotional instability, aggression and agitation; **neurological problems** such as tinnitus, hearing impairment, abnormal co-ordination and seizures, pins and needles, tremor, visual disturbances; **heart and circulatory disorders** such as high or low blood pressure, flushing, fainting, chest pain and irregular heart rhythms; **skin disorders** such as rashes, itching, hair loss, swelling, inflammation of the skin and Stevens-Johnson syndrome; **general** unwanted effects which are less likely include muscle weakness and cramps, joint and muscle pains, malaise, fatigue, fever, sweating, loss of appetite, indigestion and shortness of breath.

Do not drive or do other activities that require alertness until you know how you react to mefloquine.

Worms

Worms (*helminths*) are parasites that live part of their life in a human and part in another animal. Many worm infestations are spread in contaminated food which carries the eggs or young worms (*larvae*) because it is inadequately cooked or washed. Some, for example the hookworm, get into the body through the skin. Many worms live in the intestine, attaching themselves to the gut wall, such as the tapeworm, which feeds off the intestinal contents, and the hookworm, which feeds off the blood supply; if untreated this can lead to iron-deficiency anaemia (pages 464–5).

Some worms cause general signs of unhealthiness whilst others cause a great deal of harm. These infections need treatment. They are common in developing countries where treatment may not always be possible. The threadworm (*Enterobius vermicularis*), the most common parasitic worm in Britain, causes at most mild symptoms of itching, but nevertheless should be treated. Anthelmintic medicines are often specific for the particular worm, so your doctor should identify the parasite before treatment.

Anthelmintic treatments

Threadworm commonly affects young children because the eggs are easily spread by sucking unwashed fingers or eating food with unwashed hands. The eggs can survive in sandpits, modelling clay, and in soil. Once inside the body, the eggs develop in the upper intestines and then the adult female worm passes out to the skin around the anus where it lays eggs during the night. This causes itching and if the area is scratched, the eggs are transferred back into the body via the mouth from unwashed fingers and nails. Adult worms live for no longer than six weeks and to break their life cycle good hygiene and treatment of all the family is necessary. Taking baths, and washing hands and scrubbing nails before eating and after each visit to the toilet is therefore essential to break the chain of infection. Washing the bottom first thing in the morning will help to remove the eggs laid at night.

Threadworm infections can be treated with **mebendazole** (Vermox), the treatment of choice for adults and children over two years. Mebendazole is effective in a single dose either as a tablet or liquid, but a second dose is advisable after two to three weeks because re-infection is common. Hygiene measures alone are recommended if you are pregnant (see box overleaf). Mebendazole tablets can be bought from pharmacies (Ovex; Boots Threadworm Tablets 2 Years Plus; Pripsen Mebendazole). Mebendazole acts in the intestines where it kills the worms. It is hardly absorbed into the body and unwanted effects are minimal and self-limiting. These include abdominal pain, diarrhoea and rarely a hypersensitivity reaction. Mebendazole is also used to treat other worm infections such as roundworm, whipworm and hookworm.

Piperazine (Pripsen – on prescription or from a pharmacy) paralyses the worms in the intestines and these are then passed out with the faeces. Used for either threadworm or roundworm, Pripsen powder contains a laxative, senna, to hasten the worms' removal from the intestine. The powder is stirred into milk or water and should be drunk immediately. Threadworm infection is treated with a single dose, repeated after two weeks. Roundworm infection is treated with a single dose but then treatment can be repeated at monthly intervals for up to three months, if reinfection is a risk. Piperazine is suitable for babies over three months old, but should be avoided if you are pregnant. It should be avoided also if you have epilepsy, or poor liver or severe kidney function. All members of a household should be treated at the same time, whether or not they have symptoms, to ensure that the cycle of infection is broken. Unwanted effects include feeling or being sick, colic, diarrhoea and rarely allergic reactions such as skin rash, breathing difficulties, drowsiness or confusion. If allergic reactions are severe, contact your doctor. Piperazine may rarely cause dizziness and loss of muscular co-ordination ('worm wobble').

HOW YOU CAN HELP YOURSELF

As the adult threadworm lives for six weeks only, infections can be treated by attention to strict hygiene measures. This applies to every household member and includes the following:

- ☐ wash hands and scrub nails immediately on rising in the morning, after visiting the toilet or changing nappies, before eating and preparing food
- ☐ bathe or wash around the bottom (anus) carefully each morning
- ☐ keep finger nails short
- ☐ wear underpants at night
- ☐ change and wash underwear, nightwear and bedding (if feasible) each day
- ☐ disinfect bathroom and kitchen surfaces and vacuum carpets daily. Eggs can survive for up to two weeks on clothing, bedding and other objects.

6

HORMONES

Diabetes Obesity Thyroid disorders
Adrenal disorders Corticosteroids
Sex hormone deficiencies

Many of the body's functions are regulated by chemical messengers or *hormones* produced by a number of glands and other structures throughout the body. This is known as the **endocrine system**. Each gland produces one or more hormones to control a particular aspect of body function. Growth, sexual development and the body's control of nutrition and responses to stress are all regulated by hormones. For example, the *pancreas*, situated under the stomach next to the duodenum, produces **insulin**, which plays a key role in regulating the way the body uses carbohydrate, fat and protein. The *thyroid gland* in the neck regulates the body's *metabolism* – the chemical processes which keep the body working, for example by breaking down substances to release energy. The *adrenal glands* located on top of the kidneys produce **corticosteroids** which regulate the body's response to stress and injury and the balance of mineral salts and water. The overall functioning of the endocrine system is controlled by the *pituitary gland* in the brain.

The pituitary gland controls and regulates growth, metabolism, sexual development and reproduction through its hormones, which are responsible for activating the hormones of the other endocrine glands. The pituitary gland is partly controlled by a part of the brain called the *hypothalamus* which produces its own hormones to stimulate the pituitary. The hormones in the bloodstream feed back to regulate the pituitary and the hypothalamus. There is a continuous ebb and flow of hormones with the delicate balance maintained by the pituitary gland.

The hormone balance can be disrupted at a particular endocrine gland, for instance if the gland becomes diseased and malfunctions, or the flow of hormones secreted in the brain in the hypothalamus and the pituitary is disturbed. Most hormones are released from birth onwards but the amount varies according to the body's requirements. Other hormones are produced at particular times, for example growth hormone during childhood and teenage years and sex hormones from the start of puberty.

Diabetes

Diabetes mellitus (or 'sugar diabetes') is not a single disease, but a condition where the breakdown of sugars and starches (*carbohydrates*) in the body is permanently disordered due to lack of **insulin**. Normally, carbohydrates are broken down in the intestines to simple sugars, mostly **glucose**, which are then absorbed into the bloodstream and stored in the liver. Insulin, a hormone produced by the pancreas gland, is responsible for controlling glucose output from the liver, for transporting glucose in the blood and onwards into the body's cells. Glucose within the cells is a source of energy for the body's muscles and organs.

If you have no insulin, or too little for it to be effective, glucose cannot enter the cells and remains in the bloodstream. Blood-glucose reaches a level at which the kidneys cannot hold back the glucose and it spills into the urine. The body's cells are then starved of energy and may switch to burning fats and proteins as an energy source. When the body uses glucose for energy, the waste products are carbon dioxide and water. When fat is burnt, it produces *ketoacids* and other chemicals which can harm the body. The signs of *ketoacidosis* include feeling or being sick, weakness, stomach pains, thirst and dehydration. You also pass large quantities of urine, and *ketones* from the breakdown of fats make the breath smell of fruit. Untreated, these symptoms can lead to coma and death.

A long-term, progressive disorder, diabetes needs careful treatment and management to reduce the impact of immediate and longer-term complications that can occur. This is usually related to how long you have had the disease and how well it has been controlled. There are two main types of diabetes: **type-1 diabetes** (insulin-dependent diabetes mellitus – IDDM) and **type-2 diabetes** (non insulin-dependent diabetes mellitus – NIDDM). Type-1 diabetes occurs when there is an almost complete lack of insulin production. This affects young people most often but can occur at any age, even in infants. Regular injections of insulin are essential to maintain health. Type-2 diabetes develops when the pancreas cannot produce enough insulin and/or the body cannot use it efficiently. This occurs more often in middle-aged and older people, particularly people who are overweight. Type-2 diabetes is treated by diet and medicines taken by mouth to stimulate extra insulin production, although eventually insulin treatment may also be necessary.

Diabetes shortens life-expectancy and puts people at increased risk of a range of conditions: heart diseases, stroke, circulatory disorders, eye problems, nerve damage, infections and kidney disease. Not everyone with diabetes develops all of these conditions, but you are at greater risk than people who are not diabetic. Long-term exposure to high blood levels of glucose means that small blood vessels throughout the body eventually become damaged, resulting in tissue damage. Three areas of the body are particularly affected – the eyes, kidneys and nerves. Damage starts to appear about 10 to 20 years after diagnosis in young type-1 diabetics but can appear earlier in type-2 diabetics, especially if diabetes has remained unrecognised for a time. When diabetes is diagnosed under the age of 30 years, around a quarter to a third of these people develop kidney disease (*diabetic nephropathy*), leading to progressive kidney failure requiring dialysis or a kidney transplant. About one in three young diabetics is likely to develop visual impairment, most commonly through *retinopathy*, where the fine network of blood vessels in the retina becomes damaged. Untreated this can lead to blindness. In the past, five per cent of diabetics became blind after 30 years with the disease, but laser treatment can now preserve existing sight if it is given early enough. Nerve damage (*diabetic neuropathy*), apparent early on as a loss of vibration, sense, pain and temperature sensation in the feet, can lead to the development of foot ulcers and ultimately lower limb amputation. Nerve damage in other parts of the body can manifest as faintness or dizziness on standing up (*postural hypotension*), abnormal sweating, difficulties with bladder emptying and impotence (*erectile dysfunction*) (pages 375–6).

Type-2 diabetics are at high risk of developing heart disease, stroke and circulation problems. Damage and clots can develop in large blood vessels, leading to angina, heart attack and heart failure, also strokes and transient ischaemic attacks (see Chapter 2). Blockage of the blood vessels to lower limbs (*peripheral vascular disease*) can lead to poor circulation and pain on walking, and potentially to the development of foot ulcers and amputation. Diabetics are also more prone to infections – particularly of the bladder and skin – and to conditions such as frozen shoulder, depression, and opacity of the lens in the eye (*cataract*).

Diabetes is becoming more common in all age groups, especially in young people and children. Around 1.4 million people in the UK have diabetes and many others, possibly up to a million, may live with type-2 diabetes without knowing it. People from South Asian, African, African-Caribbean and Middle Eastern descent have a higher risk of this type of diabetes. Less affluent people and those who are overweight or obese, physically inactive or who have a family history of diabetes are at increased risk of developing diabetes. Diabetes occurs in 1 in 20 over the age of 65 years, rising to 1 in 5 over the age of 85 years.

Diabetes of either type is never classified as mild; it can have a profound impact on lifestyle, work, relationships and health. National Service Framework standards and a delivery strategy to improve services are being implemented as part of the NHS ten-year plan. The evidence suggests that if you are enabled to manage your care in partnership with healthcare professionals and with good information, then life expectancy can be increased, and illness and disability reduced. You will need regular health checks, a review of diabetic control and a management plan (see box overleaf).

TYPE-1 DIABETES

This usually occurs in young people under the age of 35 and most commonly between the ages of 10 and 16, although diabetes is starting to appear in children under five years of age. There appears to be a peak at 12 years, when a large number of hormonal changes take place in the body at the beginning of puberty. The insulin-making cells in the pancreas are destroyed by the body's own immune system, which has been triggered into action – possibly by a virus infection. Researchers are not entirely sure why the condition develops. In some cases susceptibility to the development of diabetes appears to be hereditary, but the disease itself is not carried on the genes.

HOW YOU CAN HELP YOURSELF

Learn to look after your health and control type-1 and type-2 diabetes whether you are on insulin, tablets or diet alone. You will need to see your doctor or specialist nurse for regular reviews when you are first diagnosed and then at least once a year, even if you are managing treatment well. Become an active member of the diabetes care team.

- ☐ Work with healthcare professionals to develop a care plan for good diabetes control, including personal goals for your lifestyle. Know who to contact when you need advice.
- ☐ Discuss the impact that diabetes has on your life, including work, leisure activities and driving.
- ☐ Inform the Driver and Vehicle Licensing Agency (DVLA)* and insurance company if you drive.
- ☐ Monitor your blood-glucose levels, or urine levels if appropriate, recording levels and the action taken.
- ☐ A healthy diet is essential. A dietitian can advise you about what to eat and drink, and how to control your weight.
- ☐ You should eat sensibly and regularly. You do not need to eat special, expensive diabetic foods; you can buy low-calorie drinks and foods. Eat plenty of fruit, vegetables and high-fibre foods and avoid or reduce fat. Avoid or drink alcohol in moderation.
- ☐ Exercise regularly and within your capabilities. You may need to adjust your insulin dosage when you try a new activity; ask a health professional for advice. SportEX Health* provides useful factsheets on exercise.
- ☐ Avoid smoking. Smoking adds to the complications of diabetes, particularly circulatory disorders.
- ☐ Foot care is particularly important. You should inspect your feet regularly for signs of sores, ulcers and infection. Wear well-fitting shoes and never walk barefoot. Discuss any problems with the doctor, nurse or podiatrist (chiropodist).
- ☐ Regular eye checks are essential to monitor for eye and visual problems.
- ☐ Always carry glucose tablets, a sugary drink or chocolate or some other snack to relieve 'hypo' symptoms.
- ☐ Carry a card or an identity bracelet to tell passers-by that you are diabetic, just in case you have a severe 'hypo' and lose consciousness. Note your treatment, e.g. type of insulin and dose.
- ☐ Take your diabetic treatment regularly and ensure that you do not run out of insulin and other medication. You do not pay a prescription charge unless diabetic treatment is by diet alone. Most insulin devices, pens and needles are available on prescription, but you do need to pay for blood-glucose meters and finger pricking devices.
- ☐ Join a self-help group. For example, Diabetes UK* has local branches and information on many aspects of diabetes.

Signs of insulin failure may develop swiftly over a period of two to six weeks with lethargy, blurred vision, sickness and general ill health, as well as weight loss, thirst, dehydration and a need to pass more urine (*polyuria*). These symptoms together with a high blood-glucose level are indicative of diabetes. Children developing diabetes will need life-long treatment with insulin to avoid the symptoms of ketoacidosis. They also need to maintain blood-glucose levels within specific limits, avoiding high (*hyperglycaemia*) and low (*hypoglycaemia*) blood-glucose levels to prevent complications developing (see box, pages 306–7). Attention to diet, regular exercise and an appropriate lifestyle are important. Patients and carers need to work closely with a medical team to maintain quality of life and achieve the best possible control of diabetes.

Management

The pancreas releases insulin into the bloodstream around the clock in normal situations, adjusting levels according to the amount of glucose in the blood to meet the fluctuations and demands of daily living such as eating and exercise. When insulin production becomes ineffective or stops, the body's internal insulin can be replaced with an external source, although it is difficult to copy the body's fluctuations and the exact pattern of insulin requirements. You must plan what you are going to eat every day and calculate the carbohydrate content of your food. You can then work out approximately how much insulin you need to counter the high blood-glucose levels normally produced after eating.

For everyone, diet, particularly controlling the daily intake of carbohydrate, is very important. A balanced healthy diet will be needed and dietary advice should be available. You have to take in enough carbohydrate to allow normal growth and development, but you must avoid becoming overweight. Your daily carbohydrate intake should be spread throughout the day and portions can be moved from one meal to another to achieve the best control of blood-glucose levels.

Insulin requirements vary, so the amount you need has to be carefully determined. Usually a mixture of short-acting and long-acting insulin is given: the long-acting insulin provides a background (*basal*) level while the short-acting preparation boosts insulin after meals (*bolus dose*) to deal with the additional blood-glucose.

Balancing the dose of insulin is quite a skill. Too little insulin means too much glucose remains in the blood and signs of ketoacidosis may reappear. Too much insulin and the blood-glucose will be lowered too far, causing hypoglycaemia – a 'hypo'. Signs of low blood-glucose range from irritability, bad temper and poor judgement to confusion, sweating, faintness and loss of consciousness which can happen suddenly and without warning. Blood-glucose levels must be restored as soon as possible by taking some form of sugar or glucose immediately.

TYPE-2 DIABETES

This form of diabetes often develops gradually, usually in people over the age of 40, and was therefore known as 'maturity-onset' diabetes, but it is starting to appear in younger people. Type-2 is more common than type-1 diabetes, and often occurs in overweight people. Obesity is the key factor in eight out of ten people with type-2 diabetes. It tends to run in families.

The body still produces insulin, but in too small an amount to be effective. Insulin resistance also occurs as the cells cannot take up glucose efficiently. The upset in body chemistry is less than with type-1 and you may not know that you have the condition until it is detected at a health check-up when urine is tested routinely for the presence of glucose. It is nevertheless a serious condition leading to an increased risk of conditions such as cardiovascular disease and reduced life expectancy. Early signs of this type of diabetes include thirst, increased eating and drinking (especially of sweet drinks), tiredness, blurred vision and getting up at night to pass urine. You may also lose weight, and *Candida*, normally a harmless body fungus, may grow out of control and cause infection, especially in the vagina or penis.

The illness *chronic pancreatitis* and certain medicines can both trigger type-2 diabetes. Drugs such as corticosteroids and diuretics (**thiazides** in high doses and the **furosemide** group) may cause diabetes or aggravate existing diabetes because they oppose the effect of the body's own insulin. If you take one of these medicines, you should tell any new doctor. The prescription may need to be stopped or changed. Drug-induced diabetes is usually reversible, providing the body continues to produce sufficient insulin.

Management

As with type-1 diabetes, treatment aims to relieve the immediate symptoms and to prevent long-term complications, especially heart disease, circulatory disorders and nerve damage. The first approach to treatment is weight reduction if you are overweight (pages 318–19) and changes to your diet if you do not have a weight problem. It may be unnecessary to take a medicine (oral hypoglycaemic) to control type-2 diabetes, because diet and exercise may be all that is needed to control high blood-glucose. If diet does not control blood-glucose, you may have to take an antidiabetic (oral hypoglycaemic) medicine by mouth, but diet will still be an important part of treatment. Treatment with daily injections of insulin is likely to be needed as the disease progresses.

MONITORING DIABETES

Blood-glucose levels:

- ☐ Normally, blood-glucose levels vary greatly throughout the day but usually remain within the range of 3.5–8 mmmol/litre.
- ☐ A fasting blood-glucose level of more than 7 mmol/litre or a random blood-glucose level of more than 11 mmol/litre confirms the diagnosis of diabetes mellitus if you have other diabetic symptoms. If you have no symptoms, e.g. some people with type-2 diabetes, then both tests are needed to confirm diabetes.

- ☐ Strict control of blood-glucose levels reduces the likelihood of complications, but levels fluctuate and cannot be maintained at normal levels. With diabetes, aim for levels of between 4 and 10mmol/litre for most of the time. Accept that perfect control is not possible all of the time; in any case levels vary from person to person.
- ☐ If you use insulin, monitor your blood-glucose levels because this gives a direct measure of the amount of glucose in the blood at the time of test. It helps also to detect low or high blood-glucose levels.
- ☐ Record your readings and learn what action to take. Expect peaks and troughs of blood-glucose and adjust insulin once or twice weekly, unless advised otherwise, as daily alterations to the dose are not helpful.
- ☐ If you have type-2 diabetes, frequent blood-glucose monitoring is unlikely to be necessary. Urine testing can be as helpful as can being aware of how you feel.
- ☐ Your doctor will take a blood sample to measure the amount of glycosylated haemoglobin in the blood. Glucose in the blood reacts with the haemoglobin in the red blood cells to form glycosylated haemoglobin (HbA_{1c}). Measuring the proportion of this form of haemoglobin gives an accurate indication of how well your blood-glucose has been controlled during the 6–8 weeks prior to the test. The aim is to maintain HbA_{1c} between 6.5–7.5 per cent or less (normal range 4–6 per cent).

Kidney function

You should have urine and blood tests once a year to check kidney function, to ensure that protein has not started to appear in urine. Protein in urine (*proteinuria*) is a sign that kidney function is starting to deteriorate. Treatment with an ACE inhibitor (page 110) helps to reduce this and also to control high blood pressure.

Blood pressure

The aim is to keep blood pressure as low as possible. Target readings are: systolic blood pressure less than 140mmHg; diastolic blood pressure less than 80mmHg (lower in kidney disease).

Cholesterol levels

Blood lipids, total cholesterol and triglycerides need to be measured at least once a year. Target levels are: total cholesterol less than 5mmol/litre; fasting triglyceride level 2mmol/litre.

Weight

Regular weight checks measured as Body Mass Index (BMI – page 319) will provide guidance as to whether you need to lose weight which in turn helps to control diabetes.

Eyes

Regular checks by your optometrist/ophthalmologist should detect early changes and signs of retinopathy.

All diabetics need to reduce the risk of complications, and you may also need to take other medicines – for example, a statin to regulate body fats, **aspirin** to prevent blood clotting, a blood pressure-lowering medicine to control blood pressure, and an ACE inhibitor or ACE II medicine to prevent deterioration in kidney function (pages 110–115).

Insulin

In 1889 the cause of diabetes was traced to a disorder of the pancreas gland. In 1921 two Canadian doctors, Frederick Banting and Charles Best, identified insulin as the key substance lacking in diabetics. Insulin was first tried in a human in 1922 when an extract of animal pancreas was injected. Until then, diabetes was a grave disease for which there was no cure and death was inevitable within a year or so.

Insulin is broken down by the digestive system and is therefore not effective when taken by mouth. In replacing the body's insulin, an external source of insulin must be given every day by injection. Insulin is injected under the skin (*subcutaneously*) routinely unless there is an emergency such as diabetic coma (ketoacidosis) when it is injected into a vein or muscle. External sources of insulin – from pork or occasionally beef pancreases, or genetically engineered human sequence insulins and insulin analogues – vary very slightly in their structure, but all serve the same purpose of reducing blood-glucose levels. Human sequence insulin is mainly prepared *biosynthetically* – by genetic engineering (recombinant DNA technology) using a particular type of bacterium (*Escherichia coli*) – or semi-synthetically using an enzyme to alter pork insulin. With human insulin analogues, their structure has been altered by genetic engineering to make them perform more like the body's own insulin.

Unwanted effects of insulin therapy include low blood-glucose, increased appetite and therefore weight gain; attention to diet and exercise is therefore essential. Repeatedly injecting insulin into the same site can lead to local changes in the fatty tissues (*lipodystrophy*). Overwhelming allergy to insulin preparations is very rare now; if there are problems you may need to change to another type of insulin. Local allergic reactions are also uncommon, particularly with modern preparations.

One main drawback of insulin treatment is the daily round of injections, even though needles are very fine and sharp. A **needle-free injector**, which forces the insulin dose through the skin, is an alternative to needles, for example for children or those with needle phobia. This is not completely pain-free, as some sensation will be felt and sometime bruising occurs.

Insulin pump therapy is another method for giving insulin. The insulin pump, a small device that is attached to the body on a belt or in a pocket, allows insulin to be given by continuous subcutaneous infusion via tubing and a needle inserted under the skin. A small amount of insulin is delivered constantly into the body and at meal-times you trigger additional doses of insulin to deal with peak glucose levels that occur after eating. Pump therapy appears to achieve similar results to multiple daily insulin injections (multiple-dose insulin), but allows for a more flexible lifestyle with less worry about 'hypos'. The drawbacks are that infection must be avoided at injection sites and that the injection site must be moved every 2–3 days. The National Institute for Clinical Excellence (NICE) has recommended that pump therapy should be reserved for people with type-1 diabetes in whom blood-glucose control is difficult to achieve with multiple-dose insulin, for example for someone with recurrent 'hypos' or during pregnancy. Whichever route is used, each person needs training and ongoing support on how to use insulin for the optimal control of diabetic symptoms. The evidence suggests that the complications of diabetes can be reduced with good blood-glucose control.

Researchers have looked for many years for alternative ways to give insulin, and other methods are likely to become available in the future. These include nasal, inhaled insulin and skin patches. The biggest research prize would be finding a cure for type-1 diabetes. Research in the US has shown promising results recently where type-1 diabetes in mice has been reversed by transplanting spleen cells from mice producing insulin to those with diabetes.

INSULIN PREPARATIONS

Insulin can be mixed with other substances (for example a zinc salt) which prolong its action in the body. There are three main types of insulin preparation.

Short-acting insulins, such as **soluble insulin** (e.g. Actrapid or Hypurin Porcine Neutral), act in the body within 30–60 minutes after injection, and their effect lasts up to about eight hours with peak action approximately between one and a half and four hours. A short-acting insulin should be used about 15–30 minutes before a meal as a bolus dose to deal with the increase in blood-glucose after eating. Insulin analogues **lispro** (Humalog) and **aspart** (▼Novo Rapid) can be given within 15 minutes of a meal and reach peak effect within 30–70 minutes. **Intermediate-acting insulins**, such as **isophane insulin injection** and **insulin zinc suspension**, do not begin to act until one or two hours after injection but continue to work for 16–35 hours, with a peak effect between four and 12 hours. They can be used twice daily with a short-acting insulin or once daily – for example in older people.

Short- and intermediate-acting insulins can be mixed in the same syringe, or ready-mixed preparations in a range of proportions are available (e.g. **biphasic isophane insulin**). Low blood-glucose levels can be a problem during the night because of the variability in absorption and duration of action of standard insulins. The insulin analogue, insulin **glargine** (▼Lantus), provides background or basal levels of insulin in the body over 24 hours and can reduce night-time hypoglycaemia. A short-acting insulin is also required before meals times. **Long-acting insulins**, such as **crystalline insulin zinc suspension**, can be used on its own or mixed with insulin zinc suspension. **Protamine zinc insulin** has a slower onset of action but lasts for up to about 35 hours. It is rarely used now because it binds with soluble insulin, blunting its effectiveness.

How long different insulin preparations work in the body varies from person to person. The insulin requirement for each diabetic has to be carefully assessed and this includes the type of insulin or mix of insulins, the dosage (units) and how often injections must be given. Many people can manage with just two injections a day of a mixture of short- and longer-acting insulins, but more complex regimens with multiple doses of insulin are increasingly popular because they can improve blood-glucose control (see box, pages 306–7).

If you become ill with other problems such as influenza you must continue with insulin treatment, even if you are not eating, and continue to monitor blood-glucose. Your insulin requirement may increase in feverish conditions; it also alters when you have surgery or change your type of insulin. You may need to adjust your dose if you increase or decrease the amount of exercise you take or change diet.

Injections

Insulin can be injected into the upper arms, thighs, buttocks or abdomen. It is a good idea to rotate the site of injection. Repeatedly injecting into the same site may disturb the fatty tissue under the skin and lead to swelling or pitting. Rarely some people have allergic reactions at the site of injection during the first few weeks of insulin treatment, but this is not usually troublesome and soon clears up. Insulin can be injected from a variety of devices, for example from a calibrated 100-unit syringe or from single-use disposable needles and syringes. Easy-to-carry pen injector devices (Autopen; HumaPen Ergo; Innovo; NovoPen; OptiPen Pro), for use with cartridges of insulin preparations, meter the dose needed and are now very popular. Disposable pen injectors containing prefilled mixes of biphasic isophane insulin or insulin lispro or aspart are also available. You need to know how to dispose of lancets, single-use syringes and needles safely and should have access to a sharps bin, which in turn requires safe disposal as clinical waste.

Hypoglycaemia

When you start insulin treatment your doctor or the specialist nurse will usually want you to experience the early warning effects of hypoglycaemia so that you can recognise the signs and know what action to take. Sometimes it may be helpful for a relative or friend to be taught to recognise these symptoms too in case of emergencies. If your type of insulin is changed for some reason, you may find that your awareness and warning signs of hypoglycaemia alter. It is usually necessary to adjust the dose and to monitor your progress carefully in the first few days after starting a new type of insulin. Tight control of diabetes lowers the blood-glucose level almost to the point when hypoglycaemic symptoms should occur. This can increase the frequency of hypos and reduce warning symptoms. Very severe hypoglycaemia can affect brain function.

If you feel a 'hypo' coming on you will need to eat some carbohydrate, or in a real emergency three or four lumps of sugar with a little water. Three sugar lumps or two teaspoons of sugar provides around 10 grams of glucose. Repeat this in 10–15 minutes if necessary. Alternatively, if a person is unconscious Hypostop gel (9.2g glucose per dose) can be placed inside the mouth. Your doctor may suggest that you or a relative carries an emergency supply of **glucagon**, a drug that increases blood-glucose by mobilising a stored source of sugar (glycogen) in the liver. You should take glucose or sugar after an injection of glucagon to replenish liver stores of glycogen. Glucagon can be used to treat acute hypoglycaemic symptoms in an emergency. Hospital admission will be necessary if you develop hypoglycaemia whilst taking an oral antidiabetic medicine because this effect can persist for many hours.

Driving and diabetes

If you are a car driver you will need to be particularly careful to avoid a 'hypo' while driving. Loss of warning of hypoglycaemia is quite common especially if you are dependent on insulin. You should check your blood-glucose level before you drive and every two hours on long journeys. Always carry a snack and a drink in the car so that you can stop and replenish your blood-glucose levels. If necessary share the driving with someone else, especially on longer drives. Avoid driving if you are late for a meal. You should not drive if you have lost awareness of hypoglycaemic symptoms. If you use insulin or take an antidiabetic medicine by mouth you must inform the Driver and Vehicle Licensing Agency (DVLA)★ and your insurance company that you have diabetes. If you drive heavy goods or public service vehicles and your diabetes is controlled by diet alone you must also notify the DVLA.

INSULIN

Short-acting
SOLUBLE INSULIN (NEUTRAL INSULIN)
Animal source: HYPURIN BOVINE NEUTRAL; HYPURIN PORCINE NEUTRAL; PORK ACTRAPID
Human sequence insulin: ACTRAPID; VELOSULIN; HUMULIN S; ▼INSUMAN RAPID
Human insulin analogue: INSULIN LISPRO (HUMALOG); INSULIN ASPART (▼NOVORAPID)

Intermediate- and long-acting
INSULIN ZINC SUSPENSION
Animal source: HYPURIN BOVINE LENTE
Human sequence insulin: MONOTARD; HUMULIN LENTE
CRYSTALLINE INSULIN ZINC SUSPENSION
Human sequence insulin: ULTRATARD; HUMULIN ZN
ISOPHANE INSULIN
Animal source: HYPURIN BOVINE ISOPHANE; HYPURIN PORCINE ISOPHANE; PORK INSULATARD
Human sequence insulin: INSULATARD; HUMULIN I; INSUMAN BASAL
Human insulin analogue: INSULIN GLARGINE (▼LANTUS)

Biphasic insulins
These are ready-mixed combinations of short- and a longer-acting insulin in various proportions.
BISPHASIC ISOPHANE INSULIN
Animal source: PORK MIXTARD 30; HYPURIN PORCINE 30/70 MIX

Human sequence insulin: MIXTARD 10-50 (differing proportions); HUMULIN M2-M5 (differing proportions); INSUMAN COMB 15/25/50
Human insulin analogue: BIPHASIC INSULIN LISPRO (HUMALOG MIX25 or MIX50); BIPHASIC INSULIN ASPART (▼NOVOMIX 30)

Rarely used
PROTAMINE ZINC INSULIN
Animal source: HYPURIN BOVINE PROTAMINE ZINC

Insulin is a hormone, a complex protein made in the pancreas gland. It controls blood-sugar levels and transports glucose from the bloodstream into the body's cells. Insulin is essential for health and is given to replace the body's source or to supplement it in diabetes mellitus. It is broken down by the digestive system and therefore needs to be given by injection every day. The correct dose and type of insulin have to be found for each diabetic person. Dosage may have to be adjusted according to diet, exercise and health. Too much insulin causes low blood-glucose (hypoglycaemia). Too little insulin allows too much sugar to remain in the bloodstream (hyperglycaemia) resulting in the production of waste acids and symptoms of ketoacidosis.

Before you use this medicine

Tell your doctor if you are:
☐ pregnant or planning to become pregnant – good control of diabetes is essential before conception and throughout pregnancy ☐ breast-feeding – a small amount of insulin passes through into milk, but is not harmful ☐ taking any other medicines, including vitamins and those bought over the counter.

Tell your doctor if you have or have had:
☐ adrenal, pituitary or thyroid gland problems ☐ coeliac disease ☐ liver disease or severe kidney impairment – insulin requirements reduce dose ☐ recent illness, such as severe infection ☐ allergy to insulin or any of the product ingredients.

Do not use insulin if you have low blood-glucose.

How to use this medicine

Inject the insulin dose under the skin according to the treatment plan worked out with the specialist doctor and nurse at the diabetic clinic. Vary the injection site. Before using insulin, roll the vial or pen slowly between the palms of your hands about ten times, and invert the device gently if the contents need mixing to form a uniform suspension. Check the appearance of the insulin solution each time before you inject. Information for patients providing detailed guidance should be available for all products. Test your levels of blood-glucose regularly.

Alcohol in sensible amounts can be taken – but it increases the blood-glucose lowering effect of insulin, increases weight and upsets control of diabetes. Binge drinking can lead to a severe 'hypo'.

Do not stop taking insulin suddenly or change to another type or brand of insulin or syringe without checking with your doctor or nurse. Make sure you see your doctor or specialist nurse regularly to check progress, especially when you first start insulin treatment.

If you need to have surgery, including dental work, tell the doctor or dentist that you take insulin.

Agree a plan with your doctor for missed doses, because action depends on the dose and type of insulin.

Storage Store unused insulin supplies in the refrigerator at 2–8°C, but do not freeze. If insulin has been frozen do not use it. Check use-by dates and do not use if out of date or the liquid looks lumpy, grainy or discoloured. Make sure you know what the appearance of your insulin injection should be so that you can tell if the solution has deteriorated.

Cartridges in use or carried as spare for a portable injection device may be kept at room temperature, but not exposed to excessive sunlight or heat. A device in use must not be kept in a refrigerator.

Over 65 No special requirements.

Interactions with other medicines

Some drugs can interfere with the effects of insulin. Do not take other medicines including those sold over the counter such as aspirin without checking first with your doctor, nurse or pharmacist.

The following may reduce insulin requirements:

Oral antidiabetic drugs, **monoamine-oxidase inhibitors (MAOI antidepressants)**, **non-selective beta blockers**, **ACE inhibitors**, **aspirin and alcohol** increase the risk of low blood-glucose.

Beta blockers (heart and blood pressure drugs) may mask warning signs of, and delay recovery from, low blood-glucose.

The following may increase insulin requirements:

Corticosteroids, **thyroid hormones**, **growth hormone**, **adrenaline-type drugs**, **oral contraceptives**, **danazol** and **thiazide diuretics** may increase insulin requirements.

Unwanted effects

Likely Low blood-glucose – see below.

Less likely Irritation or rash at injection site, swelling at injection site, rash, high blood-glucose – see below.

Allergy to insulin is rare. The dose and how often insulin is given to control blood-glucose are very important. You need to take action if blood-sugar levels are too low or too high.

Signs of low blood-glucose Faintness, hunger, sweating, weakness, trembling, blurred vision, confusion, headache. These symptoms mean you should take extra sugar immediately. Loss of consciousness or seizures need emergency action and medical help.

Signs of high blood-glucose Drowsiness, dry flushed skin, loss of appetite, abnormal thirst, increased urination, breath smells of fruit. You need additional short-acting insulin, contact your doctor or specialist nurse.

Medicines for type-2 diabetes

Diet, exercise and other lifestyle changes are essential for successful control in type-2 diabetes. Drug treatment is started only when diet and lifestyle measures have been tried for at least three months, and have not controlled blood-glucose adequately. If your doctor considers that a medicine is necessary it will be to augment the effect of your diet and exercise, not replace it. An antidiabetic medicine taken by mouth will usually be tried first as monotherapy, then in combination with other antidiabetic medicines. In time, insulin is also likely to be needed as the body's own insulin supplies dwindle. Insulin is also needed during times when the body is under stress, such as surgery or illness. The main groups of antidiabetic medicine taken by mouth include **metformin** (a biguanide), **sulphonylurea** drugs such as **tolbutamide**, the meglitinides such as **repaglinide**, the glitazones such as **rosiglitazone,** and **acarbose**. Generally these antidiabetic medicines are used when the body is still making some insulin.

Research supports the use of **metformin** as the antidiabetic of choice in people with type-2 diabetes who remain overweight. In use for many years, it works by reducing glucose output from the liver and by enhancing glucose uptake in muscles. Metformin does not usually cause hypo-glycaemia, unlike the sulphonylurea drugs. It can be used on its own or with other antidiabetics such as a sulphonylurea. Unwanted effects include loss of appetite, feeling or being sick and diarrhoea, which are usually transient, although at high doses (3g daily) they can be troublesome. These effects can be lessened by taking metformin tablets with or after meals. Lactic acidosis is a potential, but rare, unwanted effect of metformin and a medical emergency (page 316). Increased lactic acid is produced when the body's cells break down glucose in the absence of oxygen or when there is some other metabolic abnormality. This can lead to lactic acidosis. Metformin has the potential to cause lactic acidosis, particularly when kidney function is impaired. Alcohol or use when kidney function is impaired increases the risk of this adverse effect; metformin should not be used if you have severe liver or kidney disease.

A sulphonylurea encourages the pancreas to produce more insulin and one can be taken on its own or in combination with metformin. Most sulphonylureas are similar in effect, but they differ in how long they act in the body. **Tolbutamide** is short-acting, whereas **glibenclamide** works for over 24 hours and **chlorpropamide** acts for even longer. If these longer-acting antidiabetics cause low blood-glucose, the hypoglycaemia will be prolonged and may be hazardous. You should avoid these drugs if you are an older person or have poor liver function. Glibenclamide and chlorpropamide are best avoided if you have poor kidney function. Furthermore, chlorpropamide interacts with alcohol and for some people causes uncomfortable flushing. Tolbutamide, the oldest sulphonylurea in use, has a good safety record and is least likely to cause prolonged low levels of blood-sugar. However, the tablets are large and some people find them difficult to swallow. Other sulphonylureas include **gliclazide**, **glipizide**, **glimepiride** and **gliquidone**. A sulphonylurea medicine is usually well tolerated but gastrointestinal upsets can occur, such as feeling or being sick, diarrhoea or constipation. People taking a sulphonylurea medicine can gain weight whereas metformin helps those who are already overweight.

Repaglinide (▼NovoNorm) and **nateglinide** (▼Starlix) are new antidiabetic medicines, the meglitinides. They stimulate insulin release from the pancreas. You can take one around 30 minutes before a main meal, allowing the insulin that is released to reduce high blood-glucose levels that a diabetic experiences after a meal. They are similar to the sulphonylureas, except that they act more quickly and have a short duration of effect. Either one can be used with metformin; repaglinide can also be used on its own.

Rosiglitazone (▼Avandia) and **pioglitazone** (▼Actos) are a newer choice of drug, the glitazones. They reduce glucose output from the liver and reduce insulin resistance in muscles, which leads to reduction in blood-glucose levels. They are used mainly when a sulphonylurea and metformin in combination cannot be tolerated or is not appropriate. A glitazone may be used in combination with either metformin or a sulphonylurea. Glitazones are not yet licensed for use with both of these antidiabetic drugs as triple therapy or combined with insulin. Either glitazone can be used on its own for type-2 diabetes when metformin cannot be tolerated, but experience with using a glitazone in this way is limited. The glitazones can cause some weight gain and fluid retention. They may exacerbate or trigger heart failure.

Acarbose (Glucobay) temporarily blocks the action of intestinal enzymes responsible for breaking down foods containing starch and the sugar sucrose to glucose during the digestion process in the intestine. This delays the digestion of starch and sucrose and reduces the high blood-glucose levels after a meal. It is used either on its own or with metformin or a sulphonylurea. Acarbose does not stimulate insulin secretion, which is an advantage when the body is having difficulty producing sufficient insulin. The main unwanted side effects are flatulence, abdominal distention and diarrhoea, but if treatment is started at low doses these effects are less of a problem.

METFORMIN

METFORMIN – Tablets

GLUCOPHAGE – Tablets
METFORMIN

Metformin is an oral antidiabetic medicine which lowers high blood-glucose levels in type-2 diabetes. It is used only after dietary, exercise and lifestyle measures have failed to control blood-glucose levels. Metformin reduces glucose output from the liver and enhances glucose uptake in muscles. It acts for a short time in the body and is taken twice or three times daily. The dose can be increased gradually at the start of treatment. Metformin does not cause very low blood-glucose levels or 'hypos'. It can be taken with a sulphonylurea antidiabetic while the body can still make some insulin, or with a newer antidiabetic, a glitazone or meglitinide. It can also be taken with insulin.

Before you use this medicine

Tell your doctor if you are:
☐ pregnant – not harmful, but insulin is used during pregnancy to maintain near normal blood-glucose levels ☐ breast-feeding – not used ☐ taking any other medicines, including vitamins and those bought over the counter.

Tell your doctor if you have or have had:
☐ hypersensitivity to metformin ☐ kidney or liver disease ☐ diabetic ketoacidosis ☐ you are a heavy drinker or have acute alcohol problems ☐ heart or circulatory problems ☐ heart attack ☐ breathing difficulties ☐ severe infection (sepsis) or injury.

Avoid metformin during certain x-ray procedures or surgery – insulin will be needed.

How to use this medicine

Metformin is introduced gradually. Your doctor will give you a schedule: usually one tablet (500mg or 850mg) at breakfast for at least one week, then one tablet with breakfast and your evening meal for a further week at least, and then one tablet three times a day at breakfast, lunch and your evening meal. You will need to have blood-glucose levels measured during this time so that the dose can be adjusted.

Metformin on its own does not affect your ability to drive, but diabetes can do so and therefore care must be taken when you drive or operate machinery.

Avoid alcohol – it increases the risk of lactic acidosis, a rare unwanted effect of metformin.

Do not stop taking metformin suddenly without checking with your doctor. Your condition may worsen. If you miss a dose, take it as soon as you remember, but if your next dose is due within two hours, skip it. Do not take double the dose. If you have to have surgery, including dental work, tell the doctor or dentist that you take metformin.

Over 65 You will need regular checks for kidney function. Metformin should be avoided if kidney function is reduced.

Interactions with other medicines

X-ray contrast material containing iodine can affect kidney function. Metformin should be avoided – increased risk of lactic acidosis.

Effects on blood-glucose: Beta blockers, **corticosteroids** and **diuretics** increase blood-glucose levels. **ACE inhibitors** may decrease blood-glucose levels – metformin dose may need to be adjusted.

Unwanted effects

Likely Feeling or being sick, loss of appetite, abdominal pain, diarrhoea. Digestive system upsets usually fade with time in about two weeks, especially if metformin is introduced gradually. Diarrhoea can persist.

Less likely Metallic taste, rash, decrease in vitamin B_{12} absorption – not thought to be clinically significant.

Very rare Lactic acidosis – signs include unexpected weight loss, feeling sick with stomach pains, rapid uncontrolled breathing. Stop taking metformin and contact your doctor immediately.

Similar preparations

▼ACTOS – Tablets
PIOGLITAZONE

▼AVANDAMET – Tablets
ROSIGLITAZONE + METFORMIN

▼AVANDIA – Tablets
ROSIGLITAZONE

TOLBUTAMIDE

TOLBUTAMIDE — Tablets

Tolbutamide is an oral antidiabetic drug. It lowers high blood-glucose levels in type-2 diabetes, but is used only after dietary measures have failed to control blood-glucose. Tolbutamide must be used with a suitable diet. Like all sulphonylurea medicines, it encourages the production of insulin in the pancreas. It acts for a relatively short time in the body and rarely causes low blood-glucose levels. Tolbutamide is therefore suitable for older people. It can be used in conjunction with other oral antidiabetic drugs, such as metformin and insulin.

Before you use this medicine

Tell your doctor if you are:
☐ pregnant – tolbutamide should not be used in the first three months ☐ breast-feeding – tolbutamide should not be used ☐ taking any other medicines, including vitamins and those bought over the counter.

Tell your doctor if you have or have had:
☐ hypersensitivity to sulphonamides ☐ severe liver or kidney disease ☐ porphyria ☐ adrenal or thyroid disease ☐ diabetic ketoacidosis.

How to use this medicine

Take the tablets, either as a single dose with or immediately after the first main meal of the day or twice daily in the morning and evening.

Tolbutamide on its own does not affect your ability to drive, but diabetes can do so and therefore care must be taken when you drive or operate machinery. Avoid these activities if you have warning signs of a 'hypo'. Avoid alcohol – it may rarely cause a reaction, flushing and rapid heart beat and breathing; alcohol can also upset control of diabetes.

Do not stop taking tolbutamide suddenly without checking with your doctor. Your condition may worsen. If you miss a dose, take it as soon as you remember. If your next dose is due within two hours, take it and skip the next dose. Do not take double the dose. If you need to have surgery, including dental work, tell the doctor or dentist that you take tolbutamide.

Over 65 You may need less than the standard adult dose. Low blood-glucose is more likely. Tolbutamide may be used in mild to moderate kidney impairment in a reduced dose. It should be avoided if kidney or liver function is severely impaired.

Interactions with other medicines

Various drugs interfere with the effect of tolbutamide. Do not take other medicines including those sold over the counter without checking first with your doctor or pharmacist.

Blood-glucose lowering effects increased by:
Beta blockers
Antidepressants – monoamine-oxidase inhibitors
Antibacterials – co-trimoxazole, sulphonamides, chloramphenicol, quinolones
Antifungals – miconazole, fluconazole
Medicines for rheumatism and gout — azapropazone, sulfinpyrazone
Blood-glucose may rise with:
Corticosteroids, rifampicin, oral contraceptives, thiazide diuretics.

Unwanted effects

Likely Headache, mild digestive system upsets, e.g. feeling or being sick, constipation, diarrhoea.
Less likely Dizziness, confusion, weakness, skin rash, ringing in the ears (tinnitus), pins and needles.

Serious unwanted effects are rare: hypersensitivity reactions in the first 6–8 weeks of starting treatment, blood disorders, itching, jaundice, hepatitis and liver failure. If unwanted effects are troublesome contact your doctor. You need to take action if blood-glucose levels drop.

Signs of low blood-glucose Faintness, hunger, sweating, weakness, trembling, blurred vision, confusion, headache. These symptoms mean you should take extra sugar immediately. Loss of consciousness or seizures need emergency action and medical help.

Similar preparations

AMARYL – Tablets
GLIMEPIRIDE

DAONIL – Tablets
GLIBENCLAMIDE

DIAMICRON – Tablets
GLICLAZIDE

EUGLUCON – Tablets
GLIBENCLAMIDE

GLIBENCLAMIDE – Tablets

GLIBENESE – Tablets
GLIPIZIDE

GLICLAZIDE – Tablets

Poor choice – not recommended
CHLORPROPAMIDE – Tablets

GLIPIZIDE – Tablets

GLURENORM – Tablets
GLIQUIDONE

MINODIAB – Tablets
GLIPIZIDE

▼NOVONORM – Tablets
REPAGLINIDE

SEMI-DAONIL – Tablets
GLIBENCLAMIDE

▼STARLIX – Tablets
NATEGLINIDE

Obesity

Putting on weight is a nuisance – clothes stop fitting, it becomes harder to move around, we take up more space and our risk of developing common diseases increases. Overweight people are more likely to develop heart disease, type-2 diabetes, high blood pressure, gallstones and certain cancers, for example colon cancer and breast cancer after the menopause. Extra weight also exacerbates conditions such as arthritis (e.g. osteoarthritis of the knee), breathlessness, heartburn, breathing problems during sleep (sleep apnoea), blood clots and psychological distress including anxiety and depression.

In developed countries people gain on average nearly 1 gram of weight a day between the ages of 25 and 55 years. This tiny increase in energy intake over energy expended is equivalent to 90kcal or one chocolate digestive biscuit a day. This may not seem much, but spare energy is converted into fat which leads to weight gain. Increased food intake can lead to becoming overweight and ultimately to obesity, although the reasons why some people are more prone to excessive weight gain are not completely understood.

Weight is commonly assessed using body mass index (BMI). This is where someone's weight in kilograms is divided by the square of their height in metres i.e. kg/m^2.

The World Health Organization classifies weight in the following categories:

Weight	**BMI**
Healthy weight	18.5 to 24.9
Overweight	25 to 29.9
Obese	30 to 39.9
Severely obese	40+

For example, if you are 1.74 metres tall and weigh 82 kilograms then your BMI is 82 divided by 1.74, which gives 47.13 and divided again by 1.74 gives 27.08. Your BMI is about 27kg/m^2 and you are in the overweight range.

Obesity levels have tripled in England over the past two decades. Around a quarter of adult women and a fifth of adult men are obese and when the overweight population is added in, this amounts to about 24 million, or two-thirds of the English population. The proportion of overweight and obese children is a major cause for concern, particularly as type-2 diabetes is starting to occur in the young. Maintaining a healthy weight reduces your risk of illness and increases life expectancy. If you are overweight, losing weight can improve your quality of life and self-confidence.

The most effective way to lose weight is to eat a lower-calorie diet and take regular exercise. A balanced diet of starchy foods, which release energy more steadily (such as bread and potatoes), more fruit and vegetables (five portions a day) and less fat is a reasonable approach. Setting realistic goals in losing weight is important and your doctor, nurse or a local support group can help. Weight loss should always be gradual – about 0.5 to 1kg a week (equivalent to one bag of sugar or around 2lb) which you can achieve by eating 500 to 600 calories less a day. A weekly weigh-in can help you to monitor progress.

Once you have reached a healthier weight, eating and exercise habits need to be maintained to control weight. Diet alone is rarely effective for maintaining weight loss in the longer term, as weight is often regained. Combining weight loss with an exercise programme and/or modifying behaviour in eating habits improves the chances of sustaining weight loss. It is not that easy for some people to lose weight and if you are seriously overweight or have health risks, then treatment with a medicine to help with weight loss may be the answer. Surgery is sometimes used for people who have a BMI of 40kg/m^2 or more, or who have a BMI between 35kg/m^2 and 40kg/m^2 and who also have risk factors such as diabetes, heart disease and high blood pressure that could be helped by weight loss.

Medicines to help with weight loss

A medicine will be only part of the approach to weight loss, which requires a proper trial of diet, exercise and habit modification before you start treatment as well as a continuing programme. An anti-obesity medicine can be considered if you have a BMI of 28kg/m^2 or more, or 30kg/m^2 or more and risk factors such those outlined above. Two medicines are officially licensed for treating obesity – **orlistat** (Xenical) and **sibutramine** (▼Reductil). Orlistat works locally in the digestive system by stopping fat being absorbed into the body, whereas sibutramine works on the nervous system blocking the re-uptake of noradrenaline and serotonin (page 189). Treatment with either sibutramine or with orlistat should be used as part of a supervised programme of weight reduction where weight is regularly monitored. Combination therapy with more than one anti-obesity medicine is not recommended.

Sibutramine You need to lose at least 2kg during the first four weeks with sibutramine, then you need to have lost at least five per cent of your initial body weight (5kg for each 100kg) by three months from the start of drug treatment, in order to continue treatment. Unwanted effects of sibutramine, which can fade as treatment continues, include dry mouth, insomnia, constipation and also rapid heart beat, palpitations, flushing and raised blood pressure. Sibutramine must not be used for longer than one year. Weight gain may recur on stopping treatment.

Medicines that have been used in the past include **phentermine**, **dexfenfluramine** and **fenfluramine**, but these were associated occasionally with heart valve disease and high blood pressure in the arteries to the lungs (*pulmonary hypertension*) and are no longer recommended. Diuretics, amphetamines and hormonal treatments, for example thyroid preparations, are not recommended for helping with weight reduction. The bulking agent **methylcellulose** is claimed to reduce food intake by increasing a feeling of fullness, but there is little robust evidence to support its use in weight loss.

ORLISTAT

XENICAL – Capsules
ORLISTAT

Orlistat is a medicine which helps with weight loss by reducing fat absorption from the gut. Lipases, body chemicals that break down fats in our food, are prevented by orlistat from working in the stomach and small intestine. Just under a third of the fat that would have been absorbed into the body remains in the digestive system and passes out in stools (faeces). This dietary change leads to changes in bowel habit (more frequent), and fatty stools which may cause anal leakage and spotting on underwear. These effects can encourage people to take less fat in their diet.

Orlistat is used as part of a supervised programme of weight reduction if you have a body mass index (BMI) of 30kg/m^2 or more, or BMI 28kg/m^2 or more and risk factors such as type-2 diabetes, heart disease or high blood pressure. Treatment is started only if you have lost at least 2.5kg (5lb) in the previous month. Treatment can be continued if weight loss carries on – you must lose five per cent of your initial body weight (5kg for each 100kg) within three months, and ten per cent within six months. Treatment is not usually continued beyond a year and certainly not beyond two years.

Before you use this medicine

Tell your doctor if you are:
☐ pregnant and breast-feeding – no information on use, therefore avoid ☐ taking any other medicines, including vitamins and those bought over the counter.

Tell your doctor if you have or have had:
☐ long-term malabsorption syndrome ☐ bile duct problems, jaundice or liver disease ☐ diabetes.

How to use this medicine

Take one orlistat capsule (120mg) immediately before, during or up to one hour after each main meal. If a meal is missed or contains no fat, the dose of orlistat should be omitted. Taking more than three capsules a day does not provide further benefit. Increased fat in stools will be noticed until 1–2 days after dosing. When you stop treatment the fat in stools returns to normal within 2–3 days.

Orlistat does not affect your ability to drive or operate machinery. Alcohol does not interact with orlistat, but adds calories to your diet.

Orlistat can be stopped at anytime during the course, but preferably only after discussion with your doctor. If you miss a dose, take it within one hour of the meal, but otherwise skip it. Orlistat is not recommended for children.

Over 65 Orlistat can be used up to the age of 75 years. No special dose requirements.

Interactions with other medicines

Antidiabetic acarbose Avoid combination.
Anticoagulants such as **warfarin** Monitor INR regularly in combination with orlistat (page 151).
Immunosuppressant ciclosporin Absorption may be reduced by orlistat.
Vitamins Fat-soluble vitamins A, D, E, K and beta carotene: absorption reduced by orlistat. If vitamin supplementation is needed, avoid taking within at least two hours of orlistat or take at bedtime.

Unwanted effects

Likely Liquid oily stools, faecal urgency, loss of faecal control, flatulence.
Less likely Abdominal or rectal pain and discomfort (minimised by reducing fat in diet), headache, menstrual irregularities, anxiety, fatigue.
Rarely Hypersensitivity reactions, hepatitis.

Thyroid disorders

The thyroid gland in the neck produces several hormones that regulate the body's metabolism. *Calcitonin* is essential for a normal calcium balance. Two other hormones, *levothyroxine* (T_4) and *liothyronine* (T_3), act on all the body's cells to control the rate at which food is converted into energy. Blood levels of these two hormones are regulated by the *thyroid stimulating hormone (TSH)* produced in the pituitary gland in the brain. When blood levels of thyroid hormone rise, thyroid stimulating hormone production decreases and vice versa. Levels of these hormones can be measured and help to detect thyroid disorders. To make the hormones, the gland needs trace amounts of iodine, a mineral which is usually in plentiful supply in our diet. Different illnesses occur depending on whether too much or too little of the thyroid hormones are produced. Low blood levels of thyroid hormone T_4 cause *hypothyroidism*, but high

TSH; if the gland becomes overactive and produces high blood levels of hormones, but undetectable TSH, *hyperthyroidism* occurs.

Goitre is enlargement of the thyroid gland which may be due to abnormal growth of thyroid tissue or can be the body's response to disruption in the production of thyroid hormone.

UNDERACTIVE THYROID (HYPOTHYROIDISM)

A low level of thyroid hormones produces different illnesses depending on the person's age. If a baby is born with low levels of the hormones, it does not develop normally and will be stunted and mentally handicapped. The condition (*cretinism*) is rare and regular injections of a thyroid preparation usually establish normal development. The thyroid levels of babies are checked routinely after birth. Hypothyroidism in children delays growth and puberty.

For older people it is not certain how the disorder occurs but it may be caused by the body's own immune system attacking the thyroid gland. The illness develops slowly and is hard to recognise in its early stages, but a blood test can confirm abnormal thyroid function. Hypothyroidism is quite common, occurs more often in women than men and usually after the age of 45. Signs include tiredness, slowing of mental processes, weight increase, slower heart rate, drying and coarsening of the skin, hair loss and puffy face and eyelids. Sensitivity to cold is increased and women who are still menstruating may find that periods are heavier and prolonged or stop prematurely. The thyroid gland may enlarge and become noticeable as a swelling on the neck (*goitre*).

OVERACTIVE THYROID (HYPERTHYROIDISM)

When the thyroid gland is overactive it produces symptoms not unlike acute anxiety and it may be difficult to tell the two conditions apart. Overproduction of thyroid hormones affects all the body's cells, speeding up their functions (*metabolic rate*). Signs and symptoms of hyperthyroidism (also called *thyrotoxicosis*) include nervousness, irritability, tiredness, sweating, trembling, muscle weakness, rapid pulse and irregular heart rhythms. In more severe cases, weight loss and increased sensitivity to heat may occur. Thyroid overactivity occurs more often in women than men, particularly between the ages of 20 and 40 years. Women who are still menstruating may find that their periods are heavier, or sometimes lighter and scantier. *Graves' disease*, an autoimmune disease, is the most common form of hyperthyroidism in which an antibody develops in the body which then stimulates the thyroid gland to overproduce thyroid hormones. It tends to run in families; the risk of developing the condition is six times greater for a child of a parent with Graves' disease. The pattern of the disease fluctuates, alternating between relapse and remission and some people only ever have a single episode. Sometimes the gland may swell to produce a goitre. Thyrotoxicosis can cause an abnormal bulging of the eyes known as *exophthalmos*. The condition may be more difficult to detect in older people. Blood tests are used to measure hormone levels and to confirm the diagnosis.

Exophthalmos

Bulging eyes associated with hyperthyroidism can be uncomfortable, unsightly and even painful. It can be distressing because a person's physical appearance is altered. It occurs most commonly in women aged 20–45, and in smokers. Eye muscles become swollen and there is a build-up of fat and fluid behind the eyes, pushing the eyes outwards and leading to double vision. The severity of the condition varies but soreness, painful watering or prominence of the eyes and characteristic stare are common. In rare, severe cases sight can be threatened by pressure on the optic nerve. This needs treatment with high doses of corticosteroids (e.g. **prednisolone**) or other immunosuppressive drugs, or surgery to make more room for the eyes and the swollen muscles. Drug or surgical treatment does not affect the eye disease consistently. Once high levels of thyroid have been controlled, eye problems remain stable in the majority of people (eight out of ten), but may get worse or improve.

Your doctor will aim to preserve vision and to relieve the condition with conservative measures. Raising the head of the bed at night may prevent worsening of the fluid accumulation behind the eye. To protect the cornea at night, the eyelids can be taped and a protective patch applied. Simple eye ointment may help to prevent eyes drying out at night, while **hypromellose** eye drops can lessen the gritty sensation in the eyes during the day. Tinted glasses can reduce the unpleasant sensation from bright lights, and protect the cornea from wind and dust. Prismatic lenses in glasses will help double vision.

Medicines for thyroid disorders

HYPOTHYROIDISM

Treatment consists of replacing the body's thyroid hormone with an external source, usually **levothyroxine** (**thyroxine**) tablets containing tiny quantities equal to those the body would make normally. You will need to take tablets for the rest of your life, but this should not be difficult once a suitable dose has been established. Levothyroxine must be started at a low dose and gradually increased at two- to four-week intervals, usually supervised by a hospital doctor. Older people and those with heart disease need a smaller dose and your doctor will supervise you closely until the maintenance dose has been reached. You will need to have regular blood tests during the early stages of treatment to measure the hormone levels. At the start of levothyroxine treatment your heart may beat more rapidly as the metabolic rate increases. If you have heart disease it may cause anginal pain and muscle cramps or trigger a heart attack. Too large a dose may cause symptoms of hyperthyroidism, such as restlessness, sweating, flushing, headache and diarrhoea.

Liothyronine has a similar action to levothyroxine. Its effects develop more rapidly but it does not act for as long. Liothyronine is sometimes used by injection for treating severe hypothyroid conditions. Dried thyroid or extract of thyroid contains variable amounts of levothyroxine and liothyronine and is not recommended.

LEVOTHYROXINE

LEVOTHYROXINE — Tablets ELTROXIN — Tablets

Levothyroxine is a thyroid hormone used for replacing the body's source when the normal working of the thyroid gland is disrupted, for example treating an underactive gland (hypothyroidism). Levothyroxine also helps to relieve swelling in certain types of goitre when the thyroid gland is enlarged. It may also be used during treatment for thyroid cancer.

Replacement treatment, which must usually be taken for life, is started gradually and the dosage adjusted until the body's metabolism becomes normal. The usual dose range is 100–200 micrograms a day.

Before you use this medicine

Tell your doctor if you are:
☐ pregnant or breast-feeding – monitoring needed ☐ taking any other medicines, including vitamins and those bought over the counter.

Tell your doctor if you have or have had:
☐ heart problems ☐ high blood pressure ☐ overactive thyroid ☐ hypersensitivity to levothyroxine ☐ adrenal insufficiency ☐ diabetes mellitus ☐ diabetes insipidus (rare condition – failure of antidiuretic hormone which controls salt and water balance in the kidneys).

How to use this medicine

Take the tablet once a day, preferably before breakfast. If you are older or have heart disease, you will have a lower dose or may take a tablet on alternate days. See your doctor at least once a year for a regular check-up and blood tests to assess thyroid function.

Do not stop taking levothyroxine without talking to your doctor. Levothyroxine is replacing the body's hormone and tablets must be taken regularly or symptoms will recur. If you miss a dose take it as soon as you remember. Do not take double the dose in one day.

Over 65 You may need less than the usual adult dose.

Interactions with other medicines

Levothyroxine interacts with a number of drugs. Do not take other medicines including those sold over the counter without checking first with your doctor or pharmacist.

Oral anticoagulants such as warfarin Increased risk of bleeding with levothyroxine.

Unwanted effects

Less likely Anginal pain, irregular heart rhythm and beat, palpitations, muscle cramps, diarrhoea, vomiting, agitation, tremors, restlessness, sleeplessness, sweating, headache, muscle weakness, heat intolerance, weight loss.

Unwanted effects are unlikely but may occur at the start of treatment when your doctor is determining the dosage. If you experience the symptoms above contact your doctor.

Similar preparations

TERTROXIN — Tablets
LIOTHYRONINE

TRI-IODOTHYRONINE — Injection

HYPERTHYROIDISM

There are several possibilities for treating an overactive thyroid gland:

- ☐ treatment with an antithyroid medicine that interferes with the production of thyroid hormones
- ☐ radioactive iodine to destroy thyroid tissue and lessen the amount of hormones produced
- ☐ surgery to remove part of the gland — this may be necessary if drug treatment has failed to improve the condition or if the gland is swollen (goitre) and pressing against the wind-pipe.

Drug treatment usually lasts for a period of 12–18 months. **Carbimazole** is commonly used in the UK, but for someone who has a sensitivity reaction to it **propylthiouracil** may be needed. Both medicines interfere with the production of thyroid hormones. Treatment starts with a high dose for about four to eight weeks until hormone production is controlled. The dose is then gradually reduced and tailored to each person. About half the people taking an antithyroid medicine improve and the disease may burn out (remit) during treatment. Others may need further treatment, sometimes with alternative measures. Over-treatment may result in hypothyroidism, which must then be treated with **levothyroxine**. Sometimes a combination of a daily dose of carbimazole plus levothyroxine may be used in a 'blocking-replacement' strategy. This strategy is not suitable treatment during pregnancy, but either carbimazole or propylthiouracil can be used under close specialist supervision. Rarely, carbimazole may be associated with a defect of the skin of the scalp (*aplasia cutis*) in newborn babies but the evidence is not firmly established.

A beta blocker such as **propranolol** may be used to control symptoms at the start of treatment. It may also be used with an antithyroid drug or as part of the treatment with radioactive iodine.

CARBIMAZOLE

NEO-MERCAZOLE – Tablets

Carbimazole is an antithyroid drug which reduces thyroid hormone levels when the gland is overactive. Prolonged treatment lasts for about 18 months, during which time the disease may burn out. Carbimazole may be used in preparation for surgery (thyroidectomy) or before and after radioactive iodine treatment. Unwanted effects usually occur in the first eight weeks but improve as treatment continues. The most serious but rare adverse effect is bone-marrow depression which may lead to a blood disorder (agranulocytosis). Your doctor will ask you to report any fever, sore throat or mouth ulcers immediately.

Before you use this medicine

Tell your doctor if you are:
☐ pregnant – carbimazole may be used under very close supervision, although hyperthyroidism often remits during pregnancy ☐ breast-feeding – the baby must be carefully monitored ☐ taking any other medicines, including vitamins and those bought over the counter.

Tell your doctor if you have or have had:
☐ liver disorders ☐ hypersensitivity to carbimazole.

How to use this medicine

Take the tablets every day as directed by your doctor. At first you may take the dose two or three times a day, but once overactivity is controlled, after four to eight weeks, you may be able to take one dose a day.

Alcohol does not interfere with carbimazole's action. Do not stop taking carbimazole suddenly as symptoms may recur. Treatment is usually continued for at least six months but may be up to two years. If you miss a dose take it as soon as you remember, but skip it if it is almost time for your next dose.

Over 65 No special requirements.

Unwanted effects

Likely Feeling sick, headache, dizziness, joint pains, mild stomach upsets, skin rashes and itching.
Less likely Hair loss, muscle weakness, fever, sore throat, mouth ulcers, jaundice.

The most likely effects are common at the start of treatment but usually fade as treatment continues. Two people in 100 may develop skin rashes and itching which respond to antihistamine treatment by mouth while carbimazole treatment can be continued. Occasionally your doctor may prescribe **propylthiouracil** in place of carbimazole. **If you develop a sore throat, mouth ulcers, bruising or fever stop taking carbimazole and contact your doctor immediately as this may indicate a serious effect on blood cells (bone marrow suppression).**

Similar preparations

PROPYLTHIOURACIL — Tablets

Adrenal disorders

There are two adrenal glands, each one lying above the top of a kidney. Each adrenal gland has a centre, the *medulla*, which secretes **adrenaline** (**epinephrine**) and **noradrenaline** (**norepinephrine**), and an outer layer, the *adrenal cortex*. The medulla and cortex behave as independent glands. The release of adrenaline and noradrenaline from the medulla is controlled by the autonomic nervous system (pages 188–9). These body chemicals, which increase the heart rate and blood flow, are especially active during a wide variety of stress conditions, such as anger, fear, cold, low blood-glucose and low blood pressure. Hormone production in the adrenal cortex is mainly regulated by the *adrenocorticotrophic hormone* (ACTH) released from the pituitary gland in the brain. A feedback mechanism controls ACTH release from the hypothalamus through the level of cortical hormones circulating in the body. This mechanism controls the hypothalamic-pituitary-adrenal axis. Over 30 hormones are produced in the cortex to regulate the body's mineral salts and water balance and its response to stress and injury. There are three main groups:

- ☐ *mineralocorticoids*, such as **aldosterone**, which regulates the mineral salts in the body, acting mainly on sodium to affect the water balance within the body and in turn influence blood volume
- ☐ *glucocorticoids*, such as **hydrocortisone** (also known as **cortisol**), which regulates chemical conversion (metabolism) of carbohydrate, glucose, proteins and fats
- ☐ *sex hormones* (**androgens**, **oestrogens** and **progesterone**); the sex glands (*gonads*) are more important sites for making these hormones.

The hormones are grouped according to their main effects but some activities overlap. For example, **hydrocortisone** has mostly *glucocorticoid* activity but also some weak *mineralocorticoid* effects.

The blood level of hydrocortisone varies during the day, with higher levels in the morning and lower levels at night. This is called diurnal variation and can be important in scheduling treatment.

Disorders of the adrenal glands are relatively rare but both underactivity and overactivity can occur. Infection such as tuberculosis or the body's own immune system may be responsible for the destruction or underactivity of the gland and a tumour of the gland can cause overactivity or underactivity.

UNDERACTIVE ADRENAL GLANDS ADDISON'S DISEASE

This is a general underfunctioning of the adrenal glands which is usually fatal if untreated. Symptoms include a severe fall in blood pressure, muscle weakness, dehydration and patchy darkening (pigmention) of the skin. Both glucocorticoid and mineralocorticoid hormones have to be replaced. **Hydrocortisone** is given to replace the glucocorticoid hormones twice a day, with the higher dose in the morning and a lower dose in the evening to take account of the diurnal variation in body hydrocortisone. **Fludrocortisone** (Florinef) is usually used to replace the mineralocorticoid hormones. There are few unwanted effects from hydrocortisone because it is taken to replace the body's natural supply. If the glands have to be surgically removed (*adrenalectomy*), hydrocortisone must be replaced.

OVERACTIVE ADRENAL GLANDS

If the blood level of the body's corticoid hormones greatly increases and diurnal variation is abolished, the resulting condition is called *Cushing's syndrome*. If the disorder is due to overactivity in the part of the pituitary that produces the adrenocorticotrophic hormone (ACTH) — the hormone responsible for controlling body levels of adrenal hormones — the condition is known as *Cushing's disease*. Extra ACTH prompts the adrenal glands to make more corticoid hormones. Excess hormones lead to many changes to body function, characterised for example by muscle wasting of the limbs, thinning of the skin, moon face, increased abdominal fat and buffalo hump on the shoulders. These effects can also occur when a corticosteroid is used as drug treatment, particularly by mouth for prolonged periods (see serious unwanted effects – pages 332–4). These drug-induced Cushing's syndrome effects (*cushingoid*) are usually reversible as the dose is gradually reduced. Treatment of an overactive gland is usually by surgical means or irradiation.

Corticosteroids

Once the corticoid hormones were identified and extracted from adrenal glands, scientists were able to modify the steroid molecule to make synthetic **corticosteroids**. The term corticosteroid is used to describe the hormones produced by the cortex of the adrenal gland and also the man-made or synthetic drugs derived from these natural hormones. Some people refer to corticosteroid preparations as **'steroids'** but this may lead to confusion with **anabolic steroids**, which are synthetic derivatives of male sex hormones with limited medical usefulness; their use as body builders and tonics is quite unjustified.

Although corticosteroids are used for replacing the body's hormones in rare disorders, they are used mainly for their anti-inflammatory properties in a wide variety of conditions. Corticosteroids are used for treating disorders where the body's immune system appears to be faulty resulting in inflammation, blood disorders, allergy or rheumatic conditions. These include asthma, rheumatoid arthritis, inflammatory conditions of the bowel, skin and eyes, systemic lupus erythematosus (an autoimmune arthritis–like condition involving the skin, tissues and joints) and life-threatening disorders such as acute leukaemia. Corticosteroids are also used as an immunosuppressant following transplantation.

Each preparation varies in the balance between its *glucocorticoid* and *mineralocorticoid* effects. Glucocorticoid effects are anti-inflammatory, an effect most prized for controlling a number of serious and life-threatening conditions. Research focuses on trying to separate the anti-inflammatory and anti-allergy effects of corticosteroids from their disruptive effects on body metabolism. The corticosteroids vary in their anti-inflammatory effect; for example, **betamethasone** is very potent, but **hydrocortisone** and **cortisone** are weaker. Drugs with strong mineralocorticoid activity such as **fludrocortisone** are not used for their anti-inflammatory effect, because salt and water balance will always be disrupted.

HOW YOU CAN HELP YOURSELF

- ☐ If you use a corticosteroid routinely, you should see your doctor or nurse regularly for checks.
- ☐ **Carry a steroid treatment card if you have to take a corticosteroid for more than three weeks.** Your doctor or pharmacist can give you a card. You are unlikely to require a card for a corticosteroid used locally on the skin, in the nose or inhaled.
- ☐ Note details of the name of the corticosteroid, the dosage and length of treatment time. Keep the information up to date.
- ☐ **You must not stop taking a corticosteroid suddenly.** Your doctor will give you a schedule to reduce the dosage gradually. Always have a reserve supply of your medicine. Read and keep the patient information leaflet (PIL) which accompanies your medicine.
- ☐ If you have an illness such as diarrhoea, vomiting, a temperature or fever, continue taking your corticosteroid. Contact your doctor as you may need a higher dose during these sorts of illnesses.
- ☐ Corticosteroids taken by mouth (or by injection) can suppress the immune system, so you can be more susceptible to infections, including measles or chickenpox, and they may be more severe than usual. If you are taking a corticosteroid or have taken one in the previous three months, you should contact your doctor urgently if you have not had chickenpox and have been in contact with someone suffering from chickenpox or shingles. This also applies if you have not had measles.
- ☐ Always tell a new doctor, your dentist or any other person involved in your health care that you take a corticosteroid or that you have taken one within the last three months.

Using corticosteroids

Corticosteroids were much misused and overused as medicines when they were first introduced in the 1950s. The long-term consequences of taking cortisone by mouth for a few years, for instance to relieve painful and swollen joints in rheumatoid arthritis, did not become visible until people's backbones and hip bones began to crumble. A corticosteroid has to be taken in a much higher dose than the body's source in order to produce its anti-inflammatory effect. The beneficial anti-inflammatory effect is then also accompanied by the risk of unwanted effects. Your doctor must weigh up whether the benefits justify the unwanted effects. A corticosteroid can be life-saving.

Whenever possible a corticosteroid should be used locally – for example in enemas or eye drops, by inhalation or by direct injection into a swollen joint – rather than taken by mouth when the risk of adverse effects is greater. An inhaled corticosteroid for controlling asthma symptoms is extremely valuable. It causes few unwanted effects by this route and tiny doses are used compared with those taken by mouth. Many people with nasal symptoms during the hay fever season can expect good relief from a local corticosteroid preparation without unwanted effects (page 177).

Doses vary widely depending on the condition being treated. A corticosteroid should always be used at the lowest possible dose for the shortest length of time, particularly in children, because long-term use may affect growth. When you take a corticosteroid by mouth it is always best to take it as a single dose in the morning. This causes less *adrenal suppression* (page 333).

Pregnancy and breastfeeding – A corticosteroid is only prescribed or continued during pregnancy or breastfeeding when medically necessary. The Committee on Safety of Medicines (CSM) has reviewed the evidence for using a corticosteroid by mouth (*systemic*) during these situations and has concluded that:

- the drugs vary in their ability to reach the baby. **Betamethasone** and **dexamethasone** cross the placenta readily whereas 88 per cent of a dose of **prednisolone** is inactivated as it crosses the placenta
- there is no convincing evidence of an increased incidence of birth defects or abnormalities such as cleft palate or lip
- there is no evidence that the baby's growth slows in the womb following short courses of treatment. When treatment with a corticosteroid is prolonged or repeated, then the risk of slowed growth increases
- any adrenal suppression in the newborn baby that occurred as a result of treatment during pregnancy usually resolves and does not become a medical problem
- **prednisolone** appears in small amounts in breast milk but doses up to 40mg daily are unlikely to cause systemic effects in the baby. A baby should be monitored for signs of adrenal suppression if you have to take a higher dose.

PREDNISOLONE

PREDNISOLONE – Tablets, soluble tablets
DELTACORTRIL ENTERIC – Enteric-coated tablets
DELTASTAB Injection
MINIMS PREDNISOLONE – Single-use eye drops
PREDENEMA – Enema
PREDFOAM – Rectal foam
PRED FORTE – Eye drops
PREDSOL – Enema, suppositories, ear/eye drops

With antibiotic
PREDSOL-N – Ear/eye drops (*not recommended for eye*)
PREDNISOLONE + NEOMYCIN

Prednisolone is a corticosteroid with glucocorticoid activity used for suppressing a wide range of inflammatory and allergic disorders. Like other corticosteroids, prednisolone's actions on the body's inflammatory cells and chemical pathways are complex but include a blocking action of *prostanoids*, body chemicals that are involved in the inflammatory process. They also dampen the immune system temporarily by reducing the activity of certain white blood cells.

Short courses (less than three weeks) of treatment by mouth at low doses rarely cause serious unwanted effects. Long-term treatment or high doses by mouth can lead to unwanted effects including adrenal suppression and cushingoid effects.

Prednisolone is used locally for inflammatory bowel disease, in the eye to reduce inflammation, in joints to relieve pain and swelling, and in some cases to reduce deformity caused by arthritis. A small amount of corticosteroid can be injected locally to help conditions such as tennis or golfer's elbow or tendonitis. **If you are starting a corticosteroid by mouth, make sure you receive the manufacturer's patient information leaflet (PIL).**

Before you use this medicine

Tell your doctor if you are:
☐ pregnant or breast-feeding – page 330 ☐ taking any other medicines, including vitamins and those bought over the counter.

Tell your doctor if you have or have had:
☐ tuberculosis ☐ peptic ulcer ☐ diabetes ☐ heart disease such as heart failure or recent heart attack ☐ high blood pressure ☐ glaucoma ☐ any infection ☐ depression ☐ kidney or liver disease ☐ osteoporosis ☐ seizures (epilepsy) ☐ underactive thyroid ☐ psychiatric disorder ☐ muscle weakness with a corticosteroid.

How to use this medicine

Tablets Take the dose according to the doctor's directions either in divided doses or as a single dose in the morning after breakfast, with or after food. Sometimes you may take a double dose on alternate days. Do not take more than the dose prescribed for you.
Eye drops These are used only after visual acuity tests and checks to see that there is no infection. Your doctor should review treatment every few days. Contact your doctor if symptoms do not improve after five to seven days or the condition worsens. A corticosteroid combined with an antibiotic such as neomycin is rarely needed: you usually need one or the other.
Enema and suppositories – see Digestive system, page 81.
Corticosteroid injection into joints – see Muscle and Joints, page 394.

During prolonged courses of treatment by mouth or injection, eat food low in salt (sodium) and rich in potassium and protein.

Alcohol in small amounts should not be a problem, but it may aggravate the effect of prednisolone on the gut. Prednisolone by mouth increases the likelihood of a peptic ulcer developing with the risk of perforation.

Do not stop taking prednisolone suddenly because you may be at risk of adrenal suppression (page 333); your doctor will give you a schedule for reducing the dose gradually. Carry a steroid warning card with you if you take prednisolone by mouth or you are treated with injections (other than locally) for longer than three weeks. You are unlikely to require a card for a corticosteroid used locally on the skin, in the nose or inhaled. If you miss a dose take it as soon as you remember. If your next dose is due within six hours, take the missed dose and skip the next one.

If you need to have surgery, tell your doctor or dentist that you take a corticosteroid.

Over 65 Older people are more susceptible to the adverse effects: only use corticosteroids if absolutely necessary.

Interactions with other medicines

Various drugs interfere with the effect of prednisolone or vice versa. Do not take other medicines including those sold over the counter without checking first with your doctor or pharmacist. Interactions do not generally apply to corticosteroids used locally – on the skin, inhaled or injected into a joint.

Prednisolone antagonises the therapeutic effects of **antidiabetic medicines**, including insulin, blood pressure-lowering drugs, and diuretics.

Rifampicin or **rifabutin** (used against tuberculosis) and **antiepileptics** such as **carbamazepine**, **phenytoin**, **phenobarbital** reduce the effect of prednisolone.

Anticoagulants such as **warfarin** Effects altered by prednisolone.

Antifungal amphotericin Increased risk of low blood potassium with prednisolone.

Unwanted effects – see serious unwanted effects below, including adrenal suppression.

Serious unwanted effects occur only when prednisolone is taken systemically by mouth in high doses or by injection, or for long periods of time. The most important effects include dampening of the response to infection, metabolic changes, thinning of the bones (osteoporosis), adrenal suppression and cushingoid effects. These produce unwanted effects throughout the body, for example on the digestive system, eyes, skin, bones and muscle, mind and nerves, endocrine system and kidneys.

Similar preparations

BETAMETHASONE:
BETNELAN; BETNESOL

CORTISONE (no longer recommended)

DEFLAZACORT:
CALCORT

DEXAMETHASONE:
DECADRON

HYDROCORTISONE:
HYDROCORTISTAB; HYDROCORTONE; EFCORTESOL; SOLU-CORTEF

METHYLPREDNISOLONE:
MEDRONE; SOLU-MEDRONE; DEPO-MEDRONE

TRIAMCINOLONE:
ADCORTYL; KENALOG

SERIOUS UNWANTED EFFECTS OF CORTICOSTEROIDS

Your doctor should minimise the dose and duration of treatment by mouth to reduce the likelihood of unwanted effects developing. Some of the effects that can develop with long-term or high-dose treatment include the following.

- ☐ Increased breakdown of protein, resulting in muscle wasting and weakness: protein is also removed from skin which becomes thin and marked with purple stripes – also a delay in wound healing.
- ☐ Increased use of carbohydrate to produce heat and energy, resulting in diabetes mellitus.
- ☐ Extra sodium is retained in the body, resulting in additional water retention; this extra fluid (oedema) causes a rise in blood pressure.

☐ Upset in fat breakdown leading to deposits of fat in the face ('moon face'), on the shoulders ('buffalo hump') and on the abdomen.
☐ Lessening of the response to inflammation which may mask signs of infection.
☐ Reduced ability to fight infection (e.g. chickenpox, measles) because of a fall in the number of white blood cells. You should contact your doctor urgently if you have not had chickenpox and have been in contact with someone who has chickenpox or shingles; likewise with measles.
☐ Upset calcium balance resulting in the bones thinning and crumbling (osteoporosis); extra calcium is removed from the body via the kidneys with an increased risk of kidney stones. Destruction (*necrosis*) of the hip.
☐ Increased hair growth on the face, chest and abdomen.
☐ Eye problems including glaucoma, cataracts, corneal thinning, exacerbation of eye infections.
☐ Acne.
☐ Absence of periods in women who are menstruating.
☐ Indigestion and possible peptic ulcer with risk of perforation.
☐ Mood changes and mental disturbances, such as a heightened sense of well-being (euphoria) and depression.
☐ Reduction in the complex hormonal and nervous response to stress.

Adrenal suppression

When taking an external source of a corticosteroid for more than three weeks, the adrenal glands respond by not producing the body's usual amount of adrenal hormones. If you stop taking the external source suddenly, the body and the adrenal glands are unprepared, which can result in signs of sudden (acute) adrenal insufficiency. With long-term corticosteroid treatment the adrenal glands shut down because there is an external supply. Treatment that continues beyond three weeks must be stopped gradually, with the daily dose gently reduced. When your condition is unlikely to recur, gradual withdrawal of the corticosteroid is also recommended in circumstances when you have:

☐ recently received repeated courses, particularly for over three weeks
☐ taken a short course within one year of stopping long-term treatment
☐ received more than 40mg daily of prednisolone or equivalent dose of another corticosteroid
☐ taken repeated doses of corticosteroid in the evening
☐ other possible causes of adrenal suppression.

Withdrawal may take weeks or even months depending on the dosage and how long you have been treated with a corticosteroid. Too rapid a reduction in dose can lead to collapse and even death. The adrenal glands usually recover, but after prolonged corticosteroid treatment may function less well. This process is unnecessary with replacement therapy because hormone production is already impaired.

In times of stress, illness, infection or surgery, or while any increased demand is being made on the body's reserves, an additional dose of corticosteroid may be needed. In people with properly functioning adrenal glands, extra hormones are produced to help the body cope. If you take a corticosteroid by mouth, the body cannot respond in the normal way, so the dose must be increased to compensate during the stressful period and then gradually decreased afterwards.

Sex hormone deficiencies

Hormones play a major part in the development and maintenance of the reproductive organs. The sex hormones are mainly produced by the sex glands (*gonads*): the *ovaries* in women and the *testes* in men. The female sex hormones are **oestrogen** and **progesterone**. The male sex hormones are called **androgens**, of which **testosterone** is the most important. The male sex hormones are produced at a constant rate whereas the female hormone production varies over a 28-day cycle. The male and female sex hormones are regulated by the *gonadotrophic hormones* (*gonadotrophins*) produced by the pituitary gland. The gonadotrophic hormones stimulate the production of sex hormones, but are themselves regulated by the *gonadotrophin-releasing hormone* (GnRH) produced in another gland in the brain, the *hypothalamus*, to which the pituitary gland is attached. A complex feedback mechanism operates for most hormones so that as the blood levels of hormone rise, the hypothalamus and pituitary secrete less of their own hormones and vice versa. The situation is more complex in the female because a double feedback mechanism regulates the menstrual cycle. Sex hormone deficiencies can arise through failure of hormone production either at the hypothalamus and pituitary glands or sex glands. Medicines have been developed based on GnRH. Synthetic GnRH is known as **gonadorelin**, and the medicines derived from it are called gonadorelin analogues. These either enhance or dampen GnRH activity in the body and are used for conditions such as endometriosis, and breast cancer or prostate cancer.

FEMALE SEX HORMONES

Women's reproductive organs consist of the two ovaries, the Fallopian or uterine tubes, the womb (*uterus*), vagina and vulva. The uterus is behind the bladder and in front of the rectum, and is connected to the outside by the vagina. The inner lining of the womb is called the *endometrium*. When a girl is born, she has around a million egg-forming cells or follicles in each ovary. Many follicles die off, leaving around 300,000 at the age of 11. At the start of menstruation one or possibly two follicles start to ripen every month under the influence of the gonadotrophic hormones. The follicles produce oestrogen, which causes the development of female characteristics: breasts, pubic hair, hair under the arms and widening of the pelvis (*puberty*). Oestrogen and progesterone and synthetic derivatives are used medically to replace body hormones when they are deficient, to prevent conception, to regulate periods and to treat certain cancers.

Ovulation

Female sex hormones are produced in differing quantities over a 28-day cycle which prepares the body for fertilisation. The *follicle-stimulating hormone (FSH)* produced by the pituitary gland causes the egg cell within a follicle to ripen and stimulates oestrogen production. Under the combined influence of FSH, increased levels of oestrogen and the release of a second pituitary hormone – the *luteinising hormone* (LH) – the egg matures and *ovulation* (release of the egg) occurs. The egg is released from the follicle into the ovary and from there it passes into the Fallopian tube. Ovulation occurs in the middle of the menstrual cycle, around day 14, and sometimes causes abdominal pain. The egg travels along the Fallopian tube to the womb.

Under the influence of LH, the empty follicle produces the hormone progesterone. This circulates in blood and stops further ovulation during the cycle. The combined effect of oestrogen and progesterone during the second half of the cycle makes the lining of the womb thicken and prepare for pregnancy. If the egg is not fertilised and pregnancy does not occur, the empty follicle dies and the levels of oestrogen and progesterone fall, triggering menstruation: the egg and the thickened lining of the womb are shed with blood. The first day of blood loss is designated as day one of the cycle.

Hormone deficiency

In young women the delicate balance of sex hormones can be upset at several places in the body – the hypothalamus and pituitary glands and the ovaries. Wherever this happens, the disruption in hormonal production means that there are no monthly periods (*amenorrhoea*), and sexual development can be halted if this occurs before puberty. Tests can show the type of deficiency and your doctor can then prescribe the appropriate preparations to supplement either the gonadotrophins or oestrogen and progesterone. Other causes of periods stopping between puberty and the menopause include *polycystic ovary syndrome*, excessive loss of weight, as in the slimmer's disease *anorexia nervosa*, hard physical training, thyroid disorders, and medicines which increase levels of **prolactin**, the pituitary hormone which controls the production of breast-milk. There are no monthly periods during pregnancy and this should always be considered as a possible cause of the disrupted hormonal balance.

The menopause

As a woman grows older the egg-forming cells or follicles decrease until there are approximately 8,000 left around the age of 44. Only a few of these follicles will ripen to produce eggs and fertility gradually declines with age. As the ovaries slowly stop working, less oestrogen and progesterone are produced. At around 50 years the egg supply stops and with it monthly periods. The age at which women's periods begin and when they stop varies but it is rare for periods to continue beyond the age of 55. Each woman's levels of hormones are unique, so your body will have its own way of reacting to the hormonal changes which happen around the time of the menopause.

The menopause happens broadly in three stages:

Premenopause when you may experience irregular and more or less frequent periods, mood changes and hot flushes.

Perimenopause when periods become irregular. The date of the final period is known as the menopause. Because irregular periods make it difficult to determine this date you can only be certain your periods have stopped when you haven't had one for at least six months to a year. If periods stop before you are 50 you should allow two years to pass before you can say the menopause has occurred. Even if you have irregular periods, conception can still occur, so you will still need to use contraception until you are sure you are no longer having periods. Postmenopausal symptoms begin at this time, although two out of ten women do not have problems.

Postmenopause Hormonal changes affect the body in a number of noticeable ways. You may experience hot flushes with sweating, especially at night, and palpitations, which may interrupt sleep and lead to fatigue; vaginal and urethral dryness; mood changes; *osteoporosis* (thinning of the bones).

The main symptoms occur around the menopause but the falling level of sex hormones affects the body in many subtle ways. One effect is that up to the menopause a woman is protected against heart disease by oestrogen, but after the menopause the risk of cardiovascular disease such as heart attack or stroke increases.

– HOW YOU CAN HELP YOURSELF –

Hot flushes and sweating

- ☐ Wear several layers of light clothing so that you can peel off or put on a layer as your body temperature changes. Wear cotton as it allows the skin to breathe and air to circulate, and use cotton sheets.
- ☐ Lie on a large towel in bed so that you do not have to change the sheets every time you break out in a sweat.
- ☐ Have a tepid shower when you feel unbearably hot.
- ☐ Avoid tea, coffee, alcohol and spicy foods as these aggravate flushes.
- ☐ If you take any medicines, ask your doctor whether they could give you flushes.

Vaginal and urethral dryness The lining of the vagina becomes thin and dry. Secretions lessen and intercourse may be painful, sometimes with bleeding. There may be infection and discharge. Similar changes can occur in the bladder and the urethra, leading to cystitis (pages 280–2). You may have stress incontinence – leaking urine – when you cough, laugh or sneeze.

- ☐ Use a lubricant before intercourse.
- ☐ Regular love making, masturbation and pelvic floor muscle exercises all help to stimulate secretions and keep the vagina moist.
- ☐ If you have severe symptoms see your doctor. A vaginal oestrogen cream or hormone replacement treatment can help.
- ☐ Talk about sexual difficulties with your partner or try a counselling service.
- ☐ For stress incontinence, tone up your pelvic floor muscles: when you pass urine, pull up and back on the muscles in mid-flow to stop urine flow for a few seconds; relax, release the muscle and allow urine to flow and empty the bladder completely. When you have learnt the action you can practise these exercises at any time.

Mood changes The late forties are often the most stressful time in your life, not just because of the menopause but because there may be family, job and social changes as well.

- ☐ Find time to relax and be peaceful on your own away from children and stressful influences. Share your worries with your partner, friend or neighbour.
- ☐ Join a yoga or relaxation class. Yoga or Pilates can help you to tone muscles.
- ☐ Diet, exercise and preventing falls are important for keeping fractures at bay in older age.

Regular review Check your blood pressure; it tends to go up around the menopause. Be 'breast aware', checking regularly, particularly if you take HRT or tibolone. Go for breast screening from the age of 50 years – for more information look up *www.cancerscreening.nhs.uk/breastscreen/breastawareness.html*. Have a cervical smear regularly.

You should see your doctor if you have:

- ☐ irregular bleeding between periods around the menopause
- ☐ bleeding after more than six months without a period
- ☐ severe abdominal pain
- ☐ a dragging feeling or heaviness in the pelvis; this may mean the organs in the abdomen are beginning to drop (prolapse) because of slack muscles, a common condition which can be surgically treated
- ☐ frequent urination or inability to hold urine
- ☐ severe vaginal infection or itchiness of the vulva.

Hormone replacement therapy

The menopause is a natural occurrence for every woman. Menopausal symptoms are not life-threatening but if you have distressing symptoms which disrupt your life you may wish to take an external supply of hormones to replace the body's oestrogen and progesterone. This is called **hormone replacement therapy (HRT)** which is available as combined therapy or oestrogen-only.

Combined therapy Low doses of an oestrogen are given continuously and combined with a *progestogen* (a synthetic equivalent of progesterone) for 10 to 14 days of each month to protect the womb from changes in the endometrial lining brought about by the oestrogen, which could possibly lead to cancer. A progestogen opposes the effects of oestrogen on the womb. This type of HRT, known as *sequential combined HRT*, is taken on a monthly or three-monthly cycle which means that you continue to have regular withdrawal bleeding because of the cyclical use of progestogen. You can take oestrogen and progestogen in the same preparation, for example in a tablet or patch or as separate products. A year after your final menstrual period, that is the menopause, the choice of HRT broadens as you then have the option of taking a combined preparation of oestrogen and progestogen continuously, known as *continuous combined HRT*, which will avoid regular withdrawal bleeding.

Oestrogen-only If you have had your womb removed (see 'Surgical menopause', page 341) you can take oestrogen on its own continuously; you do not need to take a progestogen.

Before starting HRT you should discuss with your doctor the pros and cons of using it and what type of preparation you think might help. More information has become available from robust studies in the UK and in North America that have helped to place HRT use in perspective. You will need to decide for yourself whether to start HRT.

Pros: HRT relieves **menopausal and postmenopausal symptoms** – for example, hot flushes, vaginal dryness, soreness and urinary problems. If you have vaginal symptoms only, these may respond to a short course of an oestrogen cream used locally in the vagina for a few weeks. Hot flushes, vaginal symptoms and night sweats which disrupt sleep can be helped by systemic treatment – tablets, patches, gels, implants or nasal spray. HRT should be taken at the lowest dose that relieves symptoms and for the shortest length of time. Once you have started treatment it needs to be reviewed regularly – at least once a year.

HRT also helps **to prevent osteoporosis** and therefore fractures of the spine and hip (neck of femur). However, if you already have thin bones HRT cannot reverse this bone loss, but it can prevent further decline in bone density while you continue to take HRT. Although widely promoted in the past for preventing osteoporosis, HRT is no longer the preferred treatment for women because newer treatments give better results and because the risks of HRT have begun to outweigh the benefits of long-term treatment. HRT can be useful for menopausal symptoms and for preventing osteoporosis if you have had a premature menopause (perhaps because of ovarian failure or surgery). HRT is recommended up to the age of 50 years for preventing osteoporosis, but you and your doctor should review the choice of treatment. HRT for preventing osteoporosis should only be used in women over 50 years old who are unable to take other treatments, or if alternative treatments have not helped.

Cons: Evidence has been accumulating about the risk of harm from HRT. It is now known that treatment **increases the risk of certain cancers**, particularly breast cancer (see below), and of abnormal blood clots forming in the deep veins of the leg (page 148). HRT was thought to protect against heart disease, but now it appears to increase the risk, particularly in the first year of use, and offers no protective effects in the longer-term. Similarly HRT slightly increases the risk of stroke (page 144).

HRT appears to reduce the risk of colorectal cancer, decreasing the number of cases by 1 over 5 years and 2 over 10 years for every 1,000 HRT users aged 50 to 59. In women aged 60 to 69 years the number of reduced cases is estimated as 3 over 5 years and 5 to 6 over 10 years for every 1,000 HRT users.

In 2003 the CSM published summaries of two studies, the UK Million Women Study and the USA Women's Health Initiative, which looked at the long-term safety of HRT. Both studies confirm that the **risk of breast cancer** increases as follows:

- ☐ all types of HRT cause a duration-dependent increase in the risk of breast cancer. The risk starts to decline when you stop HRT and by five years, the risk reaches the same level as in women who have never taken HRT

- ☐ the increase in risk of breast cancer starts within one or two years of starting treatment and this applies to all types of HRT used
- ☐ the risk does not differ between specific preparations or routes of administration
- ☐ **tibolone**, a synthetic HRT preparation with oestrogenic and progestogenic activity, also increases the risk of breast cancer.

When the cancer risk is assessed for women aged 50–65 years, the extra number of breast cancer cases per 1,000 HRT users for *combined HRT* (oestrogen + progestogen) is estimated as 6 with 5 years' use and 19 with 10 years' use. For *oestrogen-only HRT*, the extra number of breast cancer cases is less: around one additional case with 5 years' use and 5 with 10 years' use. Doubt has also been cast about the previous observation that breast cancers that were diagnosed in HRT users were less likely to have spread compared with those in non-HRT users. Further evidence is needed to confirm this.

There is also an **increased risk of cancer of the lining of the womb** (*endometrial cancer*) if you take oestrogen on its own and have not had a hysterectomy, although taking a progestogen for 10 to 14 days each month or continuously should largely counteract this. The safety of using long-term local HRT as an oestrogen cream or pessaries in the vagina or as repeated courses is largely uncertain. Oestrogen can be absorbed from the vagina into the body, but the extent to which this happens is unknown. It appears that most local oestrogen preparations are used without the addition of progestogen systemically. The *British National Formulary* suggests that if an oestrogen cream is used long-term, then a progestogen by mouth should be taken for 12 to 14 days each month to prevent the development of endometrial abnormalities. If you use an oestrogen cream in the vagina long-term or repeatedly, you should discuss with your doctor whether you need to continue treatment, and if so, whether a progestogen systemically should be added. If you continue treatment an annual check is advised. If bleeding or spotting occurs at any time during treatment, you must see your doctor for an investigation.

There is a slightly **increased risk of ovarian cancer** if you have had a hysterectomy and take oestrogen-only HRT. The extra number of ovarian cancer cases in 1,000 oestrogen-only HRT users is around 1 with 5 years' use and 3 with 10 years' use compared with non-HRT users among women aged 50 to 69 years. For women taking combined HRT the risks of developing ovarian cancer are unknown.

Like the combined oral contraceptive, HRT **increases the risk of abnormal blood clots** forming in the deep veins of the leg or pelvis (*venous thromboembolism* – VTE). The risks are greater if you have a personal or strong family history of venous thromboembolism or of a blood clot blocking the artery to the lungs (*pulmonary embolism*), severe varicose veins, are overweight, undergoing major trauma or surgery, or if you have to lie in bed for some time because of an accident or a long illness. For women aged 50 to 59 years the extra number of VTE cases is estimated as 4 and for women aged 60 to 69 years the extra number of cases is 9 per 1,000 HRT users over a five-year period. All types of HRT preparation seem to increase the risk, which then disappears on stopping treatment.

An **increase in the risk of stroke** occurs in HRT users. For women aged 50 to 59 years about 1 extra stroke occurs which increases to 4 extra strokes for women aged 60 to 69 for every 1,000 HRT users over a five-year period.

Women can develop these conditions described above without using HRT; your risk of doing so depends on your health, lifestyle and family medical history. The extra number of cases attributed to HRT is small, particularly when compared with the health risks associated with smoking or obesity.

A group of experts on HRT from a number of European countries has now reassessed all the risks and benefits of HRT and provided new recommendations about its use. The conclusions of the group, which are endorsed by the Committee on Safety of Medicines (CSM), are as follows.

- For short-term treatment of menopausal symptoms the balance of risks and benefits is favourable – HRT therefore remains a suitable treatment option.
- For long-term use for preventing osteoporosis the balance of risks and benefits is unfavourable. HRT should only be used for preventing osteoporosis by those who are unable to take other osteoporosis prevention treatments or for whom other treatments have been unsuccessful.
- In healthy women without symptoms, the balance of risks and benefits is generally unfavourable and HRT is not recommended.

HRT is not an elixir of youth, although it has been heavily promoted as the pill that will keep women young, sexually active and free from emotional problems. Research shows that reduced oestrogen levels in the body are not responsible for psychiatric problems, and replacing the oestrogen is unlikely to cure these problems or improve quality of life. Vaginal dryness is helped by oestrogen treatment but general loss of sexual interest has more to do with relationship difficulties and other strains on life. The years leading up to the menopause are generally the most stressful in women's lives and problems need to be disentangled from the effects of the menopause.

How long should you take HRT?

The duration of treatment depends on your reasons for taking HRT and you will need to discuss these with your doctor before starting it. Menopausal symptoms fade after some time but this varies from woman to woman. If you take HRT to relieve menopausal symptoms you could try a course for 6–12 months, then stop gradually and see if troublesome symptoms return. Withdrawal from HRT can sometimes be problematic, with the return of symptoms such as hot flushes and vaginal dryness. You could restart if symptoms recur, but the increase in breast cancer risk begins within 1–2 years of starting treatment. Cyclical HRT needs to be taken if you still have periods and for up to one year after you have stopped menstruating which means you still have regular bleeds. The risks have to be balanced against the benefits. You must see your doctor for regular checks, yearly at least, to assess your health and the continuing need for treatment.

You should stop HRT immediately if any of the following occur:

- ☐ sudden severe pains in the chest
- ☐ sudden breathlessness or cough with blood spots in phlegm
- ☐ unexplained severe calf pain in one leg
- ☐ severe stomach pain
- ☐ unusual severe prolonged headache which seems to worsen
- ☐ sudden loss, or partial loss, of vision
- ☐ sudden disturbance of hearing or speech
- ☐ bad fainting attack or collapse, or unexplained seizure
- ☐ weakness or numbness suddenly affecting one side or one part of the body
- ☐ hepatitis or jaundice (yellowing of the skin or whites of the eyes)
- ☐ severe depression
- ☐ increase in blood pressure
- ☐ pregnancy.

SURGICAL MENOPAUSE

If you are under 50 and have not reached the menopause, but have a gynaecological problem such as cancer of the womb, fibroids or heavy bleeding, you may have the womb surgically removed (hysterectomy). Although your periods stop when you have a hysterectomy, you will go through the menopause later providing your ovaries have not been removed. The ovaries are important organs as they produce oestrogen and progesterone throughout your life from puberty onwards, although after the menopause levels are much reduced. Unless one or both ovaries are diseased, you should not have them removed. If they have to be removed you may experience an immediate and often severe menopause. Your doctor will then recommend hormone replacement therapy.

OESTROGEN REPLACEMENT PREPARATIONS

Natural oestrogens – **estradiol** (**oestradiol**), **estriol** (**oestriol**), or **estrone** (**oestrone**) – are generally used because they are believed to be better than synthetic alternatives. They can be taken by mouth, given as an injection or an implant, applied to the skin in a patch or gel, applied to the nose as a nasal spray or used locally in the vagina as a cream, vaginal tablets or in a ring device.

Tablets are commonly used, either as natural oestrogens alone or combined with a progestogen to oppose the effects of oestrogen. Some preparations of oestrogen with a progestogen are taken continuously whereas others, cyclical preparations, are taken for only 21 days followed by a seven-day break. Combined HRT does not provide effective contraception, nor should it be taken at the same time as an oral contraceptive. Another method of contraception should be chosen if it is needed. Discuss this with your doctor.

Implants are long-acting oestrogen preparations (estradiol implants) which are inserted under the skin, where they release the hormone over a period of months. They may be used after hysterectomy, when you do not have to take a progestogen. If you have a womb you will have to remember to take a progestogen for 10 to 13 days of the cycle. Oestrogen is broken down in the liver so not all of a dose by mouth is effective in the body. Using an implant can overcome this problem but sometimes oestrogen levels become too high and the effects cannot be stopped quickly.

A skin patch containing oestrogen releases the drug slowly through the skin (*transdermally*) into the body. This method also avoids oestrogen passing through the liver. A patch is applied once or twice weekly, either continuously or on a cyclical basis depending on the particular brand. The patch is placed on a clean, dry hairless area of unbroken skin below the waist where there is little rubbing from clothes. The plaster should not be applied on or near the breasts. It can be kept on when bathing or showering. Redness, itching and rash sometimes occur but fade when the plaster is removed, so a different site should be used each time it is changed. A number of preparations (e.g. Estracombi, Evorel, FemSeven) are complete patch systems providing oestrogen plus two weeks of progestogen per month. Otherwise, if you have a womb, progestogen tablets must be taken for 10 to 14 days of the cycle in addition to an oestrogen patch. **Skin gels** (Oestrogel; Sandrena) are also available and are applied once daily on a continuous basis; progestogen must be taken if you have a womb.

Local oestrogen cream or pessaries can be used for vaginal problems, but oestrogen passes into the bloodstream from the vagina in variable amounts. A cream should be used for a short time, say two to three weeks, repeating courses if necessary. Continuous long-term use is not recommended, particularly if you have a womb, as you will be absorbing oestrogen unopposed by a progestogen. Local oestrogen preparations include vaginal creams as estriol (Ortho-Gynest; Ovestin) or conjugated oestrogens (Premarin) and estradiol vaginal tablets (pessaries) (Vagifem). If symptoms return when you stop using the cream, your doctor may suggest trying another form of HRT. If you continue to use the cream on a long-term basis, you should take progestogen tablets too for 10 to 14 days of each month.

Estring is a vaginal ring made of silicone elastomer, which delivers a tiny dose of estradiol (7.5 micrograms over 24 hours) locally to the vagina to help vaginitis and urinary symptoms caused by atrophy and dryness after the menopause. The ring should be placed high up in the vagina and is left in place for three months. It can be removed temporarily if needed, for example if it is uncomfortable during intercourse or during treatment with other vaginal preparations. The dose of oestrogen is small and is not absorbed significantly into the blood stream. Estring is not suitable for other postmenopausal symptoms or to prevent osteoporosis. Another vaginal ring, Menoring 50, provides a significant amount of oestrogen which will be absorbed systemically; it can be used for urogenital and postmenopausal symptoms.

PROGESTERONE REPLACEMENT PREPARATIONS

A progestogen (a synthetic equivalent of progesterone) should always be used if you have a womb as it modifies some of oestrogen's effects. Oestrogen replacement on its own stimulates growth of the lining of the womb, which may lead to cancerous changes. A progestogen given for 10 to 14 days out of 28 abolishes oestrogen's effect on the womb lining. This cyclical regimen usually leads to withdrawal bleeding towards the end of the progestogen course. If you still have irregular periods, a combined preparation will help to make the cycle regular. A progestogen can also be used on a continuous basis with oestrogen, both taken throughout the 28-day cycle. This avoids monthly bleeding, although irregular bleeding may occur within the first few months of using this type of HRT. If irregular bleeding continues you must discuss this with your doctor. **Dydrogesterone**, **norethisterone**, **norgestrel**, **levonorgestrel** and **medroxyprogesterone** are commonly used in HRT preparations.

CONJUGATED OESTROGENS

PREMARIN – Tablets, vaginal cream
OESTROGEN

PREMPAK-C – Tablets
OESTROGEN + PROGESTOGEN: NORGESTREL

PREMIQUE; PREMIQUE CYCLE
OESTROGEN + PROGESTOGEN: MEDROXYPROGESTERONE

Conjugated oestrogens are a mixture of natural oestrogens (originating from pregnant mares' urine) used in low doses for replacing the body's own oestrogen supply as it dwindles at the menopause. They relieve the uncomfortable symptoms of hot flushes, night sweats and vaginal and bladder problems. Premarin is an oestrogen-only product and can be used if you do not have a womb – when a progestogen is not needed. If you have a womb you will need to take a combined preparation (Premique, Premique Cycle or Prempak-C), which contains oestrogen and a progestogen. Monthly withdrawal bleeding will occur with Prempak-C and Premique Cycle (cyclical progestogen), but not with Premique where oestrogen and progestogen are taken continuously. Premique is not started usually until at least one year after the menopause. The vaginal cream (Premarin) can be used for short periods to relieve vaginal and bladder symptoms of dryness and pain, but with long-term treatment you will also need to take a progestogen by mouth.

Before you use this medicine

Tell your doctor if you are:
□ pregnant – do not take HRT during pregnancy □ breast-feeding – high doses suppress milk flow □ taking any other medicines, including vitamins and those bought over the counter.

Tell your doctor if you have or have had:
□ high blood pressure or heart disease □ kidney disease □ diabetes □ epilepsy or migraine □ asthma □ sickle-cell anaemia □ deterioration of the hearing problem otosclerosis.

Do not take if you have or have had:
□ oestrogen-dependent cancer or breast cancer □ abnormal vaginal bleeding □ severe active liver disease □ abnormal blood clots in your veins (deep vein thrombosis) □ angina or heart attack (thromboembolic disease) □ untreated endometrial problems □ porphyria.

How to use this medicine

Before you start HRT you should have a complete physical and gynaecological check and discuss the pros and cons of treatment with your doctor. Once you have started treatment, see your doctor regularly – at least every 12 months. You should contact your doctor if you have any unusual breakthrough bleeding.
Tablets Take one tablet daily starting on the first day of your period if you are still menstruating, otherwise start at any time. With Premique Cycle and Prempak-C the oestrogen tablet is taken continuously and medoxyprogesterone or norgestrel is taken during days 15, or 17, to 28. Premique can be started at any time one year after the menopause and is taken continuously.
Vaginal cream Apply locally or insert the applicator with the measured dose into the vagina. Intravaginal treatment should be started on the fifth day of bleeding if you still have periods or otherwise as your doctor directs. Treatment should be continued for three weeks followed by one week off. For long-term treatment it is advisable to take a progestogen by mouth for 10 to 14 days of each month.

Do not stop taking this medicine suddenly as symptoms may return. Ask your doctor to give you a schedule to reduce the dose gradually. If you miss a dose take it as soon as you remember. It is very important to remember to take the progestogen tablets. If you have surgery you may need to stop taking HRT 4–6 weeks before a planned operation, although measures to prevent blood clots in the deep veins should be available in hospital.

Over 65 The lowest possible dose should be used, but there are no special requirements.

Interactions with other medicines

The low doses used in HRT are unlikely to cause significant problems. Check with your doctor or pharmacist.

Unwanted effects

Likely Feeling or being sick, abdominal cramps, fluid retention, bloating, weight gain, swollen ankles, breast tenderness or swelling, intolerance to wearing contact lenses, changes in hair growth, premenstrual-like syndrome.
Less likely Breakthrough bleeding, vaginal candidiasis, changes to sex drive, headaches, depression, irritability, pains in chest, groin, leg or calf, sudden loss of co-ordination, dizziness, weakness or numbness in arm or leg, shortness of breath, breast lumps or discharge, yellowing of the eyes or skin (jaundice), skin rash, altered blood lipids.

Effects such as feeling sick and breast tenderness usually wear off after a few weeks' treatment. If not, contact your doctor. If you have breakthrough bleeding, depression or generally feel unwell during treatment see your doctor.

Similar preparations

Oestrogen-only

AERODIOL – Nasal spray
CLIMAVAL – Tablets
ELLESTE-SOLO – Patches
ELLESTE-SOLO MX – Patches
ESTRADERM MX – Patches
ESTRADERM TTS – Patches
EVOREL – Patches
FEMATRIX – Patches
FEMSEVEN – Patches
FEMTAB – Tablets
HARMOGEN – Tablets
HORMONIN – Tablets
MENOREST – Patches
MENORING 50 – Vaginal ring
OESTROGEL – Skin gel
OVESTIN – Tablets
PROGYNOVA – Tablets
PROGYNOVA TS – Patches
SANDRENA – Skin gel
ZUMENON – Tablets

Oestrogen + progestogen (number of days of progestogen in brackets)

CLIMAGEST (12) – Tablets
CYCLO-PROGYNOVA (10) – Tablets
ELLESTE DUET (12) – Tablets
ESTRACOMBI (14) – Patches
EVOREL-PAK (12) – Oestrogen patches with progestogen tablets
EVOREL-SEQUI (14) – Patches
FEMAPAK (14) – Oestrogen patches with progestogen tablets
FEMOSTON (14) – Tablets
FEMSEVEN SEQUI (14) – Patches
FEMTAB SEQUI (12) – Tablets
NOVOFEM (12) – Tablets
NUVELLE (12) – Tablets
TRIDESTRA (14) – Tablets
TRISEQUENS (10) – Tablets

Combined continuous oestrogen and progestogen (unsuitable for use within 12 months of final menstrual period)

CLIMESSE – Tablets
ELLESTE-DUET CONTI – Tablets
EVOREL CONTI – Patches
FEMOSTON CONTI – Tablets
FEMSEVEN CONTI – Patches
FEMTAB CONTINUOUS – Tablets
INDIVINA – Tablets
KLIOFEM – Tablets
KLIOVANCE – Tablets
NUVELLE CONTINUOUS – Tablets

When oestrogen and progestogen are presented in one pack as two different medicines, you have to pay double the prescription charge. In some preparations oestrogen and progestogen are formulated in one tablet or patch, in which case only one prescription charge is due.

Tibolone (Livial) is a synthetic hormonal steroid treatment for relieving menopausal symptoms such as hot flushes and sweating. It is also used to prevent osteoporosis after the menopause, but only if you cannot take other treatments or they have not worked. Tibolone suppresses levels of gonadotrophic hormones produced in the pituitary and should not be taken until one year after the final natural period. If tibolone is taken sooner than this irregular vaginal bleeding may occur. Taken continuously tibolone does not stimulate the womb lining, so you do not have to take a progestogen to protect against disordered endometrial growth and there should be no monthly bleeding. If you do experience any vaginal bleeding, discuss this with your doctor. As with other HRT, the risk of breast cancer increases with the use of tibolone. Other unwanted effects occur occasionally and include changes in body weight, dizziness, eczema, headache, increased hair growth on the face and fluid retention.

OSTEOPOROSIS

Osteoporosis occurs when bone tissue is lost and tiny holes develop, causing the bone to become brittle and liable to break. Both men and women start to lose bone gradually from their mid-thirties onwards, but women are more at risk of developing osteoporosis. In men there may be an underlying cause, such as low testosterone levels. In women, bone is lost quite rapidly in the first few years after the menopause and the process continues gradually as you grow older. Although all bones can be affected, osteoporosis leads to an increased risk of bone fracture, particularly of the wrist, hip and spine. Bone in the spine develops cracks causing the vertebrae to collapse. This can cause severe back pain, make people shorter by several inches and lead to the characteristic rounded back.

Osteoporosis is more likely to be serious if you have one or more of the following risk factors:

- ☐ you are very thin, of lean build or have small bones
- ☐ you do not lead an active life
- ☐ you have a family history of osteoporosis
- ☐ you have had an early menopause
- ☐ you have a high daily alcohol intake
- ☐ you are a heavy smoker
- ☐ you are having or have recently had oral corticosteroid treatment
- ☐ you have certain illnesses, including myeloma (a tumour of bone-marrow cells), rheumatoid arthritis, chronic liver disease, and glandular disorders such as thyrotoxicosis and Cushing's disease
- ☐ you have a problem absorbing nutrients from the digestive system, e.g. Crohn's disease, are on a strict diet or you have had anorexia or bulimia.

Management

A balanced diet and weight-bearing exercise are both essential to keep bones healthy.

Making sure that you have enough calcium in your diet is important, together with vitamin D which aids calcium absorption from food. The recommended daily amount of calcium is 800–1,000mg (20–25mmol); one pint of milk contains about 700mg of calcium. Vitamin D is made in skin when your hands, arms and face are exposed to daylight. Some people at risk of osteoporosis may need extra calcium and vitamin D if they are frail and unable to go outside much, for example someone in a nursing home. Your doctor can prescribe a suitable calcium and vitamin D supplement. Exercise from childhood onwards is extremely important to build strong healthy bones. Regular exercise such as half an hour's daily walking, jogging or dancing can reduce bone loss. Certain exercises can help with balance, for example T'ai chi, which then helps to prevent falls and avoid fractures.

Corticosteroid treatment, such as **prednisolone** tablets 7.5mg for three months or more, increases the risk of osteoporosis; people older than 65 years are at greater risk. You will need to take preventative treatment, usually with a bisphosphonate.

Medicines for preventing and treating osteoporosis

The bisphosphonates, either **alendronate** (Fosamax) or **risedronate** (Actonel), are the drugs of choice for preventing and treating osteoporosis. The bisphosphonates are also used to treat osteoporosis as a result of prolonged corticosteroid treatment. **Disodium etidronate** (Didronel PMO) is still used if these newer drugs are not suitable.

The bisphosphonates are absorbed into bone so that the rate of bone turnover slows. They are effective, but have to be taken before food to increase absorption into the body. **Raloxifene** (▼Evista) is another drug, a selective oestrogen receptor modulator (SERM) similar to HRT but with less effect on the breasts, used to prevent or treat fractures of the spine (but not the hip) in postmenopausal women who are at increased risk of osteoporosis. Unlike HRT, raloxifene does not reduce menopausal symptoms such as hot flushes. **Calcitriol**, a vitamin D derivative, is a further alternative. **Calcitonin**, responsible for regulating bone turnover in the body via the parathyroid gland, is sometimes used by injection or nasal spray to prevent or treat postmenopausal osteoporosis. **Teriparatide** (▼Forsteo) is a new product of parathyroid hormone made by recombinant DNA technology for treating established osteoporosis after the menopause. It reduces fractures of the vertebrae in the spine, but not the hip. Teriparatide needs to be given once a day by injection under the skin and you will need to be shown how to do this. Common side effects include feeling sick, headache, dizziness and pain in the limbs.

MALE SEX HORMONES

The testes make the male sex hormones (*androgens*) under the influence of a gonadotrophic hormone produced by the pituitary gland. This occurs at puberty when the main androgen, **testosterone**, brings about sexual changes. Testosterone has *androgenic* effects which cause the voice box to enlarge and the voice to deepen, hair to grow in various parts of the body and the growth of the reproductive organs. The testes produce sperm, the male reproductive cells, at puberty and for the rest of the man's life. Testosterone also has *anabolic* effects, which cause bone and body growth and muscle development.

Sexual difficulties are rarely due to testosterone deficiency, and hormone replacement therapy for men is rarely needed. Testosterone replacement therapy is given when the body is not making its own or levels are too low. This may be due to lack of development or underdevelopment of the testes or a failure of the pituitary gland to produce a gonadotrophin to stimulate testosterone production in the testes. If puberty is delayed in a boy, a course of testosterone may be considered. However, testosterone can eventually stunt growth because it closes off the growing ends of the long bones. Hormonal treatment may therefore be given after growth is completed and always with specialist advice.

In men with low levels of testosterone, replacement therapy may help to overcome impotence and loss of sex drive, but not infertility. Men with low gonadotrophin levels because of hypothalamic-pituitary disease may have gonadotrophin treatment and this helps fertility. Testosterone replacement is usually given by long-lasting intramuscular depot injection every three to four weeks (page 34) because testosterone is broken down in the liver when it is taken by mouth. However, one preparation of testosterone (Restandol) can be effective when taken by mouth. A skin patch containing testosterone (Andropatch) or gel (▼Testogel) is an alternative way to replace the male hormone.

Additional male sex hormones will not boost testosterone levels if they are normal nor will they help impotence caused by psychological problems.

Women are sometimes treated with male hormones for certain types of cancer of the breast. Testosterone implants are sometimes used in addition to hormone replacement therapy. Male hormones given to women in large and continued doses can cause masculine features to develop.

Drugs which oppose the effect of androgens (anti-androgens) are used to treat men with cancer of the prostate. **Finasteride** (Proscar) is an anti-androgen for treating non-malignant swelling of the prostate.

7

REPRODUCTIVE AND URINARY SYSTEMS

Period problems Contraception
Bladder disorders Erectile dysfunction

The reproductive systems of both men and women are described briefly in Chapter 6.

The urinary system removes liquid waste from the body. As blood passes through the kidneys, waste products and water are filtered out and then discharged from the body at intervals. In both men and women the urinary system consists of two kidneys, each with a muscular tube, the *ureter*, running to the bladder. The bladder is a muscular storage tank for urine and can hold up to about a pint of fluid until it is convenient to empty it through the tube that leads to the outside, the *urethra*. A tight ring of sphincter muscles at the bladder outlet keeps a constant pressure on the urethra to prevent urine escaping.

Infection of the reproductive organs may be sexually transmitted but is not always so, particularly in women. In men, infection of the urinary system is uncommon because it is harder for bacteria and other organisms to gain access to the bladder and kidneys through the long urethra. A woman's urethra is shorter and the opening nearer to the vaginal and rectal openings provides easier access for infecting organisms. Bladder infections are common (see 'Cystitis', page 280). See Chapter 5 for medicines active against invading micro-organisms.

Period problems

Period problems include heavy blood loss (*menorrhagia*), painful periods (*dysmenorrhoea*) and premenstrual syndrome: physical symptoms and mood changes that occur before a period. *Endometriosis* (page 352) is a less common problem, but can cause painful periods. The menstrual cycle is usually 28 days although this can vary from woman to woman and anything from 21 to 35 days is considered normal. Hormones produced by the pituitary gland and the ovaries control and regulate the reproductive cycle and bleeding when the egg has not been fertilised.

HEAVY PERIODS – MENORRHAGIA

Continued excessive blood loss during periods can be exhausting and interfere with daily living. It is one of the commonest causes of iron deficiency anaemia in women. You may be used to the occasional heavy period but if this pattern continues you should see your doctor. The reason for heavy bleeding (menorrhagia or dysfunctional uterine bleeding) should be investigated and your doctor may ask you to keep a record of bleeding over a number of weeks, noting each day whether it is heavy, moderate or light and whether you have pain. Excessive blood loss is most commonly the result of abnormal bleeding from the womb, but there may be an underlying gynaecological reason such as endometriosis, pelvic inflammatory disease (PID), a uterine or ovarian growth or the intra-uterine contraceptive device (IUD). Hormonal imbalance such as a thyroid disorder can cause excessive bleeding and so can abnormalities of the blood clotting mechanism.

Your doctor may suggest an operation to remove or destroy the lining of the womb (*endometrium*) by a variety of surgical techniques. A combined approach to remove (*resect*) the lining of the womb (with a *loop diathermy electrode*) and destroy the tissue beneath it (with *rollerball ablation*) is often used. Alternatively one of these techniques can be used alone, or another method may be employed – *laser ablation* – where a laser is used to remove the endometrium. Removal of the womb (*hysterectomy*) is the final solution to heavy bleeding. However, there are a number of drug treatments and you may prefer to try a medicine before accepting a surgical procedure.

The **combined oral contraceptive** (oestrogen + progestogen) can reduce blood loss but is not suitable for every woman, for example if you have or have had heart disease or blood clotting problems, or if you smoke and are over the age of 35 years.

Progestogen alone taken for 21 out of 28 days is also used for treating heavy bleeding and is effective in decreasing blood loss and regulating periods. An intra-uterine progestogen device, Mirena (IUD – page 362), releases levonorgestrel in the womb and is successful in reducing heavy bleeding within 3–6 months after it has been inserted. It appears to act on the lining of the womb by decreasing inappropriate endometrial growth. Mirena is also a contraceptive.

A non-steroidal anti-inflammatory drug (NSAID) such as **mefenamic acid** (Ponstan) blocks prostaglandins and reduces bleeding as well as pain. You take the NSAID just before or as soon as menstruation starts and for as many days as bleeding is troublesome. You may be able to shorten the course and/or reduce the dose in subsequent periods. **Tranexamic acid** (Cyklokapron) is a medicine which reduces blood loss by acting on the blood clotting mechanism. It can help heavy bleeding: likely unwanted effects include feeling or being sick or diarrhoea, which usually fade when the dose is reduced. Rarely blurred or abnormal vision or colour vision disturbances occur. If eye problems develop, you should consult your doctor about stopping tranexamic acid. If you have ever had a blood clot (thrombus or embolus) you should never take tranexamic acid. **Etamsylate** (Dicynene) works in a similar way.

PAINFUL PERIODS – DYSMENORRHOEA

Painful periods can happen at any age during your reproductive life, but they are quite common during puberty when you start periods (primary dysmenorrhoea). At this stage the hormones may be unbalanced and may trigger high levels of prostaglandins in the womb which cause pain and cramps. Period pains that begin when you are older may be caused by abnormal conditions of the womb or ovaries, such as infection, fibroids or endometriosis (secondary dysmenorrhoea). You should see your doctor if period pains continue, so that any underlying problem can be investigated and treated. Smoking, for example, may increase the duration of painful periods.

Pain can be relieved with aspirin, paracetamol or an NSAID. The combined oral contraceptive stops ovulation and is effective in relieving painful periods. A progestogen on its own such as Duphaston is sometimes used, but a combined oral contraceptive is a better choice for a younger woman.

PREMENSTRUAL SYNDROME

Symptoms of premenstrual syndrome (also known as premenstrual tension) may occur for up to ten days before a period. They may vary from cycle to cycle. Psychological changes such as feelings of tension, irritability and depression and physical signs such as headache, bloating and breast tenderness are common. There may be fluid retention and other symptoms such as itching, backache and muscle and joint pains. Attacks of certain conditions, for example asthma, migraine, epilepsy and rhinitis are more frequent than at other times. Once you have had your period the symptoms disappear. The exact cause of premenstrual syndrome is unknown, but the symptoms appear to be triggered by the hormonal changes during the menstrual cycle. Severe symptoms may disrupt your life.

Your doctor may ask you to keep a record over several months of your menstrual cycle, the timing and nature of symptoms, how long they last and when your period begins. Treatment is not very satisfactory but the combined oral contraceptive sometimes seems to help. **Progestogens** have been used although there is little evidence of their value. A range of non-drug treatments including vitamins such as **pyridoxine** (vitamin B_6) and evening primrose oil have also been tried, but again there is little sound evidence to support their use in the premenstrual syndrome.

HOW YOU CAN HELP YOURSELF

PERIOD PROBLEMS

- ☐ For painful or heavy periods you may need to rest in bed with a hot water bottle.
- ☐ Take an analgesic regularly for pain relief.
- ☐ Try to avoid stressful activities just before and during your period.
- ☐ Note the dates of your periods and any unusual bleeding or symptoms.
- ☐ Do not ignore menstrual problems; if they continue for a few cycles see your doctor.
- ☐ You may like to contact one of a number of self-help groups for information and/or support – for example, the National Endometriosis Society*.

ENDOMETRIOSIS

Occasionally small pieces of the lining of the womb, the endometrium, grow in other parts of the pelvic cavity outside the womb. Most commonly growths occur on the ovary, on the surface of the womb, bladder or bowel. Each month these pieces of tissue swell and bleed, causing pain. Some blood is absorbed, but some may remain to form cysts on the ovaries or tissues may become sandwiched together with scar tissue to form adhesions. You may have severe pain just before or during the first few days of your period. Intercourse may be painful. Endometriosis sometimes leads to infertility. Specialist investigation via a laparoscope is usually necessary to confirm the diagnosis.

Treatment can be with a medicine or surgery or sometimes both. The abnormal tissue can be removed surgically; hysterectomy or removal of one or both ovaries may be necessary. Drug treatment can sometimes avoid the need for surgery, particularly in mild cases. Symptoms of endometriosis stop during pregnancy or the menopause and this observation led to the use of hormonal treatments to produce temporarily either a pseudopregnancy or 'menopause', usually for six months. The combined oral contraceptive is often first choice as unwanted effects are usually rare. A progestogen, such as **medroxyprogesterone acetate** or **norethisterone** may be used, but unwanted effects include bloating, fluid retention, weight gain, breast discomfort and skin disorders such as acne. A temporary medical menopause is brought about by using a *gonadotrophin-releasing hormone* (GnRH) such as **goserelin** (Zoladex), which first enhances and then reduces the release of pituitary hormones (FSH and LH – pages 334–5) in the brain. The normal action of oestrogen and progesterone is prevented and this reduces the endometrial growths both inside and outside the womb. Periods may stop as the ovaries also stop working during this time. The GnRH medicines, given either by monthly injection or nasal spray, are usually started in hospital, but then may be continued by your GP. Unwanted effects similar to the menopause occur which are relieved by taking HRT temporarily.

A three- to six-month course of **danazol** (Danol) or the similar **gestrinone** (Dimetriose) lowers oestrogen and progesterone hormone levels during the cycle by blocking the pituitary gonadotrophin hormones. They are used only if you do not respond to other treatments as unwanted effects limit their usefulness. These include weight gain, acne, dizziness, muscle cramps, lassitude, voice changes and extra hair growth. You must not become pregnant while taking either danazol or gestrinone; pregnancy is not usually possible with the other treatments.

MEFENAMIC ACID

MEFENAMIC ACID – Capsules, tablets, liquid for children

Mefenamic acid is a non-steroidal anti-inflammatory drug (NSAID) which relieves pain and swelling in arthritis and is used as an analgesic for relieving pain and for reducing fever in children. It is also used for relieving painful periods (primary dysmenorrhoea) and for treating excessive bleeding (menorrhagia). It acts by blocking the activity of prostaglandins, body chemicals involved in the transmission of pain. Like all NSAIDs, mefenamic acid may cause gastrointestinal upsets and should not be given to anyone with a peptic ulcer. Other NSAIDs such as **ibuprofen** can also be used for painful periods.

Before you use this medicine

Tell your doctor if you are:
☐ pregnant or breast-feeding ☐ taking any other medicines, including vitamins and those bought over the counter.

Tell your doctor if you have or have had:
☐ liver or kidney disease ☐ high blood pressure.

Do not use if you have or have had:
☐ allergy to aspirin or other NSAIDs ☐ severe kidney disease ☐ peptic ulcer or digestive disorders including inflammatory bowel disease.

How to use this medicine

Take one tablet (500mg) or one or two capsules (each 250mg) three times a day after food. (Children can be given the liquid for lowering a raised temperature but treatment should not be for longer than seven days, except for those with juvenile arthritis.)

Mefenamic acid may occasionally cause drowsiness or dizziness. If affected do not drive or operate machinery. Avoid alcohol as it may increase the risk of stomach bleeding.

Over 65 You may need less than the adult dose. Use with caution if you are dehydrated or have kidney disease.

Interactions with other medicines

NSAIDs interact with a number of different medicines. Always check with your doctor or pharmacist.
Lithium Possibility of increased blood levels and risk of toxicity.

Unwanted effects

Likely Heartburn or indigestion, feeling sick, diarrhoea.
Less likely Drowsiness, dizziness, constipation, abdominal pain or cramps, skin rash, wheezing or breathlessness.

If you develop severe diarrhoea or a skin rash while taking mefenamic acid, stop taking it and contact your doctor. You should not take mefenamic acid ever again. Contact your doctor immediately if you have bloody or black, tarry stools or vomit blood. In rare cases mefenamic acid may cause numbness or tingling arms or legs; if this happens contact your doctor.

Similar preparations

See other NSAIDs in Chapter 8.

Contraception

Contraception is the prevention of conception and pregnancy. There are several different methods: hormonal contraception, barrier methods such as the condom (sheath) or diaphragm, intrauterine devices (IUD), and, more permanently, sterilisation. The choice of contraception depends on how effective, safe and acceptable you and your partner find the method.

• *HORMONAL CONTRACEPTION* •

In 1961 the Family Planning Association* introduced the combined oral contraceptive, the 'pill', into its clinics and a new era of birth control began. The pill remains a popular, convenient method for preventing pregnancy, which is reversible and allows you to plan your family. Several million British women, particularly those who have not yet had children, choose oral contraception. There are two main types of oral contraceptives: oestrogen and progestogen combined in one tablet, the combined oral contraceptive, and the progestogen-only type. Hormonal contraception is also available as an injection, a weekly skin patch, an implant or as an intrauterine device (IUD).

• *Oral contraceptives*

The **combined oral contraceptive** containing an oestrogen and a progestogen is a most effective form of contraception, and this is the most popular type of pill for women under 30 years of age.

When an external source of oestrogen and progestogen is taken the body's hormonal control of ovulation is disrupted. The delicate balance and control between the sex hormones produced by the ovaries and the pituitary gland hormones, *follicle-stimulating hormone* (FSH) and *luteinising-hormone* (LH), produces the normal menstrual cycle and ovulation (pages 334–5). The hormones in the combined pill add to the body's supplies of oestrogen and progesterone so that the hormone levels are similar to those of pregnancy. In other words, the combined pill produces a state of 'pseudo-pregnancy'. The oestrogen content of the pill prevents the egg cell from ripening in the ovary by stopping FSH production, while the progestogen component acts on the cervix – the entrance to the womb – to form a sticky mucus plug to prevent sperm entering. Progestogen also blocks LH production.

You should use a preparation with the lowest oestrogen and progestogen content to give good cycle control and the fewest unwanted effects. Three generations of combined pills have been developed over the years. The first generation of combined pills in the early 1960s contained higher doses of oestrogen which increased the chances of a woman getting a blood clot in the deep veins of the legs, pelvis or lungs (*venous thromboembolism*). The second generation of pills contained less oestrogen, usually as ethinylestradiol, and the same types of progestogens as the first-generation pills. The third generation of pills launched in the 1980s contain lower doses of oestrogen and new forms of progestogen.

Oestrogens: ethinylestradiol is used in quantities varying from 20 to 40 micrograms (much lower doses than the first-generation pills). **Mestranol**, in Norinyl-1, is converted to ethinylestradiol in the body.

Progestogens: Older progestogens **norethisterone**, **levonorgestrel** and **etynodiol** used in the earlier-generation combined pills or alone (progestogen-only pill) may be more troublesome in terms of progestogenic effects, such as breast discomfort. Newer progestogens (**desogestrel**, **gestodene** and **norgestimate** – the third-generation pills) may have a more favourable effect on body metabolism, although desogestrel and gestodene slightly increase the risk of blood clots forming, particularly in the deep veins of the leg or pelvis – more than the older progestogens. Yet the risk of developing a blood clot with a newer progestogen is lower than with pregnancy. It is not clear whether the third newer progestogen, norgestimate, also has this effect. **Drospirenone**, the newest progestogen in a combined oral contraceptive (▼Yasmin), may cause less fluid retention.

Should you take the pill?

Taking any medicine carries some risks of harm as well as bringing benefits. When you take the pill you should understand that you are taking a medicine that will modify your body's hormonal system even though you are not unwell. Discuss with your doctor the pros and cons of taking oral contraception and of other contraceptive methods. Predictable unwanted effects such as breakthrough bleeding, fluid retention and feeling sick may lessen after the first few cycles of the pill or resolve if you switch to another preparation. However, oral contraception is not suitable for every woman and your doctor will need to check carefully that you do not have a condition that prevents you from using this form of contraception.

Pros: The combined pill is very effective as long as you take it regularly. It is convenient and does not get in the way of lovemaking. If you are a healthy non-smoker and have no risk factors such as heart disease, you may take a low-strength pill up to the age of 50. Period problems such as painful or heavy bleeding are helped by taking the combined pill. Premenstrual tension may be reduced and you are less likely to have other gynaecological disorders, for example cancer of the lining of the womb and of the ovary, ovarian cysts, tubal pregnancy (ectopic pregnancy), infections of the womb and Fallopian tubes (pelvic inflammatory disease), anaemia because of heavy periods, and non-cancerous diseases of the breast (benign breast disease).

Cons: Oestrogen increases the risk of abnormal blood clots forming, particularly in the deep veins of the legs or pelvis (venous thromboembolism). The clot may break off and travel to the heart, lungs or the blood vessels in the brain to cause conditions such as heart attack, angina or stroke and possibly death. Lower doses of oestrogen in the pill (below 50 micrograms) have reduced this risk considerably.

Progestogens also influence the formation of abnormal blood clots; the older ones (levonorgestrel, norethisterone) slightly less so than the newer ones (desogestrel and gestodene). Every year, about 5 per 100,000 healthy women not taking any oral contraceptive will develop an abnormal blood clot. In women using an oral contraceptive containing one of the older progestogens, the chance of developing a blood clot increases to about 15 per 100,000 women per year; in those using a contraceptive containing one of the newer progestogens, the chance is very slightly greater at 25 per 100,000. The chance of developing a clot also increases overall with age and if there are other risk factors for venous thromboembolism (being overweight, having varicose veins or a previous history of blood clots from any cause). However, the chance of developing a clot during pregnancy (about 60 per 100,000 pregnancies) is greater than with any combined oral contraceptive. The Committee on Safety of Medicines (CSM) now advises that, provided women are fully informed of the small risks and there are no medical reasons why they cannot take particular oral contraceptives, the decision about which to use should be based on the personal choice of the woman and the clinical judgement of her doctor.

There is also a risk of developing conditions such as high blood pressure, jaundice, cancer of the liver or gallstones. There is a small increase in the risk of developing breast cancer during the time when you take an oral contraceptive, but the risk disappears over a ten-year period once you have stopped taking the pill. The combined oral contraceptive protects against ovarian and endometrial cancer and any cancer-promoting effects have to be balanced against these well-established facts.

The combined pill should not be used if:

- ☐ you smoke 15 or more cigarettes a day and are aged at least 35 years
- ☐ you have high blood pressure – 160/100mmHg or more
- ☐ you have or have had abnormal blood clots (venous thromboembolism)
- ☐ you have or have had a stroke or ischaemic heart disease
- ☐ you have severe recurrent headaches or migraine with aura
- ☐ you have or have had breast cancer
- ☐ you have liver tumours or severe cirrhosis
- ☐ you have valvular heart disease – e.g. bacterial endocarditis, atrial fibrillation
- ☐ you have diabetes mellitus with evidence of circulatory problems or deterioration in kidneys, nerves or eyes
- ☐ you require major surgery with prolonged immobilisation due to illness or accident.

The progestogen-only pill avoids some of the risks of the combined pill and the effects of oestrogen. More commonly used by older women, it is reasonably reliable and if you take it at the same time each day its effectiveness is improved. It is convenient and does not get in the way of love-making. It can be used while breast-feeding and allows a rapid return to fertility when stopped. The risks are irregular periods, heart or circulatory disease and ovarian cysts. You should not take the progestogen-only pill if you have breast cancer currently.

Starting the pill

The **combined pill** can be started on day one of your period and is usually taken once a day for 21 days. You will then have seven days without the pill, or may have seven inactive (placebo) tablets (in every day 'ED' formulations) to take before starting the next packet of pills.

Bleeding usually occurs during this pill-free week. You will not need additional contraception unless you start the course on day four of your period or later, when ovulation may not be stopped during the first cycle. If you miss a pill, especially at the beginning or end of the packet, you are less well protected and may need to take additional contraceptive measures (see 'If you miss a pill', page 358).

The **phased combined oral contraceptive** is designed to provide a low total hormone dose and to mimic more closely the body's hormone patterns. There are two or three phases and each provides a different proportion of oestrogen and progestogen. Different phases are indicated by different-coloured tablets, and you have to take care to start with the correct tablet for day one.

The **progestogen-only pill** and long-acting progestogen-only forms can be used if you are unable to take oestrogen in the combined pill, for instance if you smoke, have high blood pressure, heart disease or have diabetes. The progestogen-only pill can provide good and effective contraception if you are approaching the menopause. Its main drawbacks are that periods may disappear or become heavy and irregular with breakthrough bleeding and you have to be conscientious in taking the pill at the same time each day (or within three hours) – see 'If you miss a pill', page 358.

HOW YOU CAN HELP YOURSELF

- ☐ Plan your contraception: discuss the matter with your doctor or visit a family planning clinic.
- ☐ Find out what the various methods are and discuss the benefits and risks.
- ☐ Give up smoking, particularly if you take the combined pill, as this will lessen the rare but serious risks of blood clots and other cardiovascular problems.
- ☐ If you take an oral contraceptive, visit your doctor regularly for blood pressure measurements and checks on your breasts and reproductive organs.
- ☐ Use a condom to protect against HIV and other sexually transmitted diseases.

Emergency contraception

If you have unprotected intercourse you had not planned, you can prevent an unintended pregnancy by taking two progestogen tablets (levonorgestrel 750 micrograms) within 72 hours (three days). Your doctor or nurse can prescribe or supply them, or if you are over 16 years of age you can buy a pack from a pharmacy. The high dose of progestogen can make you feel or be sick, but these symptoms are short-lived and rarely serious. If you are sick within three hours of taking the tablets, you can have a further course of tablets, usually with an antisickness medicine such as **domperidone,** which can be prescribed or bought from a pharmacy as Motilium 10.

This method cannot usually be used for intercourse which has taken place more than 72 hours earlier and not if you are already pregnant. It will not protect you against pregnancy during future intercourse later in the cycle and you will need to use a barrier method, such as a condom, until the next period. Your next period may be early or late. The high-dose tablets are 95 per cent effective if taken within the first 24 hours following

IF YOU MISS A PILL

Combined and phased pills

It is important to bear in mind that the critical time for loss of protection is when a pill is forgotten at the beginning or end of a cycle. The following advice is recommended by family planning organisations:

'If you forget a pill, take it as soon as you remember, and the next one at your normal time. If you are 12 or more hours late with any pill (especially the first in the packet) the pill may not work. As soon as you remember, continue normal pill taking. However, you will not be protected for the next seven days and must either not have sex or use another method such as the condom.

'If these seven days run beyond the end of your packet, start the next packet at once when you have finished the present one – do not have a gap between packets. This will mean you may not have a period until the end of two packets but this does you no harm. Nor does it matter if you see some bleeding on tablet-taking days. If you are using every day (ED) pills, miss out the seven inactive pills. If you are not sure which these are, ask your doctor or pharmacist.'

Progestogen-only pills

The following advice is recommended by family planning organisations:

'If you forget a pill, take it as soon as you remember and carry on with the next pill at the right time. If the pill was more than three hours overdue you are not protected. Continue normal pill-taking, but you must also use another method, such as the condom, for the next seven days.'

Illness: Vomiting up to three hours after taking the pill (both the combined and progestogen-only type) or very severe diarrhoea can interfere with its absorption and lessen its effectiveness. Use additional precautions, such as the condom, for any intercourse during the stomach upset and for the next seven days after recovery. If vomiting and diarrhoea occur during the time when you take your last seven tablets of a pack of combined pills, omit the pill-free interval or inactive tablets for an ED pack and continue straight on with your next pack.

unprotected intercourse, but effectiveness falls to 58 per cent by 72 hours. If pregnancy is not prevented the progestogen will not harm the baby, but there is a slightly increased risk that the baby could develop in the Fallopian tubes (an ectopic pregnancy). If you develop abdominal pains see your doctor promptly. Also you will need to see your doctor again three to four weeks after taking progestogen tablets if your period is abnormally light, heavy or brief or absent to check that you are not pregnant.

Alternatively the insertion of an *intrauterine device* (IUD) is effective if it is inserted within five days of unprotected intercourse.

COMBINED PILL

ETHINYLESTRADIOL + PROGESTOGEN

Combination preparations
ETHINYLESTRADIOL 20 MICROGRAMS:
FEMODETTE; LOESTRIN 20; MERCILON*

ETHINYLESTRADIOL 30 MICROGRAMS:
EUGYNON 30; FEMODENE*; FEMODENE ED*; LOESTRIN 30; MARVELON*; MICROGYNON 30; MICROGYNON 30 ED; MINULET*; OVRANETTE; ▼ YASMIN*

ETHINYLESTRADIOL 35 MICROGRAMS:
BREVINOR; CILEST*; NORIMIN; OVYSMEN

Patch preparation
EVRA*

Phased preparations
BINOVUM; LOGYNON; LOGYNON ED; SYNPHASE; TRIADENE*; TRI-MINULET*; TRINORDIOL; TRINOVUM

For severe acne and moderately severe hirsutism
CO-CYPRINDIOL (DIANETTE) – Tablets
ETHINYLESTRADIOL 35 MICROGRAMS + CYPROTERONE 2mg

* Contains newer progestogen

Ethinylestradiol is a synthetic female sex hormone. It is used mainly in combination with a progestogen in the combined oral contraceptive to prevent pregnancy. If taken regularly, the combined oral contraceptive offers very effective contraception.

Ethinylestradiol was used in lower doses to relieve menopausal symptoms, but other HRT preparations are now preferred. When oestradiol is combined with cyproterone as co-cyprindiol (Dianette) it is effective treatment for severe acne which has not responded to antibacterial therapy (page 447). This product is also an effective oral contraceptive.

Ethinylestradiol is a potent oestrogen and is sometimes used in the treatment of breast cancer.

Before you use this medicine

Tell your doctor if you are:
□ pregnant – the pill should not be taken as there may be a very small risk of malformation in the baby □ breast-feeding – not recommended: a progestogen-

only contraceptive can be used □ taking any other medicines, including vitamins and those bought over the counter.

Tell your doctor if you have or have had:
□ diabetes with circulatory changes □ heart disease or high blood pressure □ kidney disease □ migraine □ epilepsy or seizures □ depression □ asthma □ sickle-cell anaemia □ inflammatory bowel disease, including Crohn's disease.

Do not take if you have or have had:
□ blood clots, or a family history of these or clotting disorders □ recurrent jaundice – acute and chronic liver disease □ porphyria □ disorders of blood fats (hyperlipidaemia) □ breast or endometrial cancer □ oestrogen-dependent tumours □ severe migraine □ unexplained vaginal bleeding □ a rare skin condition (pemphigoid gestationis) during pregnancy □ certain types of jaundice (Dubin-Johnson or Rotor syndromes) □ deterioration of the ear problem otosclerosis during pregnancy.

How to use this medicine

Take the pill marked day 1 or number 1 or the correct day of the week on the first day of your period. Take one pill daily, if possible at the same time each day until you finish the 21 pills in the pack. For every day (ED) preparations you take 28 pills. If you start the pill on the first day of bleeding, you will be protected from the first day and do not need additional contraceptive measures. If you start your course of pills on the fourth day of bleeding or later, you will need to take additional precautions for seven days.

After you have taken the course of 21 pills, you have a pill-free week during which time bleeding may occur. You will probably have less bleeding and it may be a different shade of red. Sometimes bleeding occurs while you are taking the pills – this is called breakthrough bleeding or spotting which usually settles after the first few cycles. Do not stop taking the pills but mention this to your doctor or nurse when you go for a check up. For ED preparations you start a new pack as soon as you have finished the course of 28 pills.

Changing pills If you change from one combined pill to another, if possible take the first pill of your new pack on the day immediately after finishing your old pack. Bleeding will be delayed until you have finished the new course, although you may get some irregular bleeding in the meantime. You will not need additional contraception but if you take a seven-day break before starting the new pill, you will need additional contraception.

Surgical operations If you have to have surgery you may need to stop taking the combined or progestogen-only pill four weeks before major surgery or any surgery to the legs. You can usually start taking the pill at least two weeks after the operation when you have your next period and are active again. Alternatively you could continue the combined pill and request standard hospital procedures to prevent blood clots developing. If you have to lie in bed for some time because of an accident or a long illness then it is best to stop taking the pill until you are up and about. Alternatively the progestogen-only pill could be used instead.

Do not stop taking the pill unless you want to change contraception or you have decided that you want to have a baby. You should wait until you have had two periods after stopping the pill before you try to get pregnant. Ask your doctor about other contraceptive precautions to cover this time. If you become pregnant straight away, this should not be harmful. You may need to stop the pill for medical reasons (see below).

If you miss a dose, take it as soon as you remember – see 'If you miss a pill', page 358. Diarrhoea and vomiting may interfere with the absorption of the pill and reduce its effectiveness – see also page 358.

Over 65 There are similar oestrogens in hormone-replacement preparations.

Interactions with other medicines

The contraceptive effectiveness of the combined pill, including the patch, and the progestogen-only pill may be reduced by interactions with a number of medicines. Do not take other medicines without checking with your doctor, nurse or pharmacist. If you are taking long-term medication (for example, for epilepsy) you may need to take a higher-dose pill or use an alternative contraceptive method. These are the most important interactions:
Antibacterials: rifampicin and rifabutin greatly reduce the effectiveness of the pill or the patch. You will need to use additional contraceptive measures, such as condoms, while taking either of these and for four to eight weeks after stopping treatment. Other broad-spectrum antibiotics, such as **ampicillin** and **doxycycline**, may interfere with oestrogen absorption, which is a problem for short courses only. Use additional contraception for seven days after stopping treatment. If the antibiotic course lasts longer than two weeks, additional precautions become unnecessary. Your body develops resistance to this interaction.
Anticoagulants such as **warfarin** Blood thinning effect reduced by ethinylestradiol.
Ciclosporin Immunosuppressant blood levels increased by the pill.
The following medicines also reduce the pill or the patch's effectiveness.
Antidepressant St John's wort.
Antiepileptics: carbamazepine, **oxcarbazepine, phenobarbital**, **phenytoin**, **primidone** and **topiramate.**
Antifungals: griseofulvin and possibly other antifungals.
Some **antivirals** for HIV.
Bosentan for lung problems.
Modafinil for narcolepsy.

Unwanted effects

Likely Feeling or being sick, headache, breast tenderness, changes in weight, fluid retention.
Unlikely Blood clots (more common with factor V Leiden or in blood groups A, B, AB than O), changes in libido, depression, skin changes (e.g. brown patches), high blood pressure, liver disease, contact lenses may irritate.
Rare Increased sensitivity to sunlight.

Unwanted effects are usually mild and fade as you continue treatment. However, there are a number of rare adverse effects and if you have any of the following symptoms, you must stop taking your contraceptive and contact your doctor immediately:

☐ a sudden sharp or severe pain in the chest ☐ sudden shortness of breath or painful breathing ☐ unexplained cough ☐ painful or inflamed leg (e.g. calf) ☐ a crushing type of chest pain or heaviness in the chest ☐ the very first attack of migraine ☐ worsening of existing migraine ☐ sudden and unusually severe headache ☐ dizziness or fainting, quite different from anything you have had before ☐ change in normal vision or speech ☐ sudden partial or complete loss of vision ☐ weakness or numbness in one arm or leg ☐ swelling in the limbs ☐ severe depression.

Similar preparations

Combination preparations
MESTRANOL 50 MICROGRAMS:
NORINYL-1

LEVONORGESTREL

PROGESTOGEN-ONLY

Progestogen-only preparations with levonorgestrel or norgestrel
MICROVAL; NEOGEST; NORGESTON
MIRENA – Intra-uterine system

Combination preparations
EUGYNON 30; MICROGYNON 30; MICROGYNON 30 ED; OVRANETTE

Phased preparations
LOGYNON; LOGYNON ED; TRINORDIOL

Emergency contraception
LEVONELLE 2, LEVONELLE (from a pharmacy)

Levonorgestrel, or the related norgestrel, is a synthetic version of the female sex hormone progesterone. It is a single ingredient of the progestogen-only pill, a useful alternative if you cannot take the combined pill, or it is used with an oestrogen such as ethinylestradiol in the combined pill. Levonorgestrel acts on the cervix, the entrance to the womb, to form a sticky, mucuous plug making it difficult for sperm to enter. Levonorgestrel also interferes with luteinising hormone (LH) production. The progestogen-only pill may cause periods to disappear or become irregular. Breakthrough bleeding is sometimes a problem, although this often settles with long-term use. It is suitable for smokers of any age, older women and those who have unwanted effects with oestrogens.

Some progestogens similar to levonorgestrel are used in the treatment of cancers, including breast cancer.

Before you use this medicine

Tell your doctor if you are:
☐ pregnant – the pill should not be taken; there may be a very small risk of malformation in the baby ☐ breast-feeding – low doses of progestogen may pass through into the milk but are not harmful. You can take a progestogen-only pill from day 21 after your baby is born and this will protect you immediately. If you start after this time, you may need additional protection during the first 48 hours of pill-taking ☐ taking any other medicines, including vitamins and those bought over the counter.

Tell your doctor if you have or have had:
☐ diabetes with circulatory changes ☐ high blood pressure or heart or circulatory disease ☐ tubal pregnancy (ectopic pregnancy) ☐ ovarian cysts ☐ malabsorption syndromes ☐ migraine or migraine triggered by the combined pill.

Do not take if you have or have had:
☐ blood clots ☐ unexplained vaginal bleeding ☐ severe arterial disease ☐ severe liver disease ☐ itching of whole body during pregnancy or unexplained jaundice ☐ certain types of jaundice (Dubin-Johnson or Rotor syndromes) ☐ porphyria ☐ sickle cell anaemia.

How to use this medicine

Take the pill marked with the correct day of the week on the first day of your period. Take one pill daily, at the same time each day. Accurate pill-taking will improve reliability. You will be protected from the first day and do not need additional contraceptive measures. Continue taking a pill every day until you finish all the pills in the pack.

When you have finished the first pack, start your next pack the next day. Take a pill from the pack for the appropriate day of the week. Progestogen-only pills are taken without a break.

If you change from the combined pill to progestogen-only, start taking the new pill the day after completing the combined pill course so that there is no break in pill-taking.

Do not stop taking the pill unless you have decided to change contraception or you want to have a baby. You should wait until you have had two periods after stopping the pill before you try to become pregnant. Ask your doctor about other contraceptive precautions to cover this time. If you become pregnant straight away, this should not be harmful. You may need to stop the pill for medical reasons (see pages 355–6).

If you miss a dose, take it as soon as you remember and take the next one at the normal time – see 'If you miss a pill', page 358.

Over 65 There are similar progestogens in hormone replacement preparations.

Interactions with other medicines

Levonorgestrel may interact with other medicines or the effectiveness of the pill may be reduced – see also interactions for the combined pill, page 361. Do not take other medicines without checking with your doctor or pharmacist.

Unwanted effects

Likely Absent or irregular periods or changes in menstrual pattern, changes in weight, breast tenderness, swollen feet and ankles.
Less likely Feeling or being sick, headache, migraine, depression, dizziness.

If you have any of the following, stop taking the progestogen-only pill and contact your doctor;

☐ migrainous headaches develop or worsen ☐ sudden visual, hearing or perceptual disturbances ☐ painful, inflamed or swollen legs ☐ stabbing chest pains, coughing, tightness in the chest ☐ jaundice, hepatitis or itching all over ☐ significant rise in blood pressure ☐ before surgery (page 360).

Similar preparations

Progestogen-only preparations

CERAZETTE
DESOGESTREL

FEMULEN
ETYNODIOL

MICRONOR
NORETHISTERONE

NORIDAY
NORETHISTERONE

Implants

IMPLANON
ETONOGESTREL

Injections

DEPO-PROVERA
MEDROXYPROGESTERONE ACETATE

NORISTERAT
NORETHISTERONE

Combined with ethinylestradiol (oral)

BREVINOR
NORETHISTERONE

CILEST
NORGESTIMATE

Combined with ethinylestradiol (oral) continued

FEMODENE/FEMODENE ED/FEMODETTE
GESTODENE

LOESTRIN 20/LOESTRIN 30
NORETHISTERONE

MARVELON
DESOGESTREL

MERCILON
DESOGESTREL

MINULET
GESTODENE

NORIMIN
NORETHISTERONE

OVYSMEN
NORETHISTERONE

▼YASMIN
DROSPIRENONE

Phased preparations

BINOVUM
NORETHISTERONE

SYNPHASE
NORETHISTERONE

TRIADENE
GESTODENE

TRI-MINULET
GESTODENE

TRINOVUM
NORETHISTERONE

Long-acting progestogen-only contraceptives

Medroxyprogesterone acetate (Depo-Provera) injection provides three months' contraception and can be given for long-term contraception, or it may be useful as an interim measure, for example before your partner's vasectomy becomes effective. It is as effective as the combined pill, reversible and can be used without an upper age limit in smokers and for those who cannot tolerate oestrogen. **Norethisterone enantate** (Noristerat) is an oily injection which is effective for eight weeks and can be used immediately after you have had a baby. **Mirena** is an intrauterine system that releases a low dose (20 micrograms) of levonorgestrel daily into the womb. Similar in shape and size to a standard intra-uterine device, it provides up to five years' contraception. These different ways of giving progestogen provide additional contraceptive choice, particularly when long-term contraception is required. They avoid daily pill-taking, but disturb the menstrual cycle, although after a few months' use with Depo-Provera or Mirena blood-loss lessens. Transient infertility may occur after stopping treatment with Depo-Provera, but there is no evidence of permanent infertility. The contraceptive effect of Mirena and of Implanon implants is rapidly lost once taken out.

OTHER METHODS OF CONTRACEPTION

Barrier methods (condoms, diaphragms and caps) are popular now because they can protect against sexually transmitted diseases and prevent the spread of human immunodeficiency virus (HIV).

Condoms are readily available and free from the risks of hormonal contraception. The condom is very effective if used properly. However, the failure rate can be high if the condom is not applied properly to the penis and before genital contact occurs. The female condom (Femidom) offers similar protection. Training in how to use these is available at family planning clinics. Ideally two methods of contraception should be used, particularly by young people – a reliable method such as the pill, and the condom to protect against sexually transmitted infection. This is known as 'double dutch' protection.

Diaphragms and caps placed over the cervix prevent the sperm reaching the womb. The diaphragm can be inserted several hours before intercourse but must be left in place for at least six hours afterwards. The diaphragm or cap needs to be fitted for each woman and requires a little training and practice before regular use as a contraceptive.

Diaphragms and condoms are usually used with spermicides – chemicals which kill sperm cells – for additional protection. Spermicides do not give adequate protection when used alone. The effectiveness of condoms and diaphragms can be reduced if you use them with an oil-based lubricant or ointment, for example if you are using a local treatment for a candidal infection or use an oestrogen cream for menopausal symptoms. Oil-based vaginal and rectal preparations, including pessaries, ointments, creams, gels and suppositories, can damage latex rubber so that not only is contraceptive efficacy reduced but there is less protection from sexually transmitted diseases. Check with your doctor or pharmacist whether local vaginal or rectal treatment or the lubricant you use is compatible with the condom or diaphragm.

An intrauterine device (IUD) or coil is a small solid plastic device placed in the womb to prevent pregnancy. Most devices are now made of copper wound on to the stem of a plastic carrier; some have silver cores. The IUD is effective at preventing pregnancy and is suitable for women who have had children; it can now be left in place for five years before replacement with a new one. Any device fitted after the age of 40 may be safely left in place until the menopause because fertility declines with age.

The IUD is not ideal for younger women who have not had children and who may have a number of sexual partners. Its use has been associated with pelvic inflammatory disease (PID), for example with Chlamydia, and infertility. The device is usually fitted at the end of menstruation. It may cause pain and spotting between periods and heavier or prolonged bleeding for a few months but this usually lessens with time. If you find these unwanted effects unacceptable the device can be removed. The risk of infection is higher in the first 20 days following IUD insertion. You should be screened for Chlamydia, for example, before an IUD is fitted. If you experience sustained pain during the first three or four weeks with an IUD you should see your doctor urgently. An IUD should not be used if you are pregnant, have severe anaemia, very heavy periods, a history of tubal (ectopic) pregnancy, malignant tumours in the genital organs, pelvic inflammatory disease or you are having treatment which suppresses the immune system. A copper-carrying device is not suitable if you are allergic to copper.

Sterilisation of either the man or woman is popular with couples and has replaced the contraceptive pill as the most widely used method of birth control when the woman is over 30 or the family is considered complete. It is very effective contraception and difficult to reverse. The surgical procedure for either the male operation (vasectomy) or the female operation on the Fallopian tubes is straightforward, but the decision to go ahead with the method needs careful thought and discussion with your doctor.

Bladder disorders

Bladder disorders include inflammation in the bladder (*cystisis*: pages 280–2) and the urethra (*urethritis*), poor control or loss of control in passing urine (*urinary incontinence*), enlarged prostate (*benign prostatic hyperplasia*) and difficulty emptying the bladder (*urinary retention*). Infections in the bladder are usually caused by bacteria and are therefore treated with appropriate antibacterial drugs or preparations that change the acidity of urine. Signs of cystitis include the urge to keep passing urine although there is hardly anything to pass and it is painful to do so. Urethritis is inflammation or infection of the urethra, the tube that takes urine from the bladder to the outside. Urethritis is common in women after the menopause when changes to the reproductive organs may also affect the bladder and cause inflammation, frequent urination, difficult or painful urination and incontinence. Hormone replacement therapy (see Chapter 6) can help.

POOR BLADDER CONTROL

The sphincter muscles around the outlet of the bladder keep a constant pressure on the urethra and prevent urine escaping. As the volume of

TYPES OF INCONTINENCE

- ☐ **Stress incontinence** A small amount of urine leaks from your bladder as a result of even slight exertion – laughing, sneezing, coughing, jogging or lifting a heavy object – anything which exerts pressure on the abdomen to override the bladder's closure mechanism. Stress incontinence is nothing to do with psychological stress. Its main cause is the stretching and weakening of pelvic muscles which support the contents of the abdomen. This is common after childbirth and can get worse if nothing is done about it.
- ☐ **Dribble incontinence** Urine escapes gradually in drips or a thin trickle. This can be caused by severe constipation; by an overstretched bladder; or, in men, an enlarged prostate gland (which partially obstructs the urethral opening and prevents the bladder being completely emptied).
- ☐ **Urge incontinence** The bladder becomes overactive because the muscles in the bladder wall become unstable. You may need to go to the toilet frequently. The desire to pass water is so great that you cannot delay long enough to reach the toilet. This may be due to an infection – cystitis, for example – or some other irritation that makes the bladder contract involuntarily. Alternatively, you may not be able to reach the toilet in time because of an illness such as arthritis or medicines which slow your reactions or increase the volume of urine.
- ☐ **Nocturnal enuresis** Bedwetting in children who have bladder control during the day.
- ☐ **Double incontinence** Loss of control over both bowel and bladder emptying.

EXERCISES FOR PELVIC FLOOR MUSCLES

There is no need to set aside a special time or place for these exercises: they can be done sitting, standing, or even while walking.

- ☐ In a comfortable position, tighten the muscles around your back passage as if you were controlling an attack of diarrhoea. Do this several times until you are sure you have identified the correct muscles.
- ☐ Once you are familiar with the muscles gently pull them up, tightening them slowly to a count of four and then slowly relaxing them.
- ☐ When you pass urine, deliberately stop and start the flow by contracting the same muscles. Do this several times each time you pass urine – but make sure you always empty your bladder properly.

fluid increases in the bladder, stretch receptors in the bladder wall transmit this information to activate the nerves controlling the bladder. When the bladder is full, the nerves controlling urination signal the bladder muscles to contract. The sphincter muscles are then consciously relaxed to let urine out.

Urinary incontinence is the involuntary passing of urine. You find that you have no control over whether urine is passed, even if you try to stop it, or you may lose the nerve sensations that tell you the bladder is full or that urine is being passed. Whatever the cause, it can be a distressing and embarrassing problem. Urinary incontinence is a common complaint; about three million adults in Britain have a problem and many need to use an appliance or incontinence pads. Women are seven to eight times more likely to be affected than men and more than half of all women have experienced some loss of urinary control. Men, however, often accept symptoms as part of old age.

Management

Sometimes the onset of incontinence is gradual, for example in older people, but for others it can be sudden. The condition is worrying whether you lose small amounts of urine or a stream. You should see your doctor as soon as you realise you have a problem. Your doctor will ask you the following questions and it would be helpful to think about the answers and to jot them down beforehand.

- ☐ **Onset** When did the problem first start? Was it sudden or gradual?
- ☐ **Volume** Is the loss a constant dribble or an occasional flood?
- ☐ **Frequency** How often does it happen? Once a day, several times a day, or constantly?
- ☐ **Timing** Does it tend to happen more in the night or day?

Your doctor will want to find out the cause of incontinence as it can be a symptom of some underlying condition, such as an enlarged prostate (in a man). The aim is to treat the condition which should then cure or lessen

HOW YOU CAN HELP YOURSELF

- ☐ Know that incontinence is a common problem which can be investigated, treated or managed.
- ☐ Seek help and advice from your doctor, nurse or continence adviser. A physiotherapist can advise about exercises.
- ☐ A number of organisations can provide services and advice, including Age Concern*, the Disabled Living Foundation*, and the Enuresis Resource and Information Centre*.
- ☐ If you are a relative or carer of someone who is incontinent, find out as much as you can so that you can be understanding and reassuring.
- ☐ Take practical measures, such as having a commode or bedpan in every room and wearing clothing that is easily undone. The Disabled Living Foundation* can give advice on clothing.
- ☐ Do not cut down on the amount you drink as your body needs a certain amount of fluid each day. Take your fluids earlier in the day and avoid drinks late in the evening so that sleep is not disturbed.
- ☐ Take care to empty your bladder completely each time; bending forward at the waist may help.
- ☐ Keep a diary of when and how often you or the person you care for has incontinence.
- ☐ Exercise pelvic floor muscles (see box, page 367). These exercises should be routine for women after childbirth and are particularly helpful for stress incontinence.
- ☐ Make sure you know where there are toilet facilities when you are away from home.

the incontinence. If there is an infection then a course of antibiotics should help. Surgery may be necessary to correct a prolapse of the womb or to remove part or all of an enlarged prostate gland.

Sometimes there is no underlying cause; the bladder muscles simply contract, resulting in urinary frequency, urgency and sometimes incontinence. Bladder training for an over-active bladder or pelvic floor exercises for stress incontinence (women) are important treatments. Otherwise treatment with one of the following *antimuscarinic* medicines – **oxybutynin** (Ditropan; Cystrin; Lyrinel XL), **propantheline** (Pro-Banthine), **tolterodine** (Detrusitol), **propiverine** (Detrunorm) or **trospium** (▼Regurin) – may be helpful for urinary frequency and incontinence as it can lessen bladder muscle contractions and increase bladder capacity. All are similarly effective but unwanted effects can vary. Dry mouth is a common unwanted effect, although this may be less of a problem with newer modified-release preparations. Other medicines used include **flavoxate** (Urispas) or a tricyclic antidepressant, such as **imipramine** (Tofranil).

OXYBUTYNIN

OXYBUTYNIN – Tablets
CYSTRIN – Tablets
DITROPAN – Tablets, liquid
LYRINEL XL – Modified-release tablets

Oxybutynin is an antimuscarinic drug which relaxes the bladder muscles, allowing the bladder to hold more urine. It reduces the frequency of passing urine and is used for urinary incontinence, urgency and frequency in the unstable bladder. It can be used to help bladder control in conditions such as multiple sclerosis and spina bifida as well as for urge incontinence. Oxybutynin may be used, with other drug measures, for treating bedwetting in children usually aged over five years.

Before you use this medicine

Tell your doctor if you are:
☐ pregnant or breast-feeding ☐ taking any other medicines, including vitamins and those bought over the counter.

Tell your doctor if you have or have had:
☐ thyroid problems ☐ heart problems ☐ kidney or liver problems ☐ irregular heart rhythms ☐ high blood pressure ☐ enlargement of the prostate gland ☐ porphyria ☐ hiatus hernia.

Do not use if you have:
☐ obstruction of the bowel ☐ bladder outflow obstruction ☐ severe ulcerative colitis or toxic megacolon ☐ myasthenia gravis ☐ glaucoma.

How to use this medicine

Take one tablet two or three times a day. Occasionally your doctor may increase the dose to one tablet four times a day. Increasing the dose gradually reduces unwanted effects. The modified-release preparation is taken once a day and has fewer side effects.

Oxybutynin can cause drowsiness or blurred vision. Do not drive or do other activities that require alertness until you know how you react to oxybutynin. Small amounts of alcohol should not be a problem.

If you miss a dose, take it as soon as you remember, but skip it if it is almost time for your next dose. Do not take double the dose.

Your doctor should review the continuing need for treatment after six months.

Over 65 Frail older people will be more sensitive to the effects of the drug. You usually start with less than the standard adult dose.

Interactions with other medicines

Oxybutynin causes antimuscarinic unwanted effects such as dry mouth, visual disturbances and constipation. Many other medicines such as tricyclic antidepressants and phenothiazines have these effects and if two or three of these drugs are used together, unwanted effects are increased; in older people confusion is likely. Do not take other medicines without checking with your doctor or pharmacist.

Unwanted effects

Likely Dry mouth, constipation, blurred vision, feeling sick, abdominal discomfort, facial flushing, difficulty in passing urine.

Less likely Headache, incomplete emptying of the bladder, dizziness, drowsiness, dry skin, diarrhoea, irregular heart rhythms, skin problems such as rashes, reaction to the sun, local swelling, confusion, restlessness, hallucinations, seizures (rarely).

The most common unwanted effect is dry mouth, which can make you drink more and so aggravate urinary symptoms. Sucking a sweet or chewing gum will encourage saliva flow to keep the mouth comfortable.

Similar preparations

DETRUNORM – Tablets
PROPIVERINE

DETRUSITOL – Tablets, modified-release tablets
TOLTERODINE

PRO-BANTHINE – Tablets
PROPANTHELINE

▼ REGURIN – Tablets
TROSPIUM

URISPAS 200 – Tablets
FLAVOXATE

Not all cases of incontinence can be adequately controlled, and it may be necessary to use a special appliance or pads. There is a wide variety of appliances, portable urinals, collection bags for day and night use, and drainage tubes which your doctor can prescribe. The exact type of appliance depends on individual needs in different situations. For example bulky absorbent pads may be good at night, but something less obtrusive will be more appropriate during the day. There are also specially designed pants and discreet pads which can help you lead an unrestricted life. Incontinence pads are provided by local continence services free of charge to NHS patients.

Skin care is very important and the area should be kept clean and dry as far as possible to prevent sores. A barrier cream (page 425) may help after washing and drying.

Self-catheterisation is a technique that you may be able to learn and operate yourself. A catheter is a drainage tube that is inserted into the bladder to allow the urine to run out and be collected in a bag. Catheterisation is usually performed by a nurse or some other qualified person but some people with incontinence can be taught to do this for themselves. If you have incontinence or other urinary difficulties where the bladder contains a significant residual volume of urine then you may be a suitable candidate for self-catheterisation. You will need to catheterise yourself at least four times a day to prevent the bladder overfilling. The technique is not difficult, neither is it painful nor dangerous, but you will need to be taught by a doctor, continence adviser or nurse. You will also need to know how to look after the catheter and who to contact for advice at any time.

The advantages of self-catheterisation are that you can become 'dry', you can do without bulky external drainage appliances and you no longer need to remain within reach of a toilet. There should be no more smells of stale urine or embarrassing moments. Furthermore by establishing effective urinary drainage you will protect your kidneys from the effects of back pressure and urinary infection. Serious adverse effects are infrequent, especially in women. Bleeding sometimes occurs, but does not usually signify a serious problem, although you should always mention this to the nurse or doctor.

Bedwetting – nocturnal enuresis

Children usually do without nappies and gain control of their bladder function during the day by the age of two or three. Control over bladder function at night may come later, perhaps not until five or six years. Bedwetting occurs on most nights in about 15 per cent of five-year-olds and persists in as many as five per cent by the age of ten. Over 100,000 teenagers suffer from bedwetting; the Enuresis Resource and Information Centre* publishes a guide especially for this age group. If there is no underlying cause, such as a urinary tract infection, bladder training with or without the use of an enuresis alarm can be tried. An alarm system consists of a pad or mat which is placed under the child at night so that when urine is passed it completes an electric circuit, causing an alarm to sound and wake the child. After several weeks' use, the child becomes conditioned and wakes before passing urine or loses the urge to do so at night. There are also alarms that the child can wear with the detector placed in underpants and the alarm clipped to the clothing. Alarms are successful in about 65 per cent of children without any underlying cause of incontinence.

DRUGS WHICH CAN CAUSE INCONTINENCE

If you start drug treatment and experience a change in the way you urinate or defecate, ask your doctor or pharmacist if this could be caused by the drug(s). If you are already incontinent, have them regularly reviewed to check that they are not contributing to incontinence. Caffeine and alcohol may also contribute.

- ***Urinary incontinence***

Alpha blockers, e.g. **prazosin** – stress incontinence
Antimuscarinics, e.g. **atropine** – difficulty passing urine, leading to overflow
Diuretics, e.g. **furosemide** – urgency and frequency

- ***Faecal incontinence***

Opiate analgesics, e.g. **morphine**, **codeine** – leakage around constipation
Cancer treatments (chemotherapy) – diarrhoea

- ***Both***

Tricyclic antidepressants, e.g. **amitriptyline** – difficulty passing urine, leakage around constipation
Hypnotics, e.g. **benzodiazepines**, and tranquillisers, e.g. **phenothiazines** – reduced or clouded awareness, poor co-ordination

There are various alarm systems and only those conforming to Department of Health specifications or the British Standard should be used. None is available on NHS prescription but your doctor may be able to arrange one free on loan, or you can buy one.

Drug treatment of bedwetting is generally not recommended for children under seven years and is generally only used when other measures have not succeeded yet. Drug treatment and an alarm can be used together. Tricyclic antidepressant medicines such as **amitriptyline** (pages 200–203) or **imipramine** are effective, but behaviour disturbances and relapse are common after treatment stops. Unwanted effects include dry mouth, blurred vision, constipation, confusion and drowsiness; the drugs are toxic in overdosage. **Oxybutynin**, an antimuscarinic drug (page 369), may be used in children over five years; unwanted effects are similar to those of the tricyclic antidepressants. **Desmopressin** as a spray up the nose (Desmospray; Nocutil) or tablets by mouth (DDVAP; Desmotabs) is also used; unwanted effects are fewer and mild compared with the tricyclic antidepressants. The continuing need for drug treatment should be assessed by your doctor after three months – for example, by stopping treatment for one week.

INABILITY TO EMPTY THE BLADDER

Urinary retention usually occurs because the bladder muscles fail to contract sufficiently to push out all the urine. Urinary retention is a less common condition than incontinence, but causes include an enlarged prostate gland or tumour, or loss of nerve control over bladder function. Sudden and severe (acute) retention is painful and is treated by catheterisation. Your doctor will look for an underlying cause and surgery may be needed. Long-term (chronic) retention may be treated with a medicine to increase the strength of bladder muscle contraction. Drugs used include **distigmine** (Ubretid) which enhances the activity of the nerves to the bladder; **bethanechol** (Myotonine) is no longer recommended.

PROSTATE PROBLEMS

The prostate gland, a fleshy organ about the size of a large walnut, sits at the base of a man's bladder wrapped like a collar around part of the urethra. It is made of muscles and glandular tissue and during orgasm it shuts off the bladder and releases essential fluids into the semen. The prostate gland gradually enlarges in most men from middle age onwards as the cells in the gland multiply, most probably because of the continuous influence of male hormones. The enlargement is non-malignant and is known as *benign prostatic hyperplasia* (BPH). It can interfere with the flow of urine as the enlarged prostate gradually squeezes the urethra.

Many men over 60 years have an enlarged prostate but the amount of enlargement varies from man to man and you may not necessarily experience troublesome symptoms. Signs of enlarged prostate include difficulty passing water: delayed flow, stopping and starting in the middle of the flow, or straining to produce only a dribble. You may also feel an increased urge to go to the toilet. Actions such as turning on a tap or getting up in the morning may trigger the bladder so that you leak before you can get to the bathroom. Sleep may also be disrupted by visits to the toilet. Daily activities may be curtailed by the need to be in easy reach of a toilet.

If you are not distressed by your symptoms, simple lifestyle changes (reducing the quantity and timing of drinks, and training in bladder control) can help and may delay or avoid the need for further treatment. Advanced prostate trouble, however, may be painful and uncomfortable. The bladder cannot be completely emptied at each visit to the toilet, so urine left in the bladder can irritate it causing frequency and urgency, in a similar way to cystitis. In the long term the bladder wall may become deformed from the effort of straining to pass water. Incontinence may occur. Infection and back pressure on the kidneys can cause permanent damage. You may even experience a complete blockage of the urethra (*acute retention*), which requires emergency treatment to drain the bladder.

If you have urinary problems (some men have an enlarged prostate and an overactive bladder) you should discuss them with your doctor who will ask you about your symptoms and may use a scoring system to assess their severity. It will help your doctor if you can keep a diary for about a week before your appointment and note when and what you drink, when you have to go to the toilet and if possible how much urine you pass. Your doctor may then examine you to feel the size of the prostate through the rectum. Although the size of the gland bears no direct relationship to the severity of symptoms, this examination can be done to rule out other problems such as prostatic cancer. Blood and urine samples may also be needed.

Symptoms can improve spontaneously but if they interfere with your life you may need to see a urologist, a surgeon who specialises in bladder problems. The urologist will also ask you to describe your symptoms and will carry out further tests to assess whether you should have an operation, which at the moment is considered the best treatment. Watchful waiting, where no treatment is given unless your symptoms worsen, is a reasonable option. Tests include a urine test to look for infection, a urine flow test to see how fast you pass water, a blood test to assess the level of *prostate-specific antigen* (levels rise with age and sometimes in prostate cancer) and an ultrasound scan or x-ray of the bladder and kidneys.

The most popular operation, *trans-urethral resection of the prostate* (TURP), requires a general anaesthetic and amounts to a rebore of the gland. Medical treatment with an alpha blocker, which is usually tried first, include one of a range such as **alfuzosin** (Xatral), **doxazosin** (Cardura), **indoramin** (Doralese), **prazosin** (Hypovase), **tamsulosin** (Flomax) or **terazosin** (Hytrin BPH). These can relax the prostate and bladder muscles and increase urine flow. Alternatively, **finasteride** (Proscar) or **dutasteride** (▼Avodart) reduces the size of the prostate gland, which may improve symptoms while you wait for an operation or may be a useful alternative to surgery. These medicines generally produce modest improvements. Combination treatment with an alpha blocker (e.g. doxazosin) and a 5alpha-reductase inhibitor (e.g. finasteride) may give better results.

FINASTERIDE

PROSCAR – Tablets

Finasteride reduces the prostate size, improves the flow of urine and relieves other symptoms associated with benign prostatic hyperplasia. Testosterone and its more potent metabolite, dihydrotestosterone (DHT), are the male sex hormones essential for the normal development and regulation of the prostate. DHT seems to be the more active hormone and is mainly responsible for prostatic enlargement. Finasteride blocks the conversion of testosterone to DHT by inhibiting the enzyme (5alpha-reductase) responsible for this process. Benign prostatic hyperplasia develops very slowly and the process to reverse the enlargement is also gradual. Daily treatment for at least six months may be needed before symptoms improve and then only a proportion of men respond. Long-term treatment is needed to maintain any reduction in the prostate.

A low-strength finasteride tablet (▼Propecia) can be taken to assist hair growth for men with baldness problems.

Before you use this medicine

Tell your doctor if:

□ you have or have had treatment for cancer of the prostate □ your partner is pregnant or may become pregnant □ you are taking any other medicines, including vitamins and those bought over the counter.

Do not:

□ take if you are female, especially if you are or may become pregnant □ handle crushed or broken tablets if you are pregnant or may become pregnant □ give to children or young people.

How to use this medicine

Benign prostatic hyperplasia Take one tablet daily with water, with or without food. If you miss a dose, take it as soon as you remember, but skip it if it is almost time for your next dose. Do not take double the dose.

Baldness Finasteride 1mg tablet a day has to be taken continuously for three to six months before you see any results, and benefit reverses 6 to 12 months after you stop taking finasteride. It is not available on the NHS.

Over 65 No special dose requirements.

Unwanted effects

Finasteride is well tolerated. It must be taken by men only; exposure of a pregnant woman to the drug may cause abnormalities of the external genitals of a male fetus. Use a condom or other form of reliable contraception if your partner is able to become pregnant.

Likely Effects on sexual function: impotence, decreased libido and reduced volume of fluid on ejaculation; breast tenderness and enlargement; pain in the testicles; hypersensitivity reactions (rash, lip swelling).

Finasteride affects the prostate-specific antigen test.

Similar preparations

▼ AVODART – Capsules
DUTASTERIDE

Erectile dysfunction

About 1 in 10 men in the UK is consistently unable to achieve or maintain an erection during intercourse, a condition known as *erectile dysfunction* (previously referred to as impotence). Erectile dysfunction is a symptom not a disease and there may be one or more possible causes of the problem which your doctor will need to establish. Erectile function can decline as men grow older but other causes include heart and circulatory disease, high blood pressure, diabetes, neurological disorders such as multiple sclerosis, Alzheimer's disease, Parkinson's disease, HIV infection, epilepsy and spinal cord injury. These conditions or diseases enhance the decline that may occur with advancing years. Erectile dysfunction is an unwanted effect of some drugs such as **antihypertensives**, **digoxin**, **anabolic steroids**, **antidepressants**, **antipsychotics** and **benzodiazepines**. Alcohol or substance misuse and smoking also increase the likelihood of impotence. Psychological factors are occasionally the main problem but more commonly, they seem to exacerbate a pre-existing physical problem.

Treatments for erectile dysfunction have been revolutionised by the introduction of medicines that can be taken by mouth. Previously the choices included medicines given by injection, surgery or the use of vacuum pumps, which are used to create a partial vacuum around the penis, drawing blood into it. Psychosexual therapy may be helpful for some men.

Sildenafil (Viagra), the first tablet preparation (introduced in 1998), is taken about one hour before sexual activity. This new class of medicine, known as a *phosphodiesterase type-5 inhibitor* or *PDE5 inhibitor*, works by relaxing the blood vessels to the penis, increasing blood flow as you become sexually excited. Other similar preparations have been marketed – **vardenafil** (▼Levitra) and **tadalafil** (▼Cialis) – which act in the same way, although they vary in how soon they start to work and for how long they continue to have an effect. PDE5 inhibitors are not suitable for everyone and you should not take one if you take a nitrate preparation, such as **glyceryl trinitrate**, **isosorbide mono- or dinitrate** or **nicorandil** (Ikorel) for heart disease such as unstable angina, if you have low blood pressure, have had a recent stroke or heart attack, or if you have a hereditary degenerative disorder of the retina (*retinitis pigmentosa*). **Apomorphine hydrochloride** (▼Uprima), an alternative and different treatment, is dissolved in the mouth (sublingual) about 20 minutes before sexual activity. It has a short duration of action, about four hours compared with sildenafil and vardenafil (six to eight hours) and tadalafil (24 hours).

Other drug treatments for erectile dysfunction include **alprostadil injection** (Caverject; Viridal Duo) which is injected into the shaft of the penis or applied as a small pellet directly into the urethra using a special applicator (MUSE – medicated urethral system for erections). There is a small risk of the erection lasting longer than intended with alprostadil treatments; this can be dangerous, and you should seek emergency treatment if an erection lasts longer than four hours. If you use the urethral application and your partner is pregnant or may become pregnant, you should use a barrier contraceptive as alprostadil can get into the semen and may present a risk to a developing fetus.

Drug treatments for erectile dysfunction are available via the Selected List Scheme (page 18) on NHS prescription only for men with certain conditions, such as prostate cancer, kidney failure treated by dialysis or transplant, spinal cord injury, diabetes, Parkinson's disease or multiple sclerosis, or for those who were already receiving NHS treatment for erectile dysfunction on 14 September 1998. One treatment a week is generally recommended. Your doctor can write a private prescription (free of charge) if you are not in one of the recognised groups and have erectile dysfunction.

SILDENAFIL

VIAGRA – Tablets
SILDENAFIL

Sildenafil is a phosphodiesterase type-5 inhibitor (PDE5 inhibitor) which restores impaired erectile function by increasing blood flow to the penis. It will only help you to have an erection if you are sexually stimulated. Sildenafil acts indirectly on smooth muscle cells by increasing body chemicals which leads to the blood vessels relaxing in the penis. If you have heart disease your doctor will need to assess whether sildenafil or another PDE5 inhibitor is suitable for you. The main concerns are that if you have severe heart disease then sexual activity may worsen your condition or if you take sildenafil with an antianginal medicine, a nitrate, the two together can cause severe low blood pressure with the possibility of shock and circulatory collapse. Sildenafil must therefore not be taken in these situations. Sildenafil is not licensed for use in women.

Before you use this medicine

Tell your doctor if you have or have had:
☐ sickle cell anaemia ☐ cancer of the blood cells (leukaemia) or bone marrow (multiple myeloma) ☐ deformity of the penis e.g. Peyronie's disease ☐ stomach ulcer ☐ bleeding disorder e.g. haemophilia ☐ kidney or liver disease ☐ heart disease – your doctor will need to check that your heart can withstand the additional strain of sexual activity.

Do not take if you have:
☐ severe liver disease ☐ severe heart disease – unstable angina ☐ severe heart failure ☐ had a recent stroke or heart attack ☐ low blood pressure ☐ retinitis pigmentosa ☐ hypersensitivity to sildenafil.

Tell your doctor if you are taking any other medicine.

Do not take sildenafil if you take a medicine containing a nitrate or nicorandil or the recreational drug amyl nitrite ('poppers') as sildenafil will increase their effects markedly, leading to low blood pressure. Do not take sildenafil if you are using any other treatment for erectile dysfunction.

How to use this medicine

Take one tablet, usually 50mg about one hour before sexual activity is planned. Swallow the tablet whole with some water. Sildenafil works within half an hour to one hour but it will be less well absorbed into the body if you take it close to a meal.

Alcohol in large amounts can impair your ability to have an erection.

Sildenafil can cause dizziness and altered vision. Until you know how you react to it, you should avoid driving or other activities that require alertness.

You should not use sildenafil more than once a day. Taking a dose of more than 100mg does not increase sildenafil's effectiveness, but will increase unwanted effects.

Over 65 In older men and/or if you have severe impairment of kidney or liver function (e.g. cirrhosis), you should start with a low dose (25mg); the maximum recommended dose is 100mg.

Interactions with other medicines

Antianginal medicines Nitrates including **glyceryl trinitrate**, **isosorbide dinitrate** or **mononitrate** and also **nicorandil** (Ikorel) increase low blood pressure with sildenafil – these medicines must not be taken together.

Antivirals Avoid use together with **ritonavir**, a protease inhibitor for HIV – increases blood levels of sildenafil.

Alpha blockers for lowering high blood pressure or for prostate problems – avoid taking a dose of more than 25mg sildenafil within four hours of your alpha blocker.

Unwanted effects

Likely Headache, facial flushing, indigestion, dizziness, visual disturbances (e.g. increased perception of light, blue haloes, blurred vision), palpitations, nasal congestion.

Less likely Eye pain, rapid heart beat, being sick.

Rare Hypersensitivity reactions, heart attack, sudden death, irregular heart rhythm, nose bleeds, fainting, low blood pressure, prolonged erection, persistent painful erection (priapism) – a medical emergency.

Similar preparations

▼CIALIS – Tablets
TADALAFIL

▼LEVITRA – Tablets
VARDENAFIL

8

MUSCLES AND JOINTS

Osteoarthritis Rheumatoid arthritis
Gout Strains and sprains

The skeleton is the frame which encloses and protects the body's vital organs and to which muscles are attached. Over 200 bones make up the skeleton, allowing great variety of movement. The spaces between the ends of bones are joints, which are supported by strong *ligaments* and moved by the contraction of *muscles*. Muscles are connected to the skeleton at fixed points by *tendons*.

Covering the end of a bone and attached to it is a layer of tough tissue or *cartilage* which protects the bone. The greatest mobility occurs in *synovial joints* such as the knee or shoulder. In these joints the space between the adjoining ends of bones is enclosed by a strong membrane. This membrane produces *synovial fluid*, which lubricates the inside of the joint, permitting smooth movement and cushioning the bones as the joint bends, straightens or rotates.

Muscles, tendons and ligaments are tough tissues built to take the stresses and strains of body movements. However, they are subject to wear and tear with age or if used too much or too violently, for example during sporting activities. Joints also take a great deal of strain, and as you grow older the cartilage protecting the end of the bone can break down, causing pain and swelling. Disease can also affect joints to produce pain and inflammation.

Osteoarthritis

In osteoarthritis, cartilage is no longer able to repair itself and it becomes damaged and worn. The bone thickens, and bony outgrowths or 'spurs' grow around the joint. The joint may become inflamed and weakened; rarely, in severe cases it becomes deformed. The cause is not fully understood, but as you get older you are more likely to get osteoarthritis, particularly in the weight-bearing joints – the lower back, hips and knees. Osteoarthritis is more likely to develop if the joint has been used a great deal or has been damaged before, for example at work or playing sport, or if it was malformed at birth. Osteoarthritis does not normally start before the age of 50. It is more common in women.

Symptoms include pain and stiffness in the affected joint; swelling and tenderness sometimes occur. The condition may progress as the cartilage is worn away and eventually bone grates on bone; there is increasing pain and disability. Pain and stiffness are usually worse at the end of the day. The severity of osteoarthritis varies considerably from person to person, and mild forms may cause only a slight loss of cartilage with no symptoms.

HOW YOU CAN HELP YOURSELF

- ☐ Lose weight if you are overweight. Extra weight means an additional load on the weight-bearing joints and more wear and tear.
- ☐ Rest, particularly if you have osteoarthritis in a weight-bearing joint, before the pain becomes unbearable.
- ☐ Exercise. Ask your doctor what exercise you can do and how much. Gentle exercise will help to strengthen the muscles around the joint and prevent them from becoming stiff and weak. Swimming is useful – water allows you to take weight off the joints while exercising the muscles.
- ☐ See a physiotherapist in the early stages of arthritic disease rather than later. Physiotherapy teaches you the best way to keep joints mobile, strengthen muscles and adapt.
- ☐ Avoid sitting or standing in one position for long periods of time as this will make you stiff. Learn to reorganise postures and activities which seem to aggravate pain or stiffness and try to avoid them.
- ☐ Local heat may help to ease pain and stiffness. Massaging the joint helps the circulation and may give comfort.
- ☐ Walking aids, shoe insoles or 'trainers' can help to relieve the impact on affected joints.
- ☐ Find out about suitable aids and possible adaptations to your home to help you live and move about more easily. Occupational therapy in local social services departments may help. You will need a letter from your doctor.

Medicines for osteoarthritis

Arthritis treatments control and ease painful symptoms and maintain joint function, rather than cure the disease. Non-drug approaches are worth trying (see box) and may delay the need for pain relief using a medicine. The choice of medicine ranges from the simple analgesic paracetamol to a non-steroidal anti-inflammatory drug (NSAID), but local treatments with a topical NSAID (pages 382–5) or a corticosteroid injection into the arthritic joint (pages 390) may also be helpful.

Paracetamol on its own often provides effective pain relief (page 228). A dose can be taken on an occasional basis when you have infrequent pain, or regularly three or four times a day if you have pain and discomfort on most days. If paracetamol alone does not relieve the pain satisfactorily, you could take it with a low dose of an NSAID, such as **ibuprofen**, or an opioid analgesic, such as codeine (as **co-codamol**). This approach to pain relief is preferred for many osteoarthritic conditions, particularly if you are over 60.

Non-steroidal anti-inflammatory drugs (NSAIDs) are known as 'non-steroidal' drugs to distinguish them from corticosteroids, which are powerful steroidal drugs with dramatic anti-inflammatory properties (pages 382–5). An NSAID has two separate actions. In a single dose it has a similar pain-relieving activity to paracetamol and can therefore be used to ease mild or intermittent pain, for example, headaches, pain following surgery, period pains, back pain and strains and sprains (soft-tissue injury – muscles, tendons and ligaments). If taken regularly day after day, an NSAID also reduces the underlying inflammation which can make the joint swollen, hot and very painful; paracetamol does not do this. This combination of analgesic and anti-inflammatory effects makes NSAIDs particularly useful for treating pain and swelling associated with certain arthritic conditions, such as severe osteoarthritis and rheumatoid arthritis. An NSAID can also lower a raised temperature, although paracetamol is preferred because it avoids the risk of unwanted effects on the digestive system.

NSAIDs do not alter the progress of arthritic conditions but reduce inflammation and therefore pain by blocking *prostaglandin* production. Prostaglandins are body chemicals which were originally thought to have been made in the prostate gland (hence the name) but in fact are widespread throughout body tissues. They are involved as part of a cascade of body chemicals in the process of inflammation and transmission of pain, in the body's immune response and in tissue damage. Some NSAIDs known as Cox II selective inhibitors or Cox IIs, such as **meloxicam** or **rofecoxib**, have a more selective action on the enzymes (known as *cyclo-oxygenases*) that make prostaglandins, although all NSAIDs have a wide range of actions on body tissues, which explains why they can also cause an array of unwanted effects and are not suitable for everyone.

Cautions with NSAIDs

Effects on the digestive system If you have an active peptic ulcer, you should not take any type of NSAID, including selective NSAIDs (e.g. rofecoxib), because they can aggravate an ulcer, causing serious bleeding or perforation, where a hole develops in the stomach or intestine wall. These are life-threatening events and people have died from these effects, which have been worsened by taking an NSAID. Adverse effects on the gut can occur at any time during treatment, but are most common during the first month. Often the ulcer can bleed or perforate without any warning symptoms. The exception to this restricted use is when you have a serious arthritic condition (e.g. rheumatoid arthritis) and you need an NSAID to ease pain and stiffness even though you have an active ulcer. In this case your doctor must prescribe a medicine to protect the stomach and intestines (*gastroprotection*), usually with a proton pump inhibitor (e.g. **omeprazole**) or **misoprostol** (Cytotec), to prevent further injury to the stomach and intestine lining (pages 69–72).

If you have had an ulcer, bleeding or perforation in the past, but this has healed, the risk of harm remains and you should not take a non-selective NSAID (e.g. **diclofenac**). A selective NSAID, such as meloxicam or **etodolac**, or the 'coxibs' such as **celecoxib** or rofecoxib, can be taken cautiously; it has less of an effect on the gut and gastroprotection is not recommended. Your risk of harm from an NSAID increases if you are aged over 65 years, taking other medicines – such as aspirin for preventing heart attacks, an anticoagulant or corticosteroid – have other seriously debilitating illnesses or need to take an NSAID for long periods at high dosage. Again, the exception is that if you must take an NSAID in these situations, you should also have a medicine for gastroprotection (proton pump inhibitor or misoprostol).

Hypersensitivity All NSAIDs, including aspirin and the selective ones, can cause hypersensitivity or allergic reactions. If you develop wheezing, asthma symptoms, swelling, rashes (e.g. nettle rash) or acute runny nose (rhinitis), or any of these conditions worsen while you are taking an NSAID or applying one to the skin, then you should stop the NSAID. **Seek medical help immediately if these become serious anaphylactic reaction** (page 175).

Other cautions NSAIDs, including the selective ones, should be used with caution by older people and particularly by anyone who has poor kidney, liver or heart function. Many older people have some degree of kidney impairment, so an NSAID should always be used at the lowest possible dose for the shortest time to achieve an effect. If you are over 65 your doctor should avoid prescribing an NSAID for a long period if at all possible. If long-term treatment is necessary you should not have repeat prescriptions without regular check-ups. Your doctor should check your kidney function periodically if you are taking an NSAID for any length of time. You should avoid an NSAID if you are pregnant. Long-term use of some NSAIDs is associated with reduced fertility in women, but this is reversible once you stop treatment.

Unwanted effects of NSAIDs The main differences between the NSAIDs are in the severity and frequency of unwanted effects, such as indigestion, feeling sick and diarrhoea. Indigestion is common but can be lessened by taking an NSAID with or after meals; its occurrence is not linked to the development of an ulcer. NSAIDs cause their effects on the digestive system mainly through their blocking action on the prostaglandin chemicals, not through a direct effect on the gut itself. Taking enteric-coated preparations or NSAID suppositories does not avoid the risk of gut damage. Perforation, ulceration and bleeding can occur in the stomach or duodenum (see above). Other unwanted effects include headache, dizziness, vertigo, drowsiness, insomnia, increased sensitivity to sunlight (page 454), and ringing in the ears (tinnitus). Sometimes an NSAID can cause fluid to be retained in the body; one of the signs is ankle swelling. If you have heart failure (page 133) this will aggravate the problem further and your doctor would not usually prescribe an NSAID under these circumstances. The coxibs (e.g. rofe-coxib) must not be taken in severe congestive heart failure and used only cautiously if you have had heart failure, heart dysfunction (of the left ventricle) or high blood pressure. Any NSAID that causes fluid retention can increase blood pressure; it can worsen existing high blood pressure so that the risk of heart disease or stroke increases.

Taking two NSAID preparations by mouth at the same time does not increase effectiveness but it does raise the risk of unwanted effects. This includes taking ibuprofen bought over the counter for pain relief at the same time as a prescribed NSAID. Applying large amounts of a topical NSAID to the skin can lead to absorption into the body and the risk of unwanted effects.

Choice of NSAID

All NSAIDs have similar anti-inflammatory activity, but there is considerable variation in how people respond to any one NSAID. Your doctor may need to try several different NSAIDs before you find one that suits you. Most NSAIDs are rapidly absorbed and start to relieve symptoms during the first day of treatment, but sustained pain relief may not be achieved for a week and anti-inflammatory effects may take three weeks. You need to give each treatment a fair trial, so three weeks may be needed to assess activity. NSAIDs are usually taken by mouth as tablets, capsules or liquid. They are also used topically on the skin – for example, as a cream or gel for strains, sprains and bruising.

The Committee on Safety of Medicines (CSM) advises that ibuprofen is associated with the lowest risk of adverse effects on the digestive system. NSAIDs with a slightly greater or intermediate risk of gut problems include **diclofenac**, **naproxen**, **ketoprofen** and **indometacin**. **Piroxicam** seems to have an intermediate to higher risk, and **azapropazone** (Rheumox) has the highest risk. Its use is therefore restricted to rheumatoid arthritis, ankylosing spondylitis and acute gout when other NSAIDs have proved ineffective.

The selective NSAIDs cause fewer stomach and intestinal upsets than established NSAIDs. These unwanted effects are, nevertheless, still fairly common and are more likely at higher doses or when you also take aspirin for preventing heart problems. Selective NSAIDS include meloxicam (Mobic), etodolac (Lodine SR) and newer ones such as rofecoxib (Vioxx).

Aspirin, the original NSAID, is less widely used for pain relief because of its effects on the stomach which can occur at any dosage level. When taken in much higher doses (3.6g a day) aspirin has about the same anti-inflammatory effect as other NSAIDs, but at these doses aspirin is much more likely to cause unwanted effects such as stomach irritation, gastric bleeding, nausea and tinnitus.

IBUPROFEN

On prescription
IBUPROFEN – Tablets, liquid
BRUFEN – Tablets, liquid, soluble granules, modified-release tablets
FENBID – Modified-release capsules

Poor choice: combination preparation – better to use ingredients separately
CODAFEN CONTINUS – Modified-release tablets
IBUPROFEN + CODEINE

From a pharmacy/on prescription
NUROFEN FOR CHILDREN – Children's liquid (sugar-free)

Over the counter
Creams, gels and sprays for topical use:
DEEP RELIEF; FENBID; IBUGEL; IBULEVE; PROFLEX; IBUSPRAY

There are many brands of tablets, capsules and liquid for symptoms such as rheumatic and muscular pain, backache, migraine and headache, which include:
INOVEN; NUROFEN; MIGRAFEN; RELCOFEN (see also page 393).

Ibuprofen is a non-steroidal anti-inflammatory drug for relieving the swelling and pain of rheumatoid arthritis (including juvenile arthritis), ankylosing spondylitis (stiffening of the spine), osteoarthritis and other arthritic conditions. Ibuprofen blocks prostaglandin production, reduces inflammation and eases pain. It is also used for pain relief in conditions such as frozen shoulder, tendonitis, low back pain and soft tissue injuries. Ibuprofen is short-acting and has fewer unwanted effects than other NSAIDs but its anti-inflammatory effect is weaker. High doses are needed for treating rheumatoid arthritis, which may result in more serious unwanted effects; it is not suitable for inflammatory conditions such as acute gout. It reduces fever and is used as an analgesic in lower doses. Ibuprofen can be bought over the counter for pain relief in muscular and rheumatic conditions, dental pain, period pains and headache. Creams, gels and sprays are used topically for strains and sprains (soft tissue injuries).

Before you use this medicine

Tell your doctor if you are:
☐ pregnant – do not use, especially during the last three months ☐ breast-feeding – unlikely to be a problem ☐ taking any other medicines, including vitamins and those bought over the counter.

Tell your doctor if you have or have had:
☐ heart disease or high blood pressure ☐ heart failure ☐ kidney or liver disease.

Do not use if you have or have had:
☐ hypersensitivity to aspirin or other NSAIDs ☐ severe kidney disease ☐ peptic ulcer.

How to use this medicine

Take the dose three or four times daily with food or after meals. Tablet strengths include 200mg, 400mg and 600mg. Modified-release preparations may be taken once or twice daily. Granules should be dispersed in water before taking. Children with rheumatoid arthritis may take ibuprofen liquid if prescribed by a doctor. You can also buy children's preparations for reducing fever and relieving mild to moderate pain. Topical preparations are applied to the injured area three or four times daily.

Avoid alcohol as it irritates the stomach lining and increases the risk of stomach upsets. If you miss a dose, take it as soon as you remember. If your next dose is due within two hours take one dose and then skip the next.

Over 65 You may need less than the standard adult dose, especially if you have poor kidney function. If you are on long-term treatment, ask your doctor if you should have a kidney test periodically.

Interactions with other medicines

Do not take other medicines without checking with your doctor or pharmacist.
ACE inhibitors Their blood pressure-lowering effect is opposed; increased risk of kidney damage.
Analgesics Avoid taking two or more NSAIDs, including aspirin – increased risk of unwanted effects. **Ibuprofen** may reduce the cardioprotective effects of aspirin.
Antibacterials Possibly increased risk of seizures with quinolone antibiotics.

Anticoagulants Blood thinning effect of **acenocoumarol**, **warfarin** may be enhanced.
Antivirals: ritonavir increases blood levels of NSAIDs with increased risk of unwanted effects.
Diuretics Increased risk of NSAIDs' unwanted effect on kidneys.
Lithium Levels of lithium may be increased leading to toxicity.
Tacrolimus, immunosuppressant Increased risk of ibuprofen's unwanted effect on kidneys.

Unwanted effects

Likely Indigestion, heartburn, feeling or being sick, abdominal pain, diarrhoea.
Less likely Skin rashes, wheezing, breathlessness, dizziness, light-headedness, headache, hearing disturbances, ankle swelling and fluid retention, unusual bleeding or bruising, blood disorders, photosensitivity.

Contact your doctor if you develop **any** unwanted effects or if you have bloody or black, tarry faeces, stomach pains or cramps, or you vomit blood or material that looks like coffee grounds.

Similar preparations

BREXIDOL – Tablets
PIROXICAM

CLINORIL – Tablets
SULINDAC

DICLOFENAC – Tablets, injection, suppositories

DICLOMAX RETARD SR – Modified-release capsules
DICLOFENAC

DOLOBID – Tablets
DIFLUNISAL

EMFLEX – Capsules
ACEMETACIN

FELDENE – Capsules, dispersible tablets, 'melt' tablets, suppositories, gel, injection
PIROXICAM

FENBUFEN – Capsules, tablets

FENOPRON – Tablets
FENOPROFEN

FLEXIN CONTINUS – Modified-release tablets
INDOMETACIN

FROBEN – Modified-release capsules, tablets, suppositories
FLURBIPROFEN

INDOMETACIN – Capsules, suppositories, modified-release capsules

KERAL – Tablets
DEXKETOPROFEN

KETOPROFEN – Capsules

LEDERFEN – Capsules, tablets
FENBUFEN

MOBIFLEX – Tablets, injection
TENOXICAM

MOTIFENE 75mg – Modified-release capsules
DICLOFENAC

NABUMETONE – Tablets

NAPROSYN – Tablets, enteric-coated tablets
NAPROXEN

NAPROXEN – Tablets

ORUDIS – Capsules, suppositories
KETOPROFEN

ORUVAIL – Modified-release capsules, gel
KETOPROFEN

PIROXICAM – Capsules, dispersible tablets

PRESERVEX – Tablets
ACECLOFENAC

RELIFEX – Tablets, soluble tablets, liquid
NABUMETONE

RHEUMOX – Capsules, tablets
AZAPROPAZONE

SULINDAC – Tablets

SURGAM – Tablets, modified-release capsules
TIAPROFENIC ACID

SYNFLEX – Tablets
NAPROXEN

TIAPROFENIC ACID – Tablets

VOLTAROL – Tablets, modified-release tablets, dispersible tablets, injections, suppositories, gel
DICLOFENAC

VOLTAROL RAPID – Tablets
DICLOFENAC POTASSIUM

Combined with an ulcer-healing drug

ARTHROTEC – Tablets
DICLOFENAC + MISOPROSTOL

NAPRATEC – Separate tablets
NAPROXEN + MISOPROSTOL

* *Selective NSAIDs (COX IIs)*

▼ ARCOXIA - Tablets
ETORICOXIB

▼ BEXTRA – Tablets
VALDECOXIB

CELEBREX – Capsules
CELECOXIB

ECCOXOLAC – Capsules
ETODOLATE

ETODOLAC – Capsules

LODINE SR – Modified-release tablets
ETODOLAC

MOBIC – Tablets, suppositories
MELOXICAM

VIOXX – Tablets, liquid
ROFECOXIB

Nutritional supplements such as glucosamine and chondroitin may be beneficial in osteoarthritis and influence cartilage formation. Glucosamine may provide modest symptom relief if you have osteoarthritis of the knee, but the evidence for its use in other areas of the body is weak. Neither supplement is licensed as a medicine and information on long-term safety is lacking.

Injections into the knee joint

There are several products, such as Hyalgan and Synvisc, for reducing the pain of osteoarthritis in the knee. They contain a substance similar to hyaluronic acid, which is the main component of synovial fluid. They are given as a course of treatment by injection directly into the knee joint. One course may produce a small reduction in pain which can last for up to six months. After an injection there may be temporary pain, redness and swelling of the injected joint.

A corticosteroid injection into the joint may provide temporary benefit (page 390).

Rheumatoid arthritis

Rheumatoid arthritis is a disease of the whole body, not just the joints. It is an *autoimmune disease* – the body's defence mechanism, which normally protects you from infection, attacks your own tissue, including the joints. White blood cells normally recognise and attack foreign matter such as bacteria and make antibodies to fight off infection. In rheumatoid arthritis the body's immune system fails to recognise the body's own cells and turns its attack on the cells of the *synovial membrane*, causing swelling, heat and pain in the joint. If this process continues for months or years, the protective cartilage lining the bones becomes eroded, damaging the joint irreversibly.

Even within the first three to six months, bone damage may have started. All the body's joints can be affected but it is usually those of the hands, knees and feet that are involved, usually on both sides of the body.

A swollen and painful joint becomes stiff and difficult to move, and the symptoms are usually worse in the morning. Other symptoms include fever, weight loss, tiredness and anaemia. In severe cases rheumatoid arthritis involves the eyes, blood vessels, skin, heart or lungs, but this is rare. Rheumatoid arthritis affects approximately 1 per cent of the adult population and is more common in women than men. It can occur at any age, but often starts at between 30 and 50 years. You may have a mild form of the condition or it may be severe. The condition can go through dramatic ups and downs and can clear up completely. It may improve spontaneously or after a number of years 'burn out' (remit) but this is unpredictable.

The cause of rheumatoid arthritis is unclear although there is a great deal of research to find reasons as to why the body should attack its own tissues. It is not hereditary but it seems likely that some external trigger, possibly a virus or bacterium although this remains unproven, sets off the inflammatory process.

GETTING HELP

Your doctor Explain your symptoms clearly to your doctor so that together you can reach a better understanding of your problem and its treatment. See your doctor early in an attack so that treatment can be tailored to your needs. Find out what you can take for pain relief, and whether you should see a rheumatologist to discuss a strategy for managing the disease.

Rheumatoid arthritis is a disease involving the whole body, so it needs a total management plan involving other experts, surgeons, specialist nurses, physiotherapists, occupational therapists and teachers.

Self-help groups A number of organisations (for example, Arthritis Care★), provide information and advice about many aspects of arthritic diseases. Join a local branch for support from fellow sufferers.

Social services Find out if you are eligible for any allowances or benefits from the DSS. *The Disability Rights Handbook*, published by The Disability Alliance★, is a good source of information. Your local council may be able to help with a care assistant, meals on wheels and home aids or modifications.

• *OTHER DISEASES AFFECTING THE JOINTS* •

Doctors often test blood for a molecule called *rheumatoid factor* to diagnose rheumatoid arthritis. It may also be present in rare forms of arthritis where, as in rheumatoid arthritis, an active inflammation (rather than one arising from wear and tear, as in osteoarthritis) attacks the tissues. *Ankylosing spondylitis* means 'a joining up of inflamed vertebrae' and mainly affects the spine and pelvic joints, causing severe stiffening. It may be hereditary and is most common in young men. In severe cases the spine becomes fixed in a bent position, but current treatment can often prevent such disability. *Systemic lupus erythematosus* (SLE) is a rare immunological disorder which causes widespread damage; it mainly affects young women with symptoms including skin rashes, joint pains and tiredness. Other types of rheumatoid-like arthritis include *psoriatic arthritis* and *Reiter's disease*. Rare forms of arthritis that affect children known as *juvenile idiopathic arthritis* (one form is Still's disease) usually clear up after several years but may persist into adulthood.

HOW YOU CAN HELP YOURSELF

Rest and exercise Splints can be helpful, especially at night, to rest the affected joints and prevent deformity. They are best fitted by a skilled physiotherapist. Physiotherapy can help mobility and improve muscle strength. Exercising in water or swimming is beneficial; ask the physiotherapist what other exercises you can do regularly as part of the daily management of the disease.

Eat a balanced diet Special diets are not necessary, but you should eat plenty of fresh fruit and vegetables. Some people claim that avoiding certain foods is helpful. Short-term studies have shown that fish oils (for example, cod liver oil) can sometimes help inflammation and stiffness.

Weight loss will reduce the load on weight-bearing joints.

Local treatment of a painful joint can be soothing – either hot or cold. Gentle massage may also help.

Save effort Find out about suitable aids and possible adaptations to your home to help you live and move about more easily. Make sure the pharmacist supplies your medicines in containers you can open.

Surgery may be needed to correct deformities, if these develop. Knee and hip replacement operations may be an option.

Medicines for rheumatoid arthritis

Your doctor will aim to control pain, and if possible the disease process, maintain the function of joints, and prevent disability and permanent deformity. There are several approaches to treatment and no one method may be completely successful.

A simple analgesic such as paracetamol may be sufficient to relieve pain. Otherwise an NSAID (pages 382–5) can help pain, inflammation and stiffness, particularly morning stiffness, for which a modified-release preparation or suppositories at night may be used. You will need to take the NSAID regularly whether you are in pain or not because it will help to reduce and control inflammation on a long-term basis. An NSAID and paracetamol can both be used for pain relief, or a combination analgesic (pages 232–3) may be substituted for paracetamol if necessary. However, neither paracetamol nor NSAIDs slow down or stop the disease itself.

If symptoms are severe and not controlled by an NSAID, you may be given a medicine aimed at slowing the progression of the arthritis. These *antirheumatic* medicines may suppress the disease process and allow eroded cartilage to heal or at least stop further erosion. A corticosteroid may be used in specific circumstances.

DISEASE-MODIFYING DRUGS

Disease-modifying medicines are usually started by a rheumatologist and used to improve active inflammatory joint disease and also other symptoms of serious arthritic diseases. They act slowly and it may take four to six months before there is a response; sometimes the response is only partial. If one medicine does not work another type may be tried. In rheumatoid arthritis, improvement is measured by the reduction in the number of swollen and tender joints, the amount of pain (using a pain scoring method), disability and improvement in X-rays, and body chemical measures such as rheumatoid factor. These assorted medicines produce adverse effects, but with regular blood, kidney and liver tests and careful monitoring for toxicity, they can be very effective treatments. Your doctor will tell you which signs are important to report. These can include bruising, sore throat, rash or itching, and a change in vision, depending on the medicine.

Sulfasalazine (Salazopyrin) is an effective anti-inflammatory drug for rheumatoid arthritis and is also used for treating ulcerative colitis (pages 81–3). If successful, it produces a response within three to six months. Unwanted effects include rashes and gastrointestinal upsets. Serious unwanted effects are rare, but it can affect blood cells, usually in the first months of treatment, so blood and liver function tests are necessary. **Report any unexplained fever or bleeding, bruising, sore throat or malaise during treatment with sulfasalazine**.

Methotrexate affects the immune system and it can be used early in moderate to severe rheumatoid arthritis. It is taken by mouth once a week, or sometimes given by injection under the skin, and usually works within one to two months. Unwanted effects include feeling sick, diarrhoea and mouth ulcers. A vitamin supplement, folic acid by mouth, can reduce unwanted effects although this may in turn marginally reduce methotrexate's effectiveness. You should discuss this with your doctor. Blood and liver function must be monitored.

Gold compounds may be given by mouth (Ridaura) or injection (Myocrisin). Unwanted effects include diarrhoea, skin rash and adverse effects on the kidneys and blood cells. Treatment has to be stopped if serious unwanted effects occur. Gold by mouth is easy to take but slightly less effective than gold injections and often causes diarrhoea. Both forms require monthly testing of blood and urine.

Penicillamine (Distamine) has a similar action to gold. Unwanted effects occur frequently and include disturbance of taste, nausea, loss of appetite, mouth ulcers and skin rashes. These effects fade when treatment is stopped. Penicillamine also affects kidney function and blood cells.

Chloroquine (Nivaquine) and **hydroxychloroquine** (Plaquenil) are effective in moderate rheumatoid arthritis. Occasionally these drugs

ALTERNATIVE TREATMENTS

Acupuncture is the alternative therapy which is best documented in treating arthritis. It has been demonstrated to relieve pain, but cannot cure the underlying structure of a damaged joint. One theory is that it stimulates the brain to release endorphins, the body's own pain relievers. As the effect is only temporary, treatments have to be repeated regularly.

Osteopathy or **chiropractic** can provide relief of back and shoulder pain by manipulation of the spine and joints. However, it can be dangerous to have this treatment if your disease is in an active inflammatory stage, so make sure of your diagnosis before visiting a practitioner.

Herbal remedies A number of herbs have been recommended for the treatment of arthritis. Like orthodox medicines, herbal remedies can cause adverse effects and their long-term toxic effects are not always known. Herbs commonly recommended are Devil's Claw and Comfrey. Adverse effects have been demonstrated for both of these – Devil's Claw may lead to termination of pregnancy, and Comfrey has been associated with liver disease.

Homoeopathy works on the theory that substances which cause particular symptoms will cure those same symptoms if the substance is taken in an extremely dilute form. Attempts have been made to assess formally the impact of homoeopathy on arthritis, but the results have been inconclusive. Homoeopathic treatment is available on the NHS.

Other remedies Many other cures and treatments have been proposed over the years, ranging from keeping new potatoes in the pockets to aromatherapy (the external use of essential oils derived from plants). Copper bangles are popular; there is no medical evidence that they do any good, but some people find them helpful. Green-lipped mussel extract, or 'Seatone', is sold as a supplement to relieve arthritic symptoms. Unfortunately the evidence for its usefulness is not convincing.

affect the retina, which impacts on vision. You should have your eyes examined before starting treatment and then on a six-monthly basis. Immunosuppressive drugs – **azathioprine**, **ciclosporin**, or **cyclophosphamide** – are effective but are reserved for severe and disabling symptoms because of adverse effects, particularly on blood. Regular blood tests are essential. Newer medicines with similar immunosuppressive activity include **leflunomide** (▼Arava), **anakinra** (▼Kineret), **etanercept** (▼Enbrel) and **infliximab** (▼Remicade).

CORTICOSTEROIDS

A corticosteroid may be used in severe, possibly life-threatening situations. High doses have to be used to control the condition and then the corticosteroid is gradually reduced to the lowest possible maintenance dose or stopped completely.

To avoid extended use, high doses of the corticosteroid **methylprednisolone** are given by injection for three days to control the active inflammatory disease while longer-term and slower-acting treatment is started. A corticosteroid by mouth, e.g. prednisolone 7.5mg daily, may reduce joint destruction in rheumatoid arthritis of less than two years' duration. You may need treatment for two to four years and even at this low dose, osteoporosis can occur; the risk of unwanted effects have to be balanced against the benefits of corticosteroid treatment (pages 329–334). You will need to carry a steroid treatment card.

A corticosteroid used in a joint can bring relief without the adverse effects of a long-term systemic corticosteroid because the drug reaches the affected part direct and mainly acts within a confined area. A corticosteroid injected into a joint (*intra-articular*) can relieve pain, increase mobility and reduce deformity. This technique is generally used for joints such as knees, shoulders and fingers. Infected joints should not be injected as this will reduce immune defences around the joint and could lead to severe worsening of the infection. After the injection there may be a temporary increase in pain and swelling but this subsides as the corticosteroid starts to reduce inflammation.

SURGERY

In some cases, severe joint damage and pain develop despite treatment. In these cases, surgery may be advised – for example, joint replacement. Hip replacement is the most common operation; most people are discharged from hospital two to three weeks afterwards. Great improvements have been made recently in knee joint replacements: research continues into replacements for other joints such as elbows, ankles and knuckles.

Surgery can also be performed on structures around the joints: tendons may be repaired or transplanted, or synovial membranes may be cut out.

Gout

Gout is a form of arthritis caused by a disorder of the metabolism. *Uric acid*, one of the waste products of normal metabolism, leaves the body via the kidneys in urine. If its concentration becomes too high in blood, uric acid starts to form crystals which are deposited in various part of the body, most commonly in the joints of the foot (particularly the big toe), ankles, knees and hands. Crystals of uric acid also form lumps under the skin (*tophi*), often visible in the cartilage of the ear, and stones in the kidneys. The deposits of uric acid in the joints can lead to inflammation, causing intense pain which develops over a few hours. The joint quickly becomes red, swollen and extremely tender, so that any sort of pressure on the area is unbearable. Attacks of gout can recur and if untreated, the joints become damaged and eventually deformed.

The amount of uric acid increases in the body if too much is being made or if the kidneys are unable to remove it from the body adequately. The disorder can be inherited and is more common in men. Diet is an important factor and certain foods, for example red meat, sardines and offal, increase the risk of an attack. High alcohol intake is known to trigger attacks. Gout can also occur in kidney failure, in certain blood disorders and as an unwanted effect of some medicines, such as thiazide diuretics (page 100).

– HOW YOU CAN HELP YOURSELF –

- ☐ Once you have had an attack of gout it may recur. Ask your doctor whether you should have a supply of medicine to relieve an acute attack.
- ☐ Rest the affected joints.
- ☐ Reduce alcohol intake, especially beer (rich in purines). Any type of alcoholic drink can precipitate an attack of gout.
- ☐ Drink plenty of non-alcoholic fluids, especially if you are taking a medicine for preventing further attacks of gout.
- ☐ Reduce calorie and cholesterol intake. Avoid foods rich in purines (a body chemical that breaks down to uric acid) e.g. offal, some fish and shellfish, spinach. Reducing dietary intake can delay the need for medical treatment.

Medicines for gout

Medicines are used for relieving pain and inflammation in an acute attack of gout and also for the long-term control of the disease to prevent the development of joint and kidney damage. **Aspirin** and **salicylates** must not be used to treat an acute attack of gout nor during long-term control of the condition, as they can raise the uric acid levels and aggravate symptoms.

ACUTE ATTACKS

An NSAID such as **indometacin**, **diclofenac** and **naproxen** quickly relieves pain and swelling (page 382). High doses are usually prescribed for a short period to bring the acute symptoms under control. Unwanted effects are unlikely to be a problem because treatment with the NSAID is of short duration.

Colchicine, derived from the seeds of the autumn crocus, is an established treatment for relieving the acute pain and inflammation of gout. It is as effective as indometacin and can be used if you cannot tolerate an NSAID, for example, if you have heart failure or you take an anticoagulant (page 150). Unwanted effects include feeling or being sick and abdominal pain. It is toxic in higher doses, causing profuse diarrhoea, rashes and kidney damage, and these effects limit its usefulness. Colchicine is sometimes used to confirm the diagnosis of gout because it is so specific in relieving symptoms.

LONG-TERM CONTROL

If you have recurrent attacks of gout, your doctor may suggest that you take one of two types of medicine for controlling the levels of uric acid in your blood. Once you start treatment you will need to continue it indefinitely to control uric acid levels. **Allopurinol** reduces the formation of uric acid, while **sulfinpyrazone** (a *uricosuric* drug) increases its excretion. Neither drug must be started during an acute attack of gout because symptoms can be prolonged and exacerbated. Colchicine or an NSAID is given for at least one month to prevent an acute attack of gout while starting treatment with allopurinol or sulphinpyrazone for the control of high blood levels of uric acid.

ALLOPURINOL

ALLOPURINOL – Tablets ZYLORIC – Tablets

Allopurinol is used in the long-term control of gout to prevent recurrent attacks. It lowers blood levels of uric acid by inhibiting the activity of an enzyme involved in the production of uric acid. It will not relieve an acute gout attack and may even precipitate one at the beginning of treatment. Allopurinol gradually controls uric acid levels, thus preventing acute attacks of gout. It also stops uric acid stones forming in the kidneys. It can be used if kidney function is reduced, but at lower doses. It is also used to prevent high blood levels of uric acid developing with cancer treatments.

Before you use this medicine

Tell your doctor if you are:
☐ pregnant or breast-feeding ☐ taking any other medicines, including vitamins and those bought over the counter.

Tell your doctor if you have or have had:
☐ a previous reaction to allopurinol ☐ poor kidney or liver function – reduce dosage.

How to use this medicine

Take a tablet once a day, or doses over 300mg divided up to three times a day after food. The dose is increased slowly and the final dose depends on uric acid levels. Drink 2–3 litres of non-alcoholic fluids a day. Do not drive or do other activities that require alertness until you know how you react to allopurinol. It can cause drowsiness, vertigo and loss of balance. Avoid alcohol: it increases the blood levels of uric acid.

Do not stop taking this medicine without talking to your doctor. Symptoms of gout may return. If you miss a dose, take it as soon as you remember. Do not take double the dose.

Over 65 Kidney and liver function are likely to be reduced, you may need a lower dose.

Interactions with other medicines

Anticancer drugs azathioprine and **mercaptopurine** Effects are enhanced by allopurinol because it blocks their breakdown in the body.
Anticoagulants Blood-thinning effects of **warfarin** and **acenocoumarol** are possibly increased.

Unwanted effects

Likely Skin rashes, itching, red, thick or scaly skin.
Less likely Feeling or being sick, stomach pains.
Rare Hypersensitivity reactions, malaise, changes in bowel habit, headache, vertigo, drowsiness, visual and taste disturbances, numbness or tingling of hands and feet, sore throat or fever, yellow eyes or skin, hair loss.

Allopurinol is usually well tolerated. Contact your doctor if you develop a skin rash, which may occur at anytime during treatment, and especially if you have fever. The drug usually has to be stopped but your doctor may start it again cautiously if the rash was mild and fades.

Similar preparations

ANTURAN – Tablets
SULFINPYRAZONE

Strains and sprains

Injuries to soft tissues such as muscles, tendons and ligaments are common. They can occur through vigorous exercise or through repetitive use of a particular part of the body, for example, wrist strain after typing or piano playing.

Muscles ache after unaccustomed exercise, and in many sports muscles, tendons, ligaments and also bones are under great stress. Physical fitness and training parts of the body to withstand stress increase suppleness and strength and help to prevent injury. However, accidents happen – muscles, tendons or ligaments can be torn or pulled, resulting in pain for a few days, but sometimes more permanent damage. Taking vigorous exercise without building up to a suitable level of fitness may lead to injury or inflammation.

After a few days of rest most sudden injuries begin to improve and you can start gentle exercise and massage to strengthen the injured part. If the injury does not improve, see your doctor or a physiotherapist. Some injuries may need surgery. Repetitive strain injuries, such as tennis elbow, can recur and become long-term problems. They can be enormously frustrating because they prevent you from enjoying pastimes. Even with specialist treatment from a rheumatologist or physiotherapist they can remain painful.

Medicines for strains and sprains

ANALGESICS

To relieve pain a simple analgesic such as paracetamol or aspirin can be used; paracetamol has no anti-inflammatory activity (page 228). Combined analgesics (page 232) rarely have any advantage over a simple analgesic. An NSAID can be used to reduce swelling, tenderness and pain, but unwanted effects may occur (pages 380–1). However, pain relief brings the temptation to use the injured part without allowing nature to take its course during periods of enforced rest. This often leads to the injury being repeated, causing long-term symptoms.

CORTICOSTEROIDS

A local corticosteroid injection (page 390) may help injuries such as tennis or golfer's elbow – inflammation of the tendons and joint between the muscles of the forearm and the bone just above the elbow. However, the improvement following an injection does not reduce the necessity for a careful resumption of activity if renewed injury is to be avoided. In *tendinitis*, a painful and inflamed tendon, the corticosteroid is injected into the sheath surrounding the tendon. With injuries that have not responded to local corticosteroid treatment, surgery may be necessary.

HOW YOU CAN HELP YOURSELF

Use the **RICE** principle:

Rest the injured area. This helps to stop bleeding, both internal and external, and prevents further damage.
Ice – a frozen ice pack applied to the injured area can help to contain swelling. Avoid too much cold as it can burn skin. Cooling sprays are of little value.
Compression with firm bandaging, such as a crepe bandage, helps to stop internal bleeding. Avoid bandaging so tightly that you reduce the circulation to the area.
Elevation – keep the damaged limb or area raised to allow excess fluid to drain away and reduce swelling. Sports injury clinics offer a specialised service, often including physiotherapy, particularly for recent injuries.

LOCAL 'RUBS' AND LINIMENTS

Pain, whether it is on the surface of the skin or deep within the body, can be relieved by any method which causes irritation of the skin. This is known as counter-irritation and can be most comforting in injuries of the muscles, tendons and joints. *Rubefacients* are counter-irritants which produce inflammation, opening up the blood vessels to cause redness and warmth. When applying a rubefacient, massage and rubbing are the most beneficial actions, not the medicine itself. Therefore, a product that costs more – either because of some claimed property or expensive packaging (an aerosol, for example) – has no advantage over a cheaper brand in a tube or bottle. Most rubefacients (e.g. Algesal; Algipan; Transvasin) contain a salicylate such as **methyl salicylate** with menthol for a distinctive smell. When applying a rubefacient you must be careful to avoid contact with eyes, lips and other mucous membranes and inflamed or broken skin. Rubefacients are generally not suitable for children. Liniments are very harmful if accidentally swallowed; keep them well out of reach of children.

TOPICAL NSAIDs

On prescription/from a pharmacy

FELDENE – Gel*
PIROXICAM

FENBID FORTE – Gel
IBUPROFEN

IBUGEL FORTE – Gel

IBULEVE – Gel
IBUPROFEN

IBUMOUSSE – Foam*
IBUPROFEN

IBUSPRAY – Spray*
IBUPROFEN

KETOPROFEN – Gel

ORUVAIL – Gel*
KETOPROFEN

PENNSAID – Liquid
DICLOFENAC

PIROXICAM – Gel

POWERGEL – Gel
KETOPROFEN

PROFLEX – Cream*
IBUPROFEN

TRAXAM – Gel*, aerosol foam
FELBINAC

VOLTAROL EMULGEL – Gel*
DICLOFENAC

* different packs, e.g. 30g from a pharmacy.

NSAIDS APPLIED TO THE SKIN

There is no conclusive evidence that *topical* creams, gels and foams are any better than taking an NSAID by mouth, or even an analgesic such as paracetamol, but they may bring some relief. If you decide to use an NSAID on the skin, check that it is suitable for you. If you are sensitive to the effects of aspirin, ibuprofen or other NSAIDs – especially if you are asthmatic, or have had an allergic reaction or skin rash – you must not use an NSAID on the skin because it can be absorbed into the body to some degree. The amount of drug absorbed from a topical NSAID is much less (one-fifth or less) than that found in the body after taking it by mouth. Topical NSAIDs are generally well tolerated, but using an NSAID on the skin does not completely eliminate the unwanted effects which can occur with an oral NSAID. Stomach upsets such as indigestion, feeling sick, diarrhoea, headache and dizziness occasionally occur. A topical NSAID should not be used if you are pregnant or breast-feeding. Preparations contain other ingredients such as **propylene glycol** which can occasionally cause sensitisation (page 435).

The NSAID can be rubbed gently into the painful area three or four times a day; some manufacturers give a guide to how much to use. No reduction in dosage is needed for older people. Topical NSAIDs are not suitable for children. It is important to follow the dosage directions carefully because of absorption into the body.

Avoid using a topical NSAID on broken or infected skin or near the eyes, mouth and other mucous membranes, and always wash your hands after application. If the preparation gets into the eyes, rinse them immediately and thoroughly with clean water. Seek medical assistance if your eyes continue to hurt. A topical NSAID sometimes causes reddening, smarting and itching, but these effects fade on stopping treatment. A topical NSAID increases the skin's sensitivity to sunlight, and skin rashes occur occasionally. Do not use a topical NSAID under dressings, plasters or bandages which prevent air from reaching the skin (*occlusive dressings*) or apply the NSAID in the same place as other creams or ointments.

For a steady and reliable effect it is better to take an NSAID or an analgesic by mouth and/or use the RICE principle (page 394). If you need to massage the injured area, a rub or liniment may help. Combining a topical NSAID with one taken by mouth increases the risk of unwanted effects.

9

EYES, EARS, MOUTH AND THROAT

Eyes

Conjunctivitis Blepharitis Glaucoma Dry eye Contact lens problems

The eye, the organ of sight, is a sphere about 2.5cm (1 inch) in diameter, well protected above by the brow and behind by a pad of fat. Six muscles work in pairs to control the movement of each eyeball. Covering most of the eye is a tough whitish coat, the *sclera*. The *cornea* at the front forms a clear protective covering for the coloured iris and pupil and a further outer layer, the *conjunctiva*, covers the cornea and the white of the eye. The *iris* is a muscular ring which controls the inner hole, the *pupil*, through which light passes into the *lens* and then reaches the *retina*, the sensitive lining at the back of the eye, which converts light into nerve impulses. The *optic nerve* leading from the retina carries these signals to the brain, where they are interpreted as sight. The size of the pupil is regulated by the muscles of the iris. In dim light the pupil opens wide to let in as much light as possible, whereas in strong light it narrows to protect the retina from damage. Many medicines which act on the nervous system affect eyesight; for example, atropine-like drugs cause blurred vision. Tears are the eye's own cleansing and antibacterial system. Each time you blink tears wash across the cornea and conjunctiva, keeping the eye surfaces moist and clean. Tears are made in glands above the eyelid and with each blink liquid is squeezed from the gland. *Tear ducts* at the corner of the eye collect tears into a *tear sac* which then drains into the nose.

The space behind the lens is filled with a jelly-like substance called *vitreous humour* which helps to keep the eye's shape within the socket. The front part of the eye, behind the cornea and in front of the iris is filled with a watery liquid called *aqueous humour*.

Conjunctivitis

Inflammation of the conjunctiva is a common eye condition which can be caused by bacterial or viral infection or may be a symptom of allergy, especially in hay fever sufferers. Vision is not usually affected and generally reaction to light remains unchanged. If vision is affected this indicates more serious symptoms which need further investigation, for example glaucoma. Children, older people and contact lens wearers are at increased risk of eye infections. More rarely conjunctivitis develops from other causes, for example chemical irritation from eye cosmetics or an underlying problem such as thyroid disease.

An inflamed conjunctiva is red and swollen. The eye feels as if it has particles or a foreign body in it and there is a sensation of grittiness. There may also be pain although if the conjunctivitis is caused by infection this will ease as tears cleanse the conjunctiva during each day. A bacterial infection, commonly caused by the staphylococcus family, produces pus, a sticky discharge which sometimes makes it difficult to open the eyes, especially on waking. Viral conjunctivitis, which often occurs in epidemics, produces a watery discharge. You may also have a sore throat with both bacterial and viral conjunctivitis. One or both eyes may be infected and sometimes the eyelids are swollen and drooping. Allergic conjunctivitis causes redness, inflammation, itching which is sometimes severe and watery eyes.

– HOW YOU CAN HELP YOURSELF –

Eye problems are a nuisance and should never be ignored. It is difficult to distinguish between infection and allergy, so you should always ask your doctor for advice. A 'red eye' has a number of different causes; get prompt treatment especially if sight is affected or if only one eye is involved.

- ☐ If your eyes are infected, adopt strict hygienic measures to prevent the spread of infection, e.g. keep a flannel and face towel especially for your own use and wash it regularly.
- ☐ Wash your hands before and after using any eye preparations.
- ☐ Avoid using eye cosmetics until the infection has cleared up.
- ☐ Eye drop preparations should never be shared or lent to anyone: when you have finished the course of treatment, return unused amounts to the pharmacy. Never keep opened eye drop preparations for treating another infection.

Medicines for conjunctivitis

A mild eye infection may not need treatment and can clear spontaneously after a few days. Tears are cleansing, but following strict hygienic measures and bathing the eyes in cool clean water may also help. However, great care is needed in treating an eye infection yourself and if the condition does not appear to be clearing up after two days, you should consult your doctor. A bacterial infection can be treated with an antibacterial preparation applied locally to the eye, either as drops or as ointment – sometimes both are used. The active ingredient is commonly **chloramphenicol**, which acts against a wide range of bacteria. Other antibacterials for eye infections include the quinolone antibiotics **ciprofloxacin** (Ciloxan) and **ofloxacin** (Exocin) – pages 278–280 – and also **neomycin**, **framycetin**, **gentamicin** and **polymyxin B**. **Fusidic acid** (Fucithalmic) is a longer-acting gel that becomes liquid in contact with the eye. It is used twice daily when staphylococcal infections of the conjunctiva and eyelids are thought to be the cause. **Propamidine** (Brolene) is of little help in treating bacterial eye infections, although it is available from pharmacies. It is used to treat acanthamoeba keratitis (page 411). Unwanted effects such as stinging and irritation in the eye, which usually fade quickly, can occur with these preparations and sometimes systemic effects occur, for example nausea and headache with the quinolones.

APPLYING MEDICINES TO THE EYE

A medicine can be applied *topically* (direct to the affected area) in eye drops (ophthalmic solution), ointment or lotion. Sometimes a medicine such as an antimicrobial is given by injection into the conjunctiva or by mouth for severe infections that have not responded to topical treatment.

Eye drops

Just one or at most two drops of liquid are placed (instilled) in the eye per dose because this is all the eye can hold. The lower eyelid is gently pulled

WARNING

Some antibiotic preparations contain a corticosteroid (see Chapter 6: Hormones). These preparations must never be used if you have an infection or if you have 'red eye'. 'Red eye' is sometimes caused by *herpes simplex* virus, which produces an ulcer in the eye. A corticosteroid used locally in the eye may aggravate this condition and possibly lead to serious complications such as loss of vision or even loss of the eye. Furthermore, if a corticosteroid is used for more than a few weeks 'steroid glaucoma' may result in susceptible people. Following prolonged use clouding of the lens or 'steroid cataract' may occur.

The combination of a corticosteroid and an antibacterial is rarely needed.

Preparations not recommended include:

BETNESOL-N
BETAMETHASONE + NEOMYCIN

MAXITROL
DEXAMETHASONE + NEOMYCIN + POLYMYXIN B

NEO-CORTEF
HYDROCORTISONE + NEOMYCIN

PREDSOL-N
PREDNISOLONE + NEOMYCIN

SOFRADEX
DEXAMETHASONE + FRAMYCETIN + GRAMICIDIN

TOBRADEX
DEXAMETHASONE + TOBRAMYCIN

VISTA-METHASONE N
BETAMETHASONE + NEOMYCIN

down to form a pocket and the drop(s) instilled into this area. The eye should be closed for 1 to 2 minutes after instillation. Within 15 seconds the drug is diluted by tears, so it does not have long to act. For this reason some eye drops need to be used frequently and your doctor should give you precise directions, such as actual times when you need to use your drops and whether dosing should continue during the night. Longer-acting eye drop preparations are likely to become available in future as gels or suspensions, allowing once- or twice-daily dosing and greater convenience. An eye-drop dispenser, such as Opticare, that attaches to most eye drop containers makes it easier to instil drops. It is particularly useful for older people, and those with arthritic hands or poor eyesight. Your doctor can prescribe these but they are not too expensive to buy.

The drug almost always gets into the body, in variable amounts, via the blood vessels in the conjunctiva and also the tear ducts, which drain into the nose. If you lightly press a finger against the corner of the eye beside the nose after applying the drops you can keep the drug in contact with the conjunctiva for longer. After this, blow your nose to clear any drops that have reached the nasal passages. If you have to instil two different eye drop preparations at the same time you should wait five minutes before using the second. If one of the preparations stings, then use this second, so that any tears produced do not wash out the first product. Longer-acting eye drop preparations should always be used last.

When applying eye drops take care not to touch the eye or anything else with the dropper. Eyes can easily become infected through the dropper, or an infection can be transferred from one eye to the other. An eye drop preparation is sterile before it is opened, but once opened it can easily become contaminated, so a preservative is included. If you use the preparation carefully – washing your hands before applying drops, not touching the eye with the dropper and replacing the dropper in the bottle immediately after use – the drops can be used for up to one month. After this time the risk of contamination is too great.

Preservatives commonly used in eye drops include **benzalkonium chloride**, **disodium edetate**, and more rarely **thiomersal** or **phenylmercuric nitrate**. They are used in small amounts, but cause allergy in a few people. If your eye condition worsens after you have started treatment, contact your doctor – you may be allergic to one of the ingredients in the preparation.

Single-use eye drops do not contain a preservative. Each container holds a sterile dose, but must be thrown away after its first use because there is nothing in the preparation to prevent contamination once opened.

Eye ointments

Eye ointments contain the medicine in a greasy base. Preparations are sterile until opened and can be used for up to one month providing the usual hygiene measures are observed (see 'How you can help yourself', page 398). Eye ointment is generally easier to apply than drops and can be applied to the eyelids. The medicine acts for up to 15 minutes and less is absorbed into the body than with drops. Vision may be blurred immediately after applying an eye ointment and for up to half an hour after use. You should avoid driving until your vision is clear. Eye ointment does not have to be used as frequently as drops – twice-daily applications are sometimes adequate, and an eye ointment is ideal for night-time use.

Eye lotions

Solutions for washing out the eye can be used to soothe the eye or to flush out irritants or foreign bodies. Eye lotions are sterile until they are opened. A soothing lotion for use at home should not be used for longer than one month. In a first aid kit, an eye lotion such as **sodium chloride** should be used for a maximum of 24 hours after opening and not returned to the kit for future use.

CHLORAMPHENICOL

CHLORAMPHENICOL – Eye drops, eye ointment, ear drops (not recommended); capsules
CHLOROMYCETIN – Eye drops, eye ointment
KEMICETINE – Injection
MINIMS CHLORAMPHENICOL – Single-use eye drops

Chloramphenicol is an antibiotic, now mostly used topically for bacterial infections of the eye and ear. It stops bacteria from multiplying and this allows the body's own defence mechanisms to overpower any remaining infection. When taken by mouth or injected, chloramphenicol can occasionally cause serious or fatal blood disorders, so this form of treatment is reserved for life-threatening infections against which it is effective, such as typhoid fever and a certain type of meningitis. The following information applies to topical preparations only.

Before you use this medicine

Tell your doctor if you are:
☐ pregnant or breast-feeding – use during these periods does not appear to cause problems ☐ taking any other medicines, including vitamins and those bought over the counter.

Tell your doctor if you have or have had:
☐ sensitivity to any of the ingredients, such as preservatives ☐ you use contact lenses.

How to use this medicine

Eye drops Instil one or two drops into the pocket formed by gently pulling down the lower eyelid at least every two hours for the first 24 hours, reducing to four times daily as the infection is controlled. Continue to use the drops for 48 hours after the infection seems to have cleared and the eye appears normal. Do not use eye drops after one month of first opening.
Eye ointment Apply a small amount to the eye or within the lower lid three or four times daily. The ointment can be used at night and eye drops used during the day.
Ear drops Apply two or three times daily to the external ear.
If you miss a dose, apply as soon as you remember. Avoid wearing contact lenses until after you have completed the treatment. Complete the course and return any remaining medicine to a pharmacy for disposal.

Over 65 No special requirements.

Unwanted effects

Likely with eye drops Short-term stinging or burning; **with ear drops** sensitivity to the ear drop solution: around one person in ten is sensitive to propylene glycol.

If your ear condition seems to worsen, contact your doctor because you may be sensitive to the solution containing chloramphenicol. Chloramphenicol eye preparations rarely cause problems. Extremely rarely, serious or fatal blood disorders (aplastic anaemia, bone marrow depression) have been reported following the use of chloramphenicol eye preparations, but this association is not well founded. Neither the eye or ear drops are recommended for prolonged use, because the bacteria may become resistant to the antibiotic.

Similar preparations

FUCITHALMIC – Eye drops
FUSIDIC ACID

GARAMYCIN – Eye/ear drops
GENTAMICIN

GENTICIN – Eye/ear drops
GENTAMICIN

MINIMS GENTAMICIN – Single-use eye drops
GENTAMICIN

NEOMYCIN – Eye drops, eye ointment

NEOSPORIN – Eye drops
POLYMYXIN B + NEOMYCIN + GRAMICIDIN

POLYFAX – Eye ointment
POLYMYXIN B + BACITRACIN

POLYTRIM – Eye drops, eye ointment
POLYMYXIN B + TRIMETHOPRIM

SOFRAMYCIN – Eye drops, eye ointment
FRAMYCETIN

NON-BACTERIAL INFECTIONS

There is no treatment for viral conjunctivitis but this clears of its own accord in two to three weeks. Your doctor may give you an antibiotic to guard against a secondary bacterial infection. Some viral infections that may also affect the cornea, such as herpes simplex, can be treated with a specific antiviral eye preparation such as aciclovir eye ointment, pages 292–4. Fungal infections affect the cornea rather than the conjunctiva and are not common. Infection can occur after agricultural injuries in hot, humid conditions. Antifungal treatment is managed at specialist centres. Eye symptoms caused by hay fever are usually treated with one of the antihistamine eye drop preparations – **antazoline** (with **xylometazoline**, brand name Otrivine-Antistin – also from a pharmacy), **azelastine** (Optilast), **emedastine** (Emadine), **ketotifen** (Zaditen) or **levocabastine** (Livostin – also from a pharmacy). Allergic conjunctivitis can be managed with **sodium cromoglicate** eye drops, **nedocromil** (Rapitil) – pages 176–7 – or **lodoxamide** (Alomide). A corticosteroid is usually used under expert supervision, for example to reduce inflammation after an eye operation. A corticosteroid eye preparation should not be used for allergic symptoms.

Blepharitis

Blepharitis is inflammation or infection of the edge of the eyelids which makes them sore, red and itchy. There are two types: one is caused by a bacterium (*Staphylococcus*) which produces pus, ulceration and dry dandruff-like scales and the other is an eczematous condition, similar to *seborrhoeic eczema*, with greasy flakes of skin clinging to the eyelashes. Eczematous eyelids can also become infected with bacteria. Infection around an eyelash may cause a stye.

Treatment involves cleaning the eyelids very carefully and then, if there is infection, applying an antibacterial ointment regularly. In the eczematous condition the scalp and eyebrows may also be affected. If these areas are treated with a medicated shampoo, such as **ketoconazole** (Nizoral), the eyelids often improve. Styes are treated with hot compresses and an antibiotic ointment.

Glaucoma

Glaucoma is the name for a group of eye problems, commonly *acute* and *chronic glaucoma*, which can lead to loss of sight through optic nerve damage. Aqueous humour is continuously formed within the eye at the root of the iris and absorbed back into the veins via drainage channels (*trabecular meshwork*) at the junction of the cornea and the iris. The balance between the production of aqueous humour and its removal is expressed as the intra-ocular pressure or ocular tension. A certain amount of pressure is needed to keep the eye in shape and ensure normal working. Any imbalance between the formation and absorption of aqueous humour leads to increased pressure within the eye and to glaucoma. (The normal range is 12mmHg to 21mmHg; the risk increases at 30mmHg and above.) As pressure builds up, the blood vessels to the optic nerve become squashed, reducing the blood flow to the nerve. Eventually the nerve is irreversibly damaged, resulting in permanent loss of sight. Although glaucoma is usually associated with pressure that is higher than the normal range, the condition can occur when pressure is not raised. Glaucoma is a major cause of blindness but early detection and treatment with medicines or surgery can prevent irreversible damage.

You should have regular eye tests at least every two years at the optometrist, including all three glaucoma tests (see box, page 404) to monitor for any developments. Chronic glaucoma mainly affects older people – about one in 50 people aged over 40 years, rising to one in 20 by the age of 70 years. Other factors that increase risk include family history, severe short sightedness, African-Carribean origin, and possibly diabetes mellitus. Rare forms of glaucoma include secondary glaucoma (when a rise in intraocular pressure is caused by another eye condition), and developmental glaucoma that occurs in babies. Glaucoma of any type requires specialist assessment before treatment starts and your GP will refer you to an ophthalmologist.

ACUTE GLAUCOMA

Acute glaucoma (acute closed-angle glaucoma) develops suddenly and is a medical emergency. It occurs when the angle between the iris and the cornea becomes completely closed, preventing aqueous humour from draining away, and pressure from the excess fluid increases rapidly. The eye becomes red and extremely painful; you may have a headache and vomit; vision becomes blurred as the pressure distorts the cornea. You may experience warning symptoms – seeing haloes around lights – and these may occur some weeks or even months before the main attack.

Acute glaucoma needs immediate medical attention in order to prevent permanent loss of sight. Treatment includes lowering the pressure within the eye by reducing the amount of fluid with an intravenous injection of a diuretic followed by surgery or laser treatment. An operation called an *iridectomy* usually solves the problem and long-term treatment with a medicine is rarely needed. The operation involves cutting a tiny hole in the cornea and removing a strip of the iris to allow excess fluid to drain away continuously. There is a risk of the condition occurring in the other eye, so a prophylactic iridectomy is often carried out on that eye at the same time.

CHRONIC GLAUCOMA

This is the most common type of glaucoma (primary open-angle glaucoma), which develops slowly and insidiously. Fluid drains away less efficiently but the production of fluid is unaffected. More aqueous humour remains within the eye and the pressure builds up slowly and painlessly. As the optic nerve is gradually damaged the field of vision is reduced, so that eventually only a small area of central vision remains (*tunnel vision*) before sight is lost completely. Most people with glaucoma do not have symptoms until they notice some loss of vision, but by this stage the optic nerve is irreversibly damaged. Treatment can prevent further deterioration but cannot reverse damage already done. Surgery (*trabeculectomy*) or laser treatment (*trabeculoplasty*) is sometimes used to relieve chronic glaucoma.

Medicines for glaucoma

Medical treatment aims to reduce intra-ocular pressure (the lower the better), and prevent further reduction in your field of vision. Drug treatment, usually in the form of eye drops, lessens the production of aqueous humour or increases its outflow. Several different types of medicine can be used either separately or in combination. These include beta-blockers used directly in the eye, prostaglandin analogues, carbonic anhydrase inhibitors, and to a lesser extent **pilocarpine-type** (miotics) and **adrenaline-type** (sympathomimetics) drugs. Your doctor may need to add other medicines, depending on how well the intra-ocular pressure remains controlled.

A topical beta blocker, such as **timolol**, can be the first choice where people can tolerate it; it reduces the rate of production of aqueous humour within the eye, lessening pressure. A beta blocker is often useful for treating mild glaucoma, but should not be used if you are asthmatic or if you have chronic obstructive pulmonary disease, abnormally slow heartbeat, heart block or heart failure (unless this is well-controlled).

HOW YOU CAN HELP YOURSELF

- ☐ Your eyes may seem normal when glaucoma is developing, because there is no pain and your eyesight seems fine, but your vision is gradually being damaged.
- ☐ If you have a close relative with glaucoma – parent, brother or sister – take particular care to have your eyes checked regularly, particularly if you are aged over 40 years. Anyone with a family history of glaucoma is entitled to free sight tests.
- ☐ Your high street optometrist should offer you the three glaucoma tests, which together are more effective in detecting visual problems than if you have one or two of these.
- ☐ The tests involve:
    1. viewing your optic nerve by shining a light into your eye via an ophthalmoscope
    2. measuring your intraocular pressure with a tonometer
    3. assessing the visual field by showing a sequence of light spots on to a screen and asking which ones you can see (*perimetry*).

A hospital specialist will start and guide ongoing treatment. Existing damage cannot be reversed, but if glaucoma is discovered and treated early, further deterioration can be minimised.

- ☐ If you have treatment with eye drops, you will need to use them regularly every day, possibly for life. If you have to use more than one type of eye preparation at the same time of day, allow five to ten minutes between each application.
- ☐ Further help and information is available from The International Glaucoma Association★ (*www.iga.org.uk*), the Partially Sighted Society★ and the Royal National Institute for the Blind★.
- ☐ If you have glaucoma and visual defects in both eyes then you must by law inform the Drivers Medical Group at the Driver and Vehicle Licensing Agency (DVLA)★. If only one eye is affected and the other eye is normal, then you do not need to contact the DVLA.

Prostaglandin analogue eye drops **latanoprost** (Xalatan) and **travoprost** (▼Travatan) increase aqueous humour outflow. They are as effective as timolol (sometimes more so) and are increasingly used. A related prostaglandin, **bimatoprost** (▼Lumigan), has a similar effect. Latanoprost can be used initially first-line or in combination with other medicines for glaucoma, such as timolol (▼Xalacom contains **latanoprost + timolol**), while travoprost or bimatoprost are used after other eye drops have been tried or can be added to existing therapy. They can all be used once a day, usually in the evening, although the latanoprost/timolol combination is used in the morning. Unwanted effects of prostaglandin analogues include local irritation and pain in the eye, swelling of the conjunctiva, visual disturbances, and headaches. These prostaglandin analogues cause fewer systemic unwanted effects than topical beta blockers. However, one unusual effect can occur: irreversible changes to eye colour because of an increase in the brown pigment in the iris. The long-term consequences of this change are not known. Your doctor should check for any eye colour changes, particularly if you have mixed-colour irises or have treatment in one eye only. Also these medicines can darken, thicken and lengthen eye lashes.

Acetazolamide is a diuretic (carbonic anhydrase inhibitor) taken by mouth or injected into muscle to treat types of glaucoma by reducing the production of aqueous humour. Related drugs that can be used locally in the eye include **dorzolamide** (Trusopt) which is applied three times daily, and **brinzolamide** (▼Azopt), used twice or three times daily. They can be used alone or with a beta blocker. One preparation (Cosopt) combines dorzolamide and timolol and is used twice daily. Unwanted effects include changes in taste, burning sensations in the eyes, blurred vision and watering of the eyes.

Pilocarpine eye drops increase the outflow of aqueous humour by opening up the drainage channels. Local unwanted effects limit its use, particularly its miotic action of making pupil size smaller. It also affects 'accommodation', the eye's ability to focus, which results in blurred vision and brow-ache. This is particularly troublesome for people aged under 40 years and those who are short-sighted. Pilocarpine acts for about three to four hours and drops have to be instilled four times daily, although a gel formulation (Pilogel) is longer-acting and is applied at night, thus reducing blurred vision. **Dipivefrine** (Propine) converts to **adrenaline** (epinephrine) on application to the eye. It reduces the rate of production of aqueous humour as well as increasing the outflow of fluid. Adrenaline is a mydriatic: it dilates the pupil and must not be used to treat acute glaucoma, except after iridectomy. In some people, adrenaline may cause severe stinging and redness in the eye. It should be used with caution if you have blood pressure or heart disease. **Brimonidine** (Alphagan) is a more selective adrenaline-type drug which is increasingly used either with beta blocker eye drops or alone in raised intra-ocular pressure. **Apraclonidine** (Iopidine) may be used for up to one month, usually when other treatments have not controlled intra-ocular pressure adequately or after surgery.

TIMOLOL

TIMOLOL – Eye drops

COSOPT – Eye drops
TIMOLOL + DORZOLAMIDE

NYOGEL – Longer-acting eye drops
TIMOLOL

TIMOPTOL – Eye drops, single-use eye drops

TIMOPTOL-LA – Longer-acting eye drops

Timolol is a beta blocker used in the eye to reduce the pressure caused by the build up of aqueous humour (for other uses see also Chapter 2: Heart and Circulation). It is used for treating eye conditions such as chronic glaucoma; although timolol taken by mouth will reduce intra-ocular pressure, side effects may be troublesome. It lowers intra-ocular pressure by reducing the rate of production of aqueous humour. It may be used as supplementary treatment after surgery in either acute or chronic glaucoma. Longer-acting preparations can be used once a day. Although timolol is used in the eye, some of it is absorbed into the bloodstream so that effects occur throughout the body. Timolol or any other beta blocker for use in the eye should not be used if you have asthma or other breathing difficulties, heart block, heart failure or slow heartbeat (bradycardia) unless there is no alternative.

Before you use this medicine

Tell your doctor if you are:
☐ pregnant – discuss with your doctor; the effect of timolol eye drops has not been studied ☐ breast-feeding ☐ taking any other medicines, including vitamins and those bought over the counter.

Tell your doctor if you have or have had:
☐ diabetes ☐ circulation problems ☐ thyroid disorders ☐ myasthenia gravis.

Do not use if you have or have had:
☐ asthma ☐ chronic obstructive pulmonary disease ☐ heart block or uncontrolled heart failure ☐ bradycardia (slow heart beat).

How to use this medicine

Use one drop twice daily in the affected eye. See your doctor after four weeks for a check-up. If the intra-ocular pressure stabilises satisfactorily you may be able to switch to once-a-day treatment.

Do not drive or do other activities that require alertness until you know how you react to timolol. The eye drops may cause dizziness and blurred vision.

Do not stop using timolol suddenly or your condition may worsen. If you miss a dose, apply it as soon as you remember. If you are using timolol twice a day, apply the missed dose as soon as you remember, but skip it if it is nearly time for your next dose. Do not apply double the dose.

If you have to have an operation tell your doctor or dentist that you use timolol drops.

Over 65 You may be more susceptible to the systemic effects of timolol, such as increased wheezing.

Interactions with other medicines

Although timolol is used in the eye, it may be absorbed into the body and interact with medicines in the same way as a beta blocker taken by mouth (see **atenolol** drug profile, pages 107–9). Do not take other medicines without first checking with your doctor or pharmacist.

Unwanted effects

Likely In eye: stinging, burning, pain, itching, dryness, redness (including eyelids); visual changes, headache.
Less likely Allergic reactions including conjunctivitis, corneal disorders.

Timolol eye drops are rarely troublesome. Discomfort in the eyes usually fades as treatment continues. Effects throughout the body (systemic) may occur such as on the heart and circulation, breathing, digestive systems – check the atenolol drug profile, pages107–9.

Similar preparations

BETAGAN – Eye drops, single-use eye drops
LEVOBUNOLOL

BETOPTIC – Eye drops, single-use eye drops
BETAXOLOL

MINIMS METIPRANOLOL – Single-use eye drops
METIPRANOLOL

TEOPTIC – Eye drops
CARTEOLOL

ACETAZOLAMIDE

DIAMOX – Tablets, modified-release capsules, injection

Acetazolamide is a diuretic used for treating chronic glaucoma. It reduces pressure within the eye by decreasing the amount of aqueous humour produced. It is taken by mouth and can be added to other drug treatments, such as beta blocker eye drops, usually as a short-term measure when the intra-ocular pressure needs further reduction. Acetazolamide is also used before surgery in acute glaucoma. It is sometimes used with other drugs in childhood epilepsy. Acetazolamide also has an unnofficial use in preventing mountain sickness, but is no substitute for acclimatisation. Unwanted effects may be troublesome, so acetazolamide is not generally recommended for long-term treatment or for use as a diuretic (see Chapter 2: Heart and Circulation). If you take acetazolamide routinely you may need to have periodic blood tests.

Before you use this medicine

Tell your doctor if you are:
☐ pregnant – avoid acetazolamide ☐ breast-feeding ☐ taking any other medicines, including vitamins and those bought over the counter.

Tell your doctor if you have or have had:
☐ kidney disease or kidney stones ☐ adrenal gland disease (Addison's disease) ☐ diabetes ☐ liver disease ☐ problems passing urine ☐ low blood levels of sodium or potassium ☐ sensitivity to sulphonamides.

How to use this medicine

Take one tablet up to four times daily with food. The modified-release capsule can be taken once or twice a day and may be easier to remember if you have to take acetazolamide regularly.

Drink plenty of non-alcoholic fluids while you take acetazolamide to prevent kidney stones. Acetazolamide may reduce the amount of potassium in your body, so eat plenty of potassium-rich foods such as fresh fruit and vegetables (page 102).

Do not drive or do other activities that require alertness until you know how you react to acetazolamide. Avoid alcohol because it aggravates dehydration caused by acetazolamide.

Do not stop taking this medicine suddenly or your condition may worsen. If you miss a dose, take it as soon as you remember, but skip it if it is within 2 hours of your next dose. Do not take double the dose.

Over 65 You are more likely to experience unwanted effects, especially if you have severe liver impairment, urinary tract obstruction, or the body's balance of sodium and potassium is upset.

Interactions with other medicines

Lithium Acetazolamide increases the excretion of lithium from the body, leading to a fall in body lithium levels and less effectiveness.
Other diuretics, especially thiazides, enhance the potassium-lowering effect. Avoid combinations of diuretics.
Aspirin increases the level of acetazolamide in the body and the risk of unwanted effects.
Carbamazepine Acetazolamide increases the level of carbamazepine, with increased risk of unwanted effects.
Heart drugs such as **digoxin** and other blood pressure-lowering medicines may need dosage adjustment if taken at the same time as acetazolamide.

Unwanted effects

Likely Feeling or being sick, taste disturbance, thirst, stomach upsets, drowsiness, dizziness, lethargy, increased frequency of passing urine, numbness, tingling in hands or feet.
Rare Skin rashes, increased sensitivity to sunlight, fever, sore throat, unusual bruising or bleeding, confusion, ringing or buzzing in the ears, temporary deafness.

Acetazolamide is a useful treatment for glaucoma. It is not usually given for long periods, but if it is, you will need blood tests and other tests to check kidney function and the level of salts in the body. Likely unwanted effects generally fade as treatment continues and disappear once treatment is stopped. If you feel unwell while you take acetazolamide, a sulphonamide-type drug, discuss the symptoms with your doctor. If you develop a skin rash or hearing loss, stop taking acetazolamide and contact your doctor.

Similar preparations

▼AZOPT – Eye drops
BRINZOLAMIDE

COSOPT – Eye drops
DORZOLAMIDE + TIMOLOL

TRUSOPT – Eye drops
DORZOLAMIDE

Dry eye

Dry eye or chronic soreness is a common condition, particularly in post-menopausal women and old people, and is often associated with rheumatoid arthritis. The normal composition of tears may become deficient or less tear fluid may be made. You may have a feeling of grit in the eye or heaviness or drooping of the lids. You may have a headache and difficulty in opening your eyes and there may be mucus. Symptoms usually get worse in hot or smoky environments, and in the evening. Some drugs diminish tear flow.

Treatment involves using a tear substitute and if possible, avoiding situations that make your eyes worse. 'Artificial tear' drops are viscous: they thicken tear film and reduce tear drainage, but do not cure the condition. **Hypromellose** is widely used for tear deficiencies : drops are usually used hourly at first to bring symptoms under control and then at least four times a day. A synthetic polyacrylic acid, **carbomer** (Gel Tears;

Liposic; Viscotears) remains in the eye for longer than conventional artificial tear drops. The addition of **acetylcysteine**, a mucolytic, to hypromellose is useful when tears are stringy and viscous, but it causes stinging. A lubricating eye ointment (Lacri-Lube; Lubri-Tears) causes temporary visual disturbance but may be useful at night. Drops containing **phenylephrine** (Isopto Frin) add little to the effect of hypromellose and are not recommended. Many tear substitutes contain a preservative which can cause a local allergic reaction. If this happens you may have to use a single-use preparation without a preservative, such as **hydroxyethylcellulose** (Artificial Tears), or hypromellose (Artelac SDU) or **sodium chloride** solution, but these need more frequent application. Sodium chloride is also useful for soothing eyes if you are a contact lens wearer or to facilitate their removal.

One bottle of eye drops used four times daily for both eyes should last four weeks and then be discarded. Your doctor can prescribe these products or you can buy them at a pharmacy, some at less than the prescription charge.

'ARTIFICIAL TEAR' DROPS

Active ingredient	*Product name*	*Preservative*
HYPROMELLOSE	HYPROMELLOSE EYE-DROPS	benzalkonium
	ISOPTO ALKALINE	benzalkonium
	ISOPTO PLAIN	benzalkonium
HYPROMELLOSE + DEXTRAN '70'	TEARS NATURALE	benzalkonium + disodium edetate
ACETYLCYSTEINE + HYPROMELLOSE	ILUBE	benzalkonium + disodium edetate
HYDROXYETHYLCELLULOSE	MINIMS ARTIFICIAL TEARS	none (single-use)
▼CARMELLOSE	CELLUVISC	none (single-use)
LIQUID PARAFFIN + LANOLIN DERIVATIVES	LACRI-LUBE (ointment)	none
	LUBRI-TEARS (ointment)	none
POLYVINYL ALCOHOL	HYPOTEARS	benzalkonium + disodium edetate
	LIQUIFILM TEARS	benzalkonium + disodium edetate
	LIQUIFILM TEARS (preservative free)	none
	SNO TEARS	benzalkonium + disodium edetate
CARBOMER	VISCOTEARS	cetrimide + disodium edetate
	VISCOTEARS	none (single-use)
	GEL TEARS	benzalkonium
POVIDONE	OCULOTECT	none (single-use)
SODIUM CHLORIDE SOLUTION	MINIMS SODIUM CHLORIDE	none (single-use)

**benzalkonium = benzalkonium chloride*

Contact lens problems

A contact lens is a small, paper-thin, shaped piece of transparent material which is placed in the eye to correct short- or long-sightedness. Many people wear contact lenses instead of glasses, for cosmetic reasons or because it helps in sporting activities. Contact lenses can also be used for treating certain eye disorders and hiding unsightly eyes. Ideally, the lens material should not interfere with the oxygen supply to the cornea and the eye's lens, or with the usual working of the eye, such as tear secretion.

Contact lenses are broadly referred to as soft or rigid, and both types now allow varying amounts of oxygen to reach the cornea. The soft type (*hydrophilic*) are flexible and fit the shape of the eye, covering the whole of the iris. They are popular and different types are available that can be worn on a daily, bi-weekly, monthly or continuous-wear basis. Rigid lenses, the original contact lenses, are smaller and cover the pupil up to the iris. Materials used for rigid lenses (*hard* or *gas permeable*) have been improved to allow more oxygen to pass through. Rigid lenses take longer to get used to, but are good for correcting specific types of sight problems, for example those from irregular-shaped eyes. The original, *non gas-permeable* rigid lenses which did not allow any oxygen to pass through are no longer recommended. Contact lenses and their cases, that is the contact lens system, must be cared for meticulously with regular disinfection and cleaning. Poor disinfection and cleaning routines mean that the eyes, and therefore sight, are at increased risk of complications, for example from microbial contamination.

COMPLICATIONS

A contact lens is a foreign body in intimate contact with the eye and can cause complications. Any type of lens can damage the cornea causing problems such as pain, infection, foreign body sensation or discharge. If you get any problems with your lenses you should see an optician or ophthalmologist as soon as possible. Both types of lenses can cause complications. Most injuries arise from problems with the lenses including scratches, deformation and contamination. Research has shown that good lens hygiene is crucial in reducing the incidence of complications such as eye infections including the rare, but sight-threatening corneal infection Acanthamoeba keratitis. Acanthamoeba is a protozoa (page 294) – a microscopic organism that lives freely in soil and water. It is a potential hazard if non-sterile solutions, such as tap water or distilled water, are used to rinse, store or lubricate lenses. Infection with this organism is difficult to treat either with medicines or surgery, so preventing contamination is important. This and other microbial contamination is associated with ineffective lens cleaning/disinfection, and with contamination of the lens case or the eyes or lenses with tap water. Infection is also associated with irregular disinfection, trauma and swimming while wearing lenses (goggles are recommended for protection). Choosing the correct care products for your type of lens is essential as contamination can occur, for example using the one-step hydrogen peroxide disinfection solution which is less effective than the two-step version. It is important to discard contact lens solutions four weeks after opening because the preservatives become less effective and microbial growth can occur. Looking after your lenses carefully and cleaning them regularly in appropriate solutions for the lens system is essential. Check that your eyes are clear and comfortable and your vision is good each morning and evening.

Contact lenses are usually inserted daily, but high-water-content soft lenses and some hard lenses allow so much oxygen to get through to the cornea that they can be worn for up to three months. However, these extended-wear lenses are much more likely to cause infection with bacteria, fungi or viruses, tissue damage and inflammation. Most opticians would recommend shorter periods of wear for these particular lenses, especially if the lenses are worn just for convenience or cosmetic reasons.

LENSES AND MEDICINES

If you need to use eye drops or ointment you should not wear your lenses during the course of treatment, unless your lenses are for a medical purpose or your doctor says you may leave them in. Some medicines can spoil hydrophilic soft lenses and unless eye drops are known to be safe to use with these lenses, you must take them out before starting treatment and not wear them again until treatment has stopped. Eye drops may be used with rigid corneal contact lenses.

The plastic used for many hydrophilic contact lenses interacts with some preservatives used in eye drop preparations. This may cause irritation in the eye. **Benzalkonium chloride** is a common preservative and is unsuitable with all soft lenses. **Thiomersal** does not usually cause problems, **chlorhexidine** is satisfactory for some lenses and **phenylmercuric acetate** or **nitrate** is usually acceptable for short periods.

Some medicines that you take by mouth make it uncomfortable for you to wear contact lenses, for example:

- ☐ oral contraceptives (particularly higher oestrogen content)
- ☐ drugs that reduce tears e.g. atropine-like drugs, antihistamines, phenothiazines, tricyclic antidepressants, some beta blockers and diuretics
- ☐ drugs that increase tears, e.g. **hydralazine**
- ☐ drugs that reduce blink rate, e.g. antihistamines, hypnotics.

Others may discolour lenses – for example **rifampicin** and **sulfasalazine** – or be absorbed by the lens from tears: **aspirin** can cause irritation for example.

Ears

Middle-ear infection Glue ear
Outer-ear problems Wax

There are three parts to the ear. The outer ear is the visible part; the middle and inner ear are within the head protected by the skull. The outer ear flap (*pinna*) is mainly made of cartilage. It funnels sound along the ear canal to the eardrum (*tympanic membrane*), which separates the outer ear from the middle and inner ear. The middle ear contains three tiny bones within an air-filled cavity. The *eustachian tube* runs from the middle ear to the back of the throat, allowing pressure in the middle ear to be the same as the outside air pressure. The inner ear contains the organs of balance (*cochlea*) and of hearing (*labyrinth*).

Middle-ear infection

Middle-ear infection (*acute otitis media*) is common, especially in young children. Symptoms include earache, pain, fever, vomiting and temporary deafness. The middle ear can easily become infected if you have a nose or throat infection because bacteria or viruses gain access to it via the eustachian tube. A common cause of earache is a build-up of mucus in the ear after a cold. Viral infections have to run their course and are usually less serious than bacterial infections, which can be treated with antibiotics such as **amoxicillin** or **erythromycin**. Unless treated, pus from a bacterial infection may accumulate in the middle ear until the pressure builds up and the ear drum bursts or perforates. If the ear drum does burst, it will heal after the infection has cleared. Hearing may be impaired permanently. It is sometimes difficult for your doctor to tell whether your infection is caused by bacteria or a virus. Many middle-ear infections are caused by viruses that do not respond to antibiotics and will usually clear up with time. Many doctors now suggest a 'wait and see' approach with middle ear infections, particularly if you do not have fever or feel unwell. Research has shown that about three-quarters of ear infections improve within three days without an antibiotic and that an antibiotic does not shorten the duration of the illness. Having an antibiotic, just in case, means that you are exposed unnecessarily to its unwanted effects, such as feeling or being sick and diarrhoea. Pain can be relieved with either **paracetamol** or **ibuprofen**. If symptoms worsen during the 'wait and see' period then an antibiotic is likely to be needed.

Local treatment with ear drops applied to the outer ear does not help acute middle-ear problems. **Choline salicylate** (Audax) is a mild analgesic but is of doubtful value when applied to the ear. An analgesic taken by mouth gives better pain relief.

Glue ear

Glue ear (*otitis media with effusion* or *serous otitis media*) is the commonest cause of childhood deafness and affects at least one pre-school child in ten. Fluid that forms in the middle ear usually drains away but does not do so if it becomes thick and sticky; the cause of this is unknown. The transmission of sound through the middle ear is affected and hearing is impaired. Although it often follows middle-ear infection, there may be no history of ear problems at all. Poor ventilation of the middle ear via the eustachian tube may contribute, as may recurrent tonsillitis and adenoid trouble. A child with a cleft palate or Down's syndrome is particularly likely to have glue ear. Glue ear can interfere with the acquisition of normal speech and learning.

Sometimes glue ear improves spontaneously; about a quarter of the children who develop glue ear in their first year improve and half the children who develop it between the ages of one and four do. The condition improves in the summer but relapses again in the winter. Glue ear is less common in children aged over six years and in such cases often resolves of its own accord. However, at whatever age you suspect that your child has a hearing problem you should discuss your concerns with your doctor. Your child may be underperforming at school and behind in social development because of persistent deafness. Very rarely, hearing may become permanently impaired.

If glue ear is suspected your doctor may refer you to a specialist because of the risk of permanent damage to middle-ear function and impaired language development. Otherwise a period of watchful waiting, depending on the child's age and development and the severity of hearing loss, may be suggested.

Treatment with any medicine is not generally helpful. An antibiotic will only help where there is infection. There is little evidence that decongestants or antihistamines are helpful, although these preparations have been popular. Decongestants such as **pseudoephedrine** (Sudafed; Galpseud) may cause irritability, sleep disturbance and even hallucinations. Antihistamines cause daytime drowsiness and unsteadiness. Other things that you can do for your child include talking clearly and more loudly than usual, attracting your child's attention before speaking and shutting out background sound such as TV. Avoid exposure to tobacco smoke as this is a risk factor for glue ear, and raise awareness with your child's teachers.

Surgery for glue ear is now common, particularly for children aged between five and eight years. The surgeon is likely to insert *grommets* and/or to remove the *adenoids* if hearing is significantly impaired and does not improve within a few months. Grommets are tiny tubes inserted through the eardrum to allow fluid to drain into the outer ear. After a few months the grommet normally falls out and the ear drum heals.

Grommets that fall out need not be replaced unless symptoms recur. The child may swim, but not dive because water may get into the middle ear and possibly cause infection. Some doctors recommend using moulded earplugs and a swimming cap to cover the ears.

Outer-ear problems

The ear canal is lined with very fine skin covered with tiny hairs. Glands in the skin produce an oily fluid which combines with cells shed from the outermost layer of skin to form a covering of wax. The hairs catch dust and dirt which are then trapped in the wax; this is part of the ear's protective mechanisms against invading microbes.

Inflammation of the outer ear canal (*otitis externa*) is an eczema-like skin reaction. If the skin becomes broken, for example from scratching, bacteria or fungi may cause infection. The ear may itch and be quite painful; there may be some discharge and hearing may be impaired temporarily. These symptoms are similar to those of a middle-ear infection and it will be important to see your doctor for correct diagnosis.

HOW YOU CAN HELP YOURSELF

- ☐ The ear has its own self-cleansing mechanism, so avoid using cotton buds to clean out the wax. Wax is continuously produced and moves along the ear canal to the outer ear where it is removed with routine washing.
- ☐ If you develop an ear problem see your doctor.
- ☐ With outer ear problems, if the ear becomes itchy, try not to scratch it as this will encourage infection. Keep the ear canal dry and prevent soap or shampoo from getting in.
- ☐ If you have treatment, ask someone to help you apply the ear drops.
- ☐ Regular swimmers are more likely to get outer-ear problems because water breaks down the ear's protective and cleansing mechanisms. Use well-fitting ear plugs or petroleum jelly to protect the ears.

Applying ear drops

It may be difficult for you to put ear drops into your own ear so ask someone to help you. Three to four drops should be instilled into the ear canal without the dropper touching the ear. Drops are hard to keep in the ear for any length of time, so you should lie down on your side with the affected ear facing upwards for ten minutes after the solution has been instilled to allow time for the ear drops to take effect. Pressing the area in front of the ear a few times will help to get the drops into the deeper part of the ear. If there is a discharge, this should be gently mopped up. Cotton wool in the ear can prevent drainage but if you need to use some, place it in loosely and renew it frequently.

Medicines for the outer ear

If the ear is itchy and inflamed, but not infected, treatment involves using ear drops that are either astringent – causing the tissue to contract – such as **aluminium acetate**, or anti-inflammatory (a corticosteroid), both of which will help to clean the ear and soothe the inflammation. There is no evidence that one treatment is better than another. **Acetic acid** solution is active against both bacteria and fungi and useful for mild problems. An acetic acid spray solution (EarCalm) can be bought from a pharmacy.

The outer ear may be full of debris and discharge and this will need gently removing. Drops can then be instilled or, alternatively, a piece of ribbon gauze soaked in the drops can be placed gently into the ear canal. A corticosteroid such as **betamethasone** (Betnesol; Vista-Methasone) or **prednisolone** (Predsol) reduces itching and irritation but should not be used for prolonged periods as it may increase the likelihood of infection. If the ear is infected your doctor may give you ear drops containing an anti-infective drug such as **neomycin** or **framycetin**. The drops can be used for about one week but prolonged use may encourage the growth of bacteria which are resistant to the drug or allow the fungal infection to develop. **Chloramphenicol** ear drops may be used but they contain **propylene glycol** which causes sensitivity in about one person in ten. Ear drops containing an anti-infective and a corticosteroid may be used when the skin is infected as well as inflamed and eczematous. Compound anti-infective preparations containing several antibiotics, a corticosteroid, and sometimes an antifungal drug, are not recommended. An acute (sudden and severe) infection, such as a boil, may need treatment with an antibiotic by mouth, for example **flucloxacillin** or **erythromycin**.

The Committee on Safety of Medicines has told doctors that the risk of drug-induced deafness with **framycetin**, **gentamicin** or **neomycin** is increased if any of them is used in the outer ear when the ear drum has

ANTI-INFECTIVE PREPARATIONS

Anti-infective only

CANESTEN
CLOTRIMAZOLE

GARAMYCIN
GENTAMICIN

GENTICIN
GENTAMICIN

Not recommended

CHLORAMPHENICOL – High risk of sensitivity

Anti-infective with corticosteroid

AUDICORT
NEOMYCIN + TRIAMCINOLONE

BETNESOL-N
NEOMYCIN + BETAMETHASONE

GENTISONE HC
GENTAMICIN + HYDROCORTISONE

LOCORTEN-VIOFORM
CLIOQUINOL + FLUMETASONE

NEO-CORTEF
NEOMYCIN + HYDROCORTISONE

OTOMIZE
NEOMYCIN + DEXAMETHASONE

PREDSOL-N
NEOMYCIN + PREDNISOLONE

VISTA-METHASONE N
NEOMYCIN + BETAMETHASONE

Compound preparations: not recommended

OTOSPORIN
SOFRADEX
TRI-ADCORTYL OTIC

perforated. If you think your ear drum might be damaged, tell your doctor before he prescribes ear drops. Some specialists use these ear drops cautiously for treating severe middle-ear infections when the ear drum is perforated. The infection itself can impair hearing and your doctor will weigh the risks and benefits of using this type of preparation in the middle ear.

Wax

Wax provides a protective layer over the skin of the outer ear. It is a normal bodily secretion and does not need removing unless it is blocking the ear canal and drum and causing deafness or irritation.

The ear can be unblocked by using wax-softening drops. Sometimes using these drops for a few days may loosen the wax sufficiently to unblock the ear. Alternatively you may need to have the ear syringed with warm water by your doctor or practice nurse. If the wax is hard and impacted in the ear, using a wax-softening preparation before syringing will make the wax come out more easily.

A simple remedy is recommended – such as olive oil, almond oil or sodium bicarbonate ear drops. Any of these is effective and can be bought over the counter for less than the prescription charge. The oil can be warmed before use and you will need someone to help you put the drops into the ear. Lie with the affected ear uppermost for five to ten minutes afterwards. A small plug of cotton wool, coated in vaseline at the end to be inserted into the ear, may help to retain some of the fluid after treatment. Oil and wax may seep out, especially during sleep, and pillows can be protected with an old towel. Use the drops twice a day for three to four days.

Some brand name preparations contain solvents that may irritate the skin of the outer ear and should be avoided. Also, these preparations for removing wax are no better than simple oils and are generally more expensive. They include Cerumol; Exterol; Molcer; Otex; Waxsol.

Mouth and throat

Mouth ulcers Thrush
Sore throat Dry mouth

The mouth is the starting point of the digestive system. A *mucous membrane*, which secretes a slimy substance, lines the mouth, gums, palate and throat; saliva enters the mouth from glands beneath the tongue and near the ears. Special skin on the tongue contains most of the taste buds. The roof of the mouth consists of a hard (bony) palate and a soft (muscular) palate. At the back lie the *tonsils* and the *pharynx* – when these are inflamed they cause a sore throat (*tonsillitis* or *pharyngitis*). *Laryngitis* is inflammation of the vocal chords, which causes a sore throat along with hoarseness, loss of voice and a cough.

Mouth ulcers

Mouth ulcers are sore, swollen areas where the skin has broken in the mucous membrane in the mouth. At least three quarters of mouth ulcers are *minor aphthous ulcers* – these are not serious and do not point to any underlying disorder, but are painful and recur from time to time. Their cause is unknown. Women have mouth ulcers more frequently than men and they occur most commonly between the ages of 10 and 40. A day or two before the ulcer or ulcers break out part of your mouth may feel sore or burnt; pain and inflammation increase, particularly when you eat. The ulcers, up to five in number, are round or oval-shaped and whitish to yellow in the centre; the surrounding skin is red and swollen. Ulcers occur most commonly on the lips, cheeks and side of the tongue.

The mouth often acts as a barometer of health, and ulceration of the mouth can point to underlying disorders. Skin disorders often start in the mouth while vitamin deficiency or blood disorders such as iron-deficiency anaemia can cause a sore mouth or ulceration. Disorders of the digestive system such as inflammatory bowel disease (Crohn's disease and ulcerative colitis) and coeliac disease may be linked to mouth ulceration. Other causes include infection, injury, reactions to medicines, cancer and radiotherapy. Badly fitting dental plates may also be a cause of ulceration in the mouth.

Aphthous ulcers clear up of their own accord although they may take up to 14 days to heal. However, if you have an ulcer or a sore mouth which persists for more than two to three weeks, you should see your doctor. The underlying condition will need treating in addition to the ulcers.

Medicines for mouth ulcers

Local treatment aims to soothe the pain of ulcers while natural healing takes place. There are many remedies, including mouthwashes, protective pastes, gels and antiseptic lozenges. All of these may relieve symptoms in some people and you will need to find a preparation that suits you. Most of these are available from a pharmacy including local corticosteroid preparations (Adcortyl in Orabase; Corlan). Good evidence exists for the effectiveness of Corsodyl, local corticosteroids, **choline salicylate** gel and **benzydamine** mouthwash.

Mouthwashes

Mouthwashes are particularly useful when the ulcers are in awkward parts of the mouth and inaccessible. Simple mouthwashes of **sodium chloride** (for a home-made version use a rounded teaspoonful of salt to a pint of water) or **compound thymol glycerin** are soothing and may relieve the pain of ulceration caused by injury such as biting the inside of your mouth or by ill-fitting dentures. The mouthwash should be made up with warm water and can be used frequently to relieve swelling and pain.

Antiseptic mouthwashes such as **chlorhexidine** (Chlorohex; Corsodyl; Eludril) or **povidone-iodine** (Betadine) help to relieve pain and may speed healing of the ulcerated area; they are anti-infective, acting against bacteria and Candida. Some need to be diluted before use; follow the directions on the container. Chlorhexidine temporarily stains teeth, dentures and tongue a brown colour, through an interaction with tannin-containing foods and drinks, such as tea, coffee and red wines. Staining can be reduced by avoiding these items, by brushing your teeth and rinsing the mouth out well before using chlorhexidine. Occasionally the teeth and fillings may have to be scaled and polished to remove the stain completely.

Benzydamine mouthwash or spray (Difflam) can relieve the discomfort of various ulcerative conditions. It reduces the symptoms of radiation-induced mouth inflammation. The mouthwash can be used without dilution but some people find this causes stinging; diluting the liquid with an equal volume of water reduces this. Numbness and tingling of the mouth may occur but are short-lived. The mouthwash is not suitable for children under 12 years, but the spray can be used.

Carbenoxolone gel or granules (Bioplex) may relieve inflammation; the granules are added to water to make a mouthwash and used three times daily and at night.

Tetracycline mouthwash, made from breaking open a capsule and stirring it into a small amount of water, is used for severe recurrent aphthous ulceration. The mouthwash is held in the mouth for 2 to 3 minutes on each occasion, three to four times a day. The use of tetracycline mouthwash is unofficial and your doctor would need to prescribe it. It is generally used for three days. Longer courses may be needed but this increases the risk of thrush developing in the mouth. Tetracycline mouthwash should not be swallowed and can stain teeth. It should not be used in children under 12 years of age.

Protective pastes

Carmellose gelatin paste or powder (Orabase; Orahesive) protects the ulcer by forming a barrier over it and in this way it relieves discomfort. A thin layer can be applied when needed, usually after meals. The paste sticks to the ulcer, but it is quite difficult to apply, especially to some less accessible parts of the mouth. Carmellose gelatin paste is also made with the corticosteroid **triamcinolone** (Adcortyl in Orabase). The paste sticks to the ulcer and allows the corticosteroid to penetrate the damaged area. A thin layer must be carefully applied, not rubbed in, two to four times a day. In addition to treating aphthous ulcers the paste can be used for sore areas of the mouth caused by dentures, provided that these areas are not infected.

Lozenges

Hydrocortisone lozenges (Corlan) are most effective if they are used just before the ulcer develops. The lozenge is allowed to dissolve slowly in contact with the ulcer four times a day. Prolonged use may allow Candida to flourish. A corticosteroid should not be used if the mouth is infected, unless the infection is already being treated.

Compound benzocaine lozenges may relieve soreness in the mouth and painful ulcers. Benzocaine is a local anaesthetic which acts as an analgesic for a short time after it has been applied. **Lidocaine** (lignocaine) lozenges or ointment are also used. When a local anaesthetic is used in the mouth care must be taken not to anaesthetise the throat before meals as this might lead to choking. Prolonged use is not recommended because itching and soreness may develop.

Gels

Preparations containing **salicylic acid** (Pyralvex) or a **salicylate**, an aspirin derivative, have some analgesic action. **Choline salicylate** (Bonjela) may provide relief for recurrent aphthous ulcers. The benefit may come from rubbing the gums or pressure of application rather than the drug. It should not be used more frequently than every three hours because excessive application or confinement under a denture irritates the mouth and may cause further ulceration. Leave at least 30 minutes in between applying the gel and reinserting the dentures. Frequent use can lead to salicylate poisoning. Gels and other topical treatments, usually containing an antiseptic and/or a local anaesthetic such as **lidocaine** can be bought over the counter for the relief of mouth ulcers and for babies' teething problems.

Thrush

Thrush is a fungal infection caused by the yeast *Candida albicans* which lives harmlessly on the body until conditions change and allow it to proliferate (see also Chapter 5: Infections). Thrush infection in the mouth is common in babies and frail old people. Some drug treatments encourage Candida to grow unchecked, for example broad-spectrum antibiotics. Any drug that dampens the body's immune system, such as an oral corticosteroid or anti-cancer treatment, will allow Candida to proliferate. Some of the dose of an inhaled corticosteroid (for preventing asthma) is deposited at the back of the throat and this can lead to candidal overgrowth. Radiotherapy treatment to the head and neck region can also allow Candida to flourish. Conditions which interfere with the immune system, including diabetes mellitus, hormone disorders, blood disorders, advanced cancer and HIV infection, make you more susceptible to candidal overgrowth.

Oral thrush affects the mucous membrane on the insides of the cheek, the palate and throat, and also the tongue. Creamy white patches (*plaques*) which look like milk curds can be seen on a reddened mucous membrane. In babies oral thrush is often associated with a face rash. Milk curds, with which Candida may sometimes be confused, occur only on the insides of the cheeks and can be easily removed from the mucous membrane. They do not cause symptoms.

Denture stomatitis is inflammation of the mucous membrane caused by dentures which then become infected with Candida. The mucosa becomes red on the palate directly under the upper denture, but often does not cause symptoms. Candidal infection is usually associated with poor dental hygiene or an ill-fitting denture. *Angular cheilitis* is painful cracking at the angles of the mouth. Folding and fissuring at the sides of the mouth may be due to reduction of facial contour after loss of teeth or wearing down of dentures. Denture stomatitis and angular cheilitis often occur together and any infection should be treated. A sore mouth and angular cheilitis can occur with the lack of iron or vitamin B_{12}.

Medicines for oral thrush

Any underlying cause of candidal overgrowth should be considered by your doctor. For example, if an antibiotic or corticosteroid (oral or inhaled) is the probable cause then it may help to reduce the dose or change treatment. With an inhaled corticosteroid, using a spacer and rinsing the mouth with water after inhalation may help. Topical treatment with an antifungal medicine such as **nystatin**, **amphotericin** or **miconazole** (pages 283–6) is effective in controlling candidal infection. Treatment must be continued for two days after the infection appears to have cleared. Combinations of these drugs are no more effective than either drug alone and may even result in reduced effectiveness. Nystatin and amphotericin act locally and are not absorbed into the body whereas miconazole also acts locally but is partly absorbed and this increases the risk of interactions with other drugs. Intermittent or prolonged treatment may be needed where the underlying cause cannot be cleared up or is unavoidable. Treatment with an antifungal (**fluconazole** or **itraconazole**) which is taken by mouth, absorbed into the body and then works locally in the mouth may also be an option.

Oral suspension

Nystatin oral suspension (brand name Nystan) or amphotericin suspension (Fungilin) is swirled around the mouth several times before swallowing, four times a day after food. Nystan suspension does not contain sugar, lactose or gluten.

Lozenges and pastilles

Nystatin pastilles (Nystan) or amphotericin lozenges (Fungilin) can be sucked four times a day after meals. They stay in contact with the infected areas for longer than the suspension; children and older people may find them more acceptable.

Oral gel

Miconazole oral gel (Daktarin) is an orange-flavoured, sugar-free gel which is applied to the affected areas four times daily after meals. The gel should be kept in the mouth for as long as possible before swallowing. For babies the gel can be put on the candidal patches using a clean finger. A small tube of gel can be bought from a pharmacy.

Denture stomatitis and angular cheilitis

Denture stomatitis can be treated with an antifungal medicine but also needs improved oral and dental hygiene. Dentures should not be worn at night, particularly when you have angular cheilitis, and should be thoroughly cleaned with a brush at the end of the day. They should be left in diluted **hypochlorite** solution (such as Milton) or water with 1 to 2ml of nystatin suspension which should be replenished nightly. The denture(s) should be rinsed in water the following morning before use. **Chlorhexidine** solution is less effective against Candida but can be used as additional treatment for short periods. The mouthwash should be used 15 minutes before the denture is re-inserted.

Treatment of angular cheilitis sometimes needs to be prolonged with an antifungal locally in the mouth or tablets, for example miconazole gel, or nystatin cream or ointment, or suspension or fluconazole capsules by mouth. New dentures which restore the facial contour and reduce the folding at the corners of the mouth may help.

Sore throat

Discomfort at the back of the mouth and throat is commonly caused by local infection. It may also be due to allergy or drying of the mucosa caused by breathing through the mouth.

A sore throat is most commonly a viral infection which will get better with time; treatment with an antibiotic will not benefit a viral infection. Sometimes a sore throat may be caused by *streptococci* bacteria, which will require a systemic antibiotic, such as penicillin for ten days, not a local preparation. If the antibiotic **ampicillin** or **amoxicillin** (pages 269–270) is given for a sore throat caused by glandular fever (a viral infection), a rash often develops, although this does not mean you are allergic to the antibiotic.

Many antiseptic lozenges, sprays and gels are available over the counter, but there is little evidence that they are of benefit for a sore throat. Sucking a medicated lozenge, for example, stimulates the flow of saliva, but the same effect can be achieved with a boiled sweet or chewing gum (sugar-free). Antiseptic preparations may sometimes irritate the mouth and cause a sore tongue and lips. Some preparations contain a local anaesthetic such as **benzocaine**; they relieve pain but may cause itching and soreness.

Antiseptic gargles

During gargling the liquid is unlikely to get to the sore part of the throat unless it is swallowed. Even if it is swallowed – and this is not recommended – there is no evidence that a gargle helps. Two soluble aspirin tablets dispersed in half a tumblerful of water can be gargled and then swallowed. However, any benefit is likely to come from the systemic effect of aspirin rather than a local one.

Mouthwashes

Mouthwashes cleanse and freshen the mouth. Simple mouthwashes such as salt or **compound sodium chloride** mouthwash or **compound thymol glycerin** are useful and inexpensive. **Hydrogen peroxide** mouthwash also has a cleansing effect. **Chlorhexidine** (Chlorohex; Corsodyl; Eludril), **hexetidine** (Oraldene), **cetylpyridinium** (Merocet) and **povidone-iodine** (Betadine) are antibacterial, but will not help a sore throat caused by a virus.

Dry mouth

Dry mouth (*xerostomia*) may be caused by certain drugs with antimuscarinic side-effects, such as antispasmodics, tricyclic antidepressants and some antipsychotic medicines. Other causes include radiation treatment to the head and neck, or damage, perhaps through disease, of the salivary glands in the mouth. If you have a persistently dry mouth, you may develop a burning or scalded sensation in the mouth; poor oral hygiene may lead to dental caries and mouth infections (particularly thrush) and dentures may be uncomfortable to wear.

A dry mouth can be relieved using simple measures, such as taking frequent sips of cool drinks or sucking pieces of ice or sugar-free sweets or gum. When these are not sufficient, an **artificial saliva** can be used. The brand Luborant can be prescribed as a spray for use in the mouth for any condition giving rise to a dry mouth. Other preparations are available on the NHS only for dry mouth associated with radiotherapy or a condition known as *sicca syndrome*. These include AS Saliva Orthana spray or lozenges, Biotene Oralbalance gel, BioXtra gel, Glandosane spray, Saliveze spray, and Salivix pastilles. For other conditions associated with dry mouth BioXtra, Saliva Orthana lozenges, Salivese spray and Salivix pastilles can also be purchased over the counter for less than the current prescription charge. SST tablets, sucked slowly when required, are available to help dry mouth symptoms that arise when salivary gland function is impaired.

Pilocarpine tablets are used for dry mouth that arises following head and neck cancer; the drug is effective only if there is still some salivary gland function remaining following radiation therapy.

10

SKIN CONDITIONS

Eczema Psoriasis Acne
Scabies Lice Sunburn
Cuts, bites and stings
Warts and verrucae Cold sores

Skin is the body's largest organ. It protects the internal organs from external injury and keeps out harmful organisms such as bacteria. Together with the tissues underneath (*subcutaneous layers*) it acts as a store for water and fat, helping to conserve the body's fluids, although some of the body's waste products leave the body via the sweat glands in the skin. Nerve endings in the skin transmit the sensations of touch, pressure, pain and temperature and warn of possible injury. Skin plays an important part in regulating body temperature.

The thin top layer of skin cells is called the *epidermis*; the deeper layer below is known as the *dermis*. The epidermis varies in thickness in different parts of the body. Eyelids have the thinnest skin while on the palms of hands and soles of feet the epidermis is thick, hard and horny. On the outer surface dead cells are continually being rubbed off and replaced by new cells which are always forming in the bottom layer of the epidermis. Skin cells live for about three weeks, gradually moving towards the surface, where they die. The rate of formation of skin cells is highest during sleep and lowest during exercise and stress. Living cells make *keratin* which toughens the skin surface and makes up hair and nails. Some of the cells in the epidermis manufacture *melanin*, a pigment that absorbs some of the ultraviolet rays from the sun and protects against their harmful effects.

When you get hot your body loses water through the *pores* in the skin and this has a cooling effect. Each pore is a tiny opening through which fluid is released from the sweat glands in the dermis. The dermis also contains blood vessels and nerve endings. *Sebaceous glands* in the dermis make a type of oil (*sebum*) which lubricates and protects your skin and hair. The roots of the short hairs which grow from most parts of the skin are contained within channels (*follicles*) in the dermis. Although there are a number of disorders that may occur specifically on the epidermis and the dermis, skin often acts as a barometer of body health. Some skin conditions are outward signs of an underlying disorder. *Dermatitis* is the general term for skin problems when the skin is inflamed.

TYPES OF SKIN PREPARATION

Small amounts of a drug can be absorbed through the skin layers when applied as topical treatment. The drug should act locally, but some – for example, when a strong corticosteroid is applied to the skin for prolonged periods – inadvertently reach further into the body and may cause systemic effects. It is just as important to think of creams and ointments as medicines as those that are taken by mouth or injected.

The drug or active ingredient can be applied to the skin in a number of ways, using different 'vehicles', such as a cream, ointment or lotion, in which the drug is either dissolved or suspended. The vehicle carries the drug but may itself have beneficial effects on the skin, affecting how moist it is and how well the drug reaches the lower layer of skin (dermis). It may well have its own mild anti-inflammatory and soothing effect.

A *barrier* preparation contains ingredients such as **dimeticone** or **zinc compounds** to keep water and irritant substances away from the skin (see box).

- ☐ **A cream** is a fat- or oil-in-water preparation. It is less greasy than an ointment, mixes well with skin secretions and is easier to apply. Many creams have an *emollient* effect (pages 429–431).
- ☐ **An ointment** is a greasy preparation often containing soft paraffin, liquid paraffin, wax or lanolin. It does not dissolve in water and lies on the surface, protecting and lubricating the skin. Some modern ointment bases also mix with water and wash off readily. Ointments are useful for long-term dry skin conditions.
- ☐ **A gel** is a jelly-like base containing the active drug. Skin gels are usually clear so that when they dry they are hardly visible on the skin surface – an advantage for facial treatment.

BARRIER PREPARATIONS

Creams

CONOTRANE
DIMETICONE + BENZALKONIUM

DIMETICONE

DRAPOLENE
BENZALKONIUM + CETRIMIDE

MEDICAID
CETRIMIDE + LIGHT LIQUID PARAFFIN + WHITE SOFT PARAFFIN

SIOPEL
DIMETICONE + CETRIMIDE + ARACHIS OIL

SUDOCREM
WOOL FAT + ZINC OXIDE

VASOGEN
DIMETICONE + CALAMINE + ZINC OXIDE

ZINC CREAM

Ointments

METANIUM
TITANIUM DIOXIDE

MORHULIN
COD-LIVER OIL + ZINC OXIDE

ZINC OINTMENT

ZINC AND CASTOR OIL OINTMENT

Aerosol spray (main ingredients shown)

SPRILON
DIMETICONE + ZINC OXIDE + WOOL ALCOHOLS

Small quantities of many of these products can be bought from a pharmacy for less than the prescription charge.

- ☐ **A lotion** is a liquid with the drug dissolved or suspended in it. It is useful for applying a drug to a large or hairy area of the body. A lotion cools by evaporation and soothes inflamed unbroken skin. A 'shake lotion' such as calamine lotion leaves a fine powder on the skin surface as it dries and is useful for encouraging scab formation.
- ☐ **A paste** contains various amounts of insoluble powders, such as starch, **zinc oxide** or **titanium dioxide**. It is a thick and stiff preparation which acts as a barrier and protects the skin surface, and is used for marked thickening and scaling of the skin which occurs in psoriasis or long-term eczema.
- ☐ **A dusting-powder** is a mixture of dry powders such as talc, which reduces friction between skin surfaces. Rarely prescribed now, dusting-powders should not be used on moist skin because they can cake and rub the area.
- ☐ **A collodion** is a thick liquid painted on to the skin and left to dry to form a flexible, protective film over the area. A collodion may be used to seal a minor cut or wound, or to hold a dissolved drug in contact with the skin for a long period.
- ☐ **An application** is a thick liquid, an emulsion or suspension for putting on skin, nails or scalp.
- ☐ **A paint** is a liquid usually applied with a brush to the skin or mucous surfaces, such as the mouth.

Eczema and dermatitis

Eczema, from a Greek word for 'boiling', is a form of dermatitis characterised by itchy, red, scaly skin. Tiny blisters may form which leave a raw surface when scratched. The skin may become infected at this stage, usually with bacteria. If you have eczema for a long time the skin eventually becomes thickened, with the outer layer constantly flaking off as scales. The terms eczema and dermatitis are now used interchangeably.

Eczema from external causes

This is also known as *contact dermatitis* and is a common skin problem.

Irritant contact eczema occurs when the skin's surface is damaged by contact with an irritant substance, for example, detergents (washing-up liquid, shampoo, washing powders), disinfectants, acids or alkalis. The skin can react immediately or after repeated contact. The hands are commonly affected, particularly in certain occupations, for example, housework, hairdressing and building work.

Allergic contact eczema can occur when the immune system reacts to an external substance which has been touched, eaten or inhaled. There are thousands of substances with the potential to trigger an immune reaction – see box opposite for some of the common culprits. A rash develops on the skin as white blood cells release substances that open up the blood vessels in the dermis, making the surrounding area hot, red and swollen or inflamed. The reaction can take several days to develop after exposure to the trigger substance. It may develop at the point of contact – for example a nickel-containing bracelet may cause a distinct reaction around the wrist – but not necessarily. You can suddenly become allergic to a substance that has not caused a problem before. Although you can treat the skin rash, the best solution will be to discover what has caused the reaction and, if possible, avoid it on future occasions.

COMMON CAUSES OF ALLERGIC CONTACT DERMATITIS

- ☐ Nickel: jewellery (even some silver and gold), zips, coins, stainless steel, arch supports in shoes, door handles
- ☐ Rubber (latex) and associated chemicals: rubber gloves, shoes, insoles, rubber boots, chemicals
- ☐ Chromium: leather watch straps, wet cement, printing work, shoes, paints
- ☐ Epoxy resins: glues, insulating materials
- ☐ Lanolin: moisturisers and cosmetic creams, some medicinal creams and ointments
- ☐ Preservatives: most cosmetics and prescribed creams
- ☐ Plants: primula, chrysanthemum, poison ivy
- ☐ Formaldehyde: crease-resistant clothes.

Eczema from internal causes

There may be a family history with these types of skin conditions, but the mechanisms are not well understood.

Atopic eczema is common in babies and children and often starts during the first year of life. It is a common skin condition affecting up to one in five schoolchildren and up to one in ten adults.

Atopy describes a predisposition to allergic reactions. This type of eczema occurs in people who are atopic and in some cases it may be associated with asthma and/or hay fever. There is often a family history of these conditions. The skin is usually affected on the face in infants, and in the elbow creases and behind the knees in children. The skin can be itchy and very dry. The condition fluctuates with periods where it worsens ('flare-ups'), and then improves. The condition improves in many children as they grow older. They can outgrow it, but occasionally the problem persists into adulthood. In some cases atopic eczema may be linked with allergy to the house dust mite or to foods – for example, cow's milk, eggs or fish.

Seborrhoeic dermatitis (eczema) is a flaking and itchy skin condition associated with a yeast (*Malassezia*) that affects children and adults. In babies the scalp and forehead are commonly involved and the skin surface appears as a heaped mass of yellowish-brown scaling, sometimes known as 'cradle cap'. Adults have a scaly scalp and severe dandruff and a rash may develop on the face around the nose, eyebrows and also the chest, under the arms and in the groin.

Venous (varicose) eczema occurs on the lower legs in association with varicose veins or previous deep vein thrombosis (page 149). The skin becomes fragile and itchy and minor scratches can lead to a leg ulcer.

Asteatotic dermatitis is usually a result of skin drying out and most commonly affects older people or those suffering from minor malnutrition. The skin on the backs of the hands and fronts of the legs dries out, giving an appearance similar to crazy paving with deep fissures. The condition is aggravated by soaps and irritant substances and by scratching.

Medicines for eczema

Treatment depends on the cause of eczema and, if an underlying cause can be found and avoided – for example, in contact dermatitis – the condition may clear up without treatment. Where no obvious cause can be established easily – for example, atopic eczema – known skin irritants, such as detergents, wool or extremes of temperature should be avoided where practical. Treatment aims to keep the skin healthy, and to prevent or treat flare-ups. Soothing skin preparations (emollients) are the mainstay of treatment to protect the skin from outside irritants and to keep moisture in (*hydrated*). A corticosteroid applied to the skin is usually used for flare-ups; they can be used intermittently and, when you know how and when to use them appropriately, they rarely cause unwanted effects.

Intense itching (*pruritus*), caused by the release of body chemicals within the skin, can be excruciating. This leads to scratching to relieve the itch, which in turn releases more body chemicals, making the itch and inflammation worse. The skin can break down and allow irritants and bacterial toxins to penetrate, which leads to further drying. Sometimes a short course of a sedative antihistamine by mouth may help if itching is intense at night (page 178). **Doxepin** (Xepin) cream, a topical version of an antidepressant, reduces itching but seems little more effective than the vehicle alone. Effects include stinging and contact allergy when applied to the skin. The drug can be absorbed into the body and may cause drowsiness. Calamine lotion is not recommended because it is not very effective.

The topical treatments **tacrolimus** (▼Protopic) and **pimecrolimus** (▼Elidel) have anti-inflammatory properties, although how they work is not fully understood. They are immunosuppressants and do not cause skin thinning. They are new treatments for atopic eczema and their safety and appropriate use are still being evaluated. They are not suitable for children under two years of age. In severe cases an immunosuppressant, such as ciclosporin, by mouth may be needed (page 441).

Tar-containing products are occasionally used for chronic eczema. For example, a **zinc paste and coal tar bandage** may be used for treating limbs with conditions such as venous eczema. **Evening primrose oil** is available as a dietary supplement; it used to be prescribed but it was not sufficiently effective in relieving eczema. Some imported herbal creams that appear to be effective for children's atopic eczema, which were marketed as steroid-free herbal remedies, have been analysed and found to contain corticosteroids.

Mild seborrhoeic dermatitis (eczema) can be treated with a course of an anti-dandruff shampoo containing **pyrithione zinc,** which is widely available to buy, or **ketoconazole** shampoo (Nizoral), which you can buy from a pharmacy or your doctor can prescribe. Coal tar shampoos are also used, for example Alphosyl 2 in 1; Polytar AF. Cradle cap is treated with an oil (e.g. olive oil) rubbed gently into the scalp to loosen the scales before shampooing with a baby shampoo.

HOW YOU CAN HELP YOURSELF

- ☐ Avoid ordinary soap, bath additives and other detergents, as these can aggravate eczema.
- ☐ Take showers or short, cool baths. Use a soap substitute, such as emulsifying ointment or aqueous cream. Apply a soothing, moisturising preparation on damp skin after bathing.
- ☐ Cotton clothes and bedding keep the body cool. Avoid wool or wool mixtures as these can irritate.
- ☐ Use a non-biological washing powder and avoid a fabric softener, if this seems to irritate.
- ☐ Keep nails short if scratching is a problem. Cover children's hands with cotton mittens at night time.
- ☐ Keep bedrooms free of dust to minimise contact with the house dust mite (see also 'Asthma', pages 154–7).
- ☐ Wear rubber or plastic gloves with cotton linings when cleaning or washing up to protect against the effects of water and detergents. Use a moisturising hand cream afterwards.
- ☐ Gentle exercise and support stockings or tights can help varicose veins and venous eczema. These measures may prevent an ulcer forming on the leg.
- ☐ Contact The National Eczema Society*, which has branches and local groups providing support and information.

SOOTHING PREPARATIONS – EMOLLIENTS

For dry, scaling skin, an *emollient* preparation can be used. Emollients, consisting of mixtures of water, fats, waxes and oils, soothe and moisten dry skin. They should be used generously and frequently at least daily; ideally three to four times a day if possible. You should apply an emollient when the skin is moist and continue treatment even after the condition begins to improve. If large areas of the body are affected then you will need around 500g of an emollient a week, and for a child around 250g. Use of an emollient is essential for atopic eczema and may reduce flare-ups and the need for a topical corticosteroid. Emollients can be applied as creams, ointments or lotions, used as soap substitutes or added to the bath (e.g. emulsifying ointment), but all have a similar function. Ointments and oily preparations usually give better results for dry skin but are greasy and messy to use. There is a wide range of preparations, from simple formulations to more complex and expensive products, but many contain white soft paraffin or liquid paraffin as a basis. Some products combine an antiseptic with an emollient but there is no evidence to support their routine use to reduce bacterial activity on the skin. Different emollients can be used – for example an ointment at night, with more cosmetically acceptable creams applied during the day. Comparisons of products have not been carried out and choice depends on which preparation suits you and your skin.

Aqueous cream is a simple, effective and inexpensive preparation. It is mainly free of ingredients that can cause sensitisation, although this can occur, particularly in children. In general, creams contain more preservatives than ointments. Fragrances and preservatives (e.g. **parabens**, **benzyl alcohol**) can worsen an existing condition by causing contact allergic dermatitis in addition to the original problem, and so may some emollient ingredients, e.g. **lanolin** – hydrous wool fat – although hypoallergenic versions of lanolin have reduced the problem. If your skin condition worsens during treatment or does not seem to clear up, you may be allergic to one of the ingredients, either the drug itself or an additive (see box).

Products with **arachis** (peanut) oil should be avoided if you are allergic to peanuts. Some evidence suggests that arachis oil in some skin products used on babies may increase the risk of peanut allergy, particularly if products are applied to oozing or crusting areas of skin.

Camphor, menthol or **phenol** are included in some preparations and may ease itchiness. **Zinc** formulations are mildly astringent and are used as barrier preparations. Urea cream is used for moisturising scaly skin and may be helpful for older people.

EMOLLIENT PREPARATIONS

Creams/gels

AQUEOUS CREAM

AVEENO
OAT (protein fraction)

CETRABEN
WHITE SOFT PARAFFIN + LIGHT LIQUID PARAFFIN

DECUBAL CLINIC
ISOPROPYL MYRISTATE + GLYCEROL + WOOL FAT + DIMETICONE

DIPROBASE
LIQUID PARAFFIN + CETOSTEARYL ALCOHOL + WHITE SOFT PARAFFIN

DOUBLEBASE GEL
ISOPROPYL MYRISTATE + LIQUID PARAFFIN

E45
LIQUID PARAFFIN + WHITE SOFT PARAFFIN + WOOL FAT (hypoallergenic)

GAMMADERM
EVENING PRIMROSE OIL

HEWLETTS CREAM
WOOL FAT + ZINC OXIDE + ARACHIS OIL + WHITE SOFT PARAFFIN

HYDROMOL
SODIUM PIDOLATE

LIPOBASE
FATTY CREAM BASE

NEUTROGENA DERMATOLOGICAL CREAM
GLYCEROL + EMOLLIENT BASE

OILATUM
LIGHT LIQUID PARAFFIN + WHITE SOFT PARAFFIN

ULTRABASE
LIQUID PARAFFIN + WHITE SOFT PARAFFIN

UNGUENTUM M
WHITE SOFT PARAFFIN + LIQUID PARAFFIN

VASELINE DERMACARE
DIMETICONE + WHITE SOFT PARAFFIN

Creams containing urea

AQUADRATE

BALNEUM PLUS

CALMURID

E45 ITCH RELIEF

EUCERIN

NUTRAPLUS

Ointments

DIPROBASE
LIQUID PARAFFIN + WHITE SOFT PARAFFIN

EMULSIFYING OINTMENT

EPADERM
YELLOW SOFT PARAFFIN + LIQUID PARAFFIN

HYDROMOL
YELLOW SOFT PARAFFIN + EMULSIFYING WAX

HYDROUS OINTMENT

KAMILLOSAN
CHAMOMILE EXTRACTS + WOOL FAT

WHITE SOFT PARAFFIN

YELLOW SOFT PARAFFIN

Lotions

KERI
MINERAL OIL + LANOLIN OIL

LACTICARE
LACTIC ACID + SODIUM PIDOLATE

VASELINE DERMACARE
DIMETICONE + LIQUID PARAFFIN + WHITE SOFT PARAFFIN

Aerosol spray (main ingredients shown)

DERMAMIST
WHITE SOFT PARAFFIN + LIQUID PARAFFIN + COCONUT OIL

Bath additives

ALPHA KERI BATH
LIQUID PARAFFIN + WOOL FAT

AVEENO
OAT (PROTEIN FRACTION)

BALNEUM (also available with tar)
SOYA OIL

DERMALO
ACETYLATED WOOL ALCOHOLS + LIQUID PARAFFIN

DIPROBATH
ISOPROPYL MYRISTATE + LIGHT LIQUID PARAFFIN

E45
CETYL DIMETICONE

EMOLLIENT MEDICINAL BATH OIL
ACETYLATED WOOL ALCOHOLS + LIQUID PARAFFIN

EURAX
ACETYLATED WOOL ALCOHOLS + LIQUID PARAFFIN

HYDROMOL EMOLLIENT
ISOPROPYL MYRISTATE + LIGHT LIQUID PARAFFIN

IMUDERM
ALMOND OIL + LIGHT LIQUID PARAFFIN

OILATUM
ACETYLATED WOOL ALCOHOLS + LIQUID PARAFFIN

Small quantities of many of these products can be bought from a pharmacy for less than the prescription charge.

Products with antiseptics (not recommended for routine use)

DERMOL 500 LOTION
BENZALKONIUM CHLORIDE + CHLORHEXIDINE + LIQUID PARAFFIN +ISOPROPYL MYRISTATE

DERMOL 200 SHOWER EMOLLIENT
BENZALKONIUM CHLORIDE + CHLORHEXIDINE + LIQUID PARAFFIN + ISOPROPYL MYRISTATE

DERMOL 600 SHOWER EMOLLIENT
BENZALKONIUM CHLORIDE + LIQUID PARAFFIN + ISOPROPYL MYRISTATE

EMULSIDERM LIQUID
BENZALKONIUM CHLORIDE + LIQUID PARAFFIN + ISOPROPYL MYRISTATE

OILATUM
BENZALKONIUM CHLORIDE + TRICLOSAN + LIGHT LIQUID PARAFFIN

CORTICOSTEROID PREPARATIONS

Corticosteroids used on the skin (topically) suppress inflammation. A topical corticosteroid (steroid) blocks the action of the substances released by white blood cells that cause redness, swelling and heat. They accelerate the healing of damaged skin and can help reduce inflammation and itching. Corticosteroids are widely used for eczematous conditions, including weeping eczemas, providing they are not infected. Their use in eczema has been by tradition rather than by thorough evaluation, but the trials that have been done suggest that over three-quarters of patients benefit from using a corticosteroid. They are recommended for short periods intermittently to manage the flare-ups associated with atopic eczema. They do not cure eczema permanently but bring relief while they are used.

Topical corticosteroids are classified into four groups according to their strength, from mild to very potent (see table, page 434). Most people with atopic eczema have mild to moderate symptoms, which can be managed by a mild or moderately potent corticosteroid. The least potent preparation should be used to control the condition. The most potent corticosteroid preparations are generally reserved for the most difficult skin conditions under specialist supervision. When used properly a topical corticosteroid rarely causes unwanted effects and you should not be afraid to use one.

Using a corticosteroid on the skin

These guidelines can help with the appropriate use of a corticosteroid skin preparation.

- ☐ Use as mild a corticosteroid as possible for as short a period as possible to gain control of your condition: for example, 3 to 7 days for an acute flare-up or 2 to 3 weeks for chronic eczema.
- ☐ At the first sign of a flare-up, start treatment.
- ☐ Hydrocortisone 1%, a mild steroid, will be adequate for most flare-ups in children with mild to moderate eczema.
- ☐ For adults, a mild corticosteroid such as hydrocortisone should be applied to the face, skin creases (*flexures*) and thin skin, such as the genitals, only on the advice of your doctor. For other parts of the body a potent corticosteroid can be used in short bursts for three days in a row, repeated every week until the flare-up settles.
- ☐ Continue to use an emollient regularly, but not at the same time of day as the corticosteroid. Once-daily application of the steroid is usually sufficient.
- ☐ Apply the corticosteroid only to the inflamed or affected area of skin; do not use it as a general emollient.
- ☐ Put a thin covering only of the preparation on the affected area of skin so that you leave a glistening surface to the skin. The label should read 'To be spread thinly'; applying large quantities will not produce a quicker or better result.
- ☐ Ask for guidance from a health professional on the amount of preparation to use. A measure from the farthest crease in the index finger to the tip for adults ('fingertip unit') provides about half a gram (0.5g or

500mg). This should be enough to cover an area of skin twice that of a flat adult hand (fingers closed). Children use less than this – ask for guidance on measuring and application.

- Do not use a corticosteroid on its own on broken or untreated infected skin.
- If your doctor prescribes a corticosteroid preparation for a particular skin condition, do not use it for any other problem.
- Do not lend your corticosteroid to anyone or borrow anyone else's preparation. If the preparation is used for the wrong skin condition, even if it looks the same, the problem could be made much worse.
- If your skin condition worsens during treatment, discuss possible reasons with your doctor. You may be allergic to one of the ingredients (see box, page 427).

Failure to respond to treatment should be discussed with your doctor. Topics you may like to review include: Is it the right preparation for my condition? Is the corticosteroid potent enough? Are there underlying factors such as a bacterial or viral infection? Have I used the corticosteroid and emollients properly? Have I inadvertently been exposed to aggravating factors such as soap or bubble bath?

Absorption of a topical corticosteroid increases when it is applied under a dressing (*occlusion*), on severely inflamed skin, on thin skin or at flexures, such as the groin. This increases the risk of unwanted effects in both the skin and the body, but can be used carefully to increase the effectiveness of a topical corticosteroid, particularly in difficult and resistant skin conditions. 'Wet wrap' dressing, where the corticosteroid is applied under an inner wet layer and then an outer dry layer of cotton tubular dressing, is effective but generally used on specialist advice only.

Corticosteroids from a pharmacy.

You can buy a mild corticosteroid, certain brands of **hydrocortisone** or **clobetasone**, at a pharmacy for less than the prescription charge, but only for specified conditions and in certain circumstances. You may not buy any product if you are pregnant, or buy those containing hydrocortisone for a child under 10 years or clobetasone for a child under 12 years of age. Hydrocortisone cream (0.1% or 1%) or ointment (1%) can be purchased to treat allergic contact dermatitis, irritant dermatitis, insect bite reactions or mild to moderate atopic eczema for up to one week. Clobetasone 0.05% can be bought for short-term treatment or control of small patches of atopic eczema, allergic contact dermatitis or irritant dermatitis. These over-the-counter corticosteroids are not to be used on the face or delicate areas or on infected or broken skin. Your pharmacist can advise you about whether a product will be suitable or whether you should see your doctor.

Unwanted effects of topical corticosteroids

When used carefully for short periods, mild or moderately potent corticosteroid preparations are rarely associated with unwanted effects. A potent corticosteroid is generally safe and may be needed for thicker areas of the skin, such as on the palms, soles or thickened and hardened parts of skin. The more potent the preparation used in non-thickened areas, the more care is needed.

Excessive or prolonged use of a potent or very potent preparation can produce changes to the skin area being treated. The commonest effect is thinning of the skin; sometimes stretch marks develop that become permanent. Fine blood vessels under the skin surface may become more prominent (*telangiectasia*) and damaged, resulting in redness and a 'broken

CORTICOSTEROID PREPARATIONS

Mild

DIODERM
HYDROCORTISONE

EFCORTELAN
HYDROCORTISONE

HYDROCORTISONE

Certain brands available from a pharmacy

MILDISON
HYDROCORTISONE

SYNALAR 1 in 10 DILUTION
FLUOCINOLONE 0.0025%

Moderately potent

BETNOVATE RD
BETAMETHASONE VALERATE 0.025%

EUMOVATE (15g tube available from a pharmacy for adults and children over 12 years)
CLOBETASONE

HAELAN
FLUDROXYCORTIDE (FLURANDRENOLONE)

MODRASONE
ALCLOMETASONE

STIEDEX LP
DESOXYMETHASONE 0.05%

SYNALAR 1 IN 4 DILUTION
FLUOCINOLINE 0.00625%

ULTRALANUM PLAIN
FLUOCORTOLONE

Potent

BETACAP
BETAMETHASONE 0.1%

BETAMETHASONE
VALERATE 0.1%

BETAMOUSSE
BETAMETHASONE VALERATE 0.12%

BETNOVATE
BETAMETHASONE VALERATE 0.1%

CUTIVATE
FLUTICASONE

DIPROSONE
BETAMETHASONE DIPROPIONATE 0.05%

ELOCON
MOMETASONE

LOCOID
HYDROCORTISONE BUTYRATE

METOSYN
FLUOCINONIDE

NERISONE
DIFLUCORTOLONE 0.1%

PROPADERM
BECLOMETHASONE

STIEDEX
DESOXMETASONE 0.25%

SYNALAR
FLUOCINOLONE 0.025%

Very potent

DERMOVATE
CLOBETASOL

HALCIDERM
HALCINONIDE

NERISONE FORTE
DIFLUCORTOLONE 0.3%

All preparations are prescription-only.

vein' appearance. Other effects include increased hair growth, skin changes, exacerbation of acne, mild loss of skin colour (depigmentation – which may be reversible), and a rash around the mouth, particularly in young women. An untreated, infected skin condition can spread and worsen. When a potent or very potent corticosteroid has been used for some time, there may be a worsening of the skin condition when you stop using the preparation abruptly. The dosage can be gradually reduced or a less potent corticosteroid used to avoid a worsening of the condition. 'Stepping down' is unlikely to be necessary when using a potent corticosteroid for short bursts intermittently. Rarely, potent and very potent corticosteroids can be absorbed through the skin and cause effects throughout the body, for example Cushing's syndrome (page 328).

SENSITISERS IN SKIN PRODUCTS

Preservatives or other ingredients in skin products are more liable to cause problems on eczematous skin than on normal skin. Tracing what has caused the skin sensitivity can be difficult. See if you can test a small amount of emollient or other product first, before it is prescribed or you buy it. The list gives some of the common ingredients found in skin products that can cause sensitisation.

- beeswax
- benzyl alcohol
- butylated hydroxyanisole
- butylated hydroxytoluene
- cetyl alcohol
- chlorocresol
- EDTA
- ethylenediamine
- fragrances
- hydroxybenzoates (parabens)
- isopropyl palmitate
- lanolin and wool fat derivatives (purified versions reduce sensitisation)
- polysorbates
- propylene glycol*
- stearyl alcohol
- sorbic acid

**Acts as an irritant more often than causing allergic sensitisation.*

ANTIBACTERIAL PREPARATIONS

The bacterium *Staphylococcus aureus* lives on and around the body and may be involved in triggering acute flare-ups of atopic eczema. An antibiotic by mouth, either **flucloxacillin** or **erythromycin**, may be prescribed if infection is obvious – that is, if there are signs of pus, weeping or crusting, or if the infection is widespread or keeps recurring. Infected eczema is sometimes treated locally with an antibacterial cream or ointment. The antibacterial in the preparation is usually an antibiotic that is not used within the body to treat other infections, so that bacteria are not exposed to it too often and do not become resistant to the drug. Examples include **mupirocin** (Bactroban), **neomycin + bacitracin** (Cicatrin) and **polymyxin** (Polyfax). Mupirocin should not be used for longer than ten days; some resistance to its effectiveness against *Staphylococcus aureus* is starting to emerge.

The antibiotic **neomycin** is used on the skin, usually in combination with another antibacterial or a corticosteroid. It is no longer recommended for use alone or for large areas of skin because it can be absorbed into the body, for example in children and older people, increasing the risk of adverse effects (e.g. impaired hearing). Neomycin can also cause an allergic skin reaction with prolonged use. As mentioned above, an antibiotic skin preparation should be used for as short a time as possible and if the disorder worsens, making the skin more red and inflamed, you should see your doctor again.

Combination preparations of a corticosteroid with an antibiotic (e.g. **fusidic acid + hydrocortisone** – Fucidin H) or antifungal (**hydrocortisone + nystatin** – Timodine) are used on the skin when infection is suspected or present. However, it is debatable as to how useful these combined topical preparations are compared with a corticosteroid on its own. If there is obvious infection, treatment with an antibiotic by mouth may be more appropriate.

If the skin is 'weeping' your doctor may recommend the use of a wet dressing or soak (for example, weak **potassium permanganate** solution) to cleanse the skin, before applying an emollient. Not all skin conditions that ooze and weep are infected, but keeping the skin area clean with usual hygienic measures is important.

Psoriasis

Psoriasis is a chronic and sometimes distressing skin condition which can recur from time to time. In healthy skin, dead cells are constantly being rubbed off from the outer layer of the epidermis and are replaced by new cells made at the base of the epidermis. In psoriasis, this process of ordered and continual renewal goes wrong and new cell production speeds up to about ten times the normal rate, so cells accumulate under the outer layer. This process is caused by an inflammatory reaction in the dermis. Skin is usually affected in patches, and these appear as raised and thick red areas, often covered by silvery scales. This is *chronic plaque psoriasis*, the most common type. The scalp, elbows, knees and knuckles are most commonly affected, although large areas of skin can be involved. Itching is a common symptom. There are other types of psoriasis, such as *guttate psoriasis* – when a sudden eruption of small raindrop-like patches occurs, often triggered two weeks after *streptococcal tonsillitis*. In three out of ten cases it can disappear after one or two months even without treatment. *Erythrodermic psoriasis* and *generalised pustular psoriasis* are severe forms involving much of the body; these need urgent specialist assessment. These conditions can be triggered on the withdrawal of topical or systemic corticosteroids. Pustular psoriasis on the hands and feet only does not lead to the severe form. Psoriasis may be accompanied by a distinctive form of arthritis.

The underlying cause of psoriasis is not known, but around two per cent of people in Britain have the condition. Psoriasis appears for the first time at any age, but commonly between the ages of 11 and 45.

It can affect anyone, but certain genes have been linked to psoriasis. If you have a genetic tendency then it appears to require a trigger to start up the condition; for example, stress, skin damage or illness.

Occasionally psoriasis may be triggered or worsened by drug treatment with one of the following medicines: **lithium**, **chloroquine**,

hydroxychloroquine, **beta blockers**, **NSAIDs**, **ACE inhibitors**. Psoriasis may not develop until the medicine has been taken for a prolonged period.

Psoriasis comes and goes for no obvious reason. The skin may look unsightly and unpleasant, but it is not infectious. The condition may clear up (*remit*) for long periods, but there is no complete cure. It can recur at any time. Psoriasis is a condition which needs advice and guidance from your doctor, specialist nurse or a dermatologist. Good management and appropriate treatments greatly improve the outlook if you have psoriasis. Non-drug measures are generally similar to those for atopic eczema (page 429). The Psoriasis Association* provides information on all aspects of the condition and offers local support groups.

Medicines for psoriasis

Treatment aims to relieve the inflammation and scaling and to lessen the area of skin involved. The choice of treatment depends on which part and how much of the body is affected, and how you tolerate the condition and its various treatments. Local treatment is the mainstay for mild to moderate psoriasis, but for more severe conditions a medicine may be given by mouth, or other specialist treatments, such as *photochemotherapy*, used.

LOCAL TREATMENT

Emollients are essential to hydrate the skin, for their effects on drying, scaling and cracking (pages 429–31). They may also have an effect in slowing abnormal skin cell production. An emollient preparation may be all that is needed in mild conditions, but is also useful added to more specific treatments. Where the disorder is more troublesome, topical treatment with **vitamin D** or **vitamin A derivatives**, **coal tar**, **salicylic acid** or **dithranol** may help. Treatments may be used individually or in combination, depending on how effective they are and how well you tolerate them; there is great variability. Treatments can also irritate the skin and must be avoided in any inflammatory phases of psoriasis. Each treatment should be assessed after four to six weeks and continued if it is effective. If it causes significant irritation, the treatment could be reduced or stopped. Controlled exposure to ultraviolet radiation (*phototherapy*) either through natural sunlight or a special lamp may help, but you should ask your doctor or specialist about this. Ultraviolet radiation is sometimes combined with tar or dithranol treatment.

Topical vitamin derivatives

Vitamin D and its derivatives (analogues) do not smell or stain and may be more acceptable and easier to use than tar or dithranol preparations. Synthetic vitamin D preparations, **calcipotriol** (Dovonex) or **tacalcitol** (Curatoderm), or **calcitriol** (▼Silkis), an active form of vitamin D, may be helpful for plaque psoriasis. They block abnormal division of skin cells. Local skin reactions may occur – itching, redness, burning, tingling and rashes – and sometimes psoriasis can be worsened. Calcipotriol is combined with a corticosteroid, betamethasone, in ▼Dovobet, but corticosteroids have a limited role in psoriasis (see page 440). The effectiveness of vitamin D preparations may decline after a few weeks' regular treatment, but if you suspend treatment for a few weeks, efficacy returns. You could alternate treatment between a vitamin D derivative and other treatment. Vitamin D and derivatives should not be used if you have a calcium metabolism disorder, such as high levels of body calcium (*hypercalcaemia*). A derivative of vitamin A, **tazarotene gel** (Zorac) can be used for mild to moderate psoriasis affecting up to ten per cent of the body surface area. It is applied once daily usually in the evening and can be used for up to 12 weeks. Unwanted effects also include itching, burning, redness and irritation. Tazarotene can cause birth deformities and must be avoided in pregnancy. Women who can become pregnant must use adequate contraception during treatment.

Tar preparations

Coal tar lessens itching and inflammation and reduces the thickness of scaly lesions. It is also mildly antiseptic. Some of the older products are still effective – for example, coal tar and salicylic acid ointment can be rubbed well into the skin and is not unpleasant despite its smell. Tar preparations can be used up to three times a day starting with a low-strength preparation. Crude coal tar contains thousands of constituents and attempts to purify it have produced less effective compounds. Newer products are, however, less messy to use and include creams, lotions and bath preparations. Examples of products include Alphosyl, Carbo-Dome, Psoriderm and Polytar. Tar products can irritate the skin and sometimes cause an acne-like rash; they should not be put on broken or very inflamed skin. Tar baths need to be combined with ultraviolet radiation to be effective. Tar products may stain the skin temporarily and clothes and bedding permanently.

Salicylic acid

This can be used to loosen and remove thick scaly patches. A low-concentration ointment is used at first and the concentration gradually increased during a course of treatment. Unwanted effects are few but salicylic acid may occasionally cause allergic rash and drying and irritation of the skin. If large skin areas are covered or salicylic acid is used for long periods, it may be absorbed into the body sufficiently to cause dizziness and tinnitus. Salicylic acid is mixed with other ingredients in topical preparations – for example, zinc, coal tar and dithranol – to increase efficacy. Scalp psoriasis can be treated with a combination of salicylic acid, coal tar and/or sulphur and left on for at least one hour or overnight before washing off; products include Cocois and Pragmatar.

Dithranol

This compound is the most effective topical preparation for treating psoriasis, but it must be used carefully because it can cause severe skin irritation and staining of the skin and clothes. It is usually applied only to the affected skin area, covered and left for one hour or less and then removed. An overnight application of dithranol paste covered by stockinette dressings is used for intensive treatment. Some people cannot tolerate dithranol preparations even at low concentrations; fair skin is more sensitive than dark skin. If it is not tolerated it must be stopped, otherwise psoriasis may worsen. Dithranol may be combined with salicylic acid or coal tar for better effect. Some branded products are easier to use and cause less staining and irritation than the traditional pastes and ointments.

DITHRANOL

On prescription/from a pharmacy – if products contain less than 1% dithranol
DITHRANOL – Ointment, paste (Lassar's paste)
DITHROCREAM – Cream
MICANOL – Cream

Combination preparations
PSORIN – Ointment
DITHRANOL + CRUDE COAL TAR + SALICYLIC ACID
PSORIN – Scalp gel
DITHRANOL + SALICYLIC ACID
Dithranol preparations can be bought from a pharmacy if the dithranol content is less than one per cent.

Dithranol is a very effective topical treatment for mild to moderate chronic plaque psoriasis of the skin and scalp. It slows the rate of production of new skin cells in the base of the epidermis. Dithranol is irritant to the skin and is used at a low strength, for example 0.1%, with the concentration gradually increased during a course of treatment, depending on individual tolerance. It must be applied only to the affected skin patches; the surrounding skin must be protected with petroleum jelly.

In more severe cases, dithranol is combined with ultraviolet radiation treatment in hospital (Ingram's method). You soak in a warm bath containing coal tar solution and after drying you are exposed to a regulated amount of ultraviolet radiation. Dithranol is applied to the affected patches and the normal skin protected by dressings. This process is repeated daily.

Before you use this medicine

Tell your doctor if you are:
☐ pregnant or breast-feeding ☐ taking any other medicines, including vitamins and those bought over the counter.

Tell your doctor if you have had:
☐ a previous reaction to dithranol.

Do not use if you have:
☐ acute or pustular psoriasis ☐ hypersensitivity to dithranol or other ingredients of preparations.

How to use this medicine

Put a thin layer of the topical preparation on the affected patches of skin or scalp and rub in once a day. Directions for contact time may vary depending on the product used. The surrounding skin can be protected with petroleum jelly. After treatment, the preparation should be removed by bathing or showering. Pastes may be difficult to remove but an oily liquid such as liquid paraffin may help. Always wash hands thoroughly after using or touching dithranol products.

Apply daily for best results. Treatment may take between four and six weeks with gradual increases in the strength of dithranol, but good effects can be achieved. If you miss a dose, apply as soon as you remember.

Over 65 No special requirements.

Interactions with other medicines

Topical treatments (for example, salicylic acid and coal tar) with dithranol increase the skin's sensitivity and may cause additional redness and irritation.

Phenothiazine antipsychotics, **griseofulvin**, **thiazide diuretics**, **sulphonamides** and **tetracycline** may occasionally increase the skin's sensitivity to light, adding to the irritant effect of dithranol.

Unwanted effects

Likely Local burning sensation, skin irritation, staining of skin, hair, clothing, bedding and bathware.
Less likely Allergic skin rash.

If skin irritation or burning sensation is severe, contact your doctor.

Dithranol is a strong irritant and not usually recommended for the face or near the eyes, the inside of the thighs, the genital region or skin-fold areas. If dithranol gets into the eyes, bathe them immediately with copious amounts of water and seek medical advice. Dithranol has a laxative effect if swallowed.

Dithranol stains skin but this disappears in two to three weeks. Fabrics, clothing and bed linen stain permanently, so old clothes and linen should be used during a course of dithranol treatment. Staining in basins and baths can be removed with bleach.

Corticosteroids

Topical preparations are not suitable for use on their own for extensive psoriasis. Corticosteroids on the skin appear to help psoriasis initially, but with continuous use their effectiveness lessens progressively. When a topical corticosteroid is stopped after prolonged treatment, the psoriasis can become much worse and difficult to manage with other preparations. A mild corticosteroid may be useful for the face and skin folds; a more potent one can be used for other parts of the body for short periods; generally specialist advice will be required. Leave a week in between finishing treatment with a topical corticosteroid and starting dithranol. Other treatments can be used with a corticosteroid but at different times of the day, unless combined in one preparation. A corticosteroid by mouth is rarely used and taken only on specialist advice.

OTHER SPECIALIST TREATMENTS

A small number of people do not benefit from topical treatment or relapse very quickly after it. If psoriasis is extensive or disabling, systemic treatment may become necessary. These various treatments are only carried out by skin specialists and under hospital supervision.

Photochemotherapy

This involves the interaction of a **psoralen** (a relatively inert drug) and long-wave ultraviolet radiation (UVA); hence the treatment is named PUVA. The drug makes the skin cells sensitive to UVA rays and the radiation stops cells dividing so quickly. Treatment is available only in specialist centres and is suitable only for certain people. Severe burning is a short-term adverse effect while long-term hazards include the development of skin cancer, accelerated ageing and cataracts if proper care is not taken to protect the eyes.

Anticancer drugs

In severe resistant cases an anticancer drug, usually **methotrexate**, may slow the rapid rate of division of new skin cells. Methotrexate is taken by mouth (10–25mg), usually once a week, and has to be carefully monitored because it can damage the liver and bone marrow. **Azathioprine** (Imuran) or **hydroxycarbamide** (Hydrea) are alternative treatments.

Ciclosporin

An immunosuppressant medicine obtained from a fungus, ciclosporin (Neoral) diminishes the body's immune response to agents that are introduced into the body, for example in organ transplantation. It is also used to treat severe resistant psoriasis or severe atopic eczema. It is taken by mouth as capsules or a liquid. Your doctor will want to check your treatment regularly because ciclosporin can damage the kidneys.

Acitretin

This preparation, derived from vitamin A, is used for severe psoriasis and other rare disorders of the skin (e.g. Darier's disease). Acitretin (Neotigason) has a marked effect on cell division and abnormally thickened skin. It is taken by mouth, often for several months, with a rest period in between courses. Acitretin has a narrow therapeutic range, so unwanted effects are common at the start of treatment. You may experience dryness and cracking of the lips and dry skin which becomes red and itchy. Nosebleeds may occur and some hair loss, although this is reversible. Sometimes the hair falls out (*alopecia*) but regrows after treatment is finished. Acitretin can cause birth deformities and must be avoided in pregnancy. Women who can become pregnant must take effective contraceptive measures for at least one month before to at least two years after a course of acitretin. You should avoid excessive exposure to sunlight and sunlamps while taking acitretin (unless supervised) because photosensitivity can occur. Acitretin should not be taken at the same time as any of the **tetracycline** antibiotics or with **methotrexate**.

Acne

Acne is a very common skin condition, especially for young people, although it can also affect adults. It affects the skin on the face, neck, back and chest. Acne is part of puberty and growing up, and few teenagers escape it completely. Over half of all young people aged 14 to18 have mild to moderate acne; slightly more boys than girls suffer and usually more severely. About two out of ten teenagers have moderate to severe problems. While the exact cause of acne is not fully understood, it seems that a combination of increased oil production in the skin, the acne bacterium and the influence of hormones contribute to acne.

Increased production of the skin's natural oil (sebum) and of dead skin cells at the base of the hair follicle leads to blockage in the hair follicle, the duct above the sebaceous gland, as sebum and skin cells move towards the skin surface. If the follicle remains open, a plug of grease can be seen, which eventually darkens because it contains melanin. This is a blackhead (*open comedone*). If the opening becomes blocked completely, the sebaceous gland enlarges and a whitehead forms (*closed comedone*). A *pustule* develops from a whitehead when a species of bacterium which usually lives harmlessly on your skin starts to grow in the sebum trapped in the duct. This triggers the body's defence mechanism and white blood cells battle with bacteria just underneath the skin, resulting in a red spot with a yellow head. Sometimes painful inflamed cysts form in severe acne, when the walls of the grease duct and sebaceous gland rupture under the skin surface. Sebaceous gland activity is regulated by hormones. *Androgens*, the male sex hormones, stimulate sebaceous gland activity, while the female sex hormones, *oestrogens*, suppress it.

HOW YOU CAN HELP YOURSELF

- ☐ Acne is part of the body changes that take place in puberty, although it may continue into adulthood. See your doctor if you develop acne and have more than just a few spots occasionally.
- ☐ Permanent scarring can occur with acne and moderate to severe conditions need medical advice and a strategy of treatment.
- ☐ Picking, squeezing and messing with spots does not help and may cause extra damage to the skin, possibly leaving a bigger spot or scar.
- ☐ Obsessive cleansing with any of the many advertised products does not improve acne. Acne is no more common on dirty skin than on clean skin. However, removing excessive grease from the skin at normal washing time helps to make the skin feel better.
- ☐ Diet does not seem to affect the course of acne. Eating chocolate has not been shown to be linked to acne. In general try to eat a healthy, balanced diet.
- ☐ If you wish to camouflage the worst areas, use a non-greasy cosmetic base. Avoid layers of grease-based preparations.
- ☐ Sensible exposure to sunlight (pages 456–7) may be helpful for some people with mild to moderate acne, although improvement is usually temporary. Some drugs, for example tetracyclines used for acne, can cause photosensitivity. Over-exposure to ultraviolet radiation carries the long-term risk of skin cancer.

Acne treatments

Acne is treated with preparations applied to the skin (topical) and with medicines taken by mouth, depending on the severity of the condition. The choice of treatment depends on whether you have blackheads and/or whiteheads predominantly or whether the skin is more reddened and inflamed. Mild acne – a few spots now and then – can be treated with local application of **benzoyl peroxide gel**, which you can buy at a pharmacy more cheaply than paying the prescription charge, if you pay one. For moderate to severe cases, you may need to combine topical treatment with an antibiotic by mouth or try another systemic treatment such as **co-cyprindiol** (Dianette – for women only). **Isotretinoin** (Roaccutane) is reserved for severe acne that is likely to scar or that has not responded to antibiotic treatment by mouth. It may be several weeks before you see the benefit from any acne treatment.

LOCAL TREATMENT

Some topical preparations, such as the antibiotic solutions, are antibacterial only while others, such as benzoyl peroxide, have a mixed action – they are antibacterial and also encourage the skin surface to peel (*keratolytic*). Blackheads, whiteheads and inflamed areas respond well to benzoyl peroxide or **azelaic acid** (Skinoren). If acne does not respond to benzoyl peroxide after two months' regular treatment then a topical antibiotic solution could be tried. A **retinoid** (vitamin A derivative) can be useful for acne that is predominantly blackheads and whiteheads. Inflammatory acne may respond to an antibiotic solution (**erythromycin** or **clindamycin**) on the skin. Nicotinamide, of the vitamin B group, can be applied twice daily to skin as a gel for inflammatory acne.

Preparations that are not recommended because evidence for their use is poor include **antiseptics**, **corticosteroids**, **sulphur**, **salicylic acid**, **resorcinol** and **abrasives**. Topical corticosteroids can cause harm and products containing them should not be used.

BENZOYL PEROXIDE

On prescription/from a pharmacy
BREVOXYL – Cream
PANOXYL – Cream, gel, lotion, skin wash

Combined preparations
BENZAMYCIN – Gel (prescription only)
BENZOYL PEROXIDE + ERYTHROMYCIN

QUINODERM – Cream, lotion
BENZOYL PEROXIDE + HYDROXYQUINOLONE

Benzoyl peroxide is used on the skin for treating acne. It can be used for controlling a few spots or moderate to severe acne, when it is often combined with systemic treatment, such as an antibiotic. Benzoyl peroxide helps to remove excess dead skin cells and to unblock the sebaceous duct and hair follicle. It also acts against the bacteria in the sebum, the skin's natural oil. It is available in strengths ranging from 2.5 per cent to 10 per cent. You would normally start with a low-to-moderate strength product (2.5 per cent or 5 per cent) and, after two weeks' treatment, increase the strength. Benzoyl peroxide bleaches coloured fabrics.

Before you use this medicine

Tell your doctor or pharmacist if you are:
☐ pregnant or breast-feeding – no restrictions on use ☐ taking any other medicines, including vitamins and those bought over the counter.

Tell your doctor if you have or have had:
☐ sensitivity to benzoyl peroxide.

How to use this medicine

Wash the affected areas and dry gently. Apply a thin covering of the cream, lotion or gel once or twice a day. Apply regularly to get the best results, unless skin irritation develops. For very sensitive skin apply every other day. See your doctor after two weeks' treatment for assessment and discuss whether you need to change the strength of the preparation.

Over 65 Not usually used by older people.

Interactions with other medicines

Tretinoin Do not apply at the same time as benzoyl peroxide. They can be used alternately, but together may cause contact dermatitis.

Unwanted effects

Likely Skin irritation, burning, redness, peeling.
Less likely itching, rash.

Keep benzoyl peroxide away from eyes, mouth and other mucous membranes. If it accidentally touches sensitive areas, wash it off immediately. If you expose your skin to strong sunlight, apply benzoyl peroxide less often. If blistering, crusting or a skin rash develops stop using benzoyl peroxide and see your doctor.

Similar preparations

DIFFERIN – Cream, gel
ADAPALENE

ISOTREX – Gel
ISOTRETINOIN

ISOTREXIN – Gel
ISOTRETINOIN + ERYTHROMYCIN

RETIN-A – Cream, gel, lotion
TRETINOIN

SKINOREN – Cream
AZELAIC ACID

Poor choice: little evidence of effectiveness:

ACNISAL – Liquid
SALICYLIC ACID

ACTINAC – Lotion
CHLORAMPHENICOL + HYDROCORTISONE + SULPHUR

BRAVISOL – Paste
ABRASIVE

ESKAMEL – Cream
SULPHUR + RESORCINOL

Vitamin A derivatives (retinoids)

Local treatment with the vitamin A derivatives **tretinoin** (Retin-A) and **isotretinoin** (Isotrex) or a related product, **adapalene** (Differin) helps acne, particularly where there are blackheads and whiteheads. Tretinoin helps to loosen dead skin cells and allows sebum to flow more freely. Your doctor can prescribe tretinoin as a cream or gel. It is applied lightly once or twice daily to the areas where spots occur, after washing. Erythromycin is combined with tretinoin (Aknemycin Plus) as a solution and also with isotretinoin (Isotrexin) as a gel. Adapalene is less irritant than the other retinoids and is anti-inflammatory.

At the start of treatment there may be some stinging and the skin may feel warm, but you should aim for slight redness, similar to that of mild sunburn. If you have sensitive skin you can use tretinoin once a day. It may be six to eight weeks before a reasonable effect is seen and you will need to be patient and persevere with treatment. During the early weeks of treatment you may find that your acne seems to get worse, as tretinoin acts on previously unseen spots developing under the skin.

You should not get tretinoin in the eyes, mouth and mucous membranes or use it on broken or eczematous skin. If tretinoin accidentally touches sensitive areas, wash it off immediately. You should not use tretinoin at the same time, or alternate it with, other peeling agents, such as benzoyl peroxide. Avoid using an ultraviolet lamp or solarium and exposing treated areas in sunlight, because tretinoin increases sensitivity to UVB light. Unwanted effects including irritation, burning and peeling occur as part of treatment, but contact your doctor if these reactions are severe or your skin becomes sore. You must not use a retinoid on the skin if you are pregnant. Vitamin A and derivatives are potential teratogens (page 49), although the risk is low with the topical preparations. Use a secure method of contraception during topical retinoid treatment.

Topical antibiotics

Products containing **tetracycline** (Topicycline), **erythromycin** (Stiemycin; Zineryt) or **clindamycin** (Dalacin T; Zindaclin) are applied once or twice daily, after washing, to the entire area, not just to the individual spots.

In mild to moderate acne, topical antibiotic treatment, which reduces bacterial action, seems to be as effective as benzoyl peroxide or tretinion, but not more so. Topical antibiotics are usually less irritant and may help if skin soreness is a problem. The solutions are alcoholic and may cause stinging at the start of treatment which usually fades with time. Tetracycline solution may stain skin yellow and mark clothing. A topical antibiotic may help if you cannot take an antibiotic by mouth, but can rarely cause sensitisation.

SYSTEMIC TREATMENT

For moderate to severe acne or if the skin condition does not improve with topical preparations, your doctor may consider a treatment by mouth. Antibiotics, hormonal treatment and a vitamin A derivative may be tried at different stages.

Antibiotics

Oxytetracycline or **tetracycline** (pages 272–4) is used to reduce the bacteria in the sebaceous ducts and glands. These antibiotics do not act against blackheads and whiteheads that are not inflamed, so topical treatment such as a retinoid (but not a topical antibiotic) must be continued. The dose for either antibiotic is 500mg twice daily, which must be taken on an empty stomach (the morning dose an hour before breakfast). If acne does not improve after the first three months, another antibiotic could be tried. The best improvement occurs between four to six months. With severe acne, antibiotic treatment may be needed for two or more years.

Doxycycline and **minocycline** are alternative tetracyclines, but probably no more effective. They are better absorbed from the gut and can be taken with food. Erythromycin is less used because the acne bacterium is becoming resistant to it. **Trimethoprim** 300mg twice daily may be used for acne that is resistant to other antibiotics. Its use is unlicensed and occurs usually only under specialist guidance. Unwanted effects can occur (pages 277–8), including digestive system upsets such as diarrhoea. If you are also taking an oral contraceptive and diarrhoea develops, additional contraception may be necessary within the first three weeks, but after that the gut bacteria develop resistance to the antibiotic and extra contraception is no longer necessary. None of the tetracyclines should be used in pregnancy because they can harm the baby's developing bones and teeth. Erythromycin can be used during pregnancy. Minocycline may sometimes cause a darkening of the skin, which may be irreversible. It can also trigger *systemic lupus erythematosus* or worsen the existing condition, and treatment must then be stopped. Tetracyclines can provoke photosensitive rashes (pages 272–4).

Hormonal treatment

The combined oral contraceptive pill can help acne because oestrogen dampens sebaceous gland activity and suppresses androgen production. However, progestogens have androgenic properties and can worsen acne, particularly if a progestogen-only contraceptive is used. A combined pill containing one of the newer progestogens (norgestimate, gestodene or desogestrel) may be less androgenic.

Co-cyprindiol (Dianette) contains **cyproterone acetate** and **ethinyloestradiol** and is used for treating women with severe acne which has not responded to prolonged treatment with an antibiotic by mouth. It is also used for moderately severe excess hairiness (*hirsutism*), a symptom of polycystic ovary syndrome, and other conditions where androgen levels may be raised in women. Co-cyprindiol is also a form of hormonal contraception and has similar unwanted effects to the combined pill. Its tendency to cause blood clots in the deep veins of the legs (page 355) is higher than if you take a low-dose combined pill.

DIANETTE

DIANETTE – Tablets
CO-CYPRINDIOL – CYPROTERONE ACETATE + ETHINYLESTRADIOL

The combination of low doses of cyproterone and ethinylestradiol in co-cyprindiol is used for treating women with severe acne which has not responded to a prolonged course of antibiotic by mouth. Androgen, the male sex hormone, is present in small but variable amounts in all women. Androgen contributes to increased sebum production in acne, which does not necessarily mean that you have abnormally high androgen levels. Cyproterone, a synthetic progestogen, blocks androgen activity while the oestrogen ethinylestradiol reduces the amount of androgen made by the body. See Chapters 6 and 7 for details of combined oral contraception. Co-cyprindiol may also help moderately severe cases of hairiness (hirsutism) because hair growth is also androgen-dependent. Dianette also acts as an oral contraceptive, but is only prescribed if you have severe acne that has not responded to oral antibiotic treatment and/or hirsutism.

Before you use this medicine

Tell your doctor if you are:
☐ pregnant – do not take as cyproterone may cause female characteristics in a male baby ☐ breast-feeding – do not take ☐ taking any other medicines, including vitamins and those bought over the counter.

Tell your doctor if you have or have had:
☐ severe liver impairment or disease ☐ blood clots (thrombosis or embolism) or deep vein thrombosis, or family history of these ☐ diabetes with circulatory problems ☐ disorders of fat (lipid) metabolism ☐ breast or endometrial cancer ☐ sickle-cell anaemia ☐ abnormal vaginal bleeding ☐ pemphigoid (herpes) gestationis during pregnancy ☐ deterioration of hearing disorder (otosclerosis) during pregnancy.

How to use this medicine

Take one tablet every day for 21 days, starting on the first day of your period. The next course is started after seven tablet-free days. Improvement in skin condition may take several months and treatment is often needed for six to nine months. Three to four months after your condition has cleared, co-cyprindiol should be stopped.

If you miss a dose, take it as soon as you remember. If you take the tablet within 12 hours of the missed dose you do not need to take additional contraceptive measures. If more than 12 hours have passed, take the most recently missed dose, ignore earlier missed tablets, but continue to take the next seven tablets on the correct days. You will need additional contraception, such as the condom, for the next seven days. If you miss tablets during the last seven days of a course, then you should start the next pack without the usual seven-day break. At the end of the second course withdrawal bleeding should occur.

Over 65 Not generally used.

Unwanted effects

(See also Combined pill, pages 359–61.)
Likely Feeling or being sick, headache, breast tenderness, changes in weight.

Less likely Blood clots – deep vein thrombosis, changes in libido, depression, skin changes, high blood pressure, liver disease, decreased tolerance to wearing contact lenses.
Rare Increased sensitivity to sunlight.

Breakthrough bleeding or 'spotting' may occur, especially during the first few cycles. You may bleed less during the withdrawal bleeds, but this is usual. If withdrawal bleeding does not occur at all, you should see your doctor. It is important to exclude pregnancy as a possible cause before continuing with treatment.

Similar preparations

Cyproterone is used for treating prostate cancer (Cyprostat) and also to reduce tumour flare after starting gonadorelin analogue treatment (page 334). Cyproterone (Androcur) is also used on its own in higher doses for treating male hypersexuality and sexual deviation.

Isotretinoin

Isotretinoin (Roaccutane), a vitamin A derivative, is used for treating very severe acne where there are disfiguring pockets of inflammation under the skin, cysts and nodules. It reduces sebum production and the build-up of dead skin cells in the hair follicle. It relieves swelling and helps the duct to unblock. Isotretinoin is used only if systemic antibacterial treatment has been unsuccessful. This drug must not be used during pregnancy and is available only as hospital treatment under the guidance of a consultant dermatologist.

One course of three to four months' treatment produces good results in the majority of people and there is a reasonable chance (one person in two) of the condition clearing completely. However, isotretinoin has some troublesome unwanted effects, such as dry mouth, mucous membranes and skin. Dryness of the skin may cause scaling, thinning, redness and itching. Dryness of the mucous membranes in the nose may result in nosebleeds and a dry throat can lead to hoarseness. There may be muscle and joint pains and hair may be lost, but it will regrow after treatment has finished. Isotretinoin occasionally causes liver enzymes and the blood level of fats to increase, so these are checked during treatment. There is concern that isotretinoin treatment may be linked to depression and possibly to suicide, but studies have not established a direct link. Having acne is depressing and it usually coincides with major hormonal and bodily changes and also life changes (e.g. going away from home to college). You will need to discuss the pros and cons of having isotretinoin treatment with your doctor and family, who can be primed to watch out for mood changes after you start this treatment.

Women must use effective contraception while taking isotretinoin and for at least one month after treatment. Your doctor will want to make sure that you are not pregnant before starting treatment.

Scabies

Scabies and lice (page 450) live in or on the skin. They are parasites spread by close contact, causing irritation and itching of the skin, an allergic response to the mite.

Scabies (*Sarcoptes scabei*) or the 'itch mite' affects people regardless of how clean or dirty they are. It spreads usually by direct skin contact between children, between sexual partners and commonly throughout a household. *Crusted scabies*, another type of scabies (formerly 'Norwegian scabies') can also be spread via bedding and clothing. Female scabies mites burrow into the skin and lay eggs just under the surface. The eggs hatch in three to four days and become adults in 10 to 14 days, to begin the cycle again. Intense itching, especially at night, usually starts one to eight weeks after the first infection. The rash most commonly affects the hands (usually between the fingers), insides of the wrists, the elbows, the feet and the genital area. The head and neck are hardly ever affected, except in babies. The intense itching leads to scratching so that the rash sometimes looks like eczema. The scratched skin may become infected with bacteria.

HOW YOU CAN HELP YOURSELF

- ☐ If you have an itchy rash, ask the advice of a pharmacist or your doctor.
- ☐ Bathing and scrubbing will not remove the mites; you will need to use an insecticide lotion.
- ☐ Scabies mites and eggs cannot live for very long away from their human host. Re-infection from clothing or bedding is not a significant risk, except with crusted scabies, but you may feel that you want to change bedding after treatment. Hot washing, dry cleaning and ironing will all kill any mites.
- ☐ Schoolchildren should be kept at home until treatment has been carried out.

Medicines for scabies

In itself the scabies mite does not cause serious health problems, unless the skin becomes infected. Scabies is unpleasant because it causes intense itching and irritation and spreads through the community if left untreated. If you have scabies it is important to treat all people with whom you are in close contact at the same time, even if they do not have symptoms. It may be eight weeks after the first infection before you have any signs of itching, and during this time you can spread the disease without knowing. Treatment is usually applied to the whole body, including the scalp, neck, face and ears, especially the skin between the fingers and toes, the genital area, the palms and soles and under the nails. Re-apply after washing any part of the body during a treatment course.

Preparations include **permethrin 5% cream** (Lyclear Dermal Cream) as first-line treatment for 8 to 12 hours or water-based lotions of

malathion 0.5% (Derbac M, Quellada M) for 24 hours; wash off after the treatment time. Water-based lotions are preferable to those containing alcohol, which can irritate broken skin. You use one of these products twice, leaving one week between each treatment. You should not have a bath before applying the lotion. A hot bath may increase the absorption of the drug into the body and so take it away from its site of action on the skin.

Itching, and sometimes skin bumps (nodules) may persist for several weeks after treatment, even though the mite has been eliminated. An emollient or mild topical corticosteroid can help to soothe persistent itching. **Crotamiton** (Eurax) is rarely used for treating scabies but may be useful for persistent itching; it should not be used on broken skin. For night-time itching a sedative antihistamine by mouth may also help.

Benzyl benzoate lotion is still sometimes used but it is irritant and smells unpleasant. It can cause stinging, itching and burning of the skin and sometimes a rash. Benzyl benzoate has to be used on two or sometimes three consecutive days without bathing or washing hands (or it must be re-applied after washing) in between applications. It is not recommended for children, for use on broken eczematous or infected skin or during breastfeeding. Preparations of **lindane** have been discontinued in the UK.

Lice

This section discusses two common types of lice: the head louse (*Pediculus humanis capitis*) and the crab (pubic) louse (*Phthirus pubis*).

Head lice are blood-sucking insects which live close to the scalp where the environment is warm and moist with plenty of food and where they can lay eggs. They attach themselves to the base of the hair by strong, crab-like claws and do not let go even during hair-washing. Lack of hygiene or long hair does not encourage lice; in fact short, clean hair makes it easier for them to reach the scalp. Head lice infestations are very common, particularly in children aged 6 to 11. However, children of all ages can become infested, as can adults, although lice are rare in adult men. Head lice spread by close contact; for example, when heads touch, the lice simply walk from one head to the other.

An adult louse is about 3mm to 4mm long and greyish in colour. It lays about six to eight eggs a day, which are yellow and shiny and are stuck firmly to the hair base. As the baby lice grow they leave the empty egg cases, the cream or whitish coloured 'nits', still attached to the hair. After seven days the louse reaches adult form and begins the egg-laying cycle. Often the first sign of infection is itching, but by this time the lice have been in the hair for several weeks. Itching is an allergic response to lice saliva, which is injected into the scalp each time the lice feed. It takes thousands of lice bites before itching develops. When you have had head lice for some time, you start to feel unwell or 'lousy' and may have a mild temperature, muscle aches and perhaps glandular swelling.

Crab (pubic) lice are commonly passed on during sexual contact. The lice are dirty-white to yellow or grey in colour and live on fluid in the tissues. Symptoms include itching and irritation in the genital area; occasionally, hair under the arms and on the legs is infected. The skin may have blue-grey spots, not raised, which if scratched may become reddish with pus.

Children may acquire lice from infected adults or other children. Their eyebrows and eyelashes sometimes become infected. **Malathion** (pages 452 to 453) and **carbaryl** kill crab lice. Malathion aqueous lotion can be used for crab lice on eyelashes. Only water-based lotions should be used because the alcohol-containing preparations cause stinging and irritation, especially on the genitals and on scratched and broken skin.

HOW YOU CAN HELP YOURSELF

- ☐ If you know there is an outbreak of lice, for example among your child's classmates, check your family's hair (including adults) for lice immediately. Favourite places for lice include the hair behind the ears, at the nape of the neck and back of the head and under a fringe. Comb the hair over a piece of white or lightly-coloured cloth or paper with an ordinary comb and then with a fine-toothed nit comb. Lice are damaged by combing and some may fall out on to the paper as pink or brown specks.
- ☐ Nits cannot be confused with dandruff. Nits are shiny and stick to the hair while dandruff is dull and flaky and falls out.
- ☐ If you find evidence of lice, use the 'bug-busting' method (see overleaf) or get an appropriate lotion from a pharmacy.
- ☐ Lice and eggs not killed during treatment do not survive for long away from the scalp or other areas of skin. Generally it is not necessary to change pillowcases and sheets after treating the infection.
- ☐ Inspection after hair washing and regular combing with a fine-toothed comb for each member of the family helps to keep hair healthy and lice-free.
- ☐ People in close physical contact with someone with crab lice should have treatment.

Medicines for lice

Malathion and carbaryl lotions kill both the lice and the eggs. **Phenothrin** liquid or lotion (Full Marks) is also effective. Water-based lotions are preferred for children, or if you have asthma or severe eczema. Shampoos or similar preparations are not recommended because they are not in contact with the insects for long enough and may be diluted too much during use to be effective. **Permethrin** (Lyclear Creme Rinse), **phenothrin** (Full Marks Mousse), **Prioderm** and **Quellada M** shampoos are therefore not sufficiently effective. Products containing **benzyl benzoate** are also less effective. Resistant strains of lice have developed to several head lice treatments in some areas. If one treatment does not work, you need to try another one. Alternative treatments, for example tea tree oil, are unproven.

Treatment for head lice should be repeated after one week to kill lice coming out of any eggs that might have survived the first treatment. None of these products should be used on a 'just in case' basis for trying to prevent lice. Only treat if lice are found, but only regular inspection and combing will prevent lice becoming residential. 'Bug busting', a non-chemical way to treat and prevent head lice, requires regular combing with a 'bug busting' comb or similar fine-toothed comb every three to four days; to eliminate lice do this meticulously on five successive occasions. After normal hair washing, a conditioner is applied to wet hair and left on the head while the hair is combed methodically in sections. Combing removes the young lice easily before they have a chance to become adults and start laying eggs. A head louse repellent containing **piperonal** (Rappell) may help to keep hair louse-free by making the hair feel cold to the lice. Its effectiveness is not yet established.

MALATHION

From a pharmacy/on prescription
DERBAC-M – Lotion (water-based)
SULEO-M – Lotion (contains alcohol)

Not recommended
PRIODERM – Lotion (contains alcohol), shampoo (not available on NHS prescription)
QUELLADA M – Lotion (water-based), shampoo

Malathion is an insecticide used for treating scabies and lice. It kills them by interfering with their nervous system. Malathion also kills the eggs. It is available as a lotion or shampoo but the lotion is a better choice. The alcohol-containing lotion is effective if you have normal skin, but is not suitable for everyone, or for treating scabies or crab lice, but the water-based lotion can be used instead. Water-based lotions are best if you have asthma or you are treating small children because the fumes from the alcohol-containing products may trigger coughing and wheezing; they may also sting broken skin and should not be used on eczematous skin.

Before you use this medicine

Tell your doctor if you are:
☐ pregnant or breast-feeding – malathion could be used ☐ taking any other medicines, including vitamins and those bought over the counter.

Tell your doctor if you have or have had:
☐ sensitivity to malathion ☐ eczema ☐ asthma.

Babies under six months – wet comb if possible; see your doctor if you have to treat with an insecticide.

How to use this medicine

For head lice Rub the lotion into dry hair, the scalp and the affected area. Avoid getting it in the eyes. Comb the hair and allow it to dry naturally. Do not use a hair dryer because heat of any sort destroys the effectiveness of the insecticide.

Leave the lotion on for 12 hours and then wash off by shampooing in the normal way. Comb wet hair with a normal comb and then with a fine-toothed comb to remove dead lice and nits.

A residue of insecticide remains on the hair for several weeks, which may help to ward off re-infection if the hair is allowed to dry naturally. Swimming in a chlorinated pool reduces any residual effect except with permethrin.

Alcohol-containing lotions are effective but must be used carefully because they are flammable. Always allow the hair to dry naturally in a well-ventilated room. Do not cover the head before the lotion has dried completely.

For pubic (crab) lice Treat the whole body, including hairy areas, with a water-based lotion. Leave the lotion on for 12 hours or overnight. Wash off or bathe in the usual way. A second treatment is necessary after one week to kill lice coming from surviving eggs.

For scabies Use the water-based lotion. Apply to the whole body from the neck down. Pay particular attention to the skin between the fingers and toes, the palms and soles. Leave on for 24 hours before washing.

Do not use malathion more than once a week or for more than three consecutive weeks.

Over 65 No special requirements.

Unwanted effects

Less likely Skin irritation, stinging (with alcoholic lotions).

If used according to the instructions, malathion rarely causes adverse effects. Contact your doctor immediately if malathion is accidentally swallowed.

Similar preparations

Prescription only

CARYLDERM – Lotion (contains alcohol), liquid (water-based)
CARBARYL

On prescription/from a pharmacy

FULL MARKS – Liquid (water-based), lotion (contains alcohol) mousse (not recommended)
PHENOTHRIN

LYCLEAR – Cream rinse 1% (not recommended), skin cream 5% for scabies
PERMETHRIN

Sunburn

Staying out for too long in strong sunlight without protecting your skin can result in redness and swelling of the skin, particularly if you are fair-skinned. People vary in their sensitivity to sunlight, with skin types ranging from very pale skin which never tans to darker skin which rarely burns, but everyone needs to be careful in the sun The sun makes you feel good and a little sunshine every day helps you to remain healthy. *Ultraviolet* (UV) rays in sunlight activate a body chemical in the skin to form vitamin D. Doctors use types of ultraviolet light, in carefully controlled doses, to suppress certain skin problems such as eczema and psoriasis.

There are three main types of UV radiation: UVA and UVB, which reach the earth and can damage your skin, and the shorter-wave UVC, which is filtered out by the atmosphere. UVB causes sunburn and delayed tanning, whereas UVA exposure results in an immediate tan, which is why it is mainly used in sunbeds. Both UVB and UVA cause skin cancer and premature ageing of the skin. UVA rays are also responsible for photosensitivity rashes triggered by sunlight in certain disorders, for example systemic *lupus erythematosus*. A sensitivity to certain drugs and the sunlight results in skin rashes and are *photosensitivity* reactions (see box below).

When UVB rays reach your skin it thickens and the pigment cells produce more *melanin*, so that the skin turns a darker colour. Melanin absorbs and scatters the sun's rays. The more melanin in the outer skin layer the better your protection, but no one is completely safe in the sun.

UVA stimulates melanin production to produce an immediate tan, but penetrates deeper into the skin than UVB. It contributes to wrinkles, yellowing and blotching, often regarded as signs of ageing. Spending too long in the sun can lead to sunburn. The skin becomes red, hot, tight and swollen as the blood vessels are injured and leak fluid; blisters may appear. The condition is usually painful and causes itching. Some days later the top layer of the skin peels. In a severe case you may feel quite unwell with dizziness, nausea, abdominal cramps, headache and muscle weakness, and sometimes you may be sick. How sunburnt you become depends on how tanned you were to start with, how long you were in the sun and the strength of the sun. You are most at risk of burning when the sun is high in the sky in the summer months or you are near the equator or at high altitudes.

DRUGS THAT CAN CAUSE PHOTOSENSITIVITY

A few drugs cause your skin to be more sensitive to sunlight. You are likely to need a high-SPF (sun protection factor) product but check with your doctor or pharmacist what precautions you should take before going out in the sun.

Antibacterials – tetracyclines, e.g. **doxycycline**, **nalidixic acid**, **sulphonamides**

Antidepressants – **amitriptyline**, **doxepin**, **imipramine**

Diuretics – **thiazides**

Drugs for irregular heartbeat – **amiodarone**

Antipsychotics – phenothiazines, e.g **chlorpromazine**, **haloperidol**

THE SUN AND SKIN CANCER

Exposure to UVB and UVA rays can lead to the development of skin cancer. Skin cancers, particularly *malignant melanoma*, *basal cell* and *squamous cell carcinomas*, are becoming increasingly common. Getting sunburnt increases your risk of developing cancer, although skin cancer is more likely to be caused by the cumulative effect of years of exposure to the sun. It can take 20 to 30 years for skin cancer to develop. Children need good protection because they are particularly susceptible to skin damage from the sun. Babies under six months are even more at risk, because their skin has not yet fully developed its natural defences.

Melanomas usually start in moles or on normal skin, but in rare cases can occur in the eye, under the fingernails or inside the body. People with fair skin are most at risk from all types of skin cancer, especially if they also have a lot of freckles and moles and burn easily. If you have had severe sunburn at least once, especially as a child, you are also more at risk. If you have already had a malignant melanoma or a member of your family has had one, you are more at risk. Skin cancers like malignant melanoma are curable if recognised and treated early. Always check yours and your family's skin using the seven-point checklist below.

Melanoma checklist

Unlike other types of skin cancer, melanoma can strike young adults. Ask yourself these questions about any worrying pigmented patches:

☐ Has there been a change in size, or is it a new patch?
☐ Has the border become irregular in shape?
☐ Does the density of black and brown vary?
☐ Is the diameter 7mm or larger?
☐ Is there inflammation?
☐ Is there bleeding, oozing or crusting?
☐ Is there itching or altered sensation?

If you can answer yes to any of these questions, you should see your doctor, who may refer you to a specialist. Yes to any of the first three questions is most likely to mean melanoma and needs urgent discussion with your doctor.

Sunburn treatments

There are a number of remedies for relieving the pain of hot, burnt skin. If sunburn is severe, with blistering or broken skin, contact a doctor.

A tepid bath or shower can take the heat out of your skin. If you have been swimming in the sea, wash off dried salt remaining on the skin because it can aggravate sunburn. Exposing your skin to the sun tends to dry it and applying an emollient or using one in the bath ('Eczema', pages 430–32) helps to conserve moisture and soothe the skin. You do not have to use a special 'aftersun' lotion – any cooling emollient lotion will do. If you develop blisters, try to avoid bursting them because of the risk of infection. Blisters may burst in a bath so you may have to forgo cooling down in this way. Take paracetamol to relieve pain. Drink plenty of non-alcoholic fluids, especially if you have severe sunburn.

Itching may be helped by an antihistamine by mouth, particularly if a sedative one is taken at night. Creams, lotions or sprays containing antihistamines or local anaesthetics should not be used on the skin because they may cause sensitisation; these include Anethaine, Anthisan, Solarcaine and Xylocaine.

SUN PROTECTION

Using a sunscreen can help protect your skin from the ravages of strong sunlight and reduce the risk of sunburn and skin cancer. Sunscreens absorb UV radiation (e.g. **para-aminobenzoic acid (PABA)**, **cinnamates**), or reflect it (e.g. **zinc oxide**, **titanium dioxide**) so that less of the damaging rays penetrate the skin. The sun protection factor (SPF), marked on all sunscreen products, is a guide to roughly how long you are protected in the sun against UVB. The SPF is the ratio between the dose of radiation required to produce just measurable redness on protected skin, to that which produces a response on unprotected skin. The higher the SPF number, the better the protection. A sunscreen should be used to decrease sun exposure while you are outdoors but you should also combine this with other measures (see box). A star rating system graded one to four indicates UVA protection. A product with four stars, the highest rating, protects against UVA and UVB; lower numbers offer greater protection to UVB than to UVA. The usefulness of this rating system, however, remains controversial because it is arbitrary and may lull you into a false sense of security in the sun.

It is a good idea to put sunscreen on before you go out in the sun, not just when you get to the beach. The sun acts the minute you are out in it,

HOW YOU CAN HELP YOURSELF

- ☐ Use a reliable sunscreen, SPF 15 or more, depending on your skin type and location. Some sunscreens can cause an allergic rash, so find out which preparation suits you best.
- ☐ Avoid the sun between 11am and 3pm. Keep in the shade whenever possible.
- ☐ Remember that UV radiation from the sun can be strong even on cool, cloudy days.
- ☐ Sand, water and snow reflect UV radiation and increase the strength of the sun. Wind enhances skin damage produced by UV rays.
- ☐ When you are swimming, the sun may be strong up to a metre under water. Wearing a T-shirt is not the answer because the sun can go through it, especially if it is white. Use a water-resistant suntan lotion before you go into the water.
- ☐ Keep babies in the shade and protected by an umbrella if possible. All children are safest wearing a hat and a sunscreen with a high SPF.
- ☐ A wide-brimmed hat and closely woven cotton clothing can make you feel more comfortable on a hot, sunny day and help to protect you from UV rays.
- ☐ Wear sunglasses as UV radiation can damage your eyes.
- ☐ Avoid sunbeds or tanning lamps: they can cause sunburn, skin damage and skin cancer. The tan they give comes from UVA and so your skin might start to show signs of ageing earlier than normal.
- ☐ Check your skin regularly and report any unusual changes promptly to your doctor.

even while you are putting on your sunscreen. Spread the sunscreen thickly and evenly; pay particular attention to the areas at the edges of your swimming costume or clothes, and to the raised and bony parts of your body. Re-apply your sunscreen at least every two hours, even high SPF products, or more often if you are swimming or sweating.

Cuts, burns, bites and stings

Cuts and scratches are commonplace, minor injuries which need simple and prompt treatment. Skin is the body's protective covering for the internal organs, keeping out harmful micro-organisms such as bacteria. If the skin is damaged or breached in any way this protection is temporarily lost until the body mechanisms repair the injury. Skin is exposed to harmful micro-organisms all the time, but few of them lead to infection. The skin is constantly renewing itself and many minor cuts and burns heal without a trace of damage, particularly in children and young people. Deeper wounds and those covering a large area should be assessed by a doctor; they may leave a scar on healing.

CUTS

The wound should be washed in mild soap and warm water to clean it. Cold water can help to stem the blood if bleeding is profuse. Dry it gently and cover with a plaster that has a pad to prevent the wound sticking to it. An antiseptic is not needed routinely unless the wound appears to be infected. Using a small, sterile dressing strip (e.g. Leukostrip; Steri-strip) to draw a wound together may be helpful for some cuts.

If the cut is deep or long or does not stop bleeding you may need to contact your doctor, as stitches may be needed. You may also need a *tetanus* injection if you last received a dose of the vaccine more than 10 years ago. The childhood course of five injections should provide life-long cover, but always check whether you need an injection for a particular situation. An injection of tetanus immunoglobulin can provide immediate cover and can be given if you are already immunised but have a wound where the risk of contamination is high, for example from stable manure. Tetanus is a bacterium which can cause serious infection. It is also known as lockjaw because it produces a toxin in the body that affects the nerves, which results in muscular spasm, typically of the face, and eventually death, if not treated. The tetanus organism is commonly found in soil and on the ground, so any deep wound or scratch (for example from an animal or a rose thorn) is likely to pick up some tetanus bacteria. Cleaning the wound is very important but may not remove all the bacteria. Keep a record of your immunisations or ask your doctor whether you need to be immunised.

Children are normally vaccinated from the age of two months, when they receive a course of three tetanus toxoids with other vaccines to protect against serious illness. A booster dose of tetanus injection should be given just before school entry at the age of five and a further boost given in the mid-teens. Many older people have not been immunised against tetanus because it was not given routinely during childhood before 1961. Next time you visit your doctor check to see whether you are protected against tetanus.

MINOR BURNS

Accidental burns and scaldings happen frequently in and around the home. Heat damages the top skin layers, causing redness, swelling and pain. Sometimes a blister forms as fluid from the surrounding tissues oozes out. First aid should include cooling the burnt area as soon as possible with cold water: submerge the burnt area for ten minutes to take as much heat away from the skin as possible. Avoid putting ice cubes on to the skin because they can stick to it and cause further injury. Pat the area dry and leave it. If only the top layer of skin is burnt it will heal with time. Use a plaster or a film dressing (e.g. Cutifilm, Melolin, Skintact) only if the damaged area is likely to be harmed if left unprotected. A plaster may stop the air circulating freely around the burn and may also delay healing. Pain can be relieved with paracetamol or ibuprofen.

If a blister forms, leave it intact because it protects the lower skin layers as they heal and prevents bacteria settling on the damaged skin and causing infection (although not all health professionals agree on this). If the skin is burnt deeply or the burn covers a large area, contact a doctor.

BITES

Animal bites can cause severe infection as bacteria in the saliva of the animal can be introduced into wounds, especially deep injuries. Clean the wound thoroughly as soon as possible after an attack. Infection with tetanus (see 'Cuts', above) is the main concern and you should see a doctor or nurse (see above) if you have not been immunised. You may also need an antibiotic.

Insect bites cause irritation, redness, swelling and itching. Some people are not troubled much by bites whereas others – children, for example – react more. Flying insects such as mosquitoes, midges and sandflies suck blood for food and introduce a substance into the skin of their victims to make it easier to get the blood. This substance causes the irritation, which wears off with time. If the bite itches and you scratch it, the skin may become infected with bacteria. Keep the area of bitten skin clean with soap and water and apply an antiseptic cream. If the bites become badly infected you will need to see your doctor, who may prescribe an antibacterial product. Although there are a number of products especially designed for relieving the irritation of insect bites, hydrocortisone cream or ointment, or an emollient (pages 429–431) is the best treatment. Skin preparations containing antihistamines or local anaesthetics are not recommended.

INSECT STINGS

For most people a sting by a wasp or bee is an unpleasant and painful event. A bee sting should be removed from the skin by scraping a blunt blade across the area. Tweezers have been recommended but may squeeze more sting (venom) into the wound. The pain fades after a few hours and the skin can be soothed with hydrocortisone. However, a small number of people are extremely sensitive to bee and wasp stings and the allergic reaction can be life-threatening (page 175). If you are allergic to bee stings you should wear an identity bracelet (e.g. MedicAlert) and be trained to use and carry a ready-filled syringe of adrenaline, for example EpiPen.

Medicines for cuts, bites and stings

ANTISEPTICS AND DISINFECTANTS

These are chemicals that kill micro-organisms or prevent them growing where they are not wanted. Antiseptics are sometimes considered to be those products which are used on the skin while the term 'disinfectant' is reserved for preparations that prevent microbial growth on objects. In practice there is considerable overlap in the way the terms are used and between products.

Some general-purpose chemicals used for disinfecting the floor can also be applied to the skin; for example **cetrimide** and **chlorhexidine** (Savlon).

Sometimes the preparations will be specially formulated for the different circumstances or sometimes you may have to dilute the product for a particular purpose. The benefits of widespread use of antiseptics and disinfectants are sometimes unclear. Some experts think that the effects of these products are no better than using soap or detergent and water and that they delay wound healing.

INSECT REPELLENTS

There are various methods for keeping blood-sucking insects away. Clothing to cover as much of the body as possible is helpful; you can also use an insect repellent on your skin or buy a gadget such as those described below.

The most effective products are based on **diethyltoluamide** (DEET or DET). The more concentrated it is, the longer it will keep insects away. Liquids are normally the cheapest means of buying a repellent; sprays are bulky and usually more expensive, but easier to apply; sticks have a lower concentration of repellent, but have the best staying power, and are easy to carry around.

DEET must be used carefully, especially on children's skin. It can cause skin irritation for some people and it can be absorbed into the body. Keep repellents well away from children; containers do not have child-resistant closures.

Of the gadgets on sale for repelling insects, electric mosquito killers give convenient protection in enclosed areas such as hotel rooms. Spray the room with an insecticide to kill any mosquitoes before going to sleep. In countries where malaria is a problem, sleep in a screened room or use bed nets treated with **permethrin** repellent. Insect coils are less effective because they must burn reliably all through the night. Candles, repellent strips and electric buzzers do not keep insects away from you and are not effective.

Warts and verrucae

Warts and verrucae are infections of the skin caused by various types of the wart virus (human *papilloma* virus). The common wart on the hands and fingers appears as raised, thickened, skin-coloured patches (*nodules*) of skin. Small, flatter-looking nodules on the hand are known as *planar* warts. On the soles of feet, warts grow into the skin layers rather than being raised above the skin because of the pressure from the body's weight. These are *plantar* warts or *verrucae*, often called verrucas. As a verruca grows larger, it eventually causes pain when weight is put on the foot.

Genital warts, caused by a different type of human papilloma virus from the common wart or verucca, are small in size and many in number. They are passed on by sexual contact and need special treatment at a hospital clinic.

Common warts and verrucae are passed on from person to person and so almost everyone is likely to get them at some stage in their lives. The virus enters the skin through small cuts and scratches, liking in particular moist, warm areas. It lives within cells of the outer skin layer and takes over cell division, making the skin grow abnormally. You may have a single wart or verruca or several. Warts and verrucae are common in children, especially those aged 12 to 16. Some people are more likely to get the virus than others, depending on their immunity to the wart virus. Some are resistant to infection and others have to develop this resistance. Once resistance has built up the wart disappears often overnight. This spontaneous disappearance of warts, usually between six months and two years after infection, accounts for some of the myths and old wives' tales about wart cures.

Medicines for warts and verrucae

Your doctor may recommend not treating a wart or verruca because it will disappear spontaneously, although this takes time. However, warts can be troublesome because they get in the way when you use your hands or fingers; a verruca may be painful. The virus is slow-growing and resistant to all attempts to remove it. Treatment of either a wart or a verruca therefore takes time and perseverance with regular application of a suitable preparation. Most products can be bought at a pharmacy, some for less than the prescription charge, or your doctor can prescribe them.

Treatment aims to reduce the size of the wart or verruca by removing the overgrown layers of skin. **Salicylic acid** softens and destroys the wart but also the surrounding skin, which should be protected during treatment. There are various preparations and choice is not critical. Most have to be used once a day and it helps to soak the affected area in warm water for five to ten minutes before applying the preparation. All products contain salicylic acid (strength varies from 11 to 50 per cent) in an ointment or liquid and include Cuplex, Duofilm, Occlusal, Salactol, Salatac, and Verrugon. The skin surrounding the wart can be protected by putting on some petroleum jelly (for example Vaseline) before carefully applying salicylic acid. Covering the wart with a waterproof plaster helps to keep the skin soft and increases the effectiveness of treatment. Dead skin can be removed by gentle rubbing with a small, fresh piece of sand paper for each application as treatment progresses.

If treatment is not successful after three months, you may want to discuss with your doctor the possibility of removing the wart with liquid nitrogen. This method of freezing the wart is not suitable for young children because it is painful and can cause blistering. However, it is usually successful and after seven to ten days the wart goes.

Podophyllum (combined with salicylic acid in Posalfilin ointment) is a suitable verruca treatment for adults and children. It is used daily. It should not be used during pregnancy or breast feeding. A ring-shaped felt corn-plaster can be placed around the verruca, with the ring enlarged by snipping away the felt if necessary. Apply a tiny amount of ointment to the verruca and cover with a waterproof plaster. After some time, when the verruca appears soft and spongy, leave it open to the air for a day or two. The verruca should drop off, but if it does not, you repeat the treatment.

Preparations containing **formaldehyde** (Veracur) and **glutaraldehyde** (Glutarol) have less predictable effects and have to be applied twice daily. Formaldehyde and glutaraldehyde may be irritant to the skin and glutaraldehyde stains it brown. An old-fashioned remedy, **silver nitrate**, has been re-introduced as a caustic pencil (AVOCA) for applying to warts and verrucas, but evidence of its effectiveness is weak.

CAUTIONS

Wart and verruca products contain caustic substances which can damage healthy skin, and after using them you must take care to wash your hands thoroughly. Never use any of the preparations on your face or the genital region. If you are diabetic you should not treat warts or verrucae with an over-the-counter preparation, but always discuss the problem with your doctor. You should also see your doctor if the wart or verruca changes size or colour, if it bleeds or itches, if you develop a wart on the face or if you have genital warts.

VERRUCAE AND SWIMMING

The wart virus is everywhere in the environment and extremely difficult to avoid. It spreads easily in the warm, moist environment of a swimming pool and changing rooms, but there is no need to stop your child from going swimming. Putting a waterproof plaster on a wart or verruca that you are treating protects it and prevents it from spreading to others. There is then no need to wear a special rubber sock. However, some doctors think that it is unnecessary to cover verrucae at all.

Cold sores

Cold sores (recurrent *herpes labialis*) are caused by the virus *herpes simplex* (type 1). Infection can be acquired at any time, but often starts in childhood or adolescence. The virus is easily spread by close contact, probably by kissing an infected person. At the first infection, the virus gets into the nerve cells of one of the facial nerves, where it lies dormant. The virus then becomes active at intervals, causing recurrent cold sores. A variety of factors such as fever, sunlight, injury to the face, stress or menstrual periods may precipitate the infection.

An attack usually begins with a tingling or smarting sensation (the *prodromal* phase). A day later a single blister or crop of blisters form on the lips or the skin close to the mouth. The blister is painful and itchy at first and then collapses into a weeping sore which eventually dries to form a scab. This phase can last between three and ten days. It is important to avoid touching the infection during an attack to prevent the virus spreading to other areas such as the eye and to other people. Sometimes the sore can become colonised by bacteria, which cause a secondary infection. Sensible hygiene measures such as regularly washing hands and avoiding kissing can help to control the spread of infection.

Medicines for cold sores

No medicine can kill the herpes simplex virus and rid the body of it, but painful cold sores can be eased with a simple analgesic by mouth and an antiviral cream applied directly to the sore. Other cold sore remedies sooth and dry the lesion.

Aciclovir cream (Zovirax, Boots Avert, Clearsore, Soothelip, Virasorb) is an antiviral medicine for treating cold sores, but treatment must be started early in the infection to produce a beneficial effect. Aciclovir can shorten the length of an attack and may even abort the blister phase, but does not reduce itching or pain. The drug enters cells infected by the virus where it stops viral DNA synthesis and prevents the virus from multiplying. The cream must be used as soon as you feel the early signs of tingling or smarting before the blister forms or immediately it has formed.

Apply a small amount of cream to the blister five times a day for five days; if healing is incomplete by this time a further five days' treatment may be needed. Aciclovir has little effect against the virus if you have already had the cold sore for more than three days, so the cream is not worth using at this stage. Aciclovir cream is generally well tolerated but a few people have experienced a brief stinging or burning sensation with its use. Other occasional unwanted effects include redness, drying and flaking of the skin in the area of treatment. Aciclovir cream must not be used in the mouth or eyes or in the vagina as it is irritant. The cream contains **propylene glycol** and should not be used if you know you are sensitive to this ingredient (page 435).

Aciclovir can be prescribed by your doctor but you can also buy a small 2g tube for cold-sore treatment from pharmacies. If you suffer from recurrent attacks of cold sores this will save the time needed to see your doctor to get a prescription. Starting treatment early is the key to managing a painful and inconvenient infection. The over-the-counter pack costs less than the current prescription charge, and one tube should be sufficient for several attacks. **Penciclovir** (Vectavir) is a new antiviral treatment for cold sores, which is available only on prescription. It is applied every two hours, during the day, for four days. **Idoxuridine in dimethyl sulfoxide** paint (Herpid) is not strong enough at five per cent concentration to be of benefit. Topical treatment sometimes has a modest effect against cold sores. You should see your doctor if infection is more severe in the mouth or nose; treatment with an antiviral by mouth (e.g. aciclovir tablets or suspension – pages 292–4) may be needed or be considered to prevent attacks recurring.

Other topical treatments for cold sores are soothing creams or lotions, which do not generally influence the progress of the infection. Preparations available over the counter include emollient antiseptic creams (Blistex; Cymex; Lypsyl). A sunscreen lipsalve may help to reduce recurrences of cold sores, particularly if sunlight triggers attacks. Lotions containing **povidone-iodine** dry up the blisters and may affect the virus's progress if applied early enough during the tingling stage. These remedies are inexpensive and widely available.

(11)

NUTRITION AND BLOOD

Anaemia Vitamin deficiencies

Food is necessary for building and maintaining the cells and tissues in your body. The three main components of food are *protein, fat* and *carbohydrates* and an average daily diet provides a mixture of these. Protein is the body's major building material and your muscles are largely made of it. Fat is laid down as a layer under the skin to help conserve body heat and is stored all through the body. It also provides energy, although it is a less accessible source than carbohydrates which, in the form of starches and sugars, are the body's main source of energy. *Fibre*, the indigestible part of plant foods, is needed for a healthy digestive system and helps to make faeces bulky and easy to pass.

Food also contains small amounts of *minerals* and *vitamins*, which are essential for maintaining many of the normal body processes. Protein, fat and carbohydrates have to be broken down (*metabolised*) to smaller components by the digestive system before they can be absorbed and used in the body (see also Chapter 1). For example, protein in food is broken down into smaller substances called *amino acids* which the body uses to build its own proteins which are essential for replacing cells, the elements of all body tissues. Each of these biochemical reactions needs an *enzyme* – a substance that promotes the body's metabolic processes – and vitamins and minerals seem to be important aids to the functioning of enzymes.

A complete lack of essential nutrients, minerals and vitamins is uncommon in people living in wealthy countries. However, deficiencies do occur and some people are particularly at risk of not getting enough minerals and vitamins. In poorer countries inadequate supplies of food lead to illness such as *kwashiorkor*, caused by lack of protein, and *beri-beri* and *scurvy*, caused by vitamin deficiences.

Anaemia

Anaemia is a disorder affecting red blood cells. It may result from insufficient or misshapen blood cells being made or from cells being destroyed too early or lost through *haemorrhage* (excessive blood loss from the body). Red blood cells are made in *bone marrow* and normally have a life of 120 days; every day around 200,000 million must be made to replace those that are lost. Like all cells in the body, the red blood cell is made up of body protein derived from amino acids in dietary protein, so an adequate diet of protein, with vitamins and minerals to help biochemical reactions, is needed. **Iron** is an essential mineral for the manufacture of haemoglobin, the pigment in red cells which carries oxygen from the lungs to the body tissues. Two vitamins from the B group, **vitamin B_{12}** and **folic acid**, are essential for building red cells from proteins. If the activity of either of these vitamins or iron is disrupted, a form of anaemia results.

IRON-DEFICIENCY ANAEMIA

Iron-deficiency anaemia develops when there is too little iron to make haemoglobin for red blood cells. Situations that lead to decreased iron in the body include blood loss, increased requirements for iron during growth or pregnancy, poor absorption from the digestive system or too low an intake of iron from diet. Iron-rich foods include liver, meat, eggs, wholemeal cereals and leafy vegetables. Iron is well absorbed from meat and liver, but less so from vegetables and hardly at all from eggs. Although you need a certain amount of iron in your daily diet, and women need about twice as much as men, the body is economical with this mineral, as iron from old red cells is re-used in the formation of new ones. Iron is stored in bone marrow, the spleen and muscles.

However, iron-deficiency anaemia is quite common. Blood loss is the most usual cause and this may occur in women with heavy periods and at childbirth. Bleeding from the digestive system, from a peptic ulcer or other damage to the stomach or intestinal wall (for example, through disease or from regular taking of aspirin or other NSAIDs) can also lead to iron-deficiency anaemia. Symptoms of anaemia include tiredness, breathlessness on exertion, palpitations, faintness and headache. You may lose the normal colour in your lips and tongue, and the linings of your eyes and your skin may look pale. Some people also develop spoon-shaped, flattened or brittle nails. Anaemia can develop rapidly with severe blood loss.

Your doctor will always want to establish what has caused anaemia. This needs to be treated and the iron-deficiency corrected and body stores replenished. You will need blood tests to determine the haemoglobin level, which is assessed against normal reference levels for men (range 13–18 g/dL) and women (range 11.5–15.5 g/dL). You should never

HOW YOU CAN HELP YOURSELF

- ☐ Eat a well-balanced diet. Your body will absorb the amount of iron that it needs.
- ☐ Eating certain foods together increases the absorption of iron – for example, fish with spinach or vitamin C in fruit juices with bran cereals.
- ☐ If you have abnormal bleeding in urine or faeces darken see your doctor. Heavy periods for a few months or bleeding after you have stopped at the menopause need discussion with the doctor.
- ☐ Avoid iron supplements that also contain other minerals such as calcium and magnesium, as these interfere with the body's absorption of iron.
- ☐ Avoid taking an iron supplement at the same time of day as eating fibre-rich foods or calcium.

attempt to treat yourself with an iron preparation or a general tonic containing iron because these may conceal other causes of anaemia; for example, lack of a B vitamin (see below). Too much iron in the body can damage the liver, heart or kidneys. There is no risk of iron overload from the food in a normal diet.

VITAMIN B_{12} AND FOLIC ACID DEFICIENCIES

Other anaemias (*megaloblastic anaemias*) can be caused by a lack of either **vitamin B_{12}** or **folic acid**, both of which are essential for building cells, especially red blood cells. Your doctor will want to establish which is lacking and how the deficiency occurred before starting treatment.

The most common type of anaemia is *pernicious anaemia* which is mainly due to faulty absorption of vitamin B_{12} (also called cyanocobalamin). Vitamin B_{12} deficiency leads not only to anaemia but also to slow, progressive, irreversible damage to the nervous system. This damage causes numbness in the hands and feet, unsteadiness, loss of memory, confusion and depression. It may take years to develop because vitamin B_{12} stores in the liver are plentiful and the body only requires tiny amounts of the vitamin for making red cells. You may be taking in adequate amounts of vitamin B_{12}, but it cannot be absorbed into the body unless it combines with another substance made in the stomach known as *intrinsic factor*. If the intrinsic factor is deficient, the body cannot use vitamin B_{12}, the *extrinsic factor*. You may develop a deficiency if you have certain bowel disorders or have had surgery to remove all or part of your stomach or small intestine.

If your doctor finds that you are lacking vitamin B_{12} it can be replaced by an external source, but due to lack of intrinsic factor it has to be given by injection. **Hydroxocobalamin**, a derivative of vitamin B_{12}, is injected, at first every few days to restore the body's supplies and then every two to three months for the rest of your life to maintain adequate levels.

Vitamin B_{12} is found in meat, fish, milk, eggs and cheese and a balanced diet normally provides this vitamin. If you are vegetarian and do not eat eggs or dairy products you may need a vitamin B_{12} supplement, but it does not need to be injected if you do not lack intrinsic factor. Breakfast cereals, soya milk and yeast extracts fortified with vitamin B_{12} are a good alternative to supplements.

Low levels of folic acid lead to anaemia at the stage when red blood cells are made in bone marrow. Signs include tiredness, loss of appetite, nausea, diarrhoea, sore mouth and tongue, and hair loss. Folic acid is found in dark green leafy vegetables, some fresh fruit, eggs, liver, yeast extract and pulses, so that a well-balanced diet should provide adequate supplies (see table, overleaf). Some diseases of the small intestine can interfere with the body's absorption of folic acid. Lack of folic acid often occurs in alcoholics, but usually because of a poor diet. Long-term treatment with certain drugs such as **methotrexate**, **trimethoprim**, **triamterene**, corticosteroids and antiepileptic medicines (e.g. **phenytoin**) can also cause deficiency.

Your doctor will want to establish the cause of your lack of folic acid before prescribing a course of tablets. Most causes of deficiency sort themselves out with time or can be readily corrected by a short course of folic acid tablets if you cannot get enough in your diet. Folic acid may worsen the condition caused by vitamin B_{12} deficiency and should never be taken on its own for treating this type of anaemia. Folic acid can mask the symptoms of vitamin B_{12} deficiency while allowing irreversible nervous system damage to occur undetected.

Pregnancy and folic acid

During pregnancy a healthy diet is important to ensure the health of the developing baby. Research has now shown that folic acid supplementation before conception and during pregnancy is essential for a woman who has previously given birth to a baby with *spina bifida* or a similar defect (*neural tube defect*) to reduce the risk of the defect recurring in the second child. Doctors recommend supplementation with a 5mg daily dose of folic acid before the start of pregnancy and until the twelfth week of pregnancy to reduce the risk of another baby being born with a neural tube defect. If you take an antiepileptic medicine there is a theoretical risk that control of the condition may be affected by folic acid. You will need to discuss folic acid supplementation with your doctor.

It is not clear how folic acid prevents neural tube defects but doctors now recommend that all women planning a pregnancy should take 400 micrograms (0.4mg) of folic acid as a daily medicinal or food supplement to prevent a first occurrence of neural tube defect. You should take a daily folic acid supplement from the time when you plan to have a baby until the twelfth week of pregnancy. If you have not taken folic acid, but suspect that you are pregnant, you should start taking folic acid at once and continue until the twelfth week of pregnancy. Eating more folate-rich foods is also important (see table overleaf). Taking folic acid in a multivitamin product is not recommended as supplementation because of the risk of taking more than the established daily amount, not just of folic acid but also of other vitamins, such as vitamin A. When buying a supplement it is important to check the amount of folic acid in each preparation because it can vary; ask your doctor or pharmacist for advice and always read the label before you buy a product.

Medicines for anaemia

If you have a definite lack of iron you can replace this loss by taking a daily dose of an iron preparation by mouth. The iron corrects anaemia in six to eight weeks but treatment is continued for a further three months to replenish the body's iron stores. Choice of iron preparation depends on how well you tolerate different products: iron salts upset the digestive system and may make you feel sick; they also have a constipating effect, particularly for older people. Iron preparations contain either *ferrous* or *ferric* salts – ferrous salts are slightly more easily absorbed then ferric, so **ferrous sulphate** tablets are often tried first.

Some iron preparations contain vitamin C to aid absorption, but in practice the advantage is minimal. Compound iron preparations containing other minerals and vitamins are not recommended. Modified-release preparations are likely to carry the iron past the first part of the intestine where iron is best absorbed, so insufficient quantities may get into the body. Unwanted effects are reduced, possibly because less iron is absorbed, but these preparations are not recommended.

USEFUL SOURCES OF FOLATE/FOLIC ACID

Food	Folate/folic acid per typical serving	Food	Folate/folic acid per typical serving
	Micrograms		Micrograms
Vegetables (boiled unless stated)		*Fruit*	
Broccoli	30	Banana	15
Brussels sprouts	100	Grapefruit	20
Cabbage	25	Orange	50
Carrots	10	Orange juice	40
Cauliflower	45		
Green beans	50	*Cereals and cereal products*	
Peas	30	White rice, boiled	5
Potatoes old	45	Brown rice, boiled	15
Potatoes new	40	Spaghetti boiled	9
Spinach	80	White bread, average (2 slices)	25
Sweet corn	10	Wholemeal bread, average (2 slices)	40
Cucumber, raw	2	Soft grain bread (fortified with folic acid)	105
Lettuce, raw	15	Cornflakes (unfortified)	3
Tomatoes, raw	15	Cornflakes (fortified with folic acid)	100
		Branflakes (unfortified)	40
		Branflakes (fortified with folic acid)	100
To ensure vegetables do not lose folate:		*Other foods*	
– eat fresh vegetables		Bovril (per cup)	95
– boil only lightly		Yeast extract (on bread)	40
		Milk, whole/semi-skimmed (one pint)	35

1 milligram = 1,000 micrograms

Although liver is a rich source of folic acid, pregnant women and those intending to become pregnant are advised not to eat liver or liver products, because its level of vitamin A may be high and the consumption of excess vitamin A carries a risk of adverse effects.

Table derived from Department of Health guidance 1992

FERROUS SULPHATE

On prescription/from a pharmacy
FERROUS SULPHATE – Tablets

Poor choice: do not deliver sufficient iron to the body
Modified-release preparations – FEOSPAN[1]; FERROGRAD; SLOW-FE

Compound preparations containing ferrous sulphate
FEFOL[1]; FERROGRAD C[1]; FERROGRAD FOLIC; SLOW-FE-FOLIC

[1] Not on NHS prescription

Ferrous sulphate is a preparation of iron, a mineral which the body needs for making haemoglobin, the pigment in red blood cells that carries oxygen from the lungs to the tissues. You usually take in sufficient iron in a well-balanced diet, but children, teenagers, and women may need more. Women lose iron through bleeding at each period, and when they give birth. Babies fed only on milk for longer than six months are also at risk of becoming iron-deficient. Vegetarians may also need iron supplements.

Before you use this medicine

Tell your doctor if you are:
☐ pregnant or breast-feeding – take under medical advice ☐ taking any other medicines, including vitamins and those bought over the counter.

Tell your doctor if you have or have had:
☐ liver disease ☐ peptic ulcer or other intestinal disease ☐ a recent blood transfusion.

Do not take if you have or have had:
☐ diseases of iron overload (haemochromatosis, haemosiderosis) ☐ thalassaemia (an inherited form of anaemia).

How to use this medicine

Treatment of anaemia Depending on the preparation, take one, two or three tablets or capsules per day. Take them with a glassful of water or fruit juice before or in between meals; this helps iron absorption, but may increase gastric irritation. If the iron tablets make you feel sick or cause stomach pains, take the dose with or after meals or ask your doctor whether you can take a lower dose
Prevention of anaemia The dosage is usually once a day.

If you miss a dose, take it as soon as you remember, but skip it if it is almost time for your next dose. Do not take double the dose.

Over 65 No special dose requirements. An iron preparation is more likely to cause constipation in an older person.

Interactions with other medicines

Various drugs reduce the absorption of iron and sometimes vice versa if the preparations are taken at the same time of day. Do not take other medicines without checking with your doctor or pharmacist. Medicines that interact include:
Antacids: magnesium trisilicate
Antibacterials: tetracycline and **ciprofloxacin**, for example
Bisphosphonates for treating bone diseases (osteoporosis)
Levodopa, **entacapone** for Parkinson's disease
Penicillamine for modifying arthritis
Zinc: trace element.

Unwanted effects

Likely Heartburn, gastric irritation, feeling sick, dark or black stools.
Less likely Stomach pains, being sick, diarrhoea and/or constipation.

It is quite usual for iron preparations to darken stools. Contact your doctor if you have severe stomach pain, cramping or soreness, or fresh blood in stools.

Iron poisoning is extremely dangerous. Always keep iron preparations out of reach of children, particularly if the product is not in a child-resistant container. In cases of accidental poisoning, especially if a child is involved,

seek emergency treatment at hospital immediately. Do not wait for symptoms to develop as these may not appear for an hour.
Early signs Diarrhoea, nausea, vomiting, cramping, sharp stomach pains.
Late signs Bluish lips, fingernails and palms; drowsiness; pale, clammy skin; unusual tiredness; weak, fast heartbeat.

Similar preparations

On prescription/from a pharmacy

FERFOLIC SV – Tablets[1]*
FERROUS GLUCONATE + FOLIC ACID (4mg) + ASCORBIC ACID

FERROUS GLUCONATE – Tablets

FERSADAY – Tablets
FERROUS FUMARATE

FERSAMAL – Tablets, liquid
FERROUS FUMARATE

GALFER – Capsules, liquid
FERROUS FUMARATE

GALFER FA – Capsules
FERROUS FUMARATE + FOLIC ACID 350 MICROGRAMS

GIVITOL[1] – Capsules (not recommended)
FERROUS FUMARATE + VITAMINS B & C

LEXPEC with IRON – Syrup
FERRIC AMMONIUM CITRATE + FOLIC ACID (2.5mg)

LEXPEC with IRON M – Syrup
FERRIC AMMONIUM CITRATE + FOLIC ACID (500 MICROGRAM)

NIFEREX – Liquid
POLYSACCHARIDE-IRON COMPLEX

PLESMET – Liquid
FERROUS GLYCINE SULPHATE

PREGADAY – Tablets
FERROUS FUMARATE + FOLIC ACID 350 MICROGRAMS

SYTRON – Liquid
SODIUM FEREDETATE

[1] Not on NHS prescription
* Higher folic acid content for preventing recurrence of neural tube defect

Vitamin deficiencies

Vitamins play an essential part in normal body functions. They help with the production of energy from food and the regulation of the metabolism. Each metabolic process involves a specific enzyme and usually a particular vitamin or mineral to aid the biochemical reaction. The body needs only tiny amounts of vitamins and minerals, but generally cannot make them. Vitamins and minerals are found in a wide variety of foods and a well-balanced diet supplies all of these.

There are 13 vitamins essential for good health: **vitamins A, C, D, E, K** and the eight B vitamins – **thiamine** (B_1), **riboflavin** (B_2), **nicotinic acid** (B_3; niacin), **pyridoxine** (B_6), **pantothenic acid**, **biotin**, **folic acid** and **vitamin B_{12}**. The B vitamins were given numbers initially, but the system is somewhat confused because they are given names as their function becomes clear. Vitamin C and the B vitamins dissolve in water within the body and any excess is usually lost in urine; vitamins A, D, E and K dissolve only in fat and are stored for long periods in the body, mainly in the liver. Fat-soluble vitamins may accumulate if you take supplements well in excess of the body's requirements and this can lead to toxicity. Vitamins are a normal and essential part of the diet, which the body extracts from food during digestion, but when vitamins are taken in a concentrated form, sometimes at high or 'mega' doses, their effect on the body is not always understood. They are classed as medicines when used to prevent, treat or cure proven deficiencies but in high doses some can produce unwanted effects. It is important to tell your doctor or pharmacist whether you take extra vitamins regularly and if so how much.

HOW MUCH DO YOU NEED?

The answers to the questions, 'How much do people need on average?', the subjective, 'How much do I need?' and the more objective, 'How much do I need to eat to be sure that I am getting enough?' are all different and vary according to age, sex and lifestyle – and individuals have different needs for nutrients and different abilities to absorb them.

No single figure provides an adequate yardstick against which individuals can judge their nutrient intake, but a well-balanced diet – including fresh fruit, vegetables, starchy foods (e.g. bread, potatoes), reduced-fat dairy foods and protein (meat, fish, soya) – will provide all the nutrients you need unless you have a condition which imposes special requirements. Some vitamins are also made in the body. For example, biotin is manufactured by intestinal bacteria, and vitamin D is produced when the skin is exposed to sunlight. The table overleaf lists the main sources of nutrients – you are only likely to be risking deficiency if your diet is almost devoid of the sources of a particular nutrient or if you eat very little food at all.

WHO NEEDS SUPPLEMENTS?

Vitamin supplements may be needed by elderly people, women who are planning pregnancy, who are pregnant or breast-feeding, some children, and for people on limited diets. Vitamins can be prescribed to treat specific deficiency states and to prevent deficiencies developing, but not as dietary supplements except for folic acid supplementation in pregnant women to prevent neural tube defects in the developing baby.

Women at risk of developing anaemia from iron and folic acid deficiency during pregnancy may also be prescribed a supplement. However, vitamin A (including fish liver oils and multivitamins with vitamin A) should not be taken during pregnancy because of its potential to cause birth defects. A breast-feeding mother needs to ensure that she takes adequate vitamins and minerals, through diet and supplement.

Babies sometimes need additional vitamins, for example vitamin E is given if the child is premature and is incorporated into infant milk formula products. Vitamin K is given routinely to babies at birth to prevent a bleeding disorder (*haemorrhagic disease*). The Department of Health recommends supplementation with vitamins A, C and D for children between the ages of one and five. Children grow rapidly at the start of adolescence and so the requirements for energy, protein, vitamins and minerals are often high. Skipping meals or snacking on inappropriate foods also contributes to a low intake of vitamins.

Vitamin supplements are rarely needed for adults or children on balanced diets who spend some time outdoors. However, supplements may be needed for those who rarely go into the sunlight (vitamin D is formed in the body by the action of sunlight on the skin), for example

VITAL VITAMINS AND MINERALS

VITAMINS	Function in body	Main sources	Signs of deficiency
A	growth, night vision, healthy skin	liver, green leafy vegetables, carrots, yellow and orange fruit and vegetables, eggs, cheese, milk	difficulty seeing in dim light; dry, rough skin; dry eyes
B_1: thiamine	release of energy from foods	potatoes, wholemeal and white bread, vegetables, milk, breakfast cereals, pulses, nuts	inflammation of the nerves (peripheral neuritis); heart failure; excess water; feeling or being sick; beri-beri; mental confusion; brain damage
B_2: riboflavin	release of energy from foods	liver, meat, milk and cheese	sore lips and cracks at corners of mouth; mouth ulcers; sore red tongue; skin rashes; burning, itching eyes; twitching eyelids; blurred vision
B: niacin or nicotinic acid equivalents	release of energy from foods	pulses, liver, meat, bread, cereal	sore, red, cracked skin (pellagra); sore tongue and mouth; stomach pains and diarrhoea; skin rashes; mental changes – anxiety, depression and dementia
B: pantothenic acid	energy production	liver, kidney, egg, peanuts, mushrooms, cheese, pears	tiredness; headache; nausea; abdominal pains; pins and needles in limbs; muscle cramps; faintness; confusion; lack of co-ordination
B_6: pyridoxine	metabolism of proteins	liver, cereals, pulses, poultry	nerve damage; skin disorders; irritability; depression; anaemia
B_{12}: cobalamin	formation of red blood cells	meat, milk, cheese and eggs	pernicious anaemia
B: folic acid	formation of red blood cells	green leafy vegetables, all fruit and vegetables have a small amount	anaemia
B: biotin	energy production from fat	liver, pork, kidneys, nuts, cauliflower, lentils, cereals	tiredness; weakness; poor appetite; depression; hair loss

VITAMINS *cont*	Function in body	Main sources	Signs of deficiency
C: ascorbic acid	healing wounds, aids iron absorption, strengthens blood vessels	citrus fruits, blackcurrants, green leafy vegetables, potatoes, tomatoes, Brussels sprouts	scurvy – aches and pains, swollen and bleeding gums, nose bleeds, weakness
D	helps body to use calcium for healthy bones and teeth	sunlight, margarine, fatty fish, eggs, butter	rickets in children – softening and abnormal growth of bones; *osteomalacia* in adults – muscle weakness, backache, bone pain and fractures
E	protects against oxidising agents	vegetable oils, nuts, eggs, butter, wholegrain cereals, green leafy vegetables	anaemia
K	formation of proteins responsible for blood clotting	vegetables, especially cabbage, Brussels sprouts, cauliflower and spinach; liver	bleeding; delayed blood clotting
MINERALS			
Calcium	builds bones and teeth; intracellular messenger	milk, cheese, sardines, yoghurt, tofu, bread	gradual weaking of the bones
Iron	prevents anaemia; essential part of many enzymes	red meat, liver, beans, dried fruits, nuts, bread	anaemia
Zinc	normal growth and development; helps cells to divide and grow; healing	meat, liver, herring, milk, turkey, wholegrain foods, pork	retarded growth; loss of appetite; skin changes; immunological abnormalities

those who are severely disabled or housebound. People who have limited diets, such as strict vegetarians and those with a poor intake of food – for example, some people who live alone or people who are dependent on alcohol or illicit drugs – may be prone to deficiency.

People often become less interested in food as sensitivity to smell and taste decreases with age. Dental problems make eating more difficult, especially with meat and raw vegetables. Physical handicaps may hinder food preparation and eating. Although elderly people do not need to eat as much as younger people, the requirements for vitamins generally remain the same.

Deficiencies of various vitamins may occur with some medical conditions – for example, liver disease and diseases of the digestive system (such as prolonged diarrhoeal illness) prevent adequate absorption of vitamins and minerals. People who are dependent on alcohol frequently develop vitamin B deficiencies and are also prone to lack of vitamin C. Some chronic diseases reduce the appetite and therefore vitamin intake. A diet deficient in fat leads to poor absorption of fat-soluble vitamins.

Some medicines increase or decrease vitamin requirements and your doctor may advise whether or not you need a supplement if you take a medicine from the following groups long-term:

- ☐ Anticoagulants – for example **warfarin** – blood thinning effect antagonised by vitamin K (in some tube or sip feeds)
- ☐ Laxatives – for example **liquid paraffin** – interfere with the absorption of fat-soluble vitamins (vitamins A, D and K)
- ☐ Cholesterol-lowering drugs, for example **colestyramine**, **colestipol**, interfere with the absorption of fat-soluble vitamins (vitamins A,D and K)
- ☐ The anti-obesity drug **orlistat** interferes with the absorption of fat-soluble vitamins (vitamins A, D and K)
- ☐ Broad-spectrum antibiotics, for example **cephalosporins**, interfere with vitamin K production in the body. **Trimethoprim** decreases folic acid.
- ☐ The antituberculosis drug **isoniazid**: vitamin B_6 (pyridoxine) supplementation required.
- ☐ Antiepileptics – for example **carbamazepine**, **phenytoin**, **phenobarbital** – vitamin D supplementation may be needed; phenytoin and **primidone** also decrease folic acid.
- ☐ **Methotrexate** for rheumatoid arthritis, psoriasis decreases folic acid.
- ☐ Blood pressure-lowering drugs, for example **thiazides**, and vitamin D together increase the risk of high blood levels of calcium.

Vitamin supplementation should always be discussed with your doctor, who can assess your situation fully and advise on which vitamins to take.

MONEY DOWN THE DRAIN?

Many people like to take a vitamin supplement as an insurance, just in case their diets are inadequate, or to give them added zest. However, taking exercise and having adequate rest and sleep can help boost your energy levels and there is little evidence that taking a vitamin supplement improves your health if you are already well nourished. The body requires small amounts of all vitamins and minerals and no more. Using mega doses of vitamins and minerals can lead to an imbalance in the body's levels. Competition between the body's absorption and nutritional systems could lead to deficiencies. For example, large doses of iron can lead to zinc deficiency, and large doses of zinc can lead to copper deficiency.

Moreover, taking very high doses of vitamins can be hazardous, especially if you take them for prolonged periods. Excessive amounts of vitamin C can cause nausea and diarrhoea; it has also been associated with kidney stones. High doses of vitamin B_6 (pyridoxine hydrochloride) can cause loss of feeling in the arms and legs; this is usually reversible, but sometimes permanent nerve damage has occurred. Iron causes gastric irritation and is poisonous in overdose. Liver is a good source of several vitamins and minerals, but too much is not good for you. Years ago, polar explorers developed drowsiness, headaches and peeling skin which eventually turned out to be caused by high levels of vitamin A stored in polar bears' livers, which they ate. The level of vitamin A in the livers of food animals has more than doubled during the last 20 years because it is added to feed to promote growth.

These examples have been highlighted recently by the UK Expert Group on Vitamins and Minerals (EVM), which reviewed data on 31 vitamins, trace elements and minerals and set safe upper limits, or provided guidance if limits could not be set. It assessed evidence on safety in particular as a result of concerns about the possible risks of taking high doses of vitamins and minerals which are sold as food supplements. The EVM concluded that in general the vitamin and mineral supplements that people take are unlikely to cause harm, but considered that some substances may have irreversible harmful effects if taken for long periods at the highest supplemental doses. The EVM referred to concerns with **beta-carotene** (especially for smokers and people who have been exposed to asbestos), **nicotinic acid**, **zinc**, **manganese** (especially for older people) and **phosphorus**. The EVM also advised that no more than 10mg a day of vitamin B_6 should be taken, unless under medical guidance, because of the potential for high doses to cause nerve damage. Yet vitamin B_6 tablets 100mg can be bought over the counter as food supplements for premenstrual problems. This highlights the problem of differences that exist regarding the appropriate dosing of vitamins and minerals – not just in the UK but also in Europe and in the United States. European Union standards may be developed, but in the meantime the EVM guidance is helpful. Until new recommendations can be agreed more widely, the Recommended Daily Amount (RDA) remains the best guide – see the labels of many vitamin and mineral products.

Reviewing your daily diet and ensuring that you include five portions of vegetables and fruit, sources of fibre, protein, and reduced-fat dairy products should provide all the vitamins and minerals your body needs (see the useful website of the Food Standards Agency at *www.food.gov.uk*).

REFERENCE SECTION

Prescription charges Use of medicines
Useful addresses Glossary

Prescription charges

The prescription charge in England and Scotland is £6.30 for each item a doctor prescribes on an NHS form. The charge usually increases each April. In Wales the prescription charge is £6.

Many patients get their medicines free so check the list below to see if you are in one of the following groups. You can also look in leaflet HC11 *Are you entitled to help with health costs?* in Post Offices, some pharmacies and GP surgeries, or look at *www.doh.gov.uk/nhscharges/hc11.htm*

Everyone must now fill in the back of the prescription form whether they pay a prescription charge or not. Exemptions and remissions from charges are as follows.

Automatically exempt:

- ☐ children under 16
- ☐ students under 19 in full-time education (in Wales under 25 years)
- ☐ men and women aged 60 and over.

Exempt but need an exemption or remission certificate – ask your doctor or pharmacist:

- ☐ expectant mothers
- ☐ mothers who have a child under one year of age or have given birth to a stillborn baby in the last 12 months
- ☐ people who have a permanent *fistula* (such as *colostomy*, *ileostomy*, *caecostomy* or *laryngostomy*) needing continuous surgical dressing or appliance
- ☐ people with disorders needing replacement treatment – diabetes mellitus (except where treatment is by diet alone), hypothyroidism, hypoparathyroidism, hypopituitarism (e.g. diabetes insipidus), Addison's disease and other forms of hypoadrenalism, myasthenia gravis
- ☐ people with epilepsy needing continuous antiepileptic treatment
- ☐ people with continuing disability (not a temporary disability) which prevents them from leaving their home except with the help of another person
- ☐ war pensioners (for medicines needed for treating disablements)
- ☐ people who have purchased a prescription prepayment certificate (FP96) pay no further charges at the point of dispensing.

People entitled to remission

- ☐ People, and their partners, receiving income support or family income-based job seeker's allowance.
- ☐ People, and their partners, getting 'new' tax credit who have:
  - annual income of £14,200 or less (see your tax credit award) and
  - working tax credit with child tax credit or
  - working tax credit which includes a disability element (see your tax credit award) or
  - child tax credit but are not eligible for working tax credit because e.g. they do not work 16 hours a week
- ☐ People, and their partners, who are named on an NHS Charges certificate HC2 via the NHS Low Income Scheme.

Prescription prepayment certificates

If you need a lot of prescriptions – for example, you require more than five items in four months, or more than 14 items a year – but cannot get them free, a 'prescription prepayment certificate' may save you money. You can buy a certificate valid for four or twelve months from the Prescription Pricing Authority (tel: 0845 850 0030) or post the application form FP95. Forms are available from pharmacies and GP surgeries.

Multiple prescription charges

On some occasions you may have to pay more than one prescription charge, although sometimes it may appear that the prescription is for only one item. This will happen if your doctor prescribes:

- ☐ different formulations of the same drug as separate prescription items – for example the antirheumatic drug indometacin prescribed in both ordinary and modified-release forms. However, for different strengths of the same drug ordered as separate prescription items at the same time, e.g. prednisolone 5mg and prednisolone 1mg, only one charge is payable
- ☐ different presentations of the same drug – e.g. Canesten Combi pack containing a pessary and cream for fungal infections
- ☐ different drugs presented in one pack – e.g. two charges for oestrogen and progestogen tablets in hormone replacement products such as Cyclo-Progynova, Prempak-C and Trisequens, or for treating osteoporosis with etidronate tablets and calcium tablets, as Didronel PMO, and three charges for eradicating the gut bacterium Helicobacter pylori with three antimicrobial drugs in one pack, e.g. Heliclear
- ☐ elastic hosiery – a pair of stockings or knee-caps is counted as two items, i.e. two prescription charges.

No charges for contraception

Prescriptions for the pill, other medicines (spermicidal gels, creams, pessaries, injections, implants) and devices such as the intra-uterine device and diaphragm for contraception are free of charge.

MEDICINES CHEAPER OVER THE COUNTER

Some medicines which your doctor can prescribe can also be bought from a pharmacy (and some from other shops) for less than the prescription charge. If you pay a prescription charge, you can save yourself time and money by buying over the counter; if you are exempt from the charge you can save only time. The quantity of medicine you need may make over-the-counter purchases dearer in the long run, but if you have a self-limiting condition, buying rather than paying the prescription charge may make sense. Very few medicines are cheaper when bought if you need large quantities for any length of time. If you have long-term treatment it is best to see your doctor routinely for a review.

If your doctor prescribes one of the following types of medicine, check that you wouldn't be better off buying it yourself. Be warned that some medicines are sold under different brand names depending on whether they are prescribed or bought: find out the generic name to avoid confusion. Many generic products are available, and these are usually the cheapest option. Some medicines available over the counter contain lower amounts of the drug, e.g. ranitidine 75mg (Zantac 75) compared with the prescribable strengths, 150mg and 300mg. Types of product not recommended have been left out of the list.

Chapter 1: Digestive System
Antacids, antispasmodics and other medicines for dyspepsia
Antidiarrhoeals – for controlling diarrhoea
Oral rehydration salts – for helping recovery from diarrhoea
Bulk-forming agents – for improving the consistency of stools in chronic diarrhoea or constipation
Laxatives
Soothing preparations for haemorrhoids

Chapter 2: Heart and Circulation
Aspirin for stroke and heart attack prevention
Potassium supplements – for people who lose a lot of potassium during diuretic treatment
Nitrates – for treating angina

Chapter 3: Breathing Problems
Antihistamines – for hay fever and other allergies
Cough suppressants
Soothing cough medicines
Nasal decongestants

Chapter 4: Mind and Nerves
Drugs for sickness, e.g. motion sickness
Pain-relievers – aspirin, paracetamol, ibuprofen, codeine in combination preparations

Chapter 5: Infections
Preparations for preventing malaria
Worm treatments
Cystitis treatments
Preparations for candidiasis

Chapter 9: Eyes, Ears, Mouth and Throat

Anti-infective and anti-inflammatory eye drops
Artificial tears
Products for removing ear wax
Preparations for mouth ulcers
Preparations for oral thrush
Mouthwashes and gargles

Chapter 10: Skin Conditions

Emollients and barrier preparations
Emulsifying ointment and aqueous cream (soap substitutes)
Anti-itching preparations
Mild corticosteroids for some skin allergies, insect bite reactions and mild-moderate eczema
Coal tar and other preparations for psoriasis and eczema
Acne preparations
Wart preparations
Scalp preparations
Antifungal preparations – for athlete's foot, etc.
Preparations for scabies and lice
Disinfectants and antiseptics
Cold sore preparations

Chapter 11: Nutrition and Blood

Mineral supplements – iron, calcium, fluoride and zinc
Individual vitamins – A, B group, C, D
Multivitamins

Use of medicines

TAKING MEDICINES

- ☐ Always follow the directions on the label carefully.
- ☐ Do not take more or less than the recommended dose and stick to the interval between doses. Taking more of a medicine will not make it work better or any faster. Taking less of a medicine or under-dosing may mean that the treatment is not effective. Discuss any concerns that you have about dosages with your doctor or pharmacist.
- ☐ Do not give your medicine to anyone else.
- ☐ Do not take medicines after the expiry date on the label.
- ☐ Check the dose on the label carefully before giving a medicine to a child and never give an adult dose unless these are the directions on the label.
- ☐ Do not give any medicines to babies under six months old without the advice of a health professional.
- ☐ If you are taking a prescription medicine and want to take an over-the-counter product as well, check with your doctor or pharmacist before using it.
- ☐ Tablets and capsules can stick in the throat and gullet: take them with plenty of water standing or sitting upright.
- ☐ If you have capsules to take, swallow them whole unless you are told to break them open.
- ☐ With liquid medicines you will usually be given a 5ml spoon for measuring the dose. Syringes for measuring quantities less than 5ml can be bought at a pharmacy or will be supplied if the dose of a prescribed medicine is less than 5ml.

STORAGE

- ☐ Always keep medicines out of children's reach. Never leave any medicine lying around, even if you think it is out of reach. Do not give empty medicine containers to a child to play with.
- ☐ Keep medicines in tightly closed containers.
- ☐ Do not transfer medicines from their original containers to different containers unless these are proper medicine-taking reminder devices. Switching containers means that you lose the original instructions and may affect the time for which the medicine can be stored.
- ☐ If it is difficult for you to open the container in which a medicine is supplied, ask your pharmacist to put it in a bottle with an ordinary top.
- ☐ Store all medicines in a cool, dry place and protect them from light; a lockable medicine cabinet is ideal. Follow any special storage instructions such as refrigeration.
- ☐ Check the use-by-dates (expiry dates) on medicines where these are printed; discard out-of-date medicines.
- ☐ If you have medicine left over after you have finished treatment, do not keep it, but return it to your local pharmacy.

DISPOSAL

- ☐ Do not hoard medicines: take unwanted supplies to your hospital or local pharmacy.
- ☐ Do not throw medicines away in the dustbin or flush them the down the toilet.

Discard medicines when:

- ☐ tablets and capsules are two years old
- ☐ tablets are chipped, cracked or have changed colour
- ☐ capsules are hard and cracked or soft or stuck together
- ☐ aspirin and aspirin-containing medicines smell of vinegar
- ☐ ointments and creams smell or look different to the original
- ☐ liquids have thickened or discoloured, or look or smell different to the original
- ☐ ointment tubes are hard or have leaked or cracked.

Useful addresses

Age Concern Cymru
4th floor, 1 Cathedral Road
Cardiff CF11 9SD
Tel: 029-2037 1566
Fax: 029-2039 9562
Email: enquiries@accymru.org.uk
Website: www.accymru.org.uk

Age Concern England
Astral House, 1268 London Road
London SW16 4ER
Tel: 020-8679 8000
Fax: 020-8765 7211
Website: www.ace.org.uk

Age Concern Northern Ireland
3 Lower Crescent
Belfast BT7 1NR
Tel: 028-9024 5729
Fax: 028-9023 5497
Email: info@ageconcernni.org
Website: www.ageconcernni.org

Age Concern Scotland
113 Rose Street
Edinburgh EH2 3DT
Tel: 0131-220 3345
Fax: 0131-220 2779
Email: enquiries@acscot.org.uk
Website:
www.ageconcernscotland.org.uk

Arthritis Care
18 Stephenson Way
London NW1 2HD
Tel: 020-7380 6500
Helplines: Freephone (0808) 800 4050 (Mon–Fri 12–4), 020-7380 6555 (Mon–Fri 10–4), 'The Source' (young people's helpline) (0808) 8080 2000 (Mon–Fri 10–2)
Fax: 020-7380 6505
Email: helpline@arthritiscare.org.uk; thesource@arthritiscare.org.uk
Website: www.arthritiscare.org.uk

BackCare
16 Elmtree Road, Teddington
Middlesex TW11 8ST
Tel: 020-8977 5474
Fax: 020-8943 5318
Email: info@backcare.org.uk
Website: www.backcare.org

British Association for Counselling and Psychotherapy (BACP)
BACP House, 35–37 Albert Street
Rugby CV21 2SG
Tel: (0870) 443 5252
Fax: (0870) 443 5161
Email: bacp@bacp.co.uk
Website: www.bacp.co.uk

British Heart Foundation
14 Fitzhardinge Street
London W1H 6DH
Tel: 020-7935 0185
Medical information line: (0845) 070 8070
Heartstart UK 020-7487 9419
Fax: 020-7486 5820
Website: www.bhf.org.uk

British Red Cross Society
9 Grosvenor Crescent
London SW1X 7EJ
Tel: 020-7235 5454
Fax: 020-7245 6315
Email: information@redcross.org.uk
Website: www.redcross.org.uk

Chest, Heart and Stroke Scotland
65 North Castle Street
Edinburgh EH2 3LT
Tel: 0131-225 6963
Fax: 0131-220 6313
Advice line: (0845) 077 6000
Email: administrator@chss.org.uk
Website: www.chss.org.uk

Diabetes UK
10 Parkway, London NW1 7AA
Tel: 020-7424 1000
Careline: (0845) 120 2960
Fax: 020-7424 1001
Email: info@diabetes.org.uk
Website: www.diabetes.org.uk

Disability Alliance
Universal House
88–94 Wentworth Street
London E1 7SA
Tel: 020-7247 8776
Fax: 020-7247 8765
Email: office.da@dial.pipex.com
Website: www.disabilityalliance.org

Disabled Living Foundation
380–384 Harrow Road
London W9 2HU
Tel: 020-7289 6111
Helpline: (0845) 130 9177
Textphone: 020-7432 8009
Fax: 020-7266 2922
Email: advice@dlf.org.uk
Website: www.dlf.org.uk

Driver and Vehicle Licensing Authority (DVLA), Drivers Medical Group
Swansea SA99 1TU
Tel: (0870) 600 0301
Fax: (01792) 761100
Website: www.dvla.gov.uk

Enuresis Resource and Information Centre (ERIC)
34 Old School House, Britannia Road
Kingswood, Bristol BS15 8DB
Tel: (0117) 960 3060
Fax: (0117) 960 0401
Email: info@eric.org.uk
Website: www.eric.org.uk

Epilepsy Action
New Anstey House, Gate Way Drive
Yeadon, Leeds LS19 7XY
Tel: (0113) 210 8800
Helpline: Freephone (0808) 800 5050
Fax: (0113) 391 0300
Email: epilepsy@epilepsy.org.uk
Website: www.epilepsy.org.uk

Epilepsy Bereaved
PO Box 112, Wantage
Oxon OX12 8XT
Tel/Fax: (01235) 772850
Bereavement support line:
(01235) 772852
Email:
epilepsybereaved@dial.pipex.com
Website: www.sudup.org

Expert Patient Programme
Tel: (0845) 606 6040
Website: www.expertpatients.nhs.uk

Family Planning Association (FPA)
2–12 Pentonville Road
London N1 9FP
Tel: 020-7837 5432
Helpline: 020-7837 4044 (Mon–Fri 9–6)
Fax: 020-7837 3042
Website: www.fpa.org.uk

Fellowship of Depressives Anonymous (FDA)
Box FDA, Self Help Nottingham
Ormiston House, 32–36 Pelham Street
Nottingham NG1 2EG
Tel: (0870) 774 4320
Fax: (0870) 774 4319
Email: fdainfo@aol.com
Website: www.depressionanon.co.uk

General Dental Council
37 Wimpole Street, London
W1G 8DQ
Tel: 020-7887 3800
Fax: 020-7224 3294
Email: information@gdc-uk.org
Website: www.gdc-uk.org

General Medical Council
178 Great Portland Street
London W1W 5JE
Tel: 020-7580 7642
Fax: 020-7915 3641
Email: gmc@gmc-uk.org
Website: www.gmc-uk.org

Health Service Ombudsman
Health Service Ombudsman for England
Millbank Tower
Millbank, London SW1P 4QP
Tel: (0845) 015 4033

Health Service Ombudsman for Wales
5th floor, Capital Tower
Greyfriars Road, Cardiff CF10 CAG
Tel: (0845) 601 0987

Scottish Public Services Ombudsman
23 Walker Street, Edinburgh
EH3 7HX
Tel: (0870) 011 5378

Website: www.ombudsman.org.uk/hse

Heartstart UK
See British Heart Foundation

IBS Network
Northern General Hospital
Sheffield S5 7AU
Tel: (0114) 261 1531
Helpline: (01543) 492192
(Mon–Fri 6–8pm, Sat 10–12 noon)
Fax: (0114) 261 0112
Website: www.ibsnetwork.org.uk
Send an SAE

Independent Complaints Advocacy Services (ICAS)
Tel: London (0845) 120 3784; South-west (0845) 120 3782; West Midlands (0845) 120 3748; North-west (0845) 120 3735; North-east (0845) 120 3732; Yorks Humberside (0845) 120 3734; Beds & Herts (0845) 456 1082; Cambs, Norfolk & Suffolk (0845) 456 1084; Essex (0845) 456 1083; Oxon, Bucks & Berks, Hants & Isle of Wight, Surrey, West & East Sussex, Kent (0845) 600 8616; Notts, Leics & Derby, Northants (0845) 650 0088
Website: www.doh.gov.uk/complaints/advocacyservice.htm

International Glaucoma Association
108C Warner Road,
London SE5 9HQ
Tel: 020-7737 3265
Fax: 020-7346 5929
Email: info@iga.org.uk
Website: www.iga.org.uk

Malaria Reference Laboratory
London School of Hygiene and Tropical Medicine
Keppel Street, London WC1E 7HT
Tel: (0906) 550 8908
Recorded advice for travellers, £1/minute

Manic Depression Fellowship (MDF)
Castle Works, 21 St George's Road
London SE1 6ES
Tel: 020-7793 2600 (Mon–Fri 10–4)
Fax: 020-7793 2639
Email: mdf@mdf.org.uk
Website: www.mdf.org.uk

Medical Advisory Service for Travellers Abroad (MASTA)
Moorfield Road
Yeadon, Leeds LS19 7BN
Tel: (0113) 238 7575
Healthline: (0906) 822 4100
Fax: (0113) 238 7501
Email: enquiries@masta.org
Website: www.masta.org

Migraine Action Association
Unit 6, Oakley Hay
Lodge Business Park
Great Folds Road, Great Oakley
Northamptonshire NN18 9AS
Tel: (01536) 461333
Fax: (01536) 461444
Email: info@migraine.org.uk
Website: www.migraine.org.uk

Migraine Trust
2nd floor, 55–56 Russell Square
London WC1B 4HP
Tel: 020-7436 1336
Fax: 020-7436 2880
Email: info@migrainetrust.org
Website: www.migrainetrust.org

MIND (National Association for Mental Health)
15–19 Broadway
London E15 4BQ
Tel: 020-8519 2122
Fax: 020-8522 1725
Email: contact@mind.org.uk
Website: www.mind.org.uk

National Association for Colitis and Crohn's Disease
4 Beaumont House
Sutton Road, St Albans
Hertfordshire AL1 5HH
Tel: (01727) 830038
Information line: (0845) 130 2233
Fax: (01727) 862550
Email: nacc@nacc.org.uk
Website: www.nacc.org.uk

National Asthma Campaign
Providence House, Providence Place
London N1 0NT
Tel: 020-7226 2260
Fax: 020-7704 0740
Helpline: (08457) 010203
(Mon–Fri 9–5)
Website: www.asthma.org.uk

National Eczema Society
Hill House, Highgate Hill
London N19 5NA
Tel: (0870) 241 3604
Fax: 020-7281 6395
Email: helpline@eczema.org
Website: www.eczema.org

National Endometriosis Society
50 Westminster Palace Gardens
London SW1P 1RR
Tel: 020-7222 2781
Fax: 020-7222 2786
Helpline: Freephone (0808) 808 2227
Email: nes@endo.org.uk
Website: www.endo.org.uk

National Institute for Clinical Excellence (NICE)
MidCity Place, 71 High Holborn
London WC1V 6NA
Tel: 020-7067 5800
Fax: 020-7067 5801
Email: nice@nice.nhs.uk
Website: www.nice.org.uk

National Society for Epilepsy (NSE)
Chesham Lane, Chalfont St Peter
Gerrards Cross,
Buckinghamshire SL9 0RJ
Tel: (01494) 601300
Fax: (01494) 871927
Website: www.epilepsynse.org.uk

Northern Ireland Chest, Heart and Stroke Association
22 Great Victoria Street
Belfast BT2 7LX
Tel: 028-9032 0184
Fax: 028-9033 3487
Advice line: (0845) 769 7299
Cardiac helpline: (0845) 601 1658
Email: mail@nichsa.com
Website: www.nichsa.com

Nursing and Midwifery Council (NMC)
23 Portland Place
London W1B 1PZ
Tel: 020-7637 7181
Fax: 020-7436 2924
Website: www.nmc-uk.org

Pain Society
The Secretariat, 21 Portland Place
London W1B 1PY
Tel: 020-7631 8870
Fax: 020-7323 2015
Email: info@painsociety.org
Website: www.painsociety.org

Parkinson's Disease Society
215 Vauxhall Bridge Road
London SW1V 1EJ
Tel: 020-7931 8080
Helpline: Freephone (0808) 800 0303
Fax: 020-7233 9908
Email: enquiries@parkinsons.org.uk
Website: www.parkinsons.org.uk

Partially Sighted Society
PO Box 322, Doncaster
South Yorks DN1 2XA
Tel: (01302) 323132
Fax: (01302) 368998
Email: info@partsight.org.uk
Website: www.eyeconditions.org.uk

Patient Advice and Liaison Services (PALS)
NHS Direct
Tel: (0845) 4647
Websites: www.nhsdirect.nhs.uk;
www.doh.gov.uk/patientadviceand
liaisonservices
Phone the above number or your local hospital, clinic, GP surgery or health centre for details of PALS in your area

Preparing Professionals for Partnership with the Public (4Ps)
4Ps Development Centre
1st Floor, Courtfield House
St Charles' Hospital, Exmoor Street
London W10 6DZ
Tel/Fax: (01296) 632351
Email: feedback@4ps.com
Website: www.4ps.com

Psoriasis Association
Milton House
7 Milton Street
Northampton NN2 7JG
Tel: (01604) 711129
Helpline: (0845) 676 0076
Fax: (01604) 792894
Website:
www.psoriasis-association.org.uk

Resuscitation Council (UK)
5th floor, Tavistock House North
Tavistock Square
London WC1H 9HR
Tel: 020-7388 4678
Fax: 020-7383 0773
Email: enquiries@resus.org.uk
Website: www.resus.org.uk

Rethink
28 Castle Street
Kingston-upon-Thames
Surrey KT1 1SS
Tel: (0845) 456 0455
Fax: 020-8547 3862
Email: info@rethink.org
Website: www.rethink.org

Royal Life Saving Society (UK)
River House, High Street, Broom
Warwickshire B50 4HN
Tel: (01789) 773994
Fax: (01789) 773995
Email: mail@rlss.org.uk
Website: www.rlss.org.uk

Royal National Institute for the Blind (RNIB)
105 Judd Street, London WC1H 9NE
Tel: 020-7388 1266
Helpline: (0845) 766 9999
Fax: 020-7388 2034
Website: www.rnib.org.uk

Royal Pharmaceutical Society of Great Britain
1 Lambeth High Street
London SE1 7JN
Tel: 020-7735 9141
Fax: 020-7735 7629
Email: enquiries@rpsgb.org.uk
Website: www.rpsgb.org.uk

St Andrew's Ambulance Association
St Andrew's House, 48 Milton Street
Glasgow G4 0HR
Tel: 0141-332 4031
Fax: 0141-332 6582
Email: firstaid@staaa.demon.co.uk
Website: www.firstaid.org.uk

St John's Ambulance
63 York Street, London W1H 1PS
Tel: 020-7258 3456
Fax: 020-7724 0968
Email: sales@london.sja.org.uk
Website: www.sja.org.uk

Samaritans
The Upper Mill, Kingston Road
Ewell, Surrey KT17 2AF
Helpline: (08457) 909090
Textphone: 020-8394 8301
Fax: 020-8394 8300
Email: jo@samaritans.org
Website: www.samaritans.org.uk

SANE
1st Floor, Cityside House
40 Adler Street London E1 1EE
Tel: 020-7375 1002
Fax: 020-7375 2162
Saneline: (0845) 767 8000
Email: info@sane.org.uk
Website: www.sane.org.uk

Schizophrenia Association of Great Britain (SAGB)
Bryn Hyfryd, The Crescent, Bangor
Gwynedd LL57 2AG
Tel: (01248) 354048
Fax: (01248) 353659
Email: info@sagb.co.uk
Website: www.sagb.co.uk

SportEX Health
86–88 Nelson Road, Wimbledon
SW19 1HX
Tel: 020-8287 3312
Fax: 020-8404 8261
Email: info@sportex.net
Website: www.sportex.net

Stroke Association
Stroke House, 240 City Road
London EC1B 2PR
Tel: 020-7566 0300
Helpline: (0845) 303 3100
Fax: 020-7490 2686
Email: info@stroke.org.uk
Website: www.stroke.org.uk
For Scotland see Chest, Heart and Stroke Scotland, *for Northern Ireland see* Northern Ireland Chest, Heart and Stroke Association

Teaching Aids at Low Cost (TALCUK)
PO Box 49, St Albans
Hertfordshire AL1 5TX
Tel: (01727) 853869
Fax: (01727) 846852
Email: info@talcuk.org
Website: www.talcuk.org

Glossary

Acute a short-lived condition that occurs suddenly and may be severe.

Agonist A drug with a stimulating effect; it increases the activity in a particular type of cell.

Antagonist A drug with an opposing action or one which binds to a cell receptor to prevent other chemicals from stimulating the cell, often called a blocker.

Anticholinergic A drug that blocks the effects of acetylcholine, a neurotransmitter. Anticholinergic drugs have many uses, including relaxing the muscles of the gut to ease irritable bowel syndrome or to prevent travel sickness and treating urinary incontinence. However, they cause many unwanted effects, such as dry mouth, visual problems and difficulty passing urine.

Antimuscarinic *see* Anticholinergic.

Astringent A substance that causes tissue to contract by reducing its ability to hold fluid.

Autoimmune A disease such as rheumatoid arthritis in which the body produces antibodies that attack its own tissues.

Chronic A long-term condition that may develop gradually. The term chronic does not imply anything about the severity of the disease.

Corticosteroids A group of drugs which are synthetic variants of the corticoid hormones produced in the adrenal glands. They are mainly used to reduce inflammation and to suppress allergic reactions and immune activity.

Diuretics A group of drugs, also known as 'water tablets', which increase the amount of water lost from the body in urine.

Dysfunction Abnormal function of any organ.

-ectomy Surgical removal: hysterectomy is removal of the womb.

Enteric coating A special coating applied to a tablet to prevent it from dissolving until it has passed through the stomach into the intestine.

Hyper … Excess or overactivity: hyperthyroidism is over-activity of the thyroid gland.

Hypersensitivity Abnormal increased reaction of the immune system to a stimulus such as an antigen or allergen.

Hypo … Lack or underactivity: hypoglycaemia is low blood-sugar.

Ischaemia Inadequate blood supply to an organ or tissue in any part of the body, generally such as to cause transient or permanent changes (pain, cell death). It is commonly caused by disease of the arteries supplying the tissues/organ, but also as a result of injury, constriction, spasm or blockage in the artery.

Kidney function is assessed by the level of body chemicals, usually urea and creatinine, that the kidneys remove routinely from the body. The degree of impairment is assessed against the normal range of values for creatinine and urea. For example, the normal values for creatinine range from 79 to 118 micromoles per litre (blood creatinine levels) but when levels rise above 150 micromoles per litre this indicates that kidney function, such as the removal of certain medicines from the body, is impaired. The higher the level of creatinine in blood the greater the degree of kidney impairment; this is divided arbitrarily into mild, moderate and severe impairment.

Local Application of a drug to a particular part of the body in order for it to act there without spreading through the bloodstream.

Metabolism The chemical reactions that occur in the body, including those which convert food into energy and essential body chemicals and those which control the release of stored energy.

Modified-release A way of formulating a medicine so that the drug is released in a controlled way over several hours. Modified-release is a term which covers sustained-, slow- and controlled-release products.

Receptor A site on the surface of a cell with particular chemical and physical properties that allow only certain chemicals to attach themselves and influence the cell's activity. For example, adrenaline acts at adreno-ceptors.

Sympathomimetic A drug which has the same stimulating effect as neurotransmitters in the sympathetic nervous system, encouraging changes such as an increase in the heart rate or widening of the airways.

Systemic An effect throughout the body, produced by any drug which is absorbed into the bloodstream.

Topical Application of a drug on the surface of the body at the site where its effect is required.

Toxic The effect of a poison (toxin), such as a chemical produced by harmful bacteria. Drugs can have a toxic effect if they are present in too high a concentration.

Vasoconstrictor A drug that narrows blood vessels.

Vasodilator A drug that widens blood vessels.

INDEX

MEDICINE RECORD SHEET

The record sheet, which you can photocopy, on the next two pages is designed to help you get hold of information about medicines and monitor the way you use them. See pages 24–6 for details. Move on to a second record sheet if you want to note information about more than three medicines, or make separate notes based on the headings.